ROUTINE URINE TESTING

Many diagnostic and laboratory tests include the direction to perform routine blood testing and/or routine urine testing. The protocol for those tests is presented here and will be cross-referenced within the many tests requiring them.

Before

PT Explain the procedure to the patient.
PT Inform the patient if food or fluid restrictions are needed.

During

Random, fresh, or spot specimen:

• Instruct the patient to urinate into an appropriate non-sterile container.

24-hour specimen:

1. Begin the 24-hour collection by discarding the first specimen.
2. Collect all urine voided during the next 24 hours.
3. Show the patient where to store the urine.
4. Keep the urine on ice or refrigerated during the collection period. Foley bags are kept in a basin of ice. Some collections require a preservative. Check with the laboratory.
5. Post the hours for the urine collection in a prominent place to prevent accidentally discarding a specimen.
6. Instruct the patient to void before defecating so that urine is not contaminated by stool.
7. Remind the patient not to put toilet paper in the urine collection container.
8. Collect the last specimen as close as possible to the end of the 24-hour period. Add this urine to the collection.

After

• Transport the specimen promptly to the laboratory.

PT = Patient teaching

ELSEVIER
MOSBY

3251 Riverport Lane
St. Louis, Missouri 63043

MOSBY'S DIAGNOSTIC AND LABORATORY TEST REFERENCE,
TWELFTH EDITION

ISBN: 978-0-323-22576-2

Notice

Knowledge and best practice in this field are constantly changing. As new research and experience broaden our understanding, changes in research methods, professional practices, or medical treatment may become necessary.

Practitioners and researchers must always rely on their own experience and knowledge in evaluating and using any information, methods, compounds, or experiments described herein. In using such information or methods they should be mindful of their own safety and the safety of others, including parties for whom they have a professional responsibility.

With respect to any drug or pharmaceutical products identified, readers are advised to check the most current information provided (i) on procedures featured or (ii) by the manufacturer of each product to be administered, to verify the recommended dose or formula, the method and duration of administration, and contraindications. It is the responsibility of practitioners, relying on their own experience and knowledge of their patients, to make diagnoses, to determine dosages and the best treatment for each individual patient, and to take all appropriate safety precautions.

To the fullest extent of the law, neither the Publisher nor the authors, contributors, or editors assume any liability for any injury and/or damage to persons or property as a matter of products liability, negligence or otherwise, or from any use or operation of any methods, products, instructions, or ideas contained in the material herein.

ISBN: 978-0-323-22576-2

Content Strategist: Jamie Randall
Content Development Manager: Jean Sims Fornango
Publishing Services Manager: Hemamalini Rajendrababu
Project Manager: Manchu Mohan
Designer: Karen Pauls/Renee Duenow

Printed in the United States of America

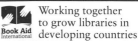

Working together
to grow libraries in
developing countries

www.elsevier.com • www.bookaid.org

Last digit is the print number:
9 8 7 6 5 4 3 2 1

MOSBY'S
DIAGNOSTIC AND LABORATORY TEST REFERENCE

Twelfth Edition

Kathleen Deska Pagana, PhD, RN
Professor Emeritus
Department of Nursing
Lycoming College
Williamsport, Pennsylvania
http://www.KathleenPagana.com
President, Pagana Keynotes & Presentations

Timothy J. Pagana, MD, FACS
Medical Director
The Kathryn Candor Lundy Breast Health Center
Susquehanna Health System
Williamsport, Pennsylvania

Theresa Noel Pagana, MD, FAAEM
Emergency Medicine Physician
Virtua Voorhees Hospital
Voorhees, New Jersey

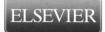

With love and adoration,
we dedicate this book to our grandchildren:

Ella Marie Gaul

Jocelyn Elizabeth Gaul

Timothy William Gaul

Justin Aquinas Gaul

Juliana Kathleen Pericci

Luke Michael Pericci

John Henry Bullen, V

The 12th edition of *Mosby's Diagnostic and Laboratory Test Reference* provides the user with an up-to-date, essential reference that allows easy access to clinically relevant laboratory and diagnostic tests. A unique feature of this handbook is its consistent format, which allows for quick reference without sacrificing the depth of detail necessary for a thorough understanding of diagnostic and laboratory testing. All tests begin on a new page and are listed in alphabetical order by their complete names. The alphabetical format is a strong feature of the book; it allows the user to locate tests quickly without first having to place them in an appropriate category or body system. The User's Guide to Test Preparation and Procedures section outlines the responsibilities of health care providers to ensure that the tests are accurately and safely performed. Use of this guide should eliminate the need for test repetition resulting from problems with patient preparation, test procedures, or collection techniques. Every feature of this book is designed to provide pertinent information in a sequence that best simulates priorities in the clinical setting.

The following information is provided, wherever applicable, for effective diagnostic and laboratory testing:

Name of test. Tests are listed by their complete names. A complete list of abbreviations and alternate test names follows each main entry.

Type of test. This section identifies whether the test is, for example, an x-ray procedure, ultrasound, nuclear scan, blood test, urine test, sputum test, or microscopic examination of tissue. This section helps the reader identify the source of the laboratory specimen or location of the diagnostic procedure.

Normal findings. Where applicable, normal values are listed for the infant, child, adult, and elderly person. Also, where appropriate, values are separated into male and female. It is important to realize that normal ranges of laboratory tests vary from institution to institution. This variability is even more obvious among the various laboratory textbooks. For this reason, we have deliberately chosen not to add a table of normal values as an appendix, and we encourage the user to check the normal values at the institution where the test is performed. This should be relatively easy because laboratory reports include normal values. Results are given in both conventional units and the International System of Units (SI units) where possible.

Possible critical values. These values give an indication of results that are well outside the normal range. These results require health care provider notification and usually result in some type of intervention. The Joint Commission is looking at the timely and reliable communication of critical laboratory values as one of its patient safety goals.

Test explanation and related physiology. This section provides a concise yet comprehensive description of each test. It includes fundamental information about the test itself, specific indications for the test, how the test is performed, what disease or disorder the various results may show, how it will affect the patient or client, and relevant pathophysiology that will enhance understanding of the test.

Contraindications. These data are crucial because they alert health care providers to patients to whom the test should not be administered. Patients highlighted in this section frequently include those who are pregnant, are allergic to iodinated or contrast dyes, or have bleeding disorders.

Potential complications. This section alerts the user to potential problems that necessitate astute assessments and interventions. For example, if a potential complication is renal failure, the implication may be to hydrate the patient before the test and force fluids after the test. A typical potential complication for many x-ray procedures is allergy to iodinated dye. Patient symptoms and appropriate interventions are described in detail.

Interfering factors. This section contains pertinent information because many factors can invalidate the test or make the test results unreliable. An important feature is the inclusion of drugs that can interfere with test results. Drugs that increase or decrease test values are always listed at the end of this section for consistency and quick access. A drug symbol (🏥) is used to emphasize these drug interferences.

Procedure and patient care. This section emphasizes the role of nurses and other health care providers in diagnostic and laboratory testing by addressing psychosocial and physiologic interventions. Patient teaching priorities are noted with a special icon (**PT**) to highlight information to be communicated to patients. For quick access to essential information, this section is divided into before, during, and after time sequences.

Before. This section addresses the need to explain the procedure and to allay patient concerns or anxieties. If patient consent is usually required, this is listed as a bulleted item.

Other important features include requirements such as fasting, obtaining baseline values, and performing bowel preparations.

During. This section gives specific directions for clinical specimen studies (e.g., urine and blood studies). Diagnostic procedures and their variations are described in a numbered, usually step-by-step format. Important information, such as who performs the test, where the study is performed, patient sensation, and duration of the procedure, is bulleted for emphasis. The duration of the procedure is very helpful for patient teaching because it indicates the time generally allotted for each study.

After. This section includes vital information that the nurse or other health care provider should heed or convey after the test. Examples include such factors as maintaining bed rest, comparing pulses with baseline values, encouraging fluid intake, and observing the patient for signs and symptoms of sepsis.

Abnormal findings. As the name implies, this section lists the abnormal findings for each study. Diseases or conditions that may be indicated by increased (▲) or decreased (▼) values are listed where appropriate.

Notes. This blank space at the end of the tests facilitates individualizing the studies according to the institution at which the test is performed. Variations in any area of the test (e.g., patient preparation, test procedure, normal values, postprocedural care) can be noted here.

This logical format emphasizes clinically relevant information. The clarity of this format allows for quick understanding of content essential to both students and health care providers. Color has been used to help locate tests and to highlight critical information (e.g., possible critical values). Color is also used in the illustrations to enhance the reader's understanding of many diagnostic procedures (e.g., bronchoscopy, fetoscopy, ERCP, pericardiocentesis, TEE). Many tables are used to simplify complex material on such topics as bioterrorism infectious agents, blood collection tubes, hepatitis testing, and protein electrophoresis. Extensive cross-referencing exists throughout the book, which facilitates understanding and helps the user tie together or locate related studies, such as hemoglobin and hematocrit.

New to this edition are standard guidelines for routine blood and urine testing located on the inside front cover for easy access. A list of abbreviations for test names is included on the book's endpapers. Appendix A includes a list of studies according to *body system.* This list may familiarize the user with other related studies the patient or client may need or the user may want to review. This should be especially useful for students and health care providers working in specialized areas. Appendix B provides a list of studies according to *test type.* This list may help the user read and learn about similarly performed tests and procedures (e.g., barium enema and barium swallow). Appendix C provides a list of blood tests used for *disease and organ panels.* Appendix D provides a list of *symbols and units of measurement.* Finally, a comprehensive index includes the names of all tests, their synonyms and abbreviations, and any other relevant terms found in the tests.

Many new studies, such as galectin-3, nicotine and metabolites, pepsinogen, and thromboelastography, have been added. All other studies have been revised and updated. Outdated studies have been eliminated.

We sincerely thank our editors for their enthusiasm and continued support. We are most grateful to the many nurses and other health care providers who made the first eleven editions of this book so successful. Thank you so much. This success validated the need for a user-friendly and quick-reference approach to laboratory and diagnostic testing.

We invite additional comments from current users of this book so that we may continue to provide useful, relevant diagnostic and laboratory test information to users of future editions.

Kathleen D. Pagana
Timothy J. Pagana
Theresa N. Pagana

contents

list of figures

Health care economics demands that laboratory and diagnostic testing be performed accurately and in the least amount of time possible. Tests should not have to be repeated because of improper patient preparation, test procedure, or specimen collection technique. The following guidelines delineate the responsibilities of health care providers to ensure safety of test procedures and accuracy of test results. Guidelines are described for the following major types of tests: blood, urine, stool, x-ray, nuclear scanning, ultrasound, and endoscopy.

Blood tests

Overview

Blood studies are used to assess a multitude of body processes and disorders. Common studies include enzymes, serum lipids, electrolyte levels, red and white blood cell counts, clotting factors, hormone levels, and levels of breakdown products (e.g., blood urea nitrogen).

Multiphasic screening machines can perform many blood tests simultaneously using a very small blood sample. The advantages of using these machines are that results are available quickly and the cost is lower when compared with individually performing each test.

Appendix C provides a list of current disease and organ panels. For example, the basic metabolic panel and the comprehensive metabolic panel have replaced the Chem-7 and Chem-12 panels. These changes are the result of federal guidelines that have standardized the nomenclature for chemistry panels.

Guidelines

- Observe universal precautions when collecting a blood specimen.
- Check whether fasting is required. Many studies, such as fasting blood sugar and cholesterol levels, require fasting for a designated period of time. Water is permitted.
- If ordered, withhold medications until the blood is drawn.
- Record the time of day when the blood test is drawn. Some blood test results (e.g., those for cortisol) vary according to a diurnal pattern, and this must be considered when blood levels are interpreted.
- In general, two or three blood tests can be done per tube of blood collected (e.g., two or three chemistry tests from one red-top tube of blood).

- Note the patient's position for certain tests (e.g., renin, because levels are affected by body position).
- Collect the blood in a properly color-coded test tube. Blood collection tubes have color-coded stoppers to indicate the presence or absence of different types of additives (preservatives and anticoagulants). A preservative prevents change in the specimen, and an anticoagulant inhibits clot formation or coagulation. Charts are available from the laboratory indicating the type of tube needed for each particular blood test. A representative chart is shown in Table **A**, p. xiv.
- Follow the recommended *order of draw* when collecting blood in tubes. Draw specimens into nonadditive (e.g., red-top) tubes before drawing them into tubes with additives. This prevents contamination of the blood specimen with additives that may cause incorrect test results. Fill the tubes in the following order:
  1. Blood culture tubes (to maintain sterility)
  2. Nonadditive tubes (e.g., red-top)
  3. Coagulation tubes (e.g., blue-top)
  4. Heparin tubes (e.g., green-top)
  5. Ethylenediaminetetraacetic acid (EDTA) tubes (e.g., lavender-top)
  6. Oxalate/fluoride tubes (e.g., gray-top)
- To obtain valid results, do not fasten the tourniquet for longer than 1 minute. Prolonged tourniquet application can cause stasis and hemoconcentration.
- Collect the blood specimen from the arm without an intravenous (IV) device, if possible. IV infusion can influence test results.
- Do not use the arm bearing a dialysis arteriovenous fistula for venipuncture unless the physician specifically authorizes it.
- Because of the risk of cellulitis, do not take specimens from the side on which a mastectomy or axillary lymph node dissection was performed.
- Follow the unit guidelines for drawing blood from an indwelling venous catheter (e.g., a triple-lumen catheter). Guidelines will specify the amount of blood to be drawn from the catheter and discarded before blood is collected for laboratory studies. The guidelines will also indicate the amount and type of solution needed to flush the catheter after drawing the blood to prevent clotting.

TABLE A   Common blood collection tubes

Top color	Additive	Purpose	Test examples
Red	Clot activator	Allows blood sample to clot Separates the serum for testing	Chemistry Bilirubin Blood urea nitrogen
Red/Black	Clot activator & gel for serum separator	Serum separator tube for serum determinatives in chemistry and serology	Chemistry, serology
Royal Blue	Heparin/ethylene-diaminetetraacetic acid (EDTA)	Provides low levels of trace elements	Trace metals, toxicology
Tan	Heparin/EDTA	Contains no lead	Lead determinatives
Purple or lavender	EDTA	Prevents blood from clotting	Hematology CBC
Gray	Oxalate/fluoride	Prevents glycolysis	Chemistry Glucose
Green	Heparin	Prevents blood from clotting when plasma needs to be tested	Chemistry Ammonia
Blue (Light)	Sodium citrate	Prevents blood from clotting when plasma needs to be tested	Prothrombin time Partial thromboplastin time
Black	Sodium citrate	Binds calcium to prevent blood clotting	Westergren erythrocyte sedimentation rate (ESR)
Yellow	Citrate dextrose	Preserves red cells	Blood cultures, blood banking studies

- Do not shake the blood specimen. Hemolysis may result from vigorous shaking and can invalidate test results. Use gentle inversions.
- Collect *blood cultures* before the initiation of antibiotic therapy. Blood cultures are often drawn when the patient manifests a fever. Often two or three cultures are taken at 30-minute intervals from different venipuncture sites.
- *Skin punctures* can be used for blood tests on capillary blood. Common puncture sites include the fingertips, earlobes, and heel surfaces. Fingertips are often used for small children, and the heel is the most commonly used site for infants.
- Ensure that the blood tubes are correctly labeled and delivered to the laboratory.
- After the specimen is drawn, apply pressure or a pressure dressing to the venipuncture site. Assess the site for bleeding.
- If the patient fasted before the blood test, reinstitute the appropriate diet.

Urine tests

Overview

Urine tests are easy to obtain and provide valuable information about many body system functions (e.g., kidney function, glucose metabolism, and various hormone levels). The ability of the patient to collect specimens appropriately should be assessed to determine the need for assistance.

Guidelines

- Observe universal precautions in collecting a urine specimen.
- Use the first morning specimen for routine urinalysis because it is more concentrated. To collect a first morning specimen, have the patient void before going to bed and collect the first urine specimen immediately upon rising.
- *Random* urine specimens can be collected at any time. They are usually obtained during daytime hours and without any prior patient preparation.
- If a *culture and sensitivity (C&S)* study is required or if the specimen is likely to be contaminated by vaginal discharge or bleeding, collect a *clean-catch* or *midstream* specimen. This requires meticulous cleansing of the urinary meatus with an antiseptic preparation to reduce contamination of the specimen by external organisms. Then the cleansing agent must be completely removed because it may contaminate

the specimen. Obtain the *midstream* collection by doing the following:

1. Have the patient begin to urinate in a bedpan, urinal, or toilet and then stop urinating. (This washes the urine out of the distal urethra.)
2. Correctly position a sterile urine container, and have the patient void 3 to 4 ounces of urine into it.
3. Cap the container.
4. Allow the patient to finish voiding.

- One-time *composite* urine specimens are collected over a period that may range anywhere from 2 to 24 hours. To collect a timed specimen, instruct the patient to void and discard the first specimen. This is noted as the *start time* of the test. Instruct the patient to save all subsequent urine in a special container for the designated period. Remind the patient to void before defecating so that urine is not contaminated by feces. Also, instruct the patient not to put toilet paper in the collection container. A preservative is usually used in the collection container. At the end of the specified time period, have the patient void and then add this urine to the specimen container, thus completing the collection process.
- Collection containers for *24-hour urine specimens* should hold 3 to 4 L of urine and have tight-fitting lids. They should be labeled with the patient's name, the starting collection date and time, the ending collection date and time, the name of the test, the preservative, and storage requirements during collection.
- Many urine collections require preservatives to maintain their stability during the collection period. Some specimens are best preserved by being kept on ice or refrigerated.
- *Urinary catheterization* may be needed for patients who are unable to void. This procedure is not preferred because of patient discomfort and the risk of patient infection.
- For patients with an *indwelling urinary catheter*, obtain a specimen by aseptically inserting a needleless syringe into the catheter at a drainage port distal to the sleeve leading to the balloon. Aspirate urine and then place it in a sterile urine container. The urine that accumulates in the plastic reservoir bag should never be used for a urine test.
- Urine specimens from infants and young children are usually collected in a disposable pouch called a *U bag*. This bag has an adhesive backing around the opening to attach to the child's perineum. After the bag is in place, check the

child every 15 minutes to see if an adequate specimen has been collected. Remove the specimen as soon as possible after the collection, and then label it and transport it to the laboratory.

Stool tests

Overview

The examination of feces provides important information that aids in the differential diagnosis of various gastrointestinal disorders. Fecal studies may also be used for microbiologic studies, chemical determinations, and parasitic examinations.

Guidelines

- Observe universal precautions in collecting a stool specimen.
- Collect stool specimens in a clean container with a fitted lid.
- Do not mix urine and toilet paper with the stool specimen. Both can contaminate the specimen and alter the results.
- Fecal analysis for occult blood, white blood cells, or qualitative fecal fat requires only a small amount of a randomly collected specimen.
- Quantitative tests for daily fecal excretion of a particular substance require a minimum of a 3-day fecal collection. This collection is necessary because the daily excretion of feces does not correlate well with the amount of food ingested by the patient in the same 24-hour period. Refrigerate specimens or keep them on ice during the collection period. Collect stool in a 1-gallon container.
- A small amount of fecal blood that is not visually apparent is termed *occult blood*. Chemical tests using commercially prepared slides are routinely used to detect fecal blood. Numerous commercial slide tests use guaiac as the indicator. These guaiac tests are routinely done on nursing units and in medical offices.
- Consider various factors (e.g., other diagnostic tests and medications) in planning the stool collection. For example, if the patient is scheduled for x-ray studies with barium sulfate, collect the stool specimen first. Various medications (e.g., tetracyclines and antidiarrheal preparations) affect the detection of intestinal parasites.
- Some fecal collections require dietary restrictions before the collection (e.g., tests for occult blood).
- Correctly label and deliver stool specimens to the laboratory within 30 minutes after collection. If you are unable to deliver the specimen within 30 minutes, it may be refrigerated for up to 2 hours.

X-ray studies

Overview

Because of the ability of x-rays to penetrate tissues, x-ray studies provide a valuable picture of body structures. X-ray studies can be as simple as a routine chest x-ray image or as complex as dye-enhanced cardiac catheterization. With the concern about radiation exposure, it is important to realize that the patient may question if the proposed benefits outweigh the risks involved.

Guidelines

- Assess the patient for any similar or recent x-ray procedures.
- Evaluate the patient for *allergies to iodine dye*. Carefully consider the following points:
  - Many types of contrast media are used in radiographic studies. For example, organic iodides and iodized oils are frequently used.
  - Allergic reactions to iodinated dye may vary from mild flushing, itching, and urticaria to severe, life-threatening anaphylaxis (evidenced by respiratory distress, drop in blood pressure, or shock). In the unusual event of anaphylaxis, the patient is treated with diphenhydramine (Benadryl), steroids, and epinephrine. Oxygen and endotracheal equipment should be on hand for immediate use.
  - The patient should always be assessed for allergies to iodine dye before it is administered. Inform the radiologist if an allergy to iodinated contrast is suspected. The radiologist may prescribe Benadryl and steroid preparation to be administered before testing. Usually, hypoallergenic nonionic contrast will be administered to allergic patients during the test.
  - After the x-ray procedure, evaluate the patient for a delayed reaction to dye (e.g., dyspnea, rashes, tachycardia, hives). This usually occurs within 2 to 6 hours after the test. Treat with antihistamines or steroids.
- Assess the patient for any evidence of dehydration or renal disease. Usually blood urea nitrogen (BUN) and creatinine tests are obtained prior to administration of iodine-containing intravenous contrast. Hydration may be required prior to the administration of iodine.
- Assess the patient for diabetes. Diabetics are particularly susceptible to renal disease caused by the administration of iodine-containing intravenous contrast. Diabetic patients who take metformin (Glucophage) or glyburide

(Micronase) are particularly susceptible to lactic acidosis and hypoglycemia. These medications may be discontinued for 1 to 4 days prior to and 1 to 2 days after the administration of iodine. Check with the x-ray department.

- Women in their childbearing years should have x-ray examinations during menses or within 10 to 14 days after the onset of menses to avoid possible exposure to a fetus.
- Pregnant women should not have x-ray procedures unless the benefits outweigh the risk of damage to the fetus.
- Note whether other x-ray studies are being planned; schedule them in the appropriate sequence. For example, x-ray examinations that do not require contrast should precede examinations that do require contrast. X-ray studies with barium should be scheduled after ultrasonography.
- Note the necessary dietary restrictions. Such studies as barium enema and intravenous pyelogram (IVP) are more accurate if the patient is kept NPO (fasting from food and liquids) for several hours before the test.
- Determine whether bowel preparations are necessary. For example, barium enemas and IVPs require bowel-cleansing regimens.
- Determine whether signed consent forms are required. These are necessary for most invasive x-ray procedures.
- Remove metal objects (e.g., necklaces, watches) because they can hinder visualization of the x-ray field.
- Patient aftercare is determined by the type of x-ray procedure. For example, a patient having a simple chest x-ray study will not require postprocedure care. However, invasive x-ray procedures involving contrast dyes (e.g., cardiac catheterization) require extensive nursing measures to detect potential complications.

Nuclear scanning

Overview

With the administration of a radionuclide and subsequent measurement of the radiation of a particular organ, functional abnormalities of various body areas (e.g., brain, heart, lung, bones) can be detected. Because the half-lives of the radioisotopes are short, only minimal radiation exposure occurs.

Guidelines

- Radiopharmaceuticals concentrate in target organs by various mechanisms. For example, some labeled compounds (e.g., hippuran) are cleared from the blood and excreted by the kidneys. Some phosphate compounds concentrate in the bone and infarcted tissue. Lung function can be studied by imaging the distribution of inhaled gases or aerosols.

- Note whether the patient has had any recent exposure to radionuclides. The previous study could interfere with the interpretation of the current study.
- Note the patient's age and current weight. This information is used to calculate the dose of radioactive substances.
- Nuclear scans are contraindicated in pregnant women and nursing mothers.
- Many scanning procedures do not require special preparation. However, a few have special requirements. For example, for bone scanning, the patient is encouraged to drink several glasses of water between the time of the injection of the isotope and the actual scanning. For some studies, blocking agents may need to be given to prevent other organs from taking up the isotope.
- For most nuclear scans, a small amount of an organ-specific radionuclide is given orally or injected intravenously. After the radioisotope concentrates in the desired area, the area is scanned. The scanning procedure usually takes place in the nuclear medicine department.
- Instruct the patient to lie still during the scanning.
- Usually encourage the patient to drink extra fluids to enhance excretion of the radionuclide after the test is finished.
- Although the amount of radionuclide excreted in the urine is very low, rubber gloves are sometimes recommended if the urine must be handled. Some hospitals may advise the patient to flush the toilet several times after voiding.

Ultrasound studies

Overview

In diagnostic ultrasonography, harmless high-frequency sound waves are emitted and penetrate the organ being studied. The sound waves bounce back to the sensor and are electronically converted into a picture of the organ. Ultrasonography is used to assess a variety of body areas, including the pelvis, abdomen, breast, heart, and pregnant uterus.

Guidelines

- Most ultrasound procedures require little or no preparation. However, the patient having a pelvic sonogram needs a full bladder, and the patient having an ultrasound examination of the gallbladder must be kept NPO before the procedure.

- Ultrasound examinations are usually performed in an ultrasound room; however, they can be performed in the patient unit.
- For ultrasound, a greasy paste is applied to the skin overlying the desired organ. This paste is used to enhance sound transmission and reception because air impedes transmission of sound waves to the body.
- Because of the noninvasive nature of ultrasonography, no special measures are needed after the study except for helping the patient remove the ultrasound paste.
- Ultrasound examinations have no radiation risk.
- Ultrasound examinations can be repeated as many times as necessary without being harmful to the patient. No cumulative effect has been seen.
- Barium has an adverse effect on the quality of abdominal studies. For this reason, schedule ultrasound of the abdomen before barium studies.
- Large amounts of gas in the bowel obstruct visualization of the bowel. This is because bowel gas is a reflector of sound.

Endoscopy procedures

Overview

With the help of a lighted, flexible instrument, internal structures of many areas of the body (e.g., stomach, colon, joints, bronchi, urinary system, and biliary tree) can be directly viewed. The specific purpose and procedure should be reviewed with the patient.

Guidelines

- Preparation for an endoscopic procedure varies according to the internal structure being examined. For example, examination of the stomach (gastroscopy) will require the passage of an instrument through the esophagus and into the stomach. The patient is kept NPO for 8 to 12 hours before the test to prevent gagging, vomiting, and aspiration. For colonoscopy, an instrument is passed through the rectum and into the colon. Therefore, the bowel must be cleansed and free of fecal material to afford proper visualization. Arthroscopic examination of the knee joint is usually done with the patient under general anesthesia, which necessitates routine preoperative care.
- Schedule endoscopic examinations before barium studies.
- Obtain a signed consent for endoscopic procedures.

- Endoscopic procedures are preferably performed by a physician in a specially equipped endoscopy room or in an operating room. However, some kinds can safely be performed at the bedside.
- Air is instilled into the bowel during colon examinations to maintain patency of the bowel lumen and to afford better visualization. This sometimes causes gas pains.
- In addition to visualization of the desired area, special procedures can be performed. Biopsies can be obtained, and bleeding ulcers can be cauterized. Also, knee surgery can be performed during arthroscopy.
- Specific postprocedure interventions are determined by the type of endoscopic examination performed. All procedures have the potential complication of perforation and bleeding. Most procedures use some type of sedation; safety precautions should be observed until the effects of the sedatives have worn off.
- After colonoscopy and similar studies, the patient may complain of rectal discomfort. A warm tub bath may be soothing.
- Usually keep the patient NPO for 2 hours after endoscopic procedures of the upper gastrointestinal system. Be certain that swallow, gag, and cough reflexes are present before permitting fluids or liquids to be ingested orally.

abdominal ultrasound (Abdominal sonogram)

Type of test   Ultrasound

Normal findings   Normal abdominal aorta, liver, gallbladder, bile ducts, pancreas, kidneys, ureters, and bladder

Test explanation and related physiology

Through the use of reflected sound waves, ultrasonography provides accurate visualization of the abdominal aorta, liver, gallbladder, pancreas, bile ducts, kidneys, ureters, and bladder. The technique of ultrasonography requires the emission of high-frequency sound waves from a transducer to penetrate the particular organ being studied. The sound waves are bounced back to the transducer and are then electronically converted into a pictorial image (Figure 1). Real-time ultrasound provides an accurate picture of the organ being studied. Doppler ultrasound provides information concerning blood flow to those organs.

The kidney is ultrasonographically evaluated to diagnose and locate renal cysts, to differentiate renal cysts from solid renal tumors, to demonstrate renal and pelvic calculi, to document hydronephrosis, to guide a percutaneously inserted needle for cyst aspiration or biopsy, and to place a nephrostomy tube. Ultrasound of the urologic tract is also used to detect malformed or ectopic kidneys and perinephric abscesses. Renal transplantation surveillance is possible with ultrasound. One advantage of a kidney sonogram over intravenous pyelography (see p. 778) is that it can be performed on patients with impaired renal function because no intravenous contrast is required.

Endourethral urologic ultrasound can also be performed through a stent that has a transducer at its end. The stent probe is placed into the urethra to examine that segment for diverticula. The stent probe can then be advanced into the bladder where the depth of a tumor into the bladder wall can be measured. With the use of wire lead guidance, the stent probe can be passed into the ureter where stones (especially those embedded into the submucosa), tumors, or extraurethral compression can be identified and localized. Finally, as the probe is advanced in the proximal ureter, renal tumors or cysts can be better delineated.

The prostate and the testes are discussed on pp. 754 and 816.

Another use of sonography is in the assessment of the abdominal aorta for aneurysmal dilation. Sonographic evidence of an aortic aneurysm greater than 5 cm or any size aneurysm that is documented to be significantly enlarging is an

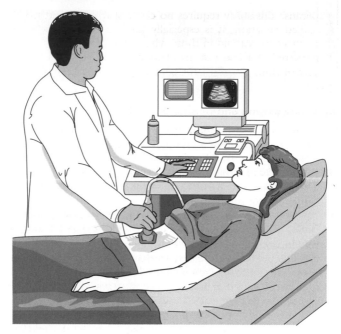

FIGURE 1 Ultrasound of the abdomen.

indication for abdominal aorta aneurysm resection. Ultrasound is also an ideal way to evaluate aneurysm patients before and after surgery.

Ultrasound is used to detect cystic structures of the *liver* (e.g., benign cysts, hepatic abscesses, and dilated hepatic ducts) and solid intrahepatic tumors (primary and metastatic). Hepatic ultrasound also can be performed intraoperatively by using a sterile probe. This technique allows for accurate location of small, nonpalpable hepatic tumors or abscesses. The *gallbladder* and *bile ducts* can be visualized and examined for evidence of gallstones, polyps, or dilation secondary to obstructive strictures or tumors. The *pancreas* is examined for evidence of tumors, pseudocysts, acute inflammation, chronic inflammation, or pancreatic abscesses. Ultrasound of the pancreas is frequently performed serially to document and demonstrate resolution of acute pancreatic inflammatory processes.

Because this study requires no contrast material and has no associated radiation, it is especially useful in patients who are allergic to contrast and in those who are pregnant. Fasting may be preferred, but it is not mandatory. (See discussion of pelvic ultrasonography [p. 697] for sonographic evaluation of pelvic organs.)

Interfering factors

- Air impedes transmission of ultrasonic waves into the body. The use of a lubricant is essential to ensure good transmission of sound waves to and from the body.
- Barium blocks transmission of ultrasonic waves. For this reason, ultrasonography of the abdomen should be performed before any barium contrast studies.
- Large amounts of gas in the bowel distort visualization of abdominal organs because bowel gas reflects sound. Likewise, ultrasonic evaluation of the lungs yields poor results.
- Obesity may affect the results of the study because sound waves are altered by fatty tissue.
- Movement causes artifacts. Some patients may need to be sedated to remain still. Uncooperative patients (especially children) may not be candidates for ultrasonography.
- Because ultrasonography requires direct contact of the transducer and the skin, it may not be possible to perform this study in postoperative patients with dressings.
- The quality of the ultrasound image and the sufficiency of the study depend to a very large part on the abilities of the ultrasound technologist performing the study.

Procedure and patient care

Before
PT Explain the procedure to the patient.
PT Tell the patient that fasting may or may not be required, depending on the organ to be examined. No fasting is required for ultrasonography of the abdominal aorta, kidney, liver, spleen, or pancreas. Fasting, however, is preferred for ultrasound of the gallbladder and bile ducts.

During
- Note the following procedural steps:
  1. The patient is placed on the ultrasonography table in the prone or supine position, depending on the organ to be studied.

2. A greasy conductive paste (coupling agent) is applied to the patient's skin. This paste is used to enhance sound wave transmission and reception.
3. A transducer is placed over the skin.
4. Pictures are taken of the reflections from the organs.

- The test is completed in approximately 20 minutes, usually by an ultrasound technologist, and is interpreted by a radiologist.

PT Tell the patient that this procedure causes no discomfort.

After

- Remove the coupling agent from the patient's skin.
- Note that if a biopsy is done, refer to biopsy of the specific organ (e.g., liver or kidney biopsy).

Abnormal findings

Kidney

Renal cysts
Renal tumor
Renal calculi
Hydronephrosis
Ureteral obstruction
Perirenal abscess
Glomerulonephritis
Pyelonephritis
Perirenal hematoma

Gallbladder

Polyps
Tumor
Gallstone

Liver

Tumor
Abscess
Intrahepatic dilated bile ducts

Pancreas

Tumor
Cysts
Pseudocysts
Abscess
Inflammation

Bile ducts

Gallstone
Dilation
Stricture
Tumor

Abdominal aorta

Aneurysm

Abdominal cavity

Ascites
Abscess

notes

acetylcholine receptor antibody panel (AChR Ab, Anti–AChR antibody)

Type of test Blood

Normal findings

ACh receptor (muscle) binding antibodies: ≤0.02 nmol/L

ACh receptor (muscle) modulating antibodies: 0 to 20% (reported as % loss of AChR)

Striational (striated muscle) antibodies: <1:60

Test explanation and related physiology

These antibodies may cause blocks in neuromuscular transmission by interfering with the binding of *acetylcholine* (ACh) to *ACh receptor* (AChR) sites on the muscle membrane, thereby preventing muscle contraction. It is this phenomenon that characterizes myasthenia gravis (MG). Antibodies to AChR occur in more than 85% of patients with acquired MG. Lower levels are seen in patients with ocular MG only. The presence of these antibodies is virtually diagnostic of MG, but a negative test does not exclude the disease. The measured titers do not correspond well with the severity of MG in different patients. In an individual patient, however, antibody levels are particularly useful in monitoring response to therapy. As the patient improves, antibody titers decrease. In adults with MG, there is at least a 20% occurrence of thymoma or other neoplasm. Neoplasms are an endogenous source of the antigens driving production of AChR autoantibodies.

There are several AChR antibodies that can be associated with MG. The AChR-*binding* antibody can activate complement and lead to loss of AChR. The AChR-*modulating* antibody causes receptor endocytosis, resulting in loss of AChR expression, which correlates most closely with clinical severity of disease. It is the most sensitive test. A positive modulating antibody test may indicate subclinical MG, contraindicating the use of curare-like drugs during surgery. The AChR-*blocking* antibody may impair binding of acetylcholine to the receptor, leading to poor muscle contraction. It is the least sensitive test (positive in only 61% of patients with MG). Not all of the antibodies impair neuromuscular transmission. For example, striational antibodies are directed at sarcomeric proteins that don't impair neuromuscular function.

Anti-striated muscle antibody (*striated muscle antibody, IgG*) titers greater than or equal to 1:80 are suggestive of myasthenia. This antibody is detectable in 30% to 40% of anti-AChR-negative patients (particularly those with bulbar symptoms only). However, striated muscle antibody can be found in rheumatic fever, myocardial infarction, and a variety of postcardiotomy states.

Interfering factors

- False-positive results may occur in patients with amyotrophic lateral sclerosis who have been treated with cobra venom.
- False-positive results may be seen in patients with penicillamine-induced or Lambert-Eaton myasthenic syndrome.
- Patients with autoimmune liver disease may have elevated results.
- ✠ Drugs that may cause *increased* levels include muscle paralytic medicines (succinylcholine) and snake venom.
- ✠ Immunosuppressive drugs may suppress the formation of these antibodies in patients with subclinical MG.

Procedure and patient care

- See inside front cover for Routine Blood Testing.
- Fasting: no
- Blood tube commonly used: red

Abnormal findings

▲ **Increased titer levels**
  Myasthenia gravis
  Ocular myasthenia gravis
  Thymoma

notes

acid phosphatase (Prostatic acid phosphatase [PAP], Tartrate-resistant acid phosphatase [TRAP])

Type of test Blood

Normal findings

Adult/elderly: 0.13-0.63 units/L (Roy, Brower, Hayden; 37 °C) or 2.2-10.5 units/L (SI units)
Child: 8.6-12.6 units/mL (30 °C)
Newborn: 10.4-16.4 units/mL (30 °C)

Test explanation and related physiology

Acid phosphatase is found in many tissues, including liver, red blood cells, bone marrow, and platelets. The highest levels are found in the prostate gland—the PAP isoenzyme. Usually (but not always) elevated levels are seen in patients with prostatic cancer that has metastasized beyond the capsule to other parts of the body, especially bone. The degree of elevation indicates the extent of disease.

Because acid phosphatase is also found at high concentrations in seminal fluid, this test can be performed on vaginal secretions to investigate alleged rape. This is now the primary use of PAP testing. High levels of acid phosphatase also exist in white blood cells (mostly monocytes and lymphocytes). They are helpful in determining the clinical course of patients with lymphoproliferative diseases and hairy cell leukemia. Acid phosphatase is a lysosomal enzyme. Therefore, lysosomal storage diseases (e.g., Gaucher disease and Niemann-Pick disease) are associated with elevated levels.

Interfering factors

- Alkaline and acid phosphatase are very similar enzymes that differ in the pH at which they are identified. Any condition associated with very high levels of alkaline phosphatase may falsely indicate high acid phosphatase levels.
- Falsely high levels of acid phosphatase may occur in males after a digital examination or after instrumentation of the prostate (e.g., cystoscopy) because of prostatic stimulation.
- ✶ Drugs that may cause *increased* levels of acid phosphatase include alglucerase, androgens (in females), and clofibrate.
- ✶ Drugs that may cause *decreased* levels include alcohol, fluorides, heparin, oxalates, and phosphates.

Procedure and patient care

- See inside front cover for Routine Blood Testing.
- Fasting: no
- Blood tube commonly used: red
- Avoid hemolysis. Red blood cells contain acid phosphatase.
- Note on the laboratory slip if the patient has had a prostatic examination or instrumentation of the prostate within the last 24 hours.
- Do *not* leave the specimen at room temperature for 1 hour or longer, because the enzyme is heat- and pH-sensitive and its activity will decrease.

Abnormal findings

▲ **Increased levels**

Prostatic carcinoma

Benign prostatic hypertrophy

Prostatitis

Multiple myeloma

Paget disease

Hyperparathyroidism

Metastasis to the bone

Sickle cell crisis

Thrombocytosis

Lysosomal disorders (e.g., Gaucher disease)

Renal diseases

Liver diseases (e.g., cirrhosis)

Rape

notes

activated clotting time (ACT, Activated coagulation time)

Type of test Blood

Normal findings 70-120 sec

Therapeutic range for anticoagulation: 150-600 sec

(Normal ranges and anticoagulation ranges vary according to type of laboratory procedure and particular therapy.)

Possible critical values Depends upon use for the test and clinical situation

Test explanation and related physiology

The ACT is primarily used to measure the anticoagulant effect of heparin or other direct thrombin inhibitors during cardiac angioplasty, hemodialysis, and cardiopulmonary bypass (CPB) surgery. This test measures the time for whole blood to clot after the addition of particulate activators. It is similar to the *activated partial thromboplastin time* (APTT, p. 693) in that it measures the ability of the *intrinsic* pathway to begin clot formation by activating factor XII (see Figure 10, p. 264). By checking the blood clotting status with ACT, the response to unfractionated heparin therapy can be monitored.

Both the APTT and the ACT can be used to monitor heparin therapy for patients during CPB. However, the ACT has several advantages over the APTT. First, the ACT is more accurate than the APTT when high doses of heparin are used for anticoagulation. This makes it especially useful during clinical situations requiring high-dose heparin, such as during CPB, when high-dose anticoagulation is necessary at levels 10 times those used for venous thrombosis. The APTT is not measurable at these high doses. The accepted goal for the ACT is 400 to 480 seconds during CPB.

Second, the ACT is both less expensive and more easily performed, even at the bedside. This allows for immediate accessibility and decreased turnaround time. The capability to perform the ACT at the point of care makes the ACT particularly useful for patients requiring angioplasty, hemodialysis, and CPB.

A nomogram is often used as a guide to reach the desired level of anticoagulation. This nomogram is used in determining the dose of protamine to neutralize the heparin upon completion of these procedures. The ACT is used in determining when it is safe to remove the vascular access upon completion of these procedures. The benefits of the *modified* ACT test are that it requires a smaller-volume blood specimen; it can be automated; it can use standardized blood/reagent mixing; and it provides faster clotting time results than the conventional ACT. The modified ACT is now being used more frequently.

Interfering factors

- The ACT is affected by biologic variables, including hypothermia, hemodilution, and platelet number and function.
- Factors affecting the pharmacokinetics of heparin (e.g., kidney or liver disease) and heparin resistance can affect ACT measurements.
- A clotted specimen can increase ACT measurements.

Procedure and patient care

- See inside front cover for Routine Blood Testing.
- Fasting: no
- Blood tube commonly used: verify with lab
- Less than 1 mL of blood is collected and placed in a machine at the bedside. When a clot forms, the ACT value is displayed.
- If the patient is receiving a continuous heparin drip, the blood sample is obtained from the arm without the intravenous catheter.
- The bleeding time will be prolonged because of anticoagulation therapy.
- Assess the patient to detect possible bleeding. Check for blood in the urine and all other excretions, and assess the patient for bruises, petechiae, and low back pain.

Abnormal findings

▲ **Increased levels**
 Heparin administration
 Clotting factor deficiencies
 Cirrhosis of the liver
 Lupus inhibitor
 Warfarin administration

▼ **Decreased levels**
 Thrombosis

notes

adrenocorticotropic hormone (ACTH, Corticotropin)

Type of test Blood

Normal findings

Adult/elderly:
  Female: 19 years and older: 6-58 pg/mL
  Male: 19 years and older: 7-69 pg/mL
Children:
  Male and female: 10-18 years: 6-55 pg/mL
  Male and female: 1 week-9 years: 5-46 pg/mL

Test explanation and related physiology

The ACTH tests the anterior pituitary gland function and provides the greatest insight into the causes of either Cushing syndrome (overproduction of cortisol) or Addison disease (underproduction of cortisol). An elaborate feedback mechanism for cortisol exists to coordinate the function of the hypothalamus, pituitary gland, and adrenal glands. ACTH is an important part of this mechanism. Corticotropin-releasing hormone (CRH) is made in the hypothalamus. This stimulates ACTH production in the anterior pituitary gland. This, in turn, stimulates the adrenal cortex to produce cortisol. The rising levels of cortisol act as negative feedback and curtail further production of CRH and ACTH.

In the patient with Cushing syndrome, an elevated ACTH level can be caused by a pituitary or a nonpituitary (ectopic) ACTH-producing tumor, usually in the lung, pancreas, thymus, or ovary. ACTH levels over 200 pg/mL usually indicate ectopic ACTH production. If the ACTH level is below normal in a patient with Cushing syndrome, an adrenal adenoma or carcinoma is probably the cause of the hyperfunction.

In patients with Addison disease, an elevated ACTH level indicates primary adrenal gland failure, as in adrenal gland destruction caused by infarction, hemorrhage, or autoimmunity; surgical removal of the adrenal gland; congenital enzyme deficiency; or adrenal suppression after prolonged ingestion of exogenous steroids. If the ACTH level is below normal in a patient with adrenal insufficiency, hypopituitarism is most probably the cause of the hypofunction.

One must be aware that there is a diurnal variation of ACTH levels that corresponds to variation of cortisol levels. Levels in evening (8 PM to 10 PM) samples are usually one half to two thirds those of morning (4 AM to 8 AM) specimens. This diurnal variation is lost when disease (especially neoplasm) affects the pituitary or adrenal glands. Likewise, stress can blunt or eliminate this normal diurnal variation.

Interfering factors

- Stress (trauma, pyrogens, or hypoglycemia) and pregnancy can increase levels.
- Recently administered radioisotope scans can affect levels.
- ✍ Drugs that may cause *increased* ACTH levels include aminoglutethimide, amphetamines, estrogens, ethanol, insulin, metyrapone, spironolactone, and vasopressin.
- ✍ Corticosteroids may *decrease* ACTH levels.

Procedure and patient care

- See inside front cover for Routine Blood Testing.
- Fasting: yes
- Blood tube commonly used: green
- Evaluate the patient for stress factors that could invalidate the test results.
- Evaluate the patient for sleep pattern abnormalities. With a normal sleep pattern, the ACTH level is the highest between 4 AM and 8 AM and the lowest around 9 PM.
- Chill the blood tube to prevent enzymatic degradation of ACTH.
- Place the specimen in ice water and send it to the chemistry laboratory immediately. ACTH is a very unstable peptide in plasma and should be stored at −20 °C to prevent artificially low values.

Abnormal findings

▲ **Increased levels**
  Addison disease (primary adrenal insufficiency)
  Cushing syndrome (pituitary-dependent adrenal hyperplasia)
  Ectopic ACTH syndrome
  Stress
  Adrenogenital syndrome (congenital adrenal hyperplasia)

▼ **Decreased levels**
  Secondary adrenal insufficiency (pituitary insufficiency)
  Cushing syndrome
  Hypopituitarism
  Adrenal adenoma or carcinoma
  Steroid administration

notes

adrenocorticotropic hormone stimulation test with cosyntropin (ACTH stimulation test, Cortisol stimulation test)

Type of test Blood

Normal findings

Rapid test: cortisol levels increase more than 7 mcg/dL above baseline

24-hour test: cortisol levels greater than 40 mcg/dL

3-day test: cortisol levels greater than 40 mcg/dL

Test explanation and related physiology

This test is performed on patients found to have an adrenal insufficiency. An increase in plasma cortisol levels after the infusion of an ACTH-like drug indicates that the adrenal gland is normal and is capable of functioning if stimulated. In that case, the cause of the adrenal insufficiency would lie within the pituitary gland (hypopituitarism, which is called secondary adrenal insufficiency). If little or no rise in cortisol levels occurs after the administration of the ACTH-like drug, the adrenal gland is the source of the problem and cannot secrete cortisol. This is called primary adrenal insufficiency (Addison disease), which may be caused by adrenal hemorrhage, infarction, autoimmunity, metastatic tumor, surgical removal of the adrenal glands, or congenital adrenal enzyme deficiency.

This test can also be used in the evaluation of patients with Cushing syndrome. Patients with Cushing syndrome caused by bilateral adrenal hyperplasia have an exaggerated cortisol elevation in response to the administration of the ACTH-like drug. Those experiencing Cushing syndrome as a result of hyperfunctioning adrenal tumors (which are usually autonomous and relatively insensitive to ACTH) have little or no increase in cortisol levels over baseline values.

Cosyntropin (Cortrosyn) is a synthetic subunit of ACTH that has the same corticosteroid-stimulating effect as endogenous ACTH in healthy persons. During this test, cosyntropin is administered to the patient, and the ability of the adrenal gland to respond is measured by plasma cortisol levels.

The *rapid stimulation test* is only a screening test. A normal response excludes adrenal insufficiency. An abnormal response, however, requires a 24-hour to 3-day prolonged ACTH stimulation test to differentiate primary insufficiency from secondary insufficiency. It should be noted that the adrenal gland can also be stimulated by insulin-induced hypoglycemia as a stressing agent. When insulin is the stimulant, cortisol and glucose levels are measured.

Interfering factors

⚫ Drugs that may cause artificially *increased* cortisol levels include corticosteroids, estrogens, and spironolactone.

Procedure and patient care

- See inside front cover for Routine Blood Testing.
- Fasting: yes
- Blood tube commonly used: red

Rapid test
- Obtain a baseline plasma cortisol level. This should be done 30 minutes before cosyntropin (ACTH-like drug) administration.
- Administer an IV injection of cosyntropin over a 2-minute period as prescribed.
- Measure plasma cortisol levels 30 and 60 minutes after drug administration.

24-hour test
- Obtain a baseline plasma cortisol level.
- Start an IV infusion of synthetic cosyntropin.
- Administer the solution as prescribed for 24 hours.
- After 24 hours, obtain another plasma cortisol level.

3-day test
- Obtain a baseline plasma cortisol level.
- Administer the prescribed dose of cosyntropin IV over an 8-hour period for 2 to 3 consecutive days.
- Measure plasma cortisol levels at 12, 24, 36, 48, 60, and 72 hours after the start of the test.

Abnormal findings

In adrenal insufficiency

Increase above normal response (secondary adrenal insufficiency)

Hypopituitarism

Exogenous steroid ingestion

Endogenous steroid production from a nonendocrine tumor

Normal or below normal response (primary adrenal insufficiency)

Addison disease

Adrenal infarction/hemorrhage

Metastatic tumor to the adrenal gland

Congenital enzyme adrenal insufficiency

Surgical removal of the adrenal gland

In Cushing syndrome

Increase above normal response

Bilateral adrenal hyperplasia

Normal or below normal response

Adrenal adenoma

Adrenal carcinoma

ACTH-producing nonadrenal tumor

Chronic steroid use

notes

adrenocorticotropic hormone stimulation test with metyrapone (ACTH stimulation test with metyrapone, Metyrapone test)

Type of test Blood; urine (24-hour)

Normal findings

Blood

11-deoxycortisol increased to >7 mcg/dL and cortisol <10 mcg/dL

Urine (24-hour)

Baseline excretion of urinary *17-hydroxycorticosteroid* (17-OCHS) more than doubled

Test explanation and related physiology

Metyrapone is a potent blocker of an enzyme involved in cortisol production. Therefore, cortisol production is reduced. When this drug is given, the resulting fall in cortisol production should stimulate pituitary secretion of ACTH by way of a negative feedback mechanism. Cortisol precursors (*11-deoxycortisol* and *17-OCHS*) can be detected in the urine or blood. This test is similar to the ACTH stimulation test with cosyntropin (see p. 13).

In patients with adrenal hyperplasia caused by pituitary overproduction of ACTH, the cortisol precursors are greatly increased, more than expected in normal patients. This is because the normal adrenal–pituitary response mechanism is still intact. No response to metyrapone occurs in patients with Cushing syndrome resulting from adrenal adenoma or carcinoma because the tumors are autonomous and therefore insensitive to changes in ACTH secretion.

This test is also used to evaluate the pituitary reserve capacity to produce ACTH. It can document that adrenal insufficiency exists as a result of pituitary disease (secondary adrenal insufficiency) rather than primary adrenal pathology.

Contraindications

• Patients with possible adrenal insufficiency
• Patients taking glucocorticosteroids

Potential complications

• Addison disease and addisonian crisis because metyrapone inhibits cortisol production
• Dizziness, sedation, allergic reaction, and bone marrow suppression

Interfering factors

- Recent administration of radioisotopes can affect results.
- ✔ Chlorpromazine interferes with the response to metyrapone and should not be administered during the testing.

Procedure and patient care

- Obtain a baseline cortisol level (see p. 301) for the blood test.
- See inside front cover for Routine Blood Testing.
- Fasting: no
- Blood tube commonly used: red or green
- See inside front cover for Routine Urine Testing.
- Obtain a baseline 24-hour urine specimen for the 17-OCHS level (see p. 541) for the urine test.

During

Blood

- Administer a prescribed dose of metyrapone at 11 PM the night before the blood sample is to be collected. Collect a venous blood sample in a red-top tube in the morning.

Urine

- Obtain a 24-hour urine specimen for the 17-OCHS level as a baseline. Then collect a 24-hour urine specimen for the 17-OCHS level during and again 1 day after the oral administration of a dose of metyrapone, which is given in 5 doses every 4 hours within 24 hours.
- Metyrapone should be administered with a glass of milk to diminish any GI side effects.

After

- Assess the patient for impending signs of addisonian crisis (muscle weakness, mental and emotional changes, anorexia, nausea, vomiting, hypotension, hyperkalemia, or vascular collapse).
- Note that addisonian crisis is a medical emergency that must be treated vigorously with replenishing steroids, reversing shock, and restoring circulation.

Abnormal findings

Increased cortisol precursors

Adrenal hyperplasia

No change in cortisol precursors

Adrenal tumor
Ectopic ACTH syndrome
Secondary adrenal insufficiency

notes

adrenal steroid precursors (Androstenediones [AD], Dehydroepiandrosterone [DHEA], Dehydroepiandrosterone sulfate [DHEA S], 11-Deoxycortisol, 17-Hydroxyprogesterone, 17-Hydroxypregnenolone, Pregnenolone)

Type of test Blood
Normal findings

		Female	Male
AD	Tanner Stage I	0.05-0.51 ng/mL	0.04-0.32 ng/mL
	Tanner Stage II	0.15-1.37 ng/mL	0.08-0.48 ng/mL
	Tanner Stage III	0.37-2.24 ng/mL	0.14-0.87 ng/mL
	Tanner Stage IV-V	0.35-2.05 ng/mL	0.27-1.07 ng/mL
DHEA	Tanner Stage I	0.14-2.76 ng/mL	0.11-2.37 ng/mL
	Tanner Stage II	0.83-4.87 ng/mL	0.37-3.66 ng/mL
	Tanner Stage III	1.08-7.56 ng/mL	0.75-5.24 ng/mL
	Tanner Stage IV-V	1.24-7.88 ng/mL	1.22-6.73 ng/mL
DHEA S	Tanner Stage I	7-209 µg/dL	7-126 µg/dL
	Tanner Stage II	28-260 µg/dL	13-241 µg/dL
	Tanner Stage III	39-390 µg/dL	32-446 µg/dL
	Tanner Stage IV-V	81-488 µg/dL	65-371 µg/dL

Test explanation and related physiology

Androstenediones (ADs, DHEA, and the sulfuric ester, DHEA S) are precursors of testosterone and estrone, and are made in the gonads and the adrenal gland. 11-Deoxycortisol, 17-hydroxyprogesterone, 17-hydroxypregnenolone, and pregnenolone are precursors of cortisol. ACTH stimulates their adrenal secretion. Children with congenital adrenal hyperplasia (CAH) have genetic mutations that cause deficiencies in the enzymes involved in the synthesis of cortisol, testosterone, aldosterone, and estrone. When defects in enzyme synthesis occur along the path of hormone synthesis, the above listed precursors exist in levels that exceed normal through the increased stimulation of ACTH. In most cases, CAH is a genetic autosomal recessive disorder.

The symptoms of the disorder depend upon which steroids are overproduced and which are deficient. As a result, CAH may present with various symptoms, including virilization of the affected female infant, signs of androgen excess in males and females, signs of sex hormone deficiency in males and females, salt-wasting crisis secondary to cortisol and aldosterone deficiency, or hormonal hypertension due to increased mineralocorticoids.

A milder, non-classic form of CAH is characterized by premature puberty, acne, hirsutism, menstrual irregularity, and infertility.

These same precursors can occur in adults due to adrenal or gonadal tumors. Patients with polycystic ovary syndrome (Stein-Leventhal syndrome) have particularly elevated levels of ADs. DHEAS levels are particularly high in patients with adrenal carcinoma.

In patients suspected of CAH, testing for a panel of steroids involved in the cortisol biosynthesis pathway may be performed to establish the specific enzyme deficiency. In most cases, basal concentrations within the normal reference interval rule out CAH. The ratio of the precursor to the final pathway product (with and without ACTH stimulation) may be used to diagnose which enzyme is deficient.

Interfering factors

- A radioactive scan performed 1 week before the test may invalidate the test results if radioimmunoassay is performed.
- Drugs that may *increase* levels of ADs include clomiphene, corticotropin, and metyrapone.
- Drugs that may *decrease* levels of ADs include steroids.

Procedure and patient care

- See inside front cover for Routine Blood Testing.
- Fasting: no
- Blood tube commonly used: serum separator or red
- PT Tell the female patient that the specimen should be collected 1 week before or after the menstrual period.
- Indicate the date of the last menstrual period (if applicable) on the laboratory form.

Abnormal findings

▲ Increased levels
Adrenal tumor
Congenital adrenal
  hyperplasia
Ectopic ACTH-producing
  tumors
Cushing syndrome (some cases)
Stein-Leventhal syndrome
Ovarian sex cord tumor

▼ Decreased levels
Gonadal failure
Primary or secondary
  adrenal insufficiency

notes

age-related macular degeneration risk analysis
(ARMD risk analysis, Y402H, and A69S)

Type of test Blood

Normal findings No mutation noted

Test explanation and related physiology

Age-related macular degeneration (ARMD) is recognized as a leading cause of blindness in the United States. Blurred or distorted vision and difficulty adjusting to dim light are common symptoms. ARMD, both wet and dry types, is considered a multifactorial disorder because it is thought to develop due to interplay between environmental (smoking) and genetic (gender, ethnicity) risk and protective (antioxidants) factors. At least two genetic variants (Y402H and A69S) have been found to be associated with an increased risk for ARMD. The Y402H and the A69S genetic variants are common polymorphisms in ARMD. An individual with two copies of the Y402H variant in the gene *CFH* and two copies of the A69S variant in the gene *LOC387715* has an approximately sixtyfold increased risk for ARMD. This is significant, given how common ARMD is in the general population.

This information can be clinically useful when making medical management decisions (for example, the use of inflammatory markers) and emphasizing to patients the benefits of smoking cessation and dietary modification. In some cases, genotype information may also assist with clinical diagnosis.

Procedure and patient care

- See inside front cover for Routine Blood Testing.
- Fasting: no
- Blood tube commonly used: lavender or yellow
- **PT** Tell the patient that results may not be available for a few weeks.

Abnormal findings

Increased risk of ARMD

notes

alanine aminotransferase (ALT, formerly Serum glutamic-pyruvic transaminase [SGPT])

Type of test Blood

Normal findings

Adult/child: 4-36 units/L at 37 °C, or 4-36 units/L (SI units)
Elderly: may be slightly higher than adult
Infant: may be twice as high as adult

Test explanation and related physiology

ALT is found predominantly in the liver; lesser quantities are found in the kidneys, heart, and skeletal muscles. Injury or disease affecting the liver parenchyma causes a release of this hepatocellular enzyme into the bloodstream, thus elevating serum ALT levels. Generally, most ALT elevations are caused by liver disease. Therefore, this enzyme is not only sensitive but also very specific in indicating hepatocellular disease. In hepatocellular disease other than viral hepatitis, the ALT/AST ratio *(DeRitis ratio)* is less than 1. In viral hepatitis, the ratio is greater than 1. This is helpful in the diagnosis of viral hepatitis.

Interfering factors

- Previous IM injections may cause elevated levels.
- ☞ Drugs that may cause *increased* ALT levels include acetaminophen, allopurinol, aminosalicylic acid (PAS), ampicillin, azathioprine, carbamazepine, cephalosporins, chlordiazepoxide, chlorpropamide, clofibrate, cloxacillin, codeine, dicumarol, indomethacin, isoniazid (INH), methotrexate, methyldopa, nafcillin, nalidixic acid, nitrofurantoin, oral contraceptives, oxacillin, phenothiazines, phenylbutazone, phenytoin, procainamide, propoxyphene, propranolol, quinidine, salicylates, tetracyclines, and verapamil.

Procedure and patient care

- See inside front cover for Routine Blood Testing.
- Fasting: no
- Blood tube commonly used: red
- Patients with liver dysfunction often have prolonged clotting times.

Abnormal findings

▲ **Increased levels**
Hepatitis
Hepatic necrosis
Hepatic ischemia
Cirrhosis
Cholestasis
Hepatic tumor
Hepatotoxic drugs
Obstructive jaundice
Severe burns
Trauma to striated muscle
Myositis
Pancreatitis
Myocardial infarction
Infectious mononucleosis
Shock

notes

aldolase

Type of test Blood

Normal findings

Adult: 3-8.2 Sibley-Lehninger units/dL or 22-59 mU/L at 37 °C
  (SI units)
Child: approximately two times the adult values
Newborn: approximately four times the adult values

Test explanation and related physiology

Serum aldolase is very similar to the enzymes aspartate aminotransferase AST (SGOT) (see p. 129) and CPK (see p. 308).
Aldolase is an enzyme used in glycolysis (breakdown of glucose).
As with AST and creatine phosphokinase, aldolase exists throughout the body in most tissues. This test is most useful for indicating muscular or hepatic cellular injury or disease. The serum
aldolase level is very high in patients with muscular dystrophies,
dermatomyositis, and polymyositis. Levels also are increased in
patients with gangrenous processes, muscular trauma, and muscular infectious diseases (e.g., trichinosis). Elevated levels are also
noted in chronic hepatitis, obstructive jaundice, and cirrhosis.

Neurologic diseases causing weakness can be differentiated
from muscular causes of weakness with this test. Normal values
are seen in patients with such neurologic diseases as poliomyelitis, myasthenia gravis, and multiple sclerosis. Elevated aldolase
levels are seen in the primary muscular disorders.

Interfering factors

- Previous IM injections may cause elevated levels.
- Strenuous exercise can cause a transient spike in aldolase.
- ☒ Drugs that may cause *increased* aldolase levels include hepato-
  toxic agents.
- ☒ Drugs that may cause *decreased* aldolase levels include
  phenothiazines.

Procedure and patient care

- See inside front cover for Routine Blood Testing.
- Fasting: verify with lab
- Blood tube commonly used: red

Abnormal findings

▲ **Increased levels**

Hepatocellular diseases
(e.g., hepatitis)

Muscular diseases
(e.g., muscular dystrophy,
dermatomyositis, and
polymyositis)

Muscular trauma (e.g., severe
crush injuries)

Muscular infections
(e.g., trichinosis)

Gangrenous processes
(e.g., gangrene of the bowel)

Myocardial infarction

▼ **Decreased levels**

Late muscular
dystrophy

Hereditary fructose
intolerance

Muscle-wasting disease

notes

aldosterone

Type of test Blood; urine (24-hour)

Normal findings

Blood

Supine: 3-10 ng/dL or 0.08-0.30 nmol/L (SI units)
Upright:
  Female: 5-30 ng/dL or 0.14-0.80 nmol/L (SI units)
  Male: 6-22 ng/dL or 0.17-0.61 nmol/L (SI units)
  Child/adolescent:
    Newborn: 5-60 ng/dL

1 week-1 year: 1-160 ng/dL	5-7 years: 5-50 ng/dL
1-3 years: 5-60 ng/dL	7-11 years: 5-70 ng/dL
3-5 years: 5-80 ng/dL	11-15 years: 5-50 ng/dL

Urine (24-hour)

2-26 mcg/24 hr or 6-72 nmol/24 hr (SI units)

Test explanation and related physiology

This test is used to diagnose hyperaldosteronism. Production of aldosterone, a hormone produced by the adrenal cortex, is regulated primarily by the renin-angiotensin system. Secondarily, aldosterone is stimulated by ACTH, low serum sodium levels, and high serum potassium levels. Aldosterone in turn stimulates the renal tubules to absorb sodium (water follows) and to secrete potassium into the urine. In this way, aldosterone regulates serum sodium and potassium levels. Because water follows sodium transport, aldosterone also partially regulates water absorption (and plasma volume).

Increased aldosterone levels are associated with primary aldosteronism, in which a tumor (usually an adenoma) of the adrenal cortex (Conn syndrome) or bilateral adrenal nodular hyperplasia causes increased production of aldosterone. Patients with primary aldosteronism characteristically have hypertension, weakness, polyuria, and hypokalemia.

Increased aldosterone levels also occur with secondary aldosteronism caused by nonadrenal conditions. These include the following:

- Renal vascular stenosis or occlusion
- Hyponatremia (from diuretic or laxative abuse) or low salt intake
- Hypovolemia
- Pregnancy or use of estrogens

- Malignant hypertension
- Potassium loading
- Edematous states (e.g., congestive heart failure, cirrhosis, nephrotic syndrome)

The aldosterone assay can be done on a 24-hour urine specimen or a plasma blood sample. The advantage of the 24-hour urine sample is that short-term fluctuations are eliminated. Plasma values are more convenient to sample, but they are affected by the short-term fluctuations.

Primary aldosteronism can be diagnosed by demonstrating very little to no rise in serum renin levels after an *aldosterone stimulation test* (using salt restriction as the stimulant). This is because aldosterone is already maximally secreted by the pathologic adrenal gland. Failure to suppress aldosterone with saline infusion (1.5 to 2 L of NSS infused between 8 AM and 10 AM, called an *aldosterone suppression test*) is further evidence of primary aldosteronism. Aldosterone can also be measured in blood obtained from adrenal venous sampling.

Interfering factors

- Strenuous exercise and stress can stimulate adrenocortical secretions and increase aldosterone levels.
- Excessive licorice ingestion can cause decreased levels because it produces an aldosterone-like effect.
- Values are influenced by posture, position, diet, diurnal variation, and pregnancy.
- If the test is performed using radioimmunoassay, recently administered radioactive medications will affect test results.
- ☒ Drugs that may cause *increased* levels include diazoxide, diuretics, hydralazine, laxatives, nitroprusside, potassium, and spironolactone.
- ☒ Drugs that may cause *decreased* levels include angiotensin-converting inhibitors (e.g., captopril), fludrocortisone, and propranolol, as well as licorice.

Procedure and patient care

- See inside front cover for Routine Blood Testing.
- Fasting: no
- Blood tube commonly used: serum separator
- PT Note that the patient is asked to be in the upright position (at least sitting) for at least 2 hours before the blood is drawn.
- PT Explain the procedure for collecting a 24-hour urine sample if urinary aldosterone is ordered. (See inside front cover for Routine Urine Testing.)

PT Give the patient verbal and written instructions regarding dietary and medication restrictions.

PT Instruct the patient to maintain a normal sodium diet (approximately 3 g/day) for at least 2 weeks before the blood or urine collection.

PT Have the patient ask the physician whether drugs that alter sodium, potassium, and fluid balance (e.g., diuretics, antihypertensives, steroids, oral contraceptives) should be withheld. Test results will be more accurate if these are suspended at least 2 weeks before either the blood or the urine test.

PT Inform the patient that renin inhibitors (e.g., propranolol) should not be taken 1 week before the test.

PT Tell the patient to avoid licorice for at least 2 weeks before the test because of its aldosterone-like effect.

During

- Occasionally, for hospitalized patients, draw the sample with the patient in the supine position *before* he or she rises.
- Obtain the specimen in the morning.
- Note that sometimes a second specimen (upright sample) is collected 4 hours later, after the patient has been up and moving.

After

- Indicate on the laboratory slip if the patient was supine or standing during the venipuncture.
- Handle the blood specimen gently. Rough handling may cause hemolysis and alter the test results.
- Transport the specimen on ice to the laboratory.

Abnormal findings

▲ **Increased levels**
Primary aldosteronism
Aldosterone-producing
   adrenal adenoma
   (Conn syndrome)
Adrenal cortical nodular
   hyperplasia
Bartter syndrome

Secondary aldosteronism
Hyponatremia
Hyperkalemia
Diuretic ingestion resulting
   in hypovolemia and
   hyponatremia
Laxative abuse
Stress
Malignant hypertension
Generalized edema
Renal arterial stenosis
Pregnancy
Oral contraceptives
Hypovolemia or hemorrhage
Cushing syndrome

▼ **Decreased levels**
Aldosterone deficiency
Renin deficiency
Steroid therapy
Addison disease
Patients on a
   high-sodium diet
Hypernatremia
Hypokalemia
Toxemia of pregnancy
Antihypertensive
   therapy

notes

alkaline phosphatase (ALP)

Type of test Blood

Normal findings

Adult: 30-120 units/L or 0.5-2.0 µKat/L
Elderly: slightly higher than adults
Child/adolescent:
    <2 years: 85-235 units/L
    2-8 years: 65-210 units/L
    9-15 years: 60-300 units/L
    16-21 years: 30-200 units/L

Test explanation and related physiology

Although ALP is found in many tissues, the highest concentrations are found in the liver, biliary tract epithelium, and bone. Detection of this enzyme is important for determining liver and bone disorders. Within the liver, ALP is present in Kupffer cells. These cells line the biliary collecting system. This enzyme is excreted into the bile. Enzyme levels of ALP are greatly increased in both extrahepatic and intrahepatic obstructive biliary disease and cirrhosis. Other liver abnormalities, such as hepatic tumors, hepatotoxic drugs, and hepatitis, cause lesser elevations in ALP levels. Reports have indicated that the most sensitive test to indicate metastatic tumor to the liver is ALP.

Bone is the most frequent extrahepatic source of ALP; new bone growth is associated with elevated ALP levels, which explains why ALP levels are high in adolescents. Pathologic new bone growth occurs with osteoblastic metastatic (e.g., breast, prostate) tumors. Paget disease, healing fractures, rheumatoid arthritis, hyperparathyroidism, and normal-growing bones are sources of elevated ALP levels as well.

Isoenzymes of ALP are sometimes used to distinguish between liver and bone diseases. The detection of isoenzymes can help differentiate the source of the pathology associated with the elevated total ALP. ALP_1 is from the liver. ALP_2 is from the bone.

Interfering factors

- Recent ingestion of a meal can increase ALP levels.
- ✗ Drugs that may cause *elevated* ALP levels include albumin made from placental tissue, allopurinol, antibiotics, azathioprine, colchicine, fluorides, indomethacin, isoniazid (INH), methotrexate, methyldopa, nicotinic acid, phenothiazine, probenecid, tetracyclines, and verapamil.

✠ Drugs that may cause *decreased* levels include arsenicals, cyanides, fluorides, nitrofurantoin, oxalates, and zinc salts.

Procedure and patient care

- See inside front cover for Routine Blood Testing.
- Fasting: no
- Blood tube commonly used: red
- Note that overnight fasting may be required for isoenzymes.
- Patients with liver dysfunction often have prolonged clotting times.

Abnormal findings

▲ Increased levels
  Cirrhosis
  Intrahepatic or extrahepatic
    biliary obstruction
  Primary or metastatic liver
    tumor
  Intestinal ischemia or
    infarction
  Metastatic tumor to the
    bone
  Healing fracture
  Hyperparathyroidism
  Paget disease of bone
  Rheumatoid arthritis
  Sarcoidosis
  Osteomalacia
  Rickets

▼ Decreased levels
  Hypothyroidism
  Malnutrition
  Milk-alkali syndrome
  Pernicious anemia
  Hypophosphatemia
  Scurvy (vitamin C
    deficiency)
  Celiac disease
  Excess vitamin B
    ingestion
  Hypophosphatasia

notes

allergy blood testing (IgE antibody test, Radioallergosorbent test [RAST])

Type of test Blood

Normal findings

Total IgE serum

Adult: 0-100 international units/mL

Child:

0-23 months: 0-13 international units/mL

2-5 years: 0-56 international units/mL

6-10 years: 0-85 international units/mL

Test explanation and related physiology

Measurement of serum IgE is an effective method to diagnose allergy and specifically identify the allergen (the substance to which the person is allergic). Serum IgE levels increase when allergic individuals are exposed to the allergen. Various classes of allergens can initiate the allergic response. They include animal dandruff, foods, pollens, dusts, molds, insect venoms, drugs, and agents in the occupational environment.

Although skin testing (see p. 33) can also identify a specific allergen, measurement of serum levels of IgE is helpful when a skin test result is questionable, when the allergen is not available in a form for dermal injection, or when the allergen may incite an anaphylactic reaction if injected. IgE is particularly helpful in cases in which skin testing is difficult (e.g., in infants or in patients with dermatographism or widespread dermatitis), and it is not always necessary to remove the patient from antihistamines, ACE inhibitors, antidepressants, or beta-blockers. The decision concerning which method to use to diagnose an allergy and to identify the allergen depends on the elapsed time between exposure to an allergen and testing, class of allergen, the age of the patient, the possibility of anaphylaxis, and the affected target organ (such as skin, lungs, or intestine). In general, allergy skin testing is the preferred method in comparison with various in vitro tests for assessing the presence of specific IgE antibodies because it is more sensitive and specific, simpler to use, and less expensive.

IgE levels, similar to provocative skin testing, are used not only to diagnose allergy but also to identify the allergen so that an immunotherapeutic regimen can be developed. Increased levels of total IgE can be diagnostic of allergic disease in general. Specific IgE blood allergy testing, however, is an in vitro test for specific IgE directed to a specific allergen. Since the development of liquid allergen preparations, the use of in vitro blood allergy testing has increased considerably. It is more accurate and safer than skin testing. There are many methods of measuring IgE. One of the older methods is the radioallergosorbent test (RAST). Immunoassay for specific IgE has replaced RAST testing.

Allergy testing of IgG antibodies can also be performed and may provide a more accurate correlation between allergen and allergic symptoms. Similar to IgE antibody testing, IgG antibody testing is often performed in "panels." For example, there are meat panels that might include IgE or IgG testing for chicken, duck, goose, and turkey. Testing a fruit panel might include IgE or IgG antibody testing for apples, bananas, peaches, and pears. Testing in panels diminishes the cost of testing. Specific allergen antibody testing can follow panel testing.

Contraindications
- Patients with multiple allergies; no information will be obtained regarding identification of the specific allergen.

Interfering factors
- Concurrent diseases associated with elevated IgG levels will cause false-negative results.

Procedure and patient care
- See inside front cover for Routine Blood Testing.
- Fasting: no
- Blood tube commonly used: serum separator
- **PT** Inform the patient that the suspected allergen will be mixed with the patient's blood specimen in the laboratory. The patient will not experience any allergic reaction by this method of testing.
- Determine if the patient has recently been treated with a corticosteroid for allergies.

Abnormal findings
Allergy-related diseases
Asthma
Dermatitis
Food allergy
Drug allergy
Occupational allergy
Allergic rhinitis
Angioedema

notes

allergy skin testing

Type of test Skin

Normal findings

<3 mm wheal diameter

<10 mm flare diameter

Test explanation and related physiology

When properly performed, skin testing is the most convenient and least expensive test for detecting allergic reactions. Skin testing provides useful confirmatory evidence when a diagnosis of allergy is suspected on clinical grounds. The simplicity, rapidity, low costs, sensitivity, and specificity explain the crucial position skin testing has in allergy testing.

In an allergic patient, immediate wheal (swelling) and flare (redness) reactions follow injection of the specific allergen (that substance to which the person is allergic). This reaction is initiated by IgE and is mediated primarily by histamine secreted from mast cells. This usually occurs in about 5 minutes and peaks at 30 minutes. In some patients a *late-phase reaction* occurs, which is highlighted by antibody and cellular infiltration into the area. This usually occurs within 1 to 2 hours.

There are three commonly accepted methods of injecting the allergen into the skin. The first method is called the *prick-puncture test* or *scratch test*. In this method, the allergen is injected into the epidermis. Life-threatening anaphylaxis reactions have not been reported with this method. The second method is called the *intradermal test*. Here the allergen is injected into the dermis (creating a skin wheal). Large local reactions and anaphylaxis have been reported with this latter method. For these two tests, the allergen placement part of the test takes about 5 to 10 minutes. The third method is called the *patch test*. This takes much longer because the patient must wear the patch for 48 hours to see if there is a delayed allergic reaction. With this method, needles are not used. Instead, an allergen is applied to a patch that is placed on the skin. It is usually done to detect whether a particular substance (e.g., latex, medications, fragrances, preservatives, hair dyes, metals, resins) is causing an allergic skin irritation, such as contact dermatitis.

Patients with dermographism (nonallergic response of redness and swelling of the skin at the site of any stimulation) develop a skin wheal with any skin irritation, even if nonallergic. In these patients, a false-positive reaction can occur with skin testing. To eliminate these sorts of false positives, a "negative control" substance consisting of just the diluent without an allergen is injected at the same time as the other skin tests are performed. Patients who are immunosuppressed because of concurrent disease or medicines may have a blunted skin reaction even in the face of allergy. This would cause false-negative results. To avoid false negatives, a "positive control" substance consisting of a histamine analogue is also injected into the forearm at the time of skin testing. This will cause a wheal and flare response even in the nonallergic patient unless the patient is immunosuppressed.

For inhalant allergens, skin tests are extremely accurate. However, for food allergies, latex allergies, drug sensitivity, and occupational allergies, skin tests are less reliable.

Contraindications
- Patients with a history of prior anaphylaxis

Potential complications
- Anaphylaxis

Interfering factors
- False-positive results may occur with dermographism.
- False-positive results may occur if the patient has a reaction to the diluent used to preserve the extract.
- False-negative results may be caused by poor-quality allergen extracts, diseases that attenuate the immune response, or improper technique.
- Infants and the elderly may have decreased skin reactivity.
- ▼ Drugs that may *decrease* the immune response of skin testing include ACE inhibitors, beta-blockers, corticosteroids, nifedipine, and theophylline.

Procedure and patient care
Before
PT Explain the procedure to the patient.
- Observe skin testing precautions:
    1. Be sure that a physician is immediately available.
    2. Evaluate the patient for dermographism.
    3. Have medications and equipment available to handle anaphylaxis.
    4. Proceed with caution in patients with current allergic symptoms.
    5. Render great detail to the injection technique.
    6. Avoid bleeding due to injection.

7. Avoid spreading of allergen solutions during the test.

8. Record the skin reaction at the proper time.

- Obtain a history to evaluate the risk of anaphylaxis.
- Identify any immunosuppressive medications the patient may be taking.
- Evaluate the patient for dermographism by rubbing the skin with a pencil eraser and looking for a wheal at the site of irritation.
- Draw up 0.05 mL of 1:1000 aqueous epinephrine into a syringe before testing in the event of an exaggerated allergic reaction.
- A negative prick-puncture test should be performed prior to an intradermal test.

During

Prick-puncture method

- A drop of the allergen solution is placed onto the volar surface of the forearm or back.
- A 25-gauge needle is passed through the droplet and inserted into the epidermal space at an angle with the bevel facing up.
- The skin is lifted up and the fluid is allowed to seep in. Excess fluid is wiped off after about a minute.

Intradermal method

- With a 25-gauge needle, the allergen solution is injected into the dermis by creating a skin wheal. In this method, the bevel of the needle faces downward. A volume of between 0.01 and 0.05 mL is injected.
- In general, the allergen solution is diluted 100- to 1000-fold before injection.

Patch method

- Clean the skin area (usually the back or arm).
- Apply the patches to the skin (as many as 20-30 can be applied).
- Instruct the patient to wear the patches for 48 hours. Tell the patient to avoid bathing or activities that cause heavy sweating.
- Tell the patient the patches will be removed at the doctor's office. Irritated skin at a patch site may indicate an allergy.

After

- Evaluate the patient for an exaggerated allergic response.
- In the event of a systemic reaction, a tourniquet should be placed above the testing site and epinephrine should be administered subcutaneously.

- With a pen, circle the area of testing and mark the allergen used.
- Read the skin test at the appropriate time.
- Skin tests are read when the reaction is mature, after about 15 to 20 minutes. Both the largest and smallest diameters of the wheal are determined. The measurements are averaged.
- The flare is measured in the same manner.
- Observe the patient for 20 to 30 minutes prior to discharge.

Abnormal findings

Allergy-related diseases
Asthma
Dermatitis
Food allergy
Drug allergy
Occupational allergy
Allergic rhinitis
Angioedema

notes

alpha$_1$-antitrypsin (A$_1$AT, AAT, Alpha$_1$-antitrypsin phenotyping)

Type of test Blood

Normal findings 85-213 mg/dL or 0.85-2.13 g/L (SI units)

Test explanation and related physiology

Serum alpha$_1$-antitrypsin (AAT) determinations should be obtained when an individual has a family history of emphysema because a familial tendency to have a deficiency of this antienzyme exists. Deficient or absent serum levels of this enzyme are found in some patients with early onset of emphysema. These people usually develop severe, disabling emphysema. A similar deficiency is seen in children with cirrhosis and other liver diseases. AAT is also an acute-phase reactant that is elevated in the face of inflammation, infection, or malignancy. It is not specific as to the source of the inflammatory process.

Deficiencies of AAT can be genetic or acquired. *Acquired* deficiencies of AAT can occur in patients with protein deficiency syndromes (e.g., malnutrition, liver disease, nephrotic syndrome, and neonatal respiratory distress syndrome). People with AAT deficiency develop severe panacinar emphysema, although it is usually more severe in the lower third of the lungs in the third or fourth decade of life.

Routine serum protein electrophoresis (see p. 760) is a good screening test for AAT deficiency because AAT accounts for about 90% of the protein in the alpha$_1$-globulin region.

Inherited AAT deficiency is associated with symptoms earlier in life than acquired AAT deficiency. Inherited AAT is also commonly associated with liver and biliary disease. Individuals of the heterozygous state have diminished or low normal serum levels of AAT. Approximately 5% to 14% of the adult population is in the heterozygous state and is considered to be at increased risk for the development of emphysema. Homozygous individuals have severe pulmonary and liver disease very early in life. AAT phenotyping is particularly helpful when blood AAT levels are suggestive but not definitive.

Interfering factors

- Serum levels of AAT increase during pregnancy.
- ✘ Drugs that may cause *increased* levels include oral contraceptives.

Procedure and patient care

- See inside front cover for Routine Blood Testing.
- Fasting: no (Verify with lab).
- Blood tube commonly used: red

PT If the results show the patient is at risk for developing emphysema, begin patient teaching. Include such factors as avoidance of smoking, infection, and inhaled irritants; proper nutrition; adequate hydration; and education about the disease process of emphysema.

Abnormal findings

▲ **Increased levels**

Acute inflammatory
  disorders
Chronic inflammatory
  disorders
Stress
Infection
Thyroid infections

▼ **Decreased levels**

Early onset of emphysema
  (in adults)
Neonatal respiratory
  distress syndrome
Cirrhosis (in children)
Low serum proteins
  (e.g., nephrotic
  syndrome, malnutrition,
  end-stage cancer,
  protein-losing
  enteropathy)

notes

alpha-fetoprotein (AFP, α_1-Fetoprotein)

Type of test Blood

Normal findings

Adult: <40 ng/mL or <40 mcg/L (SI units)

Child (<1 year): <30 ng/mL

(Ranges are stratified by weeks of gestation and vary according to laboratory.)

Test explanation and related physiology

Alpha-fetoprotein (AFP) is an oncofetal protein normally produced by the fetal liver and yolk sac. It is the dominant fetal serum protein in the first trimester of life and diminishes to very low levels by the age of 1 year. It is also normally found in very low levels in the adult.

AFP is an effective screening serum marker for fetal body wall defects. The most notable of these are neural tube defects, which can vary from a small myelomeningocele to anencephaly. If a fetus has an open body wall defect, fetal serum AFP leaks out into the amniotic fluid and is picked up by the maternal serum. AFP from fetal sources can normally be detected in the amniotic fluid or the mother's blood after 10 weeks' gestation. Peak levels occur between 16 and 18 weeks. Maternal serum reflects the changes in amniotic AFP levels. When elevated maternal serum AFP levels are identified, further evaluation with repeat serum AFP levels, amniotic fluid AFP levels, and ultrasound is warranted.

Elevated serum AFP levels in pregnancy may also indicate multiple pregnancy, fetal distress, fetal congenital abnormalities, or intrauterine death. Low AFP levels after correction for age of gestation, maternal weight, race, and presence of diabetes are found in mothers carrying a fetus with trisomy 21 (Down syndrome). See *maternal screen testing* (p. 628) and *nuchal translucency* (p. 697) for other pregnancy screening tests.

AFP is also used as a tumor marker. Increased serum levels of AFP are found in as many as 90% of patients with hepatomas. The higher the AFP level, the greater the tumor burden. A decrease in AFP is seen if the patient is responding to antineoplastic therapy. Other neoplastic conditions (e.g., nonseminomatous germ cell tumors and teratomas of the testes; yolk sac and germ cell tumors of the ovaries; and to a lesser extent Hodgkin disease, lymphoma, and renal cell carcinoma) are also associated with elevated AFP levels. With improved methods of detection, AFP can also be detected in the serum of patients with cancer of the stomach, colon, breast, or lung. Elevated AFP levels can also occur in patients with noncancerous conditions, such as cirrhosis or chronic active hepatitis.

Interfering factors

- Fetal blood contamination, which may occur during amniocentesis, can cause increased AFP levels.
- Recent administration of radioisotopes can affect values.

Procedure and patient care

- See inside front cover for Routine Blood Testing.
- Fasting: no
- Blood tube commonly used: red
- If AFP is to be performed on amniotic fluid, follow the Procedure and Patient Care for amniocentesis (see p. 52).
- Include the gestational age on the laboratory slip.

Abnormal findings

▲ **Increased maternal AFP levels**
Neural tube defects
(e.g., anencephaly,
encephalocele,
spina bifida,
myelomeningocele)
Abdominal wall defects
(e.g., gastroschisis or
omphalocele)
Multiple pregnancy
Threatened abortion
Fetal distress or
congenital anomalies
Fetal death

▼ **Decreased maternal serum AFP levels**
Trisomy 21 (Down
syndrome)
Fetal wastage

▲ **Increased nonmaternal AFP levels**

Primary hepatocellular cancer (hepatoma)

Germ cell or yolk sac cancer of the ovary

Embryonal cell or germ cell tumor of the testes

Other cancers (e.g., stomach, colon, lung, breast, or lymphoma)

Liver cell necrosis (e.g., cirrhosis or hepatitis)

notes

aluminum

Type of test   Blood

Normal findings

All ages: 0-6 ng/mL
Dialysis patients of all ages: <60 ng/mL

Test explanation and related physiology

Under normal physiologic conditions, the usual daily dietary intake of aluminum (5 to 10 mg) is completely excreted by the kidneys. Patients in renal failure (RF) lose the ability to clear aluminum and are at risk for aluminum toxicity. Aluminum-laden dialysis water and aluminum-based phosphate binder gels designed to decrease phosphate accumulation increase the incidence of aluminum toxicity in RF patients. Furthermore, the dialysis process is not highly effective at eliminating aluminum.

If aluminum accumulates, it binds to albumin and is rapidly distributed throughout the body. Aluminum overload leads to accumulation of aluminum in the brain and bone. Brain deposition has been implicated as a cause of dialysis dementia. In bone, aluminum replaces calcium and disrupts normal osteoid formation.

Serum aluminum concentrations are likely to be increased above the reference range in patients with metallic joint prosthesis. Serum concentrations >10 ng/mL in a patient with an aluminum-based implant suggest significant prosthesis wear. Chromium and other metals can be detected using similar laboratory techniques.

Interfering factors

- Special evacuated blood collection tubes are required for aluminum testing.
- Most of the common evacuated blood collection devices have rubber stoppers that are comprised of aluminum-silicate. Simple puncture of the rubber stopper for blood collection is sufficient to contaminate the specimen with aluminum.
- Gadolinium- or iodine-containing contrast media that have been administered within 96 hours can alter test results for heavy metals, including aluminum.

Procedure and patient care

- See inside front cover for Routine Blood Testing.
- Fasting: no
- Blood tube commonly used: royal blue or tan
- If the blood sample is sent to a central diagnostic laboratory, results will be available in 7 to 10 days.

Abnormal findings

▲ **Increased levels**
  Aluminum toxicity

notes

amino acid profiles (Amino acid screen)

Type of test Blood; urine

Normal findings

Normal values vary for different amino acids.

Test explanation and related physiology

Amino acids are "building blocks" of proteins, hormones, nucleic acids, and pigments. They can act as neurotransmitters, enzymes, and coenzymes. There are eight essential amino acids that must be provided to the body by the diet. The body can make the others. The essential amino acids must be transported across the gut and renal tubular lining cells. The metabolism of the essential amino acids is critical to the production of other amino acids, proteins, carbohydrates, and lipids. Amino acid levels can thereby be affected by defects in renal tubule or gastrointestinal (GI) transport of amino acids.

When there is a defect in the metabolism or transport of any one of these amino acids, excesses of their precursors or deficiencies of their "end product" amino acid are evident in the blood and/or urine. There are more than 90 diseases described that are associated with abnormal amino acid function.

Clinical manifestations of these diseases may be precluded if diagnosis is early, and appropriate dietary replacement of missing amino acids is provided. Usually, urine testing for specific amino acids is used to screen for some of these errors in amino acid metabolism and transport. Blood testing is very accurate. Federal law now requires hospitals to test all newborns for inborn errors in metabolism including amino acids. Testing is required for errors in amino acid metabolism such as phenylketonuria (PKU), maple syrup urine disease (MSUD), and homocystinuria (see newborn metabolic screening, p. 657). Testing for more rare disorders may include testing for tyrosinemia and argininosuccinic aciduria.

A few drops of blood are obtained from the heel of a newborn to fill a few circles on filter paper (Guthrie card) labeled with names of infant, parent, hospital, and primary physician. The sample is usually obtained on the second or third day of life, after protein-containing feedings (i.e., breast milk or formula) have started.

After a presumptive diagnosis is made, amino acid levels can be determined by chromatographic methods on blood or amniotic fluid. The genetic defects for many of these diseases are becoming more defined, allowing for even earlier diagnosis to be made in utero. Common examples of amino acid diseases include PKU, cystinosis, and cystic fibrosis.

Interfering factors

- The circadian rhythm affects amino acid levels. Levels are usually lowest in the morning and highest by midday.
- Pregnancy is associated with reduced levels of some amino acids.
- ✘ Drugs that may *increase* amino acids include bismuth, heparin, steroids, and sulfonamides.
- ✘ Drugs that may *decrease* some amino acid levels include estrogens and oral contraceptives.

Procedure and patient care

- See inside front cover for Routine Blood Testing.
- Fasting: yes
- Blood tube commonly used: red

Before

- Obtain a history of the patient's symptoms.
- Obtain a pedigree highlighting family members with amino acid disorders.
- **PT** A 12-hour fast is generally required before blood collection. Occasionally, a particular protein or carbohydrate load is ordered to stimulate production of a particular amino acid metabolite.

During

- Usually a 24-hour random urine specimen is required. See inside front cover for Routine Urine Testing.
- Screening is done on a spot urine using the first voided specimen in the morning.

After

- Generally, genetic counseling is provided before testing. However, acute anxiety by the patient or parents often requires emotional support immediately after obtaining a specimen.

Abnormal findings

▲ **Increased blood levels**
Specific aminoacidopathies
(e.g., PKU, maple
syrup disease)
Specific aminoacidemias
(e.g., glutaric aciduria)

▲ **Increased urine levels**
Specific aminoacidurias
(e.g., cystinuria,
homocystinuria)

▼ **Decreased blood levels**
Hartnup disease
Nephritis
Nephrotic syndromes

notes

ammonia level

Type of test Blood

Normal findings

Adult: 10-80 mcg/dL or 6-47 µmol/L (SI units)
Child: 40-80 mcg/dL
Newborn: 90-150 mcg/dL

Test explanation and related physiology

Ammonia is used to support the diagnosis of severe liver diseases (fulminant hepatitis or cirrhosis). Ammonia levels are also used in the diagnosis and follow-up of hepatic encephalopathy.

Ammonia is a by-product of protein catabolism. Most of the ammonia is made by bacteria acting on proteins present in the gut. By way of the portal vein, ammonia goes to the liver where it is normally converted into urea and then secreted by the kidneys. With severe hepatocellular dysfunction, ammonia cannot be catabolized. Furthermore, when portal blood flow to the liver is altered (e.g., in portal hypertension), ammonia cannot reach the liver to be catabolized. Ammonia levels in the blood rise. Plasma ammonia levels do not correlate well with the degree of hepatic encephalopathy. Inherited deficiencies of urea cycle enzymes, inherited metabolic disorders of organic acids, and the dibasic amino acids lysine and ornithine are a major cause of high ammonia levels in infants and adults. Finally, impaired renal function diminishes excretion of ammonia, and blood levels rise. High levels of ammonia are often associated with encephalopathy and coma.

Interfering factors

- Hemolysis increases ammonia levels because the RBCs contain about three times the ammonia content of plasma.
- Muscular exertion can increase ammonia.
- Cigarette smoking can produce significant increases in ammonia levels.
- Ammonia levels may be falsely increased if the tourniquet is too tight for a long period.
- ✘ Drugs that may cause *increased* ammonia levels include acetazolamide, alcohol, ammonium chloride, barbiturates, diuretics (e.g., loop, thiazide), narcotics, and parenteral nutrition.
- ✘ Drugs that may cause *decreased* levels include broad-spectrum antibiotics (e.g., neomycin), lactobacillus, lactulose, levodopa, and potassium salts.

Procedure and patient care
- See inside front cover for Routine Blood Testing.
- Fasting: no
- Blood tube commonly used: green
- Note that some institutions require that the specimen be sent to the laboratory in an iced container.
- Avoid hemolysis and send the specimen promptly to the laboratory.
- Many patients with liver disease have prolonged clotting times.

Abnormal findings
▲ Increased levels
Primary hepatocellular disease
Reye syndrome
Asparagine intoxication
Portal hypertension
Severe heart failure with congestive hepatomegaly
Hemolytic disease of the newborn (erythroblastosis fetalis)
Gastrointestinal bleeding with mild liver disease
Gastrointestinal obstruction with mild liver disease
Hepatic encephalopathy and hepatic coma
Genetic metabolic disorder of the urea cycle

▼ Decreased levels
Essential or malignant hypertension
Hyperornithinemia

notes

amniocentesis (Amniotic fluid analysis)

Type of test Fluid analysis

Normal findings

Weeks' gestation	Amniotic fluid volume (mL)
15	450
25	750
30-35	1500
Full term	>1500

Amniotic fluid appearance: clear; pale to straw yellow
L/S ratio: ≥2:1
Bilirubin: <0.2 mg/dL
No chromosomal or genetic abnormalities
Phosphatidylglycerol (PG): positive for PG
Lamellar body count: >30,000
Alpha-fetoprotein: dependent on gestational age and lab technique
Fetal lung maturity (FLM):
    Mature: <260 mPOL
    Transitional: 260-290 mPOL
    Immature: >290 mPOL

Test explanation and related physiology

Amniocentesis is performed on pregnant women to gather information about the fetus. The following can be evaluated by studying the amniotic fluid:
- *Fetal maturity status*, especially pulmonary maturity (when early delivery is preferred). Fetal maturity is determined by analysis of the amniotic fluid in the following manner:
  a. *Lecithin/sphingomyelin (L/S) ratio.* The L/S ratio is a measure of fetal lung maturity, which is determined by measuring the phospholipids in amniotic fluid. Lecithin is the major constituent of surfactant, an important substance required for alveolar ventilation. If surfactant is insufficient, the alveoli collapse during expiration. This may result in respiratory distress syndrome (RDS), which is a major cause of death in immature babies. In immature fetal lungs, the sphingomyelin concentration in amniotic fluid is higher than the lecithin concentration. At 35 weeks of gestation, the concentration of lecithin rapidly increases, whereas sphingomyelin concentration decreases. An L/S

ratio of 2:1 (3:1 in mothers with diabetes) or greater is a highly reliable indication that the fetal lungs and therefore the fetus are mature. In such a case, the infant would be unlikely to develop RDS after birth. As the L/S ratio decreases, the risk of RDS increases.

Lecithin concentrations can be measured directly, but offer no additional accuracy beyond the L/S ratio. As an alternative to measuring the L/S ratio, the *fetal lung maturity (FLM) test* is based on fluorescence depolarization. This test determines the ratio of surfactant to albumin to evaluate pulmonary maturity.

b. *Phosphatidylglycerol (PG).* This is a minor component (about 10%) of lung surfactant phospholipids and therefore, alone, is less accurate in measuring pulmonary maturity. However, because PG is almost entirely synthesized by mature lung alveolar cells, it is a good indicator of lung maturity. In healthy, pregnant women, PG appears in amniotic fluid after 35 weeks of gestation, and levels gradually increase until term. The simultaneous determination of the L/S ratio and the presence of PG is an excellent method of assessing fetal maturity based on pulmonary surfactant.

c. *Lamellar body count.* This test to determine fetal maturity is also based on the presence of surfactant. These lamellar bodies represent the storage form of pulmonary surfactant. Lamellar body results are calculated in units of particle density per microliter of amniotic fluid. Some researchers have recommended cutoffs of 30,000/μl and 10,000/μl to predict low and high risks for RDS, respectively. If the count is greater than 30,000, there is a 100% chance that the infant's lungs are mature enough to not experience RDS. If the lamellar body count is less than 10,000, the probability of RDS is high (67%). Values between 10,000 and 30,000/μl represent intermediate risk for RDS.

d. *Measurement of surfactant activity.* Surfactant activity is a semi-quantitative group of tests performed by determining the development and stability of foam when amniotic fluid is shaken in a solution of alcohol. This testing may be called the *tap test,* the *shake test,* or the *foam stability index test.* If a ring of bubbles forms on the surface of the solution, fetal lung maturity is indicated. If no bubbles are present, varying levels of respiratory distress syndrome are indicated.

e. *Measurement of optical density of amniotic fluid.* The measurement of amniotic fluid at 650 nm can be measured by absorbance. A denser fluid will be associated with greater lung maturity. This testing method is often used as a rapid screening test for fetal lung maturity.

- *Sex of the fetus*. Sons of mothers who are known to be carriers of X-linked recessive traits would have a 50:50 chance of inheritance.

- *Genetic and chromosomal aberrations*. Genetic and chromosomal studies performed on cells aspirated within the amniotic fluid can indicate the gender of the fetus (important in sex-linked diseases such as hemophilia) or the existence of many genetic and chromosomal aberrations (e.g., trisomy 21). See Laboratory Genetics, p. 566.

- *Fetal status affected by Rh isoimmunization*. Mothers with Rh isoimmunization may have a series of amniocentesis procedures during the second half of pregnancy to assess the level of bilirubin pigment in the amniotic fluid. The quantity of bilirubin is used to assess the severity of hemolysis in Rh-sensitized pregnancy. Amniocentesis is usually initiated at 24 to 25 weeks when hemolysis is suspected.

- *Hereditary metabolic disorders*, such as cystic fibrosis.

- *Anatomic abnormalities*, such as neural tube closure defects (myelomeningocele, anencephaly, spina bifida). Increased levels of alpha-fetoprotein (AFP) in the amniotic fluid may indicate a neural crest abnormality (see p. 39). Decreased AFP may be associated with increased risk of trisomy 21.

- *Fetal distress*, detected by meconium staining of the amniotic fluid. This is caused by relaxation of the anal sphincter. In this case, the normally colorless or pale, straw-colored amniotic fluid may be tinged with green. Other color changes may also indicate fetal distress. There are, however, more accurate and safer methods of determining fetal stress such as the fetal biophysical profile (see page 423).

- *Assessment of amniotic fluid for infection*. Amniocentesis is used to obtain fluid for bacterial culture and sensitivity when infection is suspected. This is especially helpful if premature membrane rupture is suspected. Amniotic fluid can also be obtained if viral infections that may affect the fetus are suspected during pregnancy.

- *Assessment for rupture of membranes*. Through amniocentesis, a dye can be injected into the amniotic fluid. If this same dye is found in vaginal fluid, rupture of the amniotic membrane is documented. This is sometimes referred to as the *amnio-dye test*. There are, however, more practical tests of vaginal fluid to determine membrane rupture. Most commonly, the pH of the vaginal fluid is determining using a nitrazine test strip. If the test strip turns dark or blue, amniotic fluid is present in the vagina, and membrane rupture is documented.

The timing of the amniocentesis varies according to the clinical circumstances. With advanced maternal age and if chromosomal or genetic aberrations are suspected, the test should be done early enough (at 14 to 16 weeks of gestation; at least 150 mL of fluid exists at this time) to allow a safe abortion. If information on fetal maturity is sought, performing the study during or after the 35th week of gestation is best.

Contraindications
- Patients with abruptio placentae
- Patients with placenta previa
- Patients with a history of premature labor (before 34 weeks of gestation unless the patient is receiving antilabor medication)
- Patients with an incompetent cervix or cervical insufficiency
- Patients with anhydramnios
- Patients with suspected premature labor

Potential complications
- Miscarriage
- Fetal injury
- Leak of amniotic fluid
- Infection (amnionitis)
- Abortion
- Premature labor
- Maternal hemorrhage
- Maternal Rh isoimmunization
- Amniotic fluid embolism
- Abruptio placentae
- Inadvertent damage to the bladder or intestines

Interfering factors
- Fetal blood contamination can cause false AFP elevations.
- Hemolysis of the specimen can alter results.
- Contamination of the specimen with meconium or blood may give inaccurate L/S ratios.

Procedure and patient care
Before
PT Explain the procedure to the patient. Allay any fears, and allow the patient to verbalize her concerns.
- Obtain an informed consent from the patient and her spouse.

PT Tell the patient that no food or fluid is restricted.
- Evaluate the mother's blood pressure and the fetal heart rate.
- Follow instructions regarding emptying the bladder, which depend on gestational age. Before 20 weeks of gestation, the bladder may be kept full to support the uterus. After 20 weeks, the bladder may be emptied to minimize the chance of puncture.
- Note that the placenta is localized before the study by ultrasound to permit selection of a site that will avoid placental puncture.

During
- Place the patient in the supine position.
- Note the following procedural steps:
  1. The skin overlying the chosen site is prepared and usually anesthetized locally.
  2. A needle with a stylet is inserted through the midabdominal wall and is directed at an angle toward the middle of the uterine cavity (Figure 2).
  3. The stylet is then removed and a sterile plastic syringe attached.

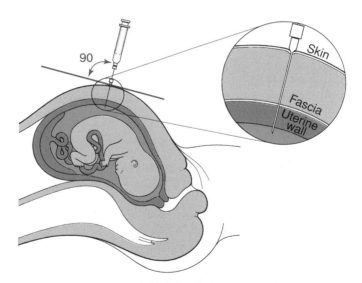

FIGURE 2 Amniocentesis. Ultrasound scanning is usually used to determine the placental site and to locate a pocket of amniotic fluid. The needle is then inserted. Three levels of resistance are felt as the needle penetrates the skin, fascia, and uterine wall. When the needle is placed within the uterine cavity, amniotic fluid is withdrawn.

4. After 5 to 10 mL of amniotic fluid is withdrawn, the needle is removed.
5. The specimen is placed in a light-resistant container to prevent breakdown of bilirubin.
6. The site is covered with an adhesive bandage.
7. If the amniotic fluid is bloody, the physician must determine whether the blood is maternal or fetal in origin. The Kleinhauer-Boetke stain will stain fetal cells pink. Meconium in the fluid is usually associated with a compromised fetus.
8. *Amniotic fluid volume* is calculated.

- Note that this procedure is performed by a physician and takes approximately 20 to 30 minutes.
- **PT** Tell the patient that the discomfort associated with amniocentesis is usually described as a mild uterine cramping that occurs when the needle contacts the uterus. Some women may complain of a pulling sensation as the amniotic fluid is withdrawn.
- Remember that many women are extremely anxious during this procedure.

After

- Place amniotic fluid in a sterile, siliconized glass container and transport it to a special chemistry laboratory for analysis. Sometimes the specimen may be sent by airmail to another commercial laboratory.
- **PT** Inform the patient that the results of this study are usually not available for more than 1 week.
- For women who have Rh-negative blood, administer RhoGAM because of the risk of isoimmunization from the fetal blood.
- Assess the fetal heart rate after the test to detect any ill effects related to the procedure. Compare this value with the preprocedure baseline value.
- **PT** If the patient felt dizzy or nauseated during the procedure, instruct her to lie on her left side for several minutes before leaving the examining room.
- Observe the puncture site for bleeding or other drainage.
- **PT** Instruct the patient to call her physician if she has any amniotic fluid loss, bleeding, temperature elevation, abdominal pain, abdominal cramping, fetal hyperactivity, or unusual fetal lethargy.

Abnormal findings

Hemolytic disease of the newborn
Rh isoimmunization
Neural tube closure defects (e.g., myelomeningocele, anencephaly, spina bifida)
Abdominal wall closure defects (e.g., gastroschisis, omphalocele)
Sacrococcygeal teratoma
Meconium staining
Immature fetal lungs
Hereditary metabolic disorders (e.g., cystic fibrosis, Tay-Sachs disease, galactosemia)
Genetic or chromosomal aberrations (e.g., sickle cell anemia, thalassemia, trisomy 21 [Down syndrome])
Sex-linked disorders (e.g., hemophilia)
Polyhydramnios
Oligohydramnios

notes

amylase

Type of test Blood; urine

Normal findings

Blood

Adult: 60-120 Somogyi units/dL or 30-220 units/L (SI units)
  Values may be slightly increased during normal pregnancy and
  in the elderly.
Newborn: 6-65 units/L

Urine (24-hour)

Up to 5000 Somogyi units/24 hr or 6.5-48.1 units/hr (SI units)

Possible critical values Blood: More than three times the
upper limit of normal (depending on the method)

Test explanation and related physiology

Serum amylase is an easily and rapidly performed test that
is commonly used to diagnose and monitor the treatment of
pancreatitis. Amylase is normally secreted from the pancreatic
acinar cell into the pancreatic duct and then into the duodenum.
Once in the intestine, it aids the catabolism of carbohydrates
to their component simple sugars. Damage to acinar cells (as
occurs in pancreatitis) or obstruction of the pancreatic duct flow
(as a result of pancreatic carcinoma) causes an outpouring of
this enzyme into the intrapancreatic lymph system and the free
peritoneum. Blood vessels draining the free peritoneum and
absorbing the lymph pick up the excess amylase. An abnormal
rise in the serum level of amylase occurs within 12 hours of the
onset of disease. Because amylase is rapidly cleared by the kidneys, serum levels return to normal 48 to 72 hours after the
initial insult. Persistent pancreatitis, duct obstruction, or pancreatic duct leak will cause persistent elevated amylase levels.

Although serum amylase is a sensitive test for pancreatic disorders, it is not specific. Other nonpancreatic diseases can cause
elevated amylase levels in the serum. For example, in a bowel
perforation, intraluminal amylase leaks into the free peritoneum
and is picked up by the peritoneal blood vessels. Also, a penetrating peptic ulcer into the pancreas will cause elevated amylase levels. Duodenal obstruction can be associated with less significant
elevations in amylase. Because salivary glands contain amylase,
elevations can be expected in patients with parotiditis (mumps).
Amylase isoenzyme testing can differentiate pancreatic from salivary hyperamylasemia.

Urine amylase levels rise after the blood levels. Several days after the onset of the disease process, serum amylase levels may be normal, but urine amylase levels are significantly elevated. Urine amylase is particularly useful in detecting pancreatitis late in the disease course.

As with serum amylase, urine amylase is sensitive but not specific for pancreatic disorders. A comparison of the renal clearance ratio of amylase with creatinine provides more specific diagnostic information than either the urine amylase level or the serum amylase level alone. When the *amylase/creatinine clearance* ratio is 5% or more, the diagnosis of pancreatitis can be made with certainty.

Interfering factors

- Serum lipemia may falsely decrease amylase levels.
- ✠ IV dextrose solutions can cause a false-negative result.
- ✠ Drugs that may cause *increased* serum amylase levels include aminosalicylic acid, aspirin, azathioprine, corticosteroids, dexamethasone, ethyl alcohol, glucocorticoids, iodine-containing contrast media, loop diuretics, methyldopa, narcotic analgesics, oral contraceptives, and prednisone.
- ✠ Drugs that may cause *decreased* levels include citrates, glucose, and oxalates.

Procedure and patient care

- See inside front cover for Routine Blood Testing.
- Fasting: no
- Blood tube commonly used: red
- See inside front cover for Routine Urine Testing.

Abnormal findings

▲ **Increased levels**

  Acute or chronic relapsing pancreatitis
  Penetrating or perforated peptic ulcer
  Necrotic or perforated bowel
  Acute cholecystitis
  Parotiditis (mumps)
  Ectopic pregnancy
  Pulmonary infarction
  Diabetic ketoacidosis
  Duodenal obstruction
  Osteogenic sarcoma
  Cryoglobulinemia
  Rheumatoid diseases

notes

amyloid beta protein precursor, soluble (sBPP)

Type of test Cerebrospinal fluid (CSF) analysis

Normal findings >450 units/L

Test explanation and related physiology

This test is used to help diagnose Alzheimer disease and other forms of senile dementia. Amyloid protein is a 42-amino-acid peptide that is broken off of a larger amyloid precursor protein (beta APP). These beta amyloid proteins have been shown to be neurotrophic and neuroprotective. Beta amyloid is deposited on the brain in the form of plaques in patients with Alzheimer disease. As a result of this deposition, levels of beta amyloid are *decreased* in the cerebrospinal fluid of patients with Alzheimer disease and other forms of dementia. Ongoing research has also focused on using CSF levels of *tau protein* as another biochemical marker for Alzheimer disease.

Recently, PET scanning with amyloid imaging has shown promise for the diagnosis of Alzheimer disease. Pittsburgh Agent B (PIB) appears to reliably detect brain amyloid due to the accumulation of A beta 42 within plaques. Studies so far have revealed high levels of amyloid retention in the brain at prodromal stages of Alzheimer disease and the possibility of discriminating Alzheimer disease from other dementia disorders by scanning with PIB. Because amyloid accumulation is one of the earliest signs of Alzheimer disease, early diagnosis may be facilitated by identifying amyloid early in the disease progression, perhaps before symptoms emerge.

Procedure and patient care

Before

PT Explain the procedure to the patient.

- Refer to the instructions for a lumbar puncture and CSF examination (see p. 596).

During

- Collect a CSF specimen as per the lumbar puncture discussion.

After

- Follow the postprocedure guidelines after a lumbar puncture.

Abnormal findings

▼ **Decreased levels**

Alzheimer disease

notes

angiotensin

A

Type of test blood

Normal findings

Angiotensin I: ≤25 pg/mL
Angiotensin II: 10-60 pg/mL

Test explanation and related physiology

Renin (page 800) is an enzyme that is released by the juxtaglomerular apparatus of the kidneys. Its release is stimulated by hypokalemia, hyponatremia, decreased renal blood perfusion, or hypovolemia. Renin stimulates the release of angiotensinogen. Angiotensin-converting enzyme (ACE) (page 60) metabolizes angiotensinogen to angiotensin I and subsequently to angiotensin II and III. Angiotensin then stimulates the release of catecholamines, antidiuretic hormone, ACTH, oxytocin, and aldosterone. Angiotensin is also a vasoconstrictor. Angiotensin is used to identify renovascular sources of hypertension. It can be measured as angiotensin I or as angiotensin II. The test is performed by direct radioimmunoassay.

Interfering factors: See renin, page 807.

Procedure and patient care

- See inside front cover for Routine Blood Testing.
- Fasting: no
- Blood tube commonly used: lavender
- **PT** Instruct the patient to maintain a normal diet with a restricted amount of sodium (~3 g/day) for 3 days before the test.
- **PT** Instruct the patient to check with a health care provider about discontinuing any medications that may interrupt renin activity.
- Record the patient's position, dietary status, and time of day on the laboratory slip.
- Place the tube of blood on ice and immediately send it to the laboratory.

Abnormal findings

▲ Increased levels
Essential hypertension
Malignant hypertension
Renovascular hypertension

▼ Decreased levels
Primary hyperaldosteronism
Steroid therapy
Congenital adrenal hyperplasia

notes

angiotensin-converting enzyme (ACE, Serum angiotensin-converting enzyme [SACE])

Type of test Blood

Normal findings 8-53 U/L

Test explanation and related physiology

ACE is used to detect and monitor the clinical course of sarcoidosis (a granulomatous disease that affects many organs, especially the lungs). It is also used to differentiate sarcoidosis from other granulomatous diseases, and to differentiate between active and dormant sarcoid disease.

Elevated ACE levels are found in a high percentage of patients with sarcoidosis. This test is used primarily in patients with sarcoidosis to evaluate the severity of disease and the response to therapy. Levels are especially high with active pulmonary sarcoidosis and can be normal with inactive (dormant) sarcoidosis. Elevated ACE levels also occur in conditions other than sarcoidosis, including Gaucher disease (a rare familial lysosomal disorder of fat metabolism), leprosy, alcoholic cirrhosis, active histoplasmosis, tuberculosis, Hodgkin disease, myeloma, scleroderma, pulmonary embolism, and idiopathic pulmonary fibrosis. ACE is elevated in the CSF of patients with neurosarcoidosis.

Interfering factors

- Patients younger than 20 years of age normally have very high ACE levels.
- Hemolysis or hyperlipidemia may falsely decrease ACE levels.
- ☛ Drugs that may cause *decreased* ACE levels include ACE inhibitor antihypertensives and steroids.

Procedure and patient care

- See inside front cover for Routine Blood Testing.
- Fasting: no
- Blood tube commonly used: red
- Note on the laboratory slip if the patient is taking steroids.

Abnormal findings

▲ Increased levels

Sarcoidosis
Gaucher disease
Tuberculosis
Leprosy
Alcoholic cirrhosis
Active histoplasmosis
Hodgkin disease
Myeloma
Idiopathic pulmonary fibrosis
Diabetes mellitus
Primary biliary cirrhosis
Amyloidosis
Hyperthyroidism
Scleroderma
Pulmonary embolism

notes

anion gap (AG, R factor)

Type of test Blood

Normal findings

16±4 mEq/L (if potassium is used in the calculation)
12±4 mEq/L (if potassium is not used in the calculation)

Test explanation and related physiology

The anion gap (AG) is the difference between the cations and the anions in the extracellular space that is routinely calculated in the laboratory (i.e., AG = [sodium + potassium] − [chloride + bicarbonate]). In some laboratories, the potassium is not measured because the level of potassium in acid/base abnormalities varies. The normal value of the AG is adjusted downward if potassium is eliminated from the equation. The AG, although not real physiologically, is created by the small amounts of anions in the blood (e.g., lactate, phosphates, sulfates, organic anions, and proteins) that are not measured.

This calculation is most often helpful in identifying the cause of metabolic acidosis. As such acids as lactic acid or ketoacids accumulate in the bloodstream, bicarbonate neutralizes them to maintain a normal pH within the blood. Mathematically, when bicarbonate decreases, the AG increases. In general, most metabolic acidotic states (excluding some types of renal tubular acidosis) are associated with an increased AG. The higher the gap is above normal, the more likely that the metabolic acidotic state is associated with the AG. Proteins can have a significant effect on AG. As albumin (usually negatively charged) increases, AG will increase.

A decreased AG is very rare but can occur when there is an increase in unmeasured (calcium or magnesium) cations. A reduction in anionic proteins (nephrotic syndrome) will also decrease AG. For example, a 1 g/dL drop in serum protein is associated with a 2.5 mEq/L drop in AG. Because the anion proteins are lost, the HCO_3 increases to maintain electrical neutrality. An increase in cationic proteins (some immunoglobulins) will also decrease AG. Except for hypoproteinemia, conditions that cause a reduced or negative AG are relatively rare compared with those associated with an elevated AG.

Interfering factors

- Hyperlipidemia may cause undermeasurement of sodium and falsely decrease AG.

- Normal values of AG vary according to different normal values for electrolytes, depending on laboratory methods of measurement.
- Drugs that *increase* AG are many. Examples include carbonic anhydrase inhibitors (e.g., acetazolamide), ethanol, methanol, and salicylate.
- Drugs that *decrease* AG are also many. Examples include acetazolamide, lithium, spironolactone, and sulindac.

Procedure and patient care

- See inside front cover for Routine Blood Testing.
- Fasting: no
- Blood tube commonly used: red or green
- If the patient is receiving an IV infusion, obtain the blood from the opposite arm.
- The sodium, potassium, chloride, and bicarbonate levels are determined by an automated multichannel analyzer. The AG is then calculated as indicated in the test explanation section.

Abnormal findings

▲ **Increased levels**
Lactic acidosis
Diabetic ketoacidosis
Alcoholic ketoacidosis
Starvation
Renal failure
Renal tubular acidosis
Increased gastrointestinal losses of bicarbonate (e.g., diarrhea or fistulae)
Hypoaldosteronism

▼ **Decreased levels**
Excess alkali ingestion
Multiple myeloma
Chronic vomiting or gastric suction
Hyperaldosteronism
Hypoproteinemia
Lithium toxicity
Bromide (cough syrup) toxicity

notes

anticardiolipin antibodies (aCL antibodies, ACA, Antiphospholipid antibodies, Lupus anticoagulant)

Type of test Blood

Normal findings

Negative:
  <23 GPL (IgG phospholipid units)
  <11 MPL (IgM phospholipid units)

Test explanation and related physiology

Anticardiolipin antibodies (immunoglobulins G and M to cardiolipin) are antiphospholipid autoantibodies that attach to phospholipids on cell membranes and can interfere with the coagulation system. *Antiphospholipid autoantibodies* include *anticardiolipin antibodies* and the *lupus anticoagulant antibody.* Phospholipid antibodies occur in patients with a variety of clinical signs and symptoms, notably thrombosis (arterial or venous), pregnancy morbidity (unexplained fetal death, premature birth, severe preeclampsia, or placental insufficiency), unexplained cutaneous circulation disturbances (livido reticularis or pyoderma gangrenosum), thrombocytopenia or hemolytic anemia, and nonbacterial thrombotic endocarditis. Phospholipid antibodies and lupus anticoagulants are found with increased frequency in patients with systemic rheumatic diseases, especially lupus erythematosus. The term *antiphospholipid syndrome (APS)* or *Hughes syndrome* is used to describe the triad of thrombosis, recurrent fetal loss, and thrombocytopenia accompanied by phospholipid antibodies or a lupus anticoagulant. These antibodies may be considered normal in the elderly person.

Interfering factors

• Patients who have or had syphilis infections can have a false-positive result.
• Transient antibodies can occur in patients with infections, AIDS, inflammation, autoimmune diseases, or cancer.
✔ False-positive results have been seen in patients who take such medications as chlorpromazine, hydralazine, penicillin, phenytoin, procainamide, and quinidine.

Procedure and patient care

• See inside front cover for Routine Blood Testing.
• Fasting: no
• Blood tube commonly used: verify with lab

Abnormal findings
▲ **Increased levels**
Systemic lupus erythematosus
Thrombosis
Thrombocytopenia
Recurrent fetal loss
Syphilis
Acute infection
Elderly persons

notes

anticentromere antibody test (Centromere antibody)

Type of test Blood

Normal findings

Negative (if positive, serum will be titrated)

Weak positive: positive at the screening titer (1:40 for human epithelial type 2 cells [HEp-2 cells]) (1:20 for kidney cells)

Moderately positive: one dilution above screening titer

Strong positive: two dilutions above screening titer

Test explanation and related physiology

A centromere is the region of the chromosome referred to as the *primary constriction* that divides the chromosome into *arms*. During cell division, the centromere exists in the *pole* of the mitotic spindle.

Anticentromere antibodies are a form of *antinuclear antibodies*. They are found in a very high percentage of patients with CREST syndrome, a variant of scleroderma. CREST syndrome is characterized by calcinosis, Raynaud phenomenon, esophageal dysfunction, sclerodactyly, and telangiectasia. Anticentromere antibodies, on the contrary, are present in only a small minority of patients with scleroderma, a disease that is difficult to differentiate from CREST syndrome. No correlation exists between antibody titer and severity of CREST syndrome.

Procedure and patient care

- See inside front cover for Routine Blood Testing.
- Fasting: no
- Blood tube commonly used: red

Abnormal findings

Positive results

CREST syndrome

notes

antichromatin antibody test (Antinucleosome antibody [anti-NCS], Antihistone antibody test [anti-HST, AHA])

Type of test Blood

Normal findings

Antinucleosome antibodies

No antibodies present in <1:20 dilution

Antihistone antibody

None detected: <1.0 units
Inconclusive: 1.0-1.5 units
Positive: 1.6-2.5 units
Strong positive: >2.5 units

Test explanation and related physiology

There are several chromatin antinuclear antibodies associated with autoimmune diseases. Nucleosome (NCS) represents the main autoantigen-immunogen in systemic lupus erythematosus (SLE), and these specific antibodies are an important marker of the disease activity. Antinucleosome (anti-NCS; antichromatin) antibodies play a key role in the pathogenesis of SLE. Nearly all patients with SLE have anti-NCS antibodies. Anti-NCS is also an antinuclear antibody (see p. 86). Anti-NCS has a sensitivity of 100% and specificity of 97% for SLE diagnosis. Anti-NCS antibodies show the highest correlation with disease activity. Anti-NCS antibodies also show strong association with renal damage (glomerulonephritis and proteinuria) associated with SLE. Anti-NCS autoantibodies are more prevalent than anti-DNA in SLE patients.

Histone antibodies are present in 20% to 55% of idiopathic SLE and 80% to 95% of drug-induced lupus erythematosus. They occur in less than 20% of other types of connective tissue diseases. This antibody is particularly helpful in identifying patients with drug-induced lupus erythematosus from drugs such as procainamide, quinidine, penicillamine, hydralazine, methyldopa, isoniazid, and acebutolol. There are several subtypes of antihistone antibodies (AHAs). In drug-induced lupus erythematosus, a specific AHA (anti-[(H2A-H2B)-DNA] IgG) is produced, while in most of the other associated diseases (rheumatoid arthritis, juvenile rheumatoid arthritis, primary biliary cirrhosis, autoimmune hepatitis, and dermatomyositis/polymyositis), the AHAs are of other varying specificities.

Procedure and patient care

- See inside front cover for Routine Blood Testing.
- Fasting: no
- Blood tube commonly used: red or gold

Abnormal findings

▲ **Increased levels**

Systemic lupus erythematosus

Drug-induced lupus erythematosus

Other autoimmune diseases

notes

A

anti–cyclic citrullinated peptide antibody (Cyclic citrullinated peptide antibody, CCP IgG anti-CCP)

Type of test Blood

Normal findings <20 units/mL

Test explanation and related physiology

Anti-CCP is known more formally as *anti–cyclic citrullinated peptide antibody*. The citrullinated peptide antigen is formed by the intermediary conversion of the amino acid ornithine to arginine. Anti-CCP appears early in the course of rheumatoid arthritis (RA). When the citrulline antibody is detected in a patient's blood, there is a high likelihood that the patient has RA. Anti-CCP is therefore useful in the diagnosis of patients with unexplained joint inflammation, especially when the traditional blood test, rheumatoid factor (RF; see p. 807), is negative or below 50 units/mL.

Many patients with early RA may not have elevation of RF, making the diagnosis difficult in the initial stage. The diagnosis of RA can be made, even if RF is negative, if the anti-CCP is elevated. This is particularly important because aggressive treatment in the early stages of RA prevents progression of joint damage. Anti-CCP may occur years before any clinical onset of arthritis or significant elevation of anti-CCP. At a cutoff of 5 units/mL, the sensitivity and specificity of anti-CCP for RA are 67.5% and 99.3%, respectively. RF has a sensitivity of 66.3% and a lower specificity (82.1%) than anti-CCP. When the two antibodies are used together, the specificity for diagnosing RA is 99.1%.

The presence of anti-CCP in RA indicates a more aggressive and destructive form of the disease. It is also a marker for disease progression. Some feel that anti-CCP–positive RA and anti-CCP–negative RA are clinically different disease entities, with the former having a far worse outcome.

Procedure and patient care

- See inside front cover for Routine Blood Testing.
- Fasting: no
- Blood tube commonly used: red

Abnormal findings

▲ **Increased levels**
   Rheumatoid arthritis

notes

antidiuretic hormone (ADH, Vasopressin)

Type of test   Blood

Normal findings

ADH: 1-5 pg/mL or 1-5 ng/L (SI units)
ADH suppression test (water load test):
    65% of water load excreted in 4 hours
    80% of water load excreted in 5 hours
    Urine osmolality (in second hour) ≤100 mmol/kg
    Urine to serum (U/S) osmolality ratio >100
    Urine specific gravity <1.003

Test explanation and related physiology

ADH, also known as *vasopressin*, is formed by the hypothalamus and is stored in the posterior pituitary gland. It controls the amount of water resorbed by the kidneys. ADH release is stimulated by an increase in serum osmolality or a decrease in intravascular blood volume. Physical stress, surgery, and even high levels of anxiety may also stimulate ADH release. With a release of ADH, more water is resorbed from the kidneys. This increases the amount of free water in the bloodstream and causes a very concentrated urine. With low ADH levels, water is allowed to be excreted, thereby producing hemoconcentration and a more dilute urine.

Diabetes insipidus (DI) results when ADH secretion is inadequate or when the kidney is unresponsive to ADH stimulation. Inadequate ADH secretion is usually associated with central neurologic abnormalities (neurogenic DI), such as trauma, tumor, inflammation of the brain (hypothalamus), or surgical ablation of the pituitary gland. Patients with DI excrete large volumes of free water within a dilute urine. Their blood is hemoconcentrated, causing them to have a strong thirst.

Primary renal diseases may make the renal collecting system less sensitive to ADH stimulation (nephrogenic DI). Again, in this instance, a dilute urine created by excretion of high volumes of free water may occur. To differentiate neurogenic DI from nephrogenic DI, a *water deprivation test (ADH stimulation test)* is performed. During this test, water intake is restricted, and urine osmolality is measured before and after vasopressin is administered. In neurogenic DI, there is no rise in urine osmolality with water restriction, but there is a rise after vasopressin administration. In nephrogenic DI, there is no rise in urine osmolality after water deprivation or vasopressin administration. The diagnosis indicated by this test can be corroborated by a serum ADH level. In neurogenic DI, ADH levels are low. In nephrogenic DI, ADH levels are high.

High serum ADH levels are also associated with the syndrome of inappropriate antidiuretic hormone (SIADH) secretion. In response to the inappropriately high level of ADH secretion, water is resorbed by the kidneys greatly in excess of normal amounts. Thus the patient becomes very hemodiluted and the urine concentrated. Blood levels of important serum ions diminish, causing severe neurologic, cardiac, and metabolic alterations. SIADH can be associated with pulmonary diseases (e.g., tuberculosis, bacterial pneumonia), severe stress (e.g., surgery, trauma), CNS tumor, or infection. Ectopic secretion of ADH from neoplasm (paraneoplastic syndrome) can cause SIADH. The most common tumors associated with SIADH include carcinomas of the lung and thymus; lymphomas; leukemia; and carcinomas of the pancreas, urologic tract, and intestine. Patients with myxedema or Addison disease also can experience SIADH. Some drugs are also known to cause SIADH (see below).

The *water load test (ADH suppression test)* is used to differentiate SIADH from other causes of hyponatremia or edematous states. Usually this test is done concomitant with measurements of urine and serum osmolality. Patients with SIADH will excrete none or very little of the water load. Furthermore, their urine osmolality will never be <100, and the urine/serum ratio is >100. Patients with other hyponatremia, edematous states, or chronic renal diseases will excrete up to 80% of the water load and will develop midrange osmolality results.

Interfering factors
- Patients with dehydration, hypovolemia, and stress may have increased ADH levels.
- Patients with overhydration, decreased serum osmolality, and hypervolemia may have decreased ADH levels.
- Use of a glass syringe or collection tube causes degradation of ADH.
- ✗ Drugs that *increase* ADH levels and may cause SIADH include acetaminophen, barbiturates, carbamazepine, cholinergic agents, cyclophosphamide, some diuretics (e.g., thiazides), estrogen, narcotics, nicotine, oral hypoglycemic agents (particularly sulfonylureas), and tricyclic or SSRI antidepressants.
- ✗ Drugs that *decrease* ADH levels include alcohol, beta-adrenergic agents, morphine antagonists, and phenytoin.

Procedure and patient care
- See inside front cover for Routine Blood Testing.
- Fasting: yes
- Blood tube commonly used: red
- Evaluate the patient for high levels of physical or emotional stress.
- Collect a venous blood sample in a *plastic* red-top tube with the patient in the sitting or recumbent position.
- The *water load* test necessitates a baseline serum sodium prior to water administration. Urine is later collected for specific gravity and osmolality. Blood is collected for osmolality.

Abnormal findings
▲ **Increased levels**
  Syndrome of inappropriate antidiuretic hormone (SIADH)
  Nephrogenic diabetes insipidus caused by primary renal diseases
  Postoperative days 1 to 3
  Severe physical stress (e.g., trauma, pain, prolonged mechanical ventilation)
  Hypovolemia
  Dehydration
  Acute porphyria

▼ **Decreased levels**
  Neurogenic (or central) diabetes insipidus
  Surgical ablation of the pituitary gland
  Hypervolemia
  Decreased serum osmolality

notes

anti-DNA antibody test (Anti–deoxyribonucleic acid antibodies, Antibody to double-stranded DNA, Anti–double-stranded DNA, Anti–ds-DNA, DNA antibody, Native double-stranded DNA)

Type of test Blood

Normal findings

Negative: <5 international units/mL
Intermediate: 5-9 international units/mL
Positive: ≥10 international units/mL

Test explanation and related physiology

The anti-DNA test is useful for the diagnosis and follow-up of systemic lupus erythematosus (SLE). This antibody is found in approximately 65% to 80% of patients with active SLE and rarely in other diseases. High titers are characteristic of SLE. Low to intermediate levels of this antibody may be found in patients with other rheumatic diseases and in those with chronic hepatitis, infectious mononucleosis, and biliary cirrhosis. The anti-DNA titer decreases with successful therapy and increases with an exacerbation of SLE, especially with the onset of lupus glomerulonephritis. The test can return to near negative with dormant SLE. This test is semi-quantitative. Therefore, small changes in antibody levels do not indicate disease activity.

The anti-DNA IgG antibody is a subtype of the *antinuclear antibodies (ANAs)* (see p. 86). If the ANAs are negative, there is no reason to test for anti-DNA antibodies. There are two types of anti-DNA antibodies. The first and most popular is the antibody against double-stranded DNA (anti–ds-DNA). The second type is the antibody against single-stranded DNA (anti–ss-DNA), which is less sensitive and specific for SLE but is positive in other autoimmune diseases. These antibody-antigen complexes that occur with autoimmune disease are not only diagnostic but are major contributors to the disease process. These complexes induce the complement system, which then may cause local or systemic tissue injury.

Interfering factors

- A radioactive scan performed within 1 week before the test may alter the test results.
- ✘ Drugs that may cause *increased* levels include hydralazine and procainamide.

Procedure and patient care

- See inside front cover for Routine Blood Testing.
- Fasting: no
- Blood tube commonly used: red

Abnormal findings

▲ **Increased levels**

Collagen vascular disease (e.g., systemic lupus erythematosus)

Chronic hepatitis

Infectious mononucleosis

Biliary cirrhosis

notes

anti–extractable nuclear antigens (Anti-ENAs, Antibodies to extractable nuclear antigens, Antihistidyl transfer synthase [anti–Jo-1], Antiribonucleoprotein [anti-RNP], Anti-Smith [anti-SM])

Type of test Blood

Normal findings Negative

Test explanation and related physiology

The anti-ENAs are used to assist in the diagnosis of systemic lupus erythematosus (SLE) and mixed connective tissue disease (MCTD) and to eliminate other rheumatoid diseases.

Anti-ENAs are a type of *antinuclear antibody* to certain nuclear antigens that consist of RNA and protein. The ENA antigen is sometimes referred to as *saline-extracted antigen.* The most common ENAs are *Smith (SM)* and *ribonucleoprotein (RNP).*

The *antinuclear Smith (anti-SM)* antibody is present in about 30% of patients with SLE and in about 8% of patients with MCTD. However, it is not present in patients with most other rheumatoid-collagen diseases.

The *antinuclear ribonucleoprotein (anti-RNP)* antibody is reported in nearly 100% of patients with MCTD and in about 25% of patients with SLE, discoid lupus, and progressive systemic sclerosis (scleroderma). In high titer, anti-RNP is suggestive of MCTD.

The *antihistidyl transfer synthase (anti–Jo-1)* antibodies occur in patients with autoimmune interstitial pulmonary fibrosis and in a minority of patients with aggressive autoimmune myositis.

There are two other antibodies to ENAs. Anti–SS-A and anti–SS-B are described on p. 96 and are used mainly in the diagnostic evaluation of Sjögren syndrome.

Procedure and patient care

- See inside front cover for Routine Blood Testing.
- Fasting: no
- Blood tube commonly used: red

Abnormal findings

▲ **Increased anti-SM antibodies**
  Systemic lupus erythematosus
▲ **Increased anti-RNP antibodies**
  Mixed connective tissue disease
  Systemic lupus erythematosus
  Discoid lupus scleroderma
▲ **Increased anti–Jo-1 antibodies**
  Pulmonary fibrosis
  Autoimmune myositis

notes

anti–glomerular basement membrane antibodies
(Anti-GBM antibody, AGBM, Glomerular basement antibody, Goodpasture antibody)

Type of test Blood; microscopic examination of tissue (lung or renal)

Normal findings

Tissue

Negative: no immunofluorescence noted on the renal or lung tissue basement membrane

Blood: EIA (enzyme immunoassay)

Negative: <20 units

Borderline: 20-100 units

Positive: >100 units

Test explanation and related physiology

This test is used to detect the presence of circulating glomerular basement membrane (GBM) antibodies commonly present in autoimmune-induced nephritis (Goodpasture syndrome).

Goodpasture syndrome is an autoimmune disease characterized by the presence of antibodies circulating against antigens in the basement membrane of the renal glomerular and the pulmonary alveoli. These immune complexes activate the complement system and thereby cause tissue injury. Patients with this problem usually display a triad of glomerulonephritis (hematuria), pulmonary hemorrhage (hemoptysis), and antibodies to basement membrane antigens. About 60% to 75% of patients with immune-induced glomerular nephritis have these pulmonary complications.

Lung or renal biopsies are required to obtain tissue on which to demonstrate these antibodies with immunohistochemical techniques. Serum assays are faster and more reliable methods for diagnosing Goodpasture syndrome, especially in patients in whom a renal or lung biopsy may be difficult or contraindicated. Furthermore, serum levels can be used in monitoring response to therapy (plasmapheresis or immunosuppression).

Procedure and patient care

- See inside front cover for Routine Blood Testing.
- Fasting: yes
- Blood tube commonly used: red
- **PT** If a lung biopsy (see p. 604) or renal biopsy (see p. 792) will be used to collect the specimen, explain these procedures to the patient.

Abnormal findings

Positive

Goodpasture syndrome
Autoimmune glomerulonephritis
Lupus nephritis

notes

anti-glycan antibodies (Crohn disease prognostic panel, Multiple sclerosis antibody panel)

Type of test Blood

Normal findings Negative

Test explanation and related physiology

Anti-glycan antibodies are immunologically directed to sugar-containing components on the surface of cells (particularly erythrocytes). Antibodies to glycans can be instigated by bacterial, fungal, and parasite infections. The use of glycan arrays for systematic screening of patients with multiple sclerosis (MS) and inflammatory bowel disease (particularly Crohn disease) has been helpful in differentiating these diseases. Furthermore, these antibodies are used to determine treatment and prognosis.

Utilizing enzyme-linked immunosorbent assays, these antibodies can be identified and quantified. Anti-*Saccharomyces cerevisiae* antibody (ASCA), anti-laminaribioside carbohydrate antibody (ALCA), anti-mannobioside carbohydrate antibody (AMCA), and anti-chitobioside carbohydrate antibody (ACCA) are used to evaluate Crohn disease and differentiate Crohn colitis from ulcerative colitis. When all are positive, Crohn disease is much more likely than ulcerative colitis.

Other anti-glycan antibodies are specific for MS patients.

Procedure and patient care

- See inside front cover for Routine Blood Testing.
- Fasting: no
- Blood tube commonly used: lavender, pink, or green

Abnormal findings

▲ **Increased levels**
  Crohn disease
  Multiple sclerosis

notes

anti-liver/kidney microsomal type 1 antibodies
(Anti-LKM-1 antibodies)

Type of test   Blood

Normal findings

≤20 units (negative)
20.1-24.9 units (equivocal)
≥25 units (positive)

Test explanation and related physiology

Autoimmune liver disease (e.g., autoimmune hepatitis and primary biliary cirrhosis) is characterized by the presence of autoantibodies, including smooth muscle antibodies (SMA) (page 93), antimitochondrial antibodies (AMA) (page 82), and anti-liver/kidney microsomal antibodies type 1 (anti-LKM-1). Subtypes of autoimmune hepatitis (AIH) are based on autoantibody reactivity patterns. For example, the presence of smooth muscle antibodies (SMAs) is consistent with the diagnosis of chronic autoimmune hepatitis. The presence of anti-liver/kidney microsomal type 1 antibodies with or without SMAs is consistent with autoimmune hepatitis type 2. The presence of antimitochondrial antibodies is consistent with primary biliary cirrhosis.

Anti-LKM-1 antibodies serve as a serologic marker for AIH type 2 and typically occur in the absence of SMAs and antinuclear antibodies. Children often have other autoantibodies (e.g., parietal cell antibodies and thyroid microsomal antibodies). These antibodies react with a short linear sequence of the recombinant antigen cytochrome monooxygenase P450 2D6. Patients with AIH type 2 more often tend to be young and female and have a severe form of disease that responds well to immunosuppressive therapy.

Patients with chronic hepatitis resulting from hepatitis C can also have elevated anti-LKM-1 antibodies. The diagnosis of autoimmune liver disease cannot be made on antibody testing alone. In many instances, autoimmune liver disease panel testing, including the antibodies discussed in the preceding paragraph, is performed. Testing is performed by semi-quantitative enzyme-linked immunosorbent assay/semi-quantitative indirect fluorescent antibody.

Procedure and patient care

- See inside front cover for Routine Blood Testing.
- Fasting: no

- Blood tube commonly used: serum separator
PT Explain the importance of performing the test in the morning.
- Blood may be sent to a reference laboratory. Results are available in about 1 week.

Abnormal findings

▲ **Increased levels**
  Autoimmune hepatitis

notes

antimitochondrial antibody (AMA)

Type of test Blood

Normal findings No antimitochondrial antibodies (AMAs) at titers >1:5 or <0.1 units

Test explanation and related physiology

The AMA is used primarily to aid in the diagnosis of primary biliary cirrhosis. AMA is an anticytoplasmic antibody directed against a lipoprotein in the mitochondrial membrane. Normally the serum does not contain AMA at a titer greater than 1:5. AMA appears in 94% of patients with primary biliary cirrhosis. This disease occurs predominantly in young and middle-aged women. It has a slow, progressive course marked by elevated liver enzymes, especially alkaline phosphatase and gamma-glutamyl transpeptidase (see pp. 29 and 452) and positive AMA. Liver biopsy (see p. 591) is usually required to confirm the diagnosis. There are subgroups of AMA. The M-2 subgroup is very specific for primary biliary cirrhosis.

Procedure and patient care

- See inside front cover for Routine Blood Testing.
- Fasting: no
- Blood tube commonly used: red

Abnormal findings

▲ Increased levels

Primary biliary cirrhosis

Chronic active hepatitis

Systemic lupus erythematosus

Syphilis

Drug-induced cholestasis

Autoimmune hepatitis (e.g., scleroderma, systemic lupus erythematosus)

Extrahepatic obstruction

Acute infectious hepatitis

notes

antimyocardial antibody (AMA)

Type of test Blood

Normal findings Negative (if positive, serum will be titrated)

Test explanation and related physiology

This test is used to detect an autoimmune source of myocardial injury and disease. Antimyocardial antibodies (AMAs) may be detected in rheumatic heart disease, cardiomyopathy, postthoracotomy syndrome, and postmyocardial infarction syndromes. This test is used both in the detection of an autoimmune cause for these conditions and for monitoring their response to treatment. Antibodies against heart muscle are also found in 20% to 40% of postcardiac surgery patients and in a smaller number of postmyocardial infarction patients. These antibodies are usually associated with a pericarditis that follows the myocardial injury associated with cardiac surgery or myocardial infarction (Dressler syndrome). AMA has also been detected with cardiomyopathy.

Procedure and patient care

- See inside front cover for Routine Blood Testing.
- Fasting: no
- Blood tube commonly used: red

Abnormal findings

▲ **Increased levels**

Rheumatic heart disease

Cardiomyopathy

Postthoracotomy syndrome

Postmyocardial infarction

Rheumatic fever

Streptococcal infection

notes

antineutrophil cytoplasmic antibody (ANCA)

Type of test Blood

Normal findings Negative

Test explanation and related physiology

ANCAs are directed against cytoplasmic components of neutrophils. This test is used to assist in the diagnosis of granulomatous vascular diseases, such as Wegener granulomatosis (WG). It also is useful in following the course of the disease, monitoring the response to therapy, and providing early detection of relapse. WG is a regional systemic vasculitis in which the small arteries of the kidneys, lungs, and upper respiratory tract (nasopharynx) are damaged by a granulomatous inflammation. Diagnosis used to be made by biopsy of clinically affected tissue. Serologic testing now plays a key role in the diagnosis of WG and other systemic vasculitis syndromes.

When ANCAs are detected with indirect immunofluorescence microscopy, two major patterns of staining are present: cytoplasmic ANCA (c-ANCA) and perinuclear ANCA (p-ANCA). Specific immunochemical assays demonstrate that c-ANCA consists mainly of antibodies to proteinase 3 (PR3), and p-ANCA consists of antibodies to myeloperoxidase (MPO). Using the antigen-specific immunochemical assay to characterize ANCA (rather than the pattern of immunofluorescence microscopy) is more specific and more clinically relevant; therefore, the terms *proteinase 3-ANCA (PR3-ANCA)* and *myeloperoxidase-ANCA (MPO-ANCA)* are used.

The PR3 autoantigen is highly specific (95% to 99%) for WG. When the disease is limited to the respiratory tract, the PR3 is positive in about 65% of patients. Nearly all patients with WG limited to the kidney do not have positive PR3. When WG is inactive, the percentage of positive PR3 drops to about 30%.

The MPO autoantigen is found in 50% of patients with WG centered in the kidney. It also occurs in patients with non-WG glomerulonephritis, such as microscopic polyangiitis (MPA). P-ANCA antibodies can also differentiate various forms of inflammatory bowel disease. See also anti-glycan antibodies, page 79. P-ANCA antibodies are found in 50% to 70% of ulcerative colitis (UC) patients, but in only 20% of Crohn disease (CD) patients.

Procedure and patient care
- See inside front cover for Routine Blood Testing.
- Fasting: no
- Blood tube commonly used: verify with lab

Abnormal findings
▲ Increased levels
  Wegener granulomatosis
  Microscopic polyarteritis
  Idiopathic crescentic glomerulonephritis
  Ulcerative colitis
  Primary sclerosing cholangitis
  Autoimmune hepatitis
  Churg-Strauss vasculitis
  Active viral hepatitis
  Crohn disease

notes

antinuclear antibody (ANA)

Type of test Blood

Normal findings Negative at 1:40 dilution

Test explanation and related physiology

ANA is a group of antinuclear antibodies used to diagnose systemic lupus erythematosus (SLE) and other autoimmune (rheumatic) diseases (Box 1). Some of the antibodies in this group are specific for SLE, and others are specific for other autoimmune diseases. ANA can be tested as a specific antibody or as a group with nonspecific antigens (Box 2). The former is more specific, but testing ANA with less specific antigens may be an excellent preliminary test for those suspected of having autoimmune diseases.

Because almost all patients with SLE develop autoantibodies, a negative ANA test excludes the diagnosis. Positive results occur in approximately 95% of patients with this disease; however, many other rheumatic diseases (see Box 1) are also associated with ANA.

ANA tests are performed using different assays (indirect immunofluorescence microscopy or enzyme-linked immunosorbent assay [ELISA]), and results are reported as a titer with a particular type of immunofluorescence pattern (when positive). Low-level titers are considered negative, while increased titers are positive and indicate an elevated concentration of antinuclear antibodies.

ANA shows up on indirect immunofluorescence as fluorescent patterns in cells that are fixed to a slide and are evaluated

---

BOX 1   Diseases associated with antinuclear antibodies

Systemic lupus erythematosus
Sjögren syndrome
Scleroderma
Raynaud disease
Rheumatoid arthritis
Dermatomyositis
Mixed connective tissue disease
Autoimmune hepatitis
Autoimmune thyroiditis
Juvenile rheumatoid arthritis
Primary biliary cirrhosis
Polymyositis

BOX 2   Antinuclear antibodies

Anti-RNA antibodies
Anti-ENA antibodies
  Antinuclear Smith (SM) antibodies
  Antinuclear RNP antibodies
  Antihistidyl antibodies
Antichromatin antibodies
  Antinucleosome antibodies
  Antihistone antibodies
  Anti-DNA antibodies
    Anti–ds-DNA antibodies
    Anti–ss-DNA antibodies
Anti–SS-A (Ro)
Anti–SS-B (La)

under a UV microscope. Different patterns are associated with a variety of autoimmune disorders. When combined with a more specific subtype of ANA (Box 2), the pattern can increase specificity of the ANA subtypes for the various autoimmune diseases (Figure 3). An example of a positive result might be: "Positive at 1:320 dilution with a homogeneous pattern."

As the disease becomes less active because of therapy, the ANA titers can be expected to fall (Table 1). In this text, the more commonly used ANA subtypes are separately discussed. About 95% of SLE patients have a positive ANA test result. If a

TABLE 1   Autoimmune disease and positive ANAs

Autoimmune disease	Positive antibodies
SLE	ANA, SLE prep, ds-DNA, ss-DNA, anti-DNP, SS-A
Drug-induced SLE	ANA
Sjögren syndrome	RF, ANA, SS-A, SS-B
Scleroderma	ANA, Scl-70, RNA, ds-DNA
Raynaud disease	ACA, Scl-70
Mixed connective tissue disease	ANA, RNP, RF, ss-DNA
Rheumatoid arthritis	RF, ANA, RANA, RAP
Primary biliary cirrhosis	AMA
Thyroiditis	Antimicrosomal, antithyroglobulin
Chronic active hepatitis	ASMA

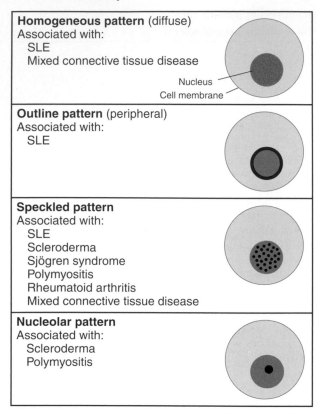

Homogeneous pattern (diffuse)
Associated with:
  SLE
  Mixed connective tissue disease

Nucleus
Cell membrane

Outline pattern (peripheral)
Associated with:
  SLE

Speckled pattern
Associated with:
  SLE
  Scleroderma
  Sjögren syndrome
  Polymyositis
  Rheumatoid arthritis
  Mixed connective tissue disease

Nucleolar pattern
Associated with:
  Scleroderma
  Polymyositis

FIGURE 3 Patterns of immunofluorescent staining of antinuclear antibodies and the diseases with which they are associated.

patient also has symptoms of SLE (e.g., arthritis, rash, autoimmune thrombocytopenia), then he or she probably has SLE.

Interfering factors

- ☛ Drugs that may cause a false-positive ANA test include acetazolamide, aminosalicylic acid, chlorprothixene, chlorothiazides, griseofulvin, hydralazine, penicillin, phenylbutazone, phenytoin sodium, procainamide, streptomycin, sulfonamides, and tetracyclines.
- ☛ Drugs that may cause a false-negative test include steroids.

Procedure and patient care

- See inside front cover for Routine Blood Testing.
- Fasting: no
- Blood tube commonly used: red

Abnormal findings

▲ **Increased levels**
  Systemic lupus erythematosus
  Rheumatoid arthritis
  Chronic hepatitis
  Periarteritis (polyarteritis) nodosa
  Dermatomyositis
  Scleroderma
  Infectious mononucleosis
  Raynaud disease
  Sjögren syndrome
  Other immune diseases
  Leukemia
  Myasthenia gravis
  Cirrhosis

notes

antiparietal cell antibody (APCA)

Type of test   Blood

Normal findings   Negative

Test explanation and related physiology

Parietal cells exist in the proximal stomach and produce hydrochloric acid and intrinsic factor. Intrinsic factor is necessary for the absorption of vitamin B_{12} (see p. 986). Antiparietal cell antibodies (APCAs) are found in nearly 90% of patients with pernicious anemia. Nearly 60% of these patients also have antiintrinsic factor antibodies. It is thought that these antibodies contribute to the destruction of the gastric mucosa in these patients. APCA is also found in patients with atrophic gastritis, gastric ulcers, and gastric cancer.

APCA is present in other autoimmune-mediated diseases, such as thyroiditis, myxedema, juvenile diabetes, Addison disease, and iron-deficiency anemia. Nearly 10% to 15% of the normal population has APCA. As one ages, the incidence of having APCA increases (especially in relatives of patients with pernicious anemia).

APCA can cross-react with other antibodies, especially anticellular and antithyroid antibodies. Titer levels greater than 1:240 are considered positive.

Procedure and patient care

- See inside front cover for Routine Blood Testing.
- Fasting: no
- Blood tube commonly used: red

Abnormal findings

▲ Increased levels

   Pernicious anemia
   Atrophic gastritis
   Hashimoto thyroiditis
   Myxedema
   Insulin-dependent diabetes mellitus
   Addison disease

notes

antiscleroderma antibody (Scl-70 antibody, Scleroderma antibody, RNA polymerase III antibody)

Type of test Blood

Normal findings Negative

Test explanation and related physiology

This antibody is diagnostic for scleroderma (progressive systemic sclerosis [PSS]) and is present in 45% of patients with that disease. Scl-70 antibody is an *antinuclear antibody* (see p. 86). PSS is a multisystem disorder characterized by inflammation with subsequent fibrosis of the small blood vessels in skin and visceral organs, including the heart, lungs, kidneys, and gastrointestinal tract. A collagen-like substance is also deposited into the tissue of these organs. In general, the higher the titer of Scl-70 antibody, the more likely that PSS exists and the more active the disease is. As the disease becomes less active because of therapy, the Scl-70 antibody titers can be expected to fall.

The absence of this antibody does not exclude the diagnosis of PSS. The antibody is rather specific for PSS but is occasionally seen in other autoimmune diseases (e.g., systemic lupus erythematosus, mixed connective tissue disease, Sjögren syndrome, polymyositis, and rheumatoid arthritis).

RNA polymerase III antibodies are found in 11% to 23% of patients with PSS. PSS patients who are positive for RNA polymerase III antibodies form a distinct serologic subgroup and usually do not have any of the other antibodies typically found in PSS patients, such as anticentromere (p. 66) or anti-Scl70. PSS patients with anti-RNA polymerase III have an increased risk of the diffuse cutaneous form of scleroderma, with a high likelihood of skin involvement and hypertensive renal disease. A positive result supports a possible diagnosis of PSS. This autoantibody is strongly associated with diffuse cutaneous scleroderma and with an increased risk of acute renal crisis. A negative result indicates no detectable IgG antibodies to RNA polymerase III, but does not rule out the possibility of PSS (11% to 33% sensitivity).

Interfering factors

☛ Drugs that may cause *increased* levels include aminosalicylic acid, isoniazid, methyldopa, penicillin, propylthiouracil, streptomycin, and tetracycline.

Procedure and patient care

- See inside front cover for Routine Blood Testing.
- Fasting: no
- Blood tube commonly used: red

Abnormal findings

Positive results

Scleroderma
CREST syndrome

notes

anti–smooth muscle antibody (ASMA)

Type of test Blood

Normal findings No anti–smooth muscle antibodies (ASMAs) at titers >1:20

Test explanation and related physiology

The ASMA is used primarily to aid in the diagnosis of autoimmune chronic active hepatitis (CAH), which has also been referred to as *lupoid* CAH. ASMA is an *anticytoplasmic antibody* directed against actin, a cytoskeletal protein. Normally the serum does not contain ASMA at a titer greater than 1:20. ASMA is the most commonly recognized autoantibody in the setting of CAH. It appears in 70% to 80% of patients with CAH. Some types of CAH do not have positive ASMA antibodies.

ASMA is not specific for CAH and can be positive in patients with viral infections, malignancy, multiple sclerosis, primary biliary cirrhosis, and *Mycoplasma* infections. Usually the titer of ASMA is low in these diseases. With CAH, the titer is usually higher than 1:160. The titers are not helpful in prognosis, nor do they indicate disease response to therapy.

Procedure and patient care

- See inside front cover for Routine Blood Testing.
- Fasting: no
- Blood tube commonly used: red

Abnormal findings

▲ Increased levels

Chronic active hepatitis

Mononucleosis hepatitis

Primary biliary cirrhosis

Viral hepatitis

Multiple sclerosis

Malignancy

Intrinsic asthma

notes

antispermatozoal antibody (Sperm agglutination and inhibition, Sperm antibodies, Antisperm antibodies, Infertility screen)

Type of test Fluid analysis; blood

Normal findings <50% binding

Test explanation and related physiology

The antispermatozoal antibody test is an infertility test used to detect the presence of sperm antibodies. Antibodies directed toward sperm antigens can result in diminished fertility. This test is used in the evaluation of an infertile couple usually after a post-coital test is positive. For fertilization to occur, the sperm head must first attach to the *zona pellucida* of the egg. Sperm antibodies interfere with this binding. Although there is consensus that these antibodies play a role in infertility, the percentage of sperm that must be bound by antibodies before fertility is adversely affected is less clear. IgA antisperm antibodies attached to the sperm tail are associated with poor motility and poor penetration of cervical mucus. IgG antisperm antibodies are associated with blockage of sperm-ovum fusion. Semen and serum may contain sperm antibodies. Semen is the preferred specimen type for males. In cases where semen production may present difficulties, a serum specimen can be tested instead. Serum is the preferred specimen type in females.

Positives are reported as percentage of sperm with positive bindings, the class of antibody involved (IgG, IgA, and IgM), and the site of binding (head, midpiece, tail, and/or tail tip). Greater than 50% binding is usually required to significantly lower a patient's fertility.

Not only is this test indicated for male infertility studies, it is also used as a follow-up test when sperm agglutination is noted in the ejaculate. It is also used in men with a history of testicular trauma, biopsy, vasectomy reversal, genital tract infection, or obstructive lesions of the male ductal system. Antisperm antibodies may be found in the blood of men with blocked efferent ducts of the testes (a common cause of low sperm counts or poor sperm mobility) and in 30% to 70% of men who have had a vasectomy. Resorption of sperm from the blocked ducts results in the formation of autoantibodies to sperm as a result of sperm antigens interacting with the immune system. High titers of IgG autoantibodies are often associated with postvasectomy degeneration of the testes, which explains why 50% of males remain infertile after successful repair of a previous vasectomy.

Procedure and patient care

- See inside front cover for Routine Blood Testing.
- Fasting: no
- Blood tube commonly used: red

Sperm specimen

PT Inform the man that a semen specimen should be collected after avoiding ejaculation for at least 3 days.

- Give the male patient the proper container for the sperm collection.

PT If the specimen is to be collected at home, be certain the patient is told that it must be taken to the laboratory for testing within 2 hours after collection.

- Collect venous blood samples from both the male and the female patient.
- For a vaginal mucus specimen, collect 1 mL of cervical mucus and place it in a plastic vial.

PT Instruct the couple on when and how to obtain the test results.

Abnormal findings

Infertility
Blocked efferent ducts in the testes
Vasectomy
Testicular trauma

notes

anti–SS-A (Ro), anti–SS-B (La), and anti–SS-C antibodies (Anti-Ro, Anti-La, Sjögren antibodies)

Type of test   Blood

Normal findings

SS-A (Ro) antibodies, IgG
   <1 U (negative)
   ≥1 U (positive)
SS-B (La) antibodies, IgG
   <1 U (negative)
   ≥1 U (positive)

Test explanation and related physiology

These three antinuclear antibodies are considered anti–extractable nuclear antigens (see p. 75) and are used to diagnose Sjögren syndrome. Ro, La, and SS-C antibodies are subtypes of *antinuclear antibodies (ANAs)*; they react to nuclear antigens extracted from human B lymphocytes. Ro and La result in a speckled immunofluorescent pattern when seen in the UV microscope (see Figure 3, p. 88). Sjögren syndrome is an immunogenic disease characterized by progressive destruction of the lacrimal and salivary exocrine glands, leading to mucosal and conjunctival dryness. This disease can occur by itself (primary) or in association with other autoimmune diseases, such as systemic lupus erythematosus (SLE), rheumatoid arthritis (RA), and scleroderma. In the latter case, it is referred to as secondary Sjögren syndrome.

Anti–SS-A antibodies may be found in approximately 60% to 70% of patients with primary Sjögren syndrome. Anti–SS-B antibodies may be found in approximately half of patients with primary Sjögren syndrome. When anti–SS-A and anti–SS-B antibodies are both positive, Sjögren syndrome can be diagnosed. These antibodies are only occasionally found when secondary Sjögren syndrome is associated with RA. In fact, anti–SS-B is found only in primary Sjögren syndrome. However, anti–SS-C is positive in about 75% of patients with RA or patients with RA and secondary Sjögren syndrome. Therefore, these antibodies are also useful in differentiating primary from secondary Sjögren syndrome.

Anti–SS-A can also be found in 25% of patients with SLE. This is particularly useful in ANA-negative cases of SLE because these antibodies are present in the majority of such patients. Anti–SS-B is rarely found in SLE, however. In general, the higher the titer of anti-SS antibodies, the more likely that Sjögren syndrome exists and the more active the disease is. As Sjögren syndrome becomes less active with therapy, the anti-SS antibody titers can be expected to fall.

Procedure and patient care

- See inside front cover for Routine Blood Testing.
- Fasting: no
- Blood tube commonly used: red

Abnormal findings

Positive

Sjögren syndrome
Rheumatoid arthritis
ANA-negative systemic lupus erythematosus
Neonatal lupus

notes

antithrombin activity and antigen assay (Antithrombin III [AT-III] activity/assay, Functional antithrombin III assay, Heparin cofactor, Immunologic antithrombin III, Serine protease inhibitor)

Type of test   Blood

Normal findings

Antithrombin activity:
   Newborn: 35% to 40%
   >6 months to adult: 80% to 130%
Antithrombin antigen assay:
   Plasma: >50% of control value
   Serum: 15% to 34% lower than plasma value
   Immunologic: 17-30 mg/dL
   Functional: 80% to 120%
Values vary according to laboratory methods.

Test explanation and related physiology

AT-III is an alpha$_2$ globulin produced in the liver. It inhibits the serine proteases involved in coagulation (II, X, IX, XI, XII). In normal homeostasis, coagulation results from a balance between AT-III and thrombin. A deficiency of AT-III increases coagulation or the tendency toward thrombosis. A hereditary deficiency of AT-III is characterized by a predisposition toward thrombus formation. This is passed on as an autosomal dominant abnormality. Individuals with hereditary AT-III deficiency typically develop thromboembolic events in their early twenties. These thrombotic events are usually venous.

Acquired AT-III deficiency may be seen in patients with cirrhosis, liver failure, advanced carcinoma, nephrotic syndrome, disseminated intravascular coagulation (DIC), protein-losing enteropathies, and acute thrombosis. AT-III is also decreased as much as 30% in pregnant women and women who take estrogens. Antithrombin activity testing is ordered, along with other tests for hypercoagulable disorders (e.g., protein C and protein S, and lupus anticoagulant), when a patient has been experiencing recurrent venous thrombosis. Antithrombin should be measured after a blood clot has been treated and resolved as both the presence of the clot and the therapy used to treat it will affect antithrombin results.

AT-III provides most of the anticoagulant effect of heparin. Heparin increases antithrombin activity by 1000-fold. Patients who are deficient in AT-III may be heparin resistant and require unusually high doses for an anticoagulation effect. In general, patients respond to heparin if more than 60% of normal AT-III levels exist.

There are two tests for AT-III. The first is a *functional* assay and measures AT-III activity. The second quantifies the AT-III antigen. The antithrombin activity test is performed before the antigen test to evaluate whether the total amount of functional antithrombin activity is normal. Antithrombin activity is the primary (screening) antithrombin assay. If antithrombin activity is normal, AT-III is not the cause of the hypercoagulable state. If antithrombin activity is abnormal, antithrombin antigen should be quantified.

Asymptomatic individuals with an antithrombin deficiency should receive prophylactic anticoagulation to increase their antithrombin levels before any medical/surgical interventions in which inactivity increases the risk of thrombosis. Increased levels of AT-III are not usually considered a problem and may occur in patients with acute hepatitis, obstructive jaundice, vitamin K deficiency, and kidney transplantation.

Antithrombin studies are also used as an adjunct in the diagnosis and management of carbohydrate-deficient glycoprotein syndromes (CDGSs) because defective glycosylation of this AT-III in individuals with CDGSs will cause hypercoagulation. Deficient AT-III may also contribute to recurrent miscarriages.

Antithrombin activity testing is also used to monitor treatment of antithrombin deficiency disorders by infusion of antithrombin concentrates.

Interfering factors

- Drugs that may cause *increased* levels include anabolic steroids, androgens, oral contraceptives (containing progesterone), and sodium warfarin.
- Drugs that may cause *decreased* levels include fibrinolytics, heparin, L-asparaginase, and oral contraceptives (containing estrogen).

Procedure and patient care

- See inside front cover for Routine Blood Testing.
- Fasting: no
- Blood tube commonly used: light blue or red
- Patients receiving heparin therapy may develop a hematoma at the venipuncture site.

Test results and clinical significance

▲ **Increased levels**
  Kidney transplant
  Acute hepatitis
  Obstructive jaundice
  Vitamin K deficiency

▼ **Decreased levels**
  Disseminated intravascular
    coagulation (DIC)
  Hypercoagulation states (e.g.,
    deep vein thrombosis)
  Hepatic disorders
    (especially cirrhosis)
  Nephrotic syndrome
  Protein-wasting diseases
    (malignancy)
  Hereditary familial
    deficiency of AT-III

notes

antithyroglobulin antibody (Thyroid autoantibody, Thyroid antithyroglobulin antibody, Thyroglobulin antibody)

Type of test Blood

Normal findings <116 IU/mL

Test explanation and related physiology

This test is used as a marker for autoimmune thyroiditis and related diseases. Thyroglobulin autoantibodies bind thyroglobulin (Tg), which is a major thyroid-specific protein that plays a crucial role in thyroid hormone synthesis, storage, and release. Tg remains in the thyroid follicles until hormone production is required. Tg is not secreted into the systemic circulation under normal circumstances. However, follicular destruction through inflammation (Hashimoto thyroiditis or chronic lymphocytic thyroiditis and autoimmune hypothyroidism), hemorrhage (nodular goiter), or rapid disordered growth of thyroid tissue (as may be observed in Graves disease or follicular cell-derived thyroid neoplasms) can result in leakage of Tg into the bloodstream. This results in the formation of autoantibodies to Tg in some individuals.

The anti-Tg test is usually performed in conjunction with the antithyroid peroxidase antibody test (see p. 102). When this is done, the specificity and sensitivity are greatly increased.

Interfering factors

- Normal individuals, especially elderly women, may have anti-Tg antibodies.

Procedure and patient care

- See inside front cover for Routine Blood Testing.
- Fasting: no
- Blood tube commonly used: red

Abnormal findings

▲ Increased levels

Hashimoto thyroiditis

Rheumatoid arthritis

Rheumatoid-collagen disease

Pernicious anemia

Thyrotoxicosis

Hypothyroidism

Thyroid carcinoma

Myxedema

Autoimmune hemolytic anemia

notes

antithyroid peroxidase antibody (Anti-TPO, TPO-Ab, Antithyroid microsomal antibody, Thyroid autoantibody)

Type of test Blood

Normal findings Titer <9 IU/mL

Test explanation and related physiology

This test is primarily used in the differential diagnosis of thyroid diseases. Thyroid microsomal antibodies are commonly found in patients with various thyroid diseases. They are present in 70% to 90% of patients with Hashimoto thyroiditis. Microsomal antibodies are produced in response to microsomes escaping from the thyroid epithelial cells surrounding the thyroid follicle. These escaped microsomes then act as antigens and stimulate the production of antibodies. These immune complexes initiate inflammatory and cytotoxic effects on the thyroid follicle. This test is often performed in conjunction with the antithyroglobulin antibody test, which greatly increases the specificity and sensitivity.

Although many different thyroid diseases are associated with elevated antimicrosomal antibody levels, the most frequent is chronic thyroiditis (Hashimoto thyroiditis in adults and lymphocytic thyroiditis in children and young adults). Both of these chronic inflammatory diseases have been associated with other autoimmune (collagen-vascular) diseases.

The most sensitive assay for antimicrosomal antibodies is the antithyroid peroxidase (anti-TPO) antibody. Anti-TPO is present in almost all patients with Hashimoto thyroiditis; in more than 70% of those with Graves disease; and, to a variable degree, in patients with nonthyroid autoimmune disease. Anti-TPO correlates with the degree of lymphocytic infiltrations (inflammation) in the thyroid. Among healthy people, 5% to 10% have elevated anti-TPO levels.

Procedure and patient care

- See inside front cover for Routine Blood Testing.
- Fasting: no
- Blood tube commonly used: red

Abnormal findings

▲ **Increased levels**
   Hashimoto thyroiditis
   Rheumatoid arthritis
   Rheumatoid-collagen disease
   Pernicious anemia
   Thyrotoxicosis
   Hypothyroidism
   Thyroid carcinoma
   Myxedema

notes

apolipoproteins

Type of test   Blood

Normal findings

Apo A-I

Adult/elderly:
  Male: 75-160 mg/dL
  Female: 80-175 mg/dL
Child:
  Newborn:
    Male: 41-93 mg/dL
    Female: 38-106 mg/dL
  6 months-4 years:
    Male: 67-167 mg/dL
    Female: 60-148 mg/dL
  5-17 years: 83-151 mg/dL

Apo B

Adult/elderly:
  Male: 50-125 mg/dL
  Female: 45-120 mg/dL
Child:
  Newborn: 11-31 mg/dL
  6 months-3 years: 23-75 mg/dL
  5-17 years:
    Male: 47-139 mg/dL
    Female: 41-132 mg/dL

Apo A-I/Apo B ratio

Male: 0.85-2.24
Female: 0.76-3.23

Lipoprotein (a)

Caucasian (5th-95th percentiles):
  Male: 2.2-49.4 mg/dL
  Female: 2.1-57.3 mg/dL
African American (5th-95th percentiles):
  Male: 4.6-71.8 mg/dL
  Female: 4.4-75 mg/dL

Test explanation and related physiology

This test is used to evaluate the risk of atherogenic heart and peripheral vascular diseases. These proteins are indicators of atherogenic risks much like high-density lipoprotein (HDL), low-density lipoprotein (LDL), and very-low-density lipoprotein (VLDL). Apolipoproteins are the protein part of lipoproteins (e.g., HDL, LDL). In general, apolipoproteins play an important role in lipid transport in the lymphatic and circulatory systems. They act as enzyme cofactors in lipoprotein synthesis. Apolipoproteins also act as receptor ligands to improve transport of fat particles in the cell. Apolipoprotein synthesis in the liver is controlled by many factors, including dietary composition, hormones (e.g., insulin, glucagon, thyroxin, estrogens, androgens), alcohol intake, and various drugs (e.g., statins, niacin, fibric acids).

There are several types of apolipoproteins, including apo A-I, apo B, and apo E. *Apolipoprotein A (apo A)* is the major polypeptide component of HDL. Low levels of apo A are associated with increased risk of coronary or peripheral artery disease (CPAD). Elevated levels may protect against CPAD.

Apo B is the major polypeptide component of LDL and chylomicrons. Apo B makes cholesterol soluble for deposition in the arterial wall. Forty percent of the protein portion of VLDL is composed of apo B. Familial hypercholesterolemia type B is caused by mutations in the apo B gene.

Lp(a) (referred to as *lipoprotein little a*) is a heterogeneous group of lipoproteins consisting of an apo A molecule attached to an apo B molecule. An increased level of Lp(a) may be an independent risk factor for atherosclerosis and is particularly harmful to the endothelium. Serum concentrations of Lp(a) appear to be largely related to genetic factors; diet and statin drugs do not have a major impact on Lp(a) levels. Niacin does lower Lp(a) levels, however. Measurement of serum Lp(a) may contribute to a more comprehensive risk assessment in high-risk patients.

Apolipoprotein E (apo E) is involved in cholesterol transport. Through genotyping, three alleles for apo E have been identified: E2, E3, and E4. Each person gets an allele from each parent. E3/3 is the normal. E2/2 is found rarely and is associated with type III hyperlipidemia. E4/4 or E4/3 is associated with high LDL levels. The apo E4 gene has been proposed as a risk factor for Alzheimer disease. Apo E2 and E4 are associated with increased triglycerides.

Lp-PLA2 is a lipase enzyme located on the surface of circulating LDL. This protein is atherogenic.

Interfering factors

Apo A-I

- Physical exercise may increase apo A-I levels.
- Smoking may decrease levels.
- Diets high in carbohydrates or polyunsaturated fats may decrease apo A-I levels.
- Drugs that may *increase* apo A-I levels include carbamazepine, estrogens, ethanol, lovastatin, niacin, oral contraceptives, phenobarbital, pravastatin, and simvastatin.
- Drugs that may *decrease* apo A-I levels include androgens, beta-blockers, diuretics, and progestins.

Apo B

- Diets high in saturated fats and cholesterol may increase apo B levels.
- Drugs that may *increase* apo B levels include androgens, beta-blockers, diuretics, ethanol abuse, and progestins.
- Drugs that may *decrease* apo B levels include cholestyramine, estrogen (postmenopausal women), lovastatin, neomycin, niacin, simvastatin, and thyroxine.

Lipoprotein (a)

- Drugs that may *decrease* Lp(a) include estrogens, neomycin, niacin, and stanozolol.

Procedure and patient care

- See inside front cover for Routine Blood Testing.
- Fasting: yes (12-14 hours).
- Blood tube commonly used: red.
- PT Inform the patient that smoking is prohibited before the test.

Abnormal findings

▲ **Increased apo A-I**
Familial
hyperalphalipoproteinemia
Pregnancy
Weight reduction

▼ **Decreased apo A-I**
Coronary artery disease
Ischemic coronary disease
Myocardial infarction
Familial
hypoalphalipoproteinemia
Fish eye disease
Uncontrolled diabetes
mellitus
Tangier disease
Nephrotic syndrome
Chronic renal failure
Cholestasis
Hemodialysis

▲ **Increased apo B**
Hyperlipoproteinemia (types
IIa, IIb, IV, V)
Nephrotic syndrome
Pregnancy
Hemodialysis
Biliary obstruction
Coronary artery disease
Diabetes mellitus
Hypothyroidism
Anorexia nervosa
Renal failure

▼ **Decreased apo B**
Tangier disease
Hyperthyroidism
Malnutrition
Inflammatory joint disease
Chronic pulmonary disease
Weight reduction
Chronic anemia
Reye syndrome

▲ **Increased Lp(a)**
Premature coronary artery
disease
Stenosis of cerebral arteries
Uncontrolled diabetes mellitus
Severe hypothyroidism
Familial hypercholesterolemia
Chronic renal failure
Estrogen depletion
Apo E-4 gene
Alzheimer disease

▼ **Decreased Lp(a)**
Alcoholism
Malnutrition
Chronic hepatocellular
disease

notes

Apt test (Downey test, Qualitative fetal hemoglobin stool test, Stool for swallowed blood)

Type of test Stool

Normal findings

No fetal blood present.
Maternal blood may be present.

Test explanation and related physiology

Blood in the stool of a newborn must be rapidly evaluated. Furthermore, some serious diseases present as rectal bleeding in the newborn. Much more commonly, however, newborns may simply be defecating maternal blood that was swallowed during birth or breastfeeding.

The Apt test is performed on the stool specimen to differentiate maternal from fetal blood in the stool. Fetal hemoglobin is resistant to denaturation; adult hemoglobin (hemoglobin A) is not. This test can be performed on stool, a stool-stained diaper, amniotic fluid, or vomitus.

Procedure and patient care

Before

PT Explain the procedure to the newborn's parents.
- Assess the vital signs of the newborn with possible intestinal bleeding.

During

- Obtain an adequate stool or vomitus specimen.
- In the laboratory, 1% NaOH is added to the specimen. Vomitus (and sometimes stool) is diluted and centrifuged first. Maternal blood turns brown; newborn blood stays red or pink.

After

- If maternal blood is present, reassure the parents and examine the mother for nipple erosion and/or cracking.
- If newborn blood is present, begin close observation and support during further diagnostic procedures.

Abnormal findings

Active gastrointestinal bleeding
Necrotizing enterocolitis

notes

arterial blood gases (ABGs, blood gases)

A

Type of test Blood

Normal findings

pH

Adult/child: 7.35-7.45
Newborn: 7.32-7.49
2 months-2 years: 7.34-7.46
pH (venous): 7.31-7.41

Pco_2

Adult/child: 35-45 mm Hg
Child <2 years: 26-41 mm Hg
Pco_2 (venous): 40-50 mm Hg

HCO_3

Adult/child: 21-28 mEq/L
Newborn/infant: 16-24 mEq/L

Po_2

Adult/child: 80-100 mm Hg
Newborn: 60-70 mm Hg
Po_2 (venous): 40-50 mm Hg

O_2 saturation

Adult/child: 95%-100%
Elderly: 95%
Newborn: 40%-90%

O_2 content

Arterial: 15-22 vol %
Venous: 11-16 vol %

Base excess: 0±2 mEq/L

Alveolar to arterial O_2 difference: <10 mm Hg

Possible critical values

pH: <7.25, >7.55
Pco_2: <20, >60
HCO_3: <15, >40
Po_2: <40
O_2 saturation: 75% or lower
Base excess: ±3 mEq/L

Test explanation and related physiology

Measurement of ABGs provides valuable information in assessing and managing a patient's respiratory (ventilation) and metabolic (renal) acid/base and electrolyte homeostasis. It is also used to assess adequacy of oxygenation. ABGs are used to monitor patients on ventilators, to monitor critically ill nonventilator patients, to establish preoperative baseline parameters, and to enlighten electrolyte therapy.

pH

The pH is inversely proportional to the actual hydrogen ion concentration. Therefore, as the hydrogen ion concentration decreases, the pH increases, and vice versa. The pH is a measure of alkalinity (pH >7.4) and acidity (pH <7.35). In respiratory or metabolic alkalosis, the pH is elevated; in respiratory or metabolic acidosis, the pH is decreased (Table 2).

Pco_2

The Pco_2 is a measure of the partial pressure of CO_2 in the blood. Pco_2 is a measurement of ventilation capability. The faster and more deeply one breathes, the more CO_2 is blown off and Pco_2 levels drop. Therefore, Pco_2 is referred to as the *respiratory* component in acid-base determination because this value is controlled primarily by the lungs. As the CO_2 level increases, the pH decreases. The CO_2 level and the pH are inversely proportional. The Pco_2 in the blood and cerebrospinal fluid is a major stimulant to the breathing center in the brain. As Pco_2 levels rise, breathing is stimulated. If Pco_2 levels rise too high, breathing cannot keep up with the demand to blow off or ventilate. As Pco_2 levels rise further, the brain is depressed and ventilation decreases further, causing coma.

The Pco_2 level is elevated in primary respiratory acidosis and is decreased in primary respiratory alkalosis (Table 2). Because the lungs compensate for primary metabolic acid/base derangements, Pco_2 levels are affected by metabolic disturbances as well. In metabolic acidosis, the lungs attempt to compensate by blowing off CO_2 to raise pH. In metabolic alkalosis, the lungs attempt to compensate by retaining CO_2 to lower pH (Table 3).

Bicarbonate (HCO_3) or CO_2 content

Most of the CO_2 content in the blood is HCO_3. The bicarbonate ion is a measure of the *metabolic (renal/kidney)* component of the acid-base equilibrium. It is regulated by the kidneys. This ion can be measured directly by the bicarbonate value or indirectly by the CO_2 content (see p. 208). As the HCO_3 level

TABLE 2   Normal values for arterial blood gases and abnormal values in uncompensated acid-base disturbances

Acid-base disturbances	pH	Pco₂ (mm Hg)	HCO₃ (mEq/L)	Common causes
None (normal values)	7.35-7.45	35-45	22-26	
Respiratory acidosis	↓	↑	Normal	Respiratory depression (drugs, central nervous system trauma) Pulmonary disease (pneumonia, chronic obstructive pulmonary disease, respiratory underventilation)
Respiratory alkalosis	↑	↓	Normal	Hyperventilation (emotions, pain, respirator overventilation)
Metabolic acidosis	↓	Normal	↓	Diabetes, shock, renal failure, intestinal fistula
Metabolic alkalosis	↑	Normal	↑	Sodium bicarbonate overdose, prolonged vomiting, nasogastric drainage

TABLE 3   Acid-base disturbances and compensatory mechanisms

Acid-base disturbance	Mode of compensation
Respiratory acidosis	Kidneys will retain increased amounts of HCO_3 to increase pH.
Respiratory alkalosis	Kidneys will excrete increased amounts of HCO_3 to lower pH.
Metabolic acidosis	Lungs blow off CO_2 to raise pH.
Metabolic alkalosis	Lungs retain CO_2 to lower pH.

increases, the pH also increases; therefore, the relationship of bicarbonate to pH is directly proportional. HCO_3 is elevated in metabolic alkalosis and decreased in metabolic acidosis (Table 3). The kidneys also are used to compensate for primary respiratory acid-base derangements. For example, in respiratory acidosis, the kidneys attempt to compensate by resorbing increased amounts of HCO_3. In respiratory alkalosis, the kidneys excrete HCO_3 in increased amounts to lower pH. (See Table 3.)

Po_2

This is an indirect measure of the oxygen content of arterial blood. Po_2 is a measure of the tension (pressure) of oxygen dissolved in the plasma. This pressure determines the force of O_2 to diffuse across the pulmonary alveoli membrane. The Po_2 level is decreased in patients who:

- Are unable to oxygenate the arterial blood because of O_2 diffusion difficulties (e.g., pneumonia)
- Have premature mixing of venous blood with arterial blood (e.g., in congenital heart disease)
- Have underventilated and overperfused pulmonary alveoli (pickwickian syndrome or patients with significant atelectasis)

O_2 saturation

Oxygen saturation is an indication of the percentage of hemoglobin saturated with O_2. When 92% to 100% of the hemoglobin carries O_2, the tissues are adequately provided with O_2, assuming normal O_2 dissociation. As the Po_2 level decreases, the percentage of hemoglobin saturation also decreases. When the Po_2 level drops below 60 mm Hg, small decreases in the Po_2 level cause large decreases in the percentage of hemoglobin saturated with O_2. At O_2 saturation levels of 70% or lower, the tissues are unable to extract enough O_2 to carry out their vital functions.

O_2 saturation is calculated by the blood gas machine using the following formula:

$$\text{Percentage of } O_2 \text{ saturation} = 100 \times \frac{\text{Volume of } O_2 \text{ content Hgb}}{\text{Volume of } O_2 \text{ Hgb capacity}}$$

Pulse oximetry is a noninvasive method of determining O_2 saturation (p. 673).

O_2 content

This is a calculated number that represents the amount of O_2 in the blood. The formula for calculation is

$$O_2 \text{ content} = O_2 \text{ saturation} \times \text{Hgb} \times 1.34 + Po_2 \times 0.003$$

Nearly all O_2 in the blood is bound to hemoglobin. O_2 content decreases with the same diseases that diminish Po_2.

Base excess/deficit

This number is calculated by the blood gas machine by using the pH, Pco_2, and hematocrit. It represents the amount of buffering anions in the blood. HCO_3 is the largest of these. Others include hemoglobin, proteins, and phosphates. Base excess is a way to take all these anions into account when determining acid/base treatment based on the *metabolic* component. Negative base excess (deficit) indicates a metabolic acidosis (e.g., lactic acidosis). A positive base excess indicates metabolic alkalosis or compensation to prolonged respiratory acidosis.

Alveolar (A) to arterial (a) O_2 difference (A-a gradient)

This is a calculated number that indicates the difference between alveolar (A) O_2 and arterial (a) O_2. The normal value is less than 10 mm Hg (torr). If the A-a gradient is abnormally high, there is either a problem in diffusing O_2 across the alveolar membrane (thickened edematous alveoli) or unoxygenated blood is mixing with the oxygenated blood.

Contraindications

- Patients with a negative Allen test
- Patients with arteriovenous fistula proximal to the site of proposed access
- Patients with severe coagulopathy

Potential complications

- Occlusion of the artery used for access
- Penetration of other important structures anatomically juxtaposed to the artery (e.g., nerve)

Interfering factors

- O_2 saturation can be falsely increased with the inhalation of carbon monoxide.
- ☛ Respiration can be inhibited by sedatives or narcotics.

Procedure and patient care

Before

PT Explain the procedure to the patient.

PT Tell the patient that an arterial puncture is associated with more discomfort than a venous puncture.

- Notify the laboratory before drawing ABGs so that the necessary equipment can be calibrated before the blood sample arrives.
- Perform the *Allen test* to assess collateral circulation.
- To perform the Allen test, make the patient's hand blanch by obliterating both the radial and the ulnar pulses, and then release the pressure over the ulnar artery only. If flow through the ulnar artery is good, flushing will be seen immediately. The Allen test is then positive, and the radial artery can be used for puncture.
- If the Allen test is negative (no flushing), repeat it on the other arm.
- If both arms give a negative result, choose another artery for puncture.

During

- Note that arterial blood can be obtained from any area of the body where strong pulses are palpable, usually from the radial, brachial, or femoral artery.
- Cleanse the arterial site.
- Use a small gauge needle to collect the arterial blood in an air-free heparinized syringe.
- After drawing blood, remove the needle and apply pressure to the arterial site for 3 to 5 minutes.
- Expel any air bubbles in the syringe.
- Cap the syringe and gently rotate to mix the blood and heparin.
- Note that an arterial puncture is performed by laboratory technicians, respiratory-inhalation therapists, nurses, or physicians in approximately 10 minutes.

After

- Place the arterial blood on ice and immediately take it to the chemistry laboratory for analysis.

- Apply pressure or a pressure dressing to the arterial puncture site for 3 to 5 minutes to avoid hematoma formation.
- Assess the puncture site for bleeding. Remember that an artery rather than a vein has been stuck.

Abnormal findings

▲ **Increased pH (alkalosis)**
Metabolic alkalosis
Hypokalemia
Hypochloremia
Chronic and high-volume gastric suction
Chronic vomiting
Aldosteronism
Mercurial diuretics
Respiratory alkalosis
Chronic heart failure
Cystic fibrosis
Carbon monoxide poisoning
Pulmonary emboli
Shock
Acute and severe pulmonary diseases
Anxiety neuroses
Pain
Pregnancy

▼ **Decreased pH (acidosis)**
Metabolic acidosis
Ketoacidosis
Lactic acidosis
Severe diarrhea
Renal failure

Respiratory acidosis
Respiratory failure

▲ **Increased P_{CO_2}**
Chronic obstructive pulmonary disease (COPD) (bronchitis, emphysema)
Oversedation
Head trauma
Overoxygenation in a patient with COPD
Pickwickian syndrome

▼ **Decreased P_{CO_2}**
Hypoxemia
Pulmonary emboli
Anxiety
Pain
Pregnancy

▲ **Increased HCO_3**
Chronic vomiting
Chronic and high-volume
  gastric suction
Aldosteronism
Use of mercurial diuretics
Chronic obstructive
  pulmonary disease

▲ **Increased Po_2, increased O_2 content**
Polycythemia
Increased inspired O_2
Hyperventilation

▼ **Decreased HCO_3**
Chronic and severe
  diarrhea
Chronic use of loop
  diuretics
Starvation
Diabetic ketoacidosis
Acute renal failure

▼ **Decreased Po_2, decreased O_2 content**
Anemias
Mucus plug
Bronchospasm
Atelectasis
Pneumothorax
Pulmonary edema
Adult respiratory
  distress syndrome
Restrictive lung disease
Atrial or ventricular
  cardiac septal defects
Emboli
Inadequate O_2
  in inspired air
  (suffocation)
Severe hypoventilation
  (e.g., oversedation,
  neurologic somnolence)

notes

arteriography (Angiography)

Type of test   X-ray with contrast dye

Normal findings   Normal arterial vasculature

Test explanation and related physiology

With the injection of radiopaque contrast material into arteries, blood vessels can be visualized to determine arterial anatomy or vascular disease. With a catheter usually placed through the femoral artery and into the desired artery, radiopaque contrast is rapidly injected while x-ray images are obtained. Blood flow dynamics, arterial occlusive disease, or vascular anomalies are easily seen. With the use of *digital subtraction angiography (DSA)*, bony structures can be obliterated from the picture. Coronary arteriography is described under cardiac catheterization (see p. 214).

Renal angiography permits evaluation of renal artery blood flow dynamics. Arteriosclerotic narrowing (stenosis) of the renal artery is best demonstrated with this study. The angiographic location of the stenotic area is helpful if considering surgical repair of stenting.

Lower extremity arteriography allows for accurate identification and location of occlusions within the abdominal aorta and lower extremity arteries. Total or near-total occlusion of the flow of dye is seen in arteriosclerotic vascular occlusive disease. Emboli are seen as total occlusions of the artery. Arterial traumas, such as lacerations or intimal tears (laceration of the inner arterial lining), likewise appear as total or near-total obstruction of the flow of dye. Unusual arterial disorders, such as Buerger disease and fibromuscular dysplasia, have the classic arterial *beading*, which is pathognomonic.

Arterial vascular balloon dilation and stenting can be performed if a short-segment arterial stenosis is identified. In these instances, the wire is placed through the angiocatheter into the area of narrowing. A balloon catheter is inserted over the wire. The dilating balloon is inflated, and the arteriosclerotic plaque is gently and persistently dilated, and can then be stented.

With angiography, there is always a concern that the arterial puncture site may not seal, leading to a pseudoaneurysm. More recently, vascular closure products have been used to quickly seal femoral artery punctures following catheterization procedures. This allows for early ambulation and hospital discharge. The injection of these materials on the vascular entrance site creates a mechanical seal by sandwiching the arteriotomy between a bio-absorbable anchor and a collagen sponge, which dissolve within 60 to 90 days.

Contraindications

The following represent relative contraindications. If the information/therapy is necessary to obtain through arteriography, appropriate steps can be taken to reduce risks in these patients. As in all diagnostic testing, the risks must be weighed against the benefits.

- Patients with allergies to shellfish or iodinated dye
- Patients who are uncooperative or agitated
- Patients who are pregnant, unless the benefits outweigh the risks
- Patients with renal disorders, because iodinated contrast is nephrotoxic
- Patients with a bleeding propensity
- Patients with unstable cardiac disorders
- Patients who are dehydrated, because they are especially susceptible to dye-induced renal failure

Potential complications

- Allergic reaction to iodinated dye
- Hemorrhage from the arterial puncture site
- Arterial embolism from dislodgment of an arteriosclerotic plaque
- Soft tissue infection around the puncture site
- Renal failure, especially in elderly patients who are chronically dehydrated or have a mild degree of renal failure
- Dissection of the intimal lining of the artery causing complete or partial arterial occlusion
- Pseudoaneurysm development as a result of failure of the puncture site to seal
- Lactic acidosis may occur in patients who are taking metformin. The metformin should not be taken the day of the test to prevent this complication.

Procedure and patient care

Before

PT Explain the procedure to the patient. Allay any fears and allow the patient to verbalize concerns.

- Obtain written and informed consent for this procedure.

PT Inform the patient that a warm flush may be felt when the dye is injected.

- Assess the possibility of allergies to iodinated dye.

- Determine if the patient has been taking anticoagulants.
- Keep the patient NPO for 2 to 8 hours before testing.
- Mark the site of the patient's peripheral pulses with a pen before arterial catheterization. This will permit assessment of the peripheral pulses after the procedure.
- If the patient does not have peripheral pulses before arteriography, document that fact so that arterial occlusion will not be suspected on the postangiogram assessment.
- Ensure that the appropriate renal function studies are normal.
- If the patient has diminished renal function, provide IV hydration to minimize further renal damage.
- **PT** Instruct the patient to void before the study because the iodinated dye can act as an osmotic diuretic.
- **PT** Inform the patient that bladder distention may cause some discomfort during the study.

During
- Note the following preprocedure steps:
  1. The patient may be sedated before being taken to the angiography room, which is usually within the radiology department.
  2. The patient is placed on the x-ray table in the supine position.
  3. If the femoral artery is to be used, the groin is shaved, prepared as per protocol, and draped in a sterile manner.
  4. The femoral artery is cannulated, and a wire is threaded up that artery and into or near the opening of the desired artery to be examined.
  5. A catheter is then placed over the wire. The wire and catheter are placed under fluoroscopic visualization. Because the catheter and wire have curled tips at their ends, they can be manipulated directly into the artery to be studied. The wire is removed.
  6. Through the catheter, iodinated contrast material is injected by the use of an automated injector at a preset, controlled rate. This occurs over several seconds.
  7. Cinefluoroscopy is used to visualize the injection in real time.
- Note that this procedure is usually performed by an angiographer (radiologist) in approximately 1 hour.
- **PT** During the dye injection, remind the patient that an intense, burning flush may be felt throughout the body but lasts only a few seconds.
- **PT** Tell the patient that the most significant discomfort is the groin puncture that was necessary for arterial access.

PT Remind the patient of the discomfort of lying on a hard x-ray table for a long period.

After

- After x-ray studies are completed, remove the catheter and apply a pressure dressing to the puncture site.
- Monitor the patient's vital signs for indications of hemorrhage.
- Assess the peripheral arterial pulse in the extremity used for vascular access and compare it with the preprocedure baseline.
- Observe the arterial puncture site frequently for signs of bleeding or hematoma.
- Maintain pressure at the puncture site with a 1- to 2-lb sandbag or an IV bag.
- Keep the patient on bed rest for up to 8 hours after the procedure to allow for complete sealing of the arterial puncture site. If a vascular closure product is used, the patient may ambulate within 2 hours.
- Note and compare the color and temperature of the extremity with that of the uninvolved extremity.
- Notify the physician if the patient has severe, continuous pain.

PT Instruct the patient to drink fluids to prevent dehydration caused by the diuretic action of the dye.

- Evaluate the patient for delayed allergic reaction to the dye.

PT Instruct the patient to report any signs of numbness, tingling, pain, or loss of function in the involved extremity.

Abnormal findings

Arteriography of the peripheral vascular system

Arteriosclerotic occlusion

Embolus occlusion

Primary arterial diseases (e.g., fibromuscular dysplasia, Buerger disease)

Aneurysm

Kidney arteriography

Atherosclerotic narrowing of the renal artery

Fibrodysplasia of the renal artery

Renal vascular causes of hypertension

notes

arthrocentesis with synovial fluid analysis

Type of test Fluid analysis

Normal findings

Appearance	Clear, straw colored, no blood
RBC	None
WBC	0-150/mm^3
WBC differential	
Neutrophils	7%
Lymphocytes	24%
Monocytes	48%
Macrophages	10%
Glucose	Equal to fasting blood glucose
Protein	1-3 dL
LDH	<25 mg/dL
Uric acid	6-8 mg/dL
Gram stain	Negative

Test explanation and related physiology

Arthrocentesis is performed to establish the diagnosis of joint infection, arthritis, crystal-induced arthritis (gout and pseudo-gout), synovitis, or neoplasms involving the joint. This procedure is also used to identify the cause of joint inflammation or effusion and to inject antiinflammatory medications (usually corticosteroids) into a joint space.

Arthrocentesis is performed by inserting a sterile needle into the joint space of the involved joint to obtain synovial fluid for analysis. Synovial fluid is a liquid found in small amounts within the joints. Aspiration (withdrawal of the fluid) may be performed on any major joint, such as the knee, shoulder, hip, elbow, wrist, or ankle.

The fluid sample is examined microscopically and chemically. A Gram stain and culture of the fluid is usually performed. Normal joint fluid is clear, straw colored, and quite viscous because of the hyaluronic acid, which acts as a lubricant. Viscosity is reduced in patients with inflammatory arthritis. Viscosity can be roughly estimated by forcing some synovial fluid from a syringe. Fluid of normal viscosity forms a "string" more than 5 cm long; fluid of low viscosity as seen in inflammation drips in a manner similar to water.

The *mucin clot test* correlates with the viscosity and is an estimation of hyaluronic acid-protein complex integrity. This test is performed by adding acetic acid to joint fluid. The formation of a tight, ropy clot indicates qualitatively good mucin and the presence of adequate molecules of intact hyaluronic acid. Hyaluronic acid can be directly quantified by enzyme-linked immunoabsorbent assay. The mucin clot is poor in quality and quantity in the presence of an inflammatory joint disease, such as rheumatoid arthritis (RA). By itself, synovial fluid should not spontaneously form a fibrin clot (clot without the addition of acetic acid) because normal joint fluid does not contain fibrinogen. If, however, bleeding into the joint (from trauma or injury) has occurred, the synovial fluid will clot.

The synovial fluid glucose value is usually within 10 mL/dL of the fasting serum glucose value. For proper interpretation, the synovial fluid glucose and serum glucose samples should be drawn simultaneously after the patient has fasted for 6 hours. The synovial fluid glucose level falls with increasing severity of inflammation. Although lowest in septic arthritis (the synovial fluid glucose value may be <50% of the serum glucose value), a low synovial glucose level also may be seen in patients with rheumatoid arthritis. The synovial fluid is also tested for protein, uric acid, and lactate levels. Increased uric acid levels indicate gout. Increased protein and lactate levels indicate bacterial infection or inflammation.

Cell counts are also performed on the synovial fluid. Normally the joint fluid contains less than 150 WBCs/mm^3 and 2000 RBCs/mL. An increased WBC count with a high percentage of neutrophils (over 75%) supports the diagnosis of acute bacterial infectious arthritis. Leukocytes can also occur in other conditions, such as acute gouty arthritis and rheumatoid arthritis. The differential WBC count, however, will indicate monocytosis or lymphocytosis with these later-mentioned diseases.

Bacterial and fungal cultures are usually requested and performed when infection is suspected. The administration of antibiotics before arthrocentesis may diminish growth of bacteria from synovial fluid cultures and confound results. Smears for acid-fast stains for tubercle bacilli are also performed on the synovial fluid. Synovial fluid is also examined under polarized light for the presence of crystals, which permits differential diagnosis between gout and pseudogout. (The calcium pyrophosphate dihydrate crystals of pseudogout are birefringent [blue on red background] when examined with a polarized light microscope.)

The synovial fluid is also analyzed for complement levels (page 277). Complement levels are decreased in patients with systemic lupus erythematosus, rheumatoid arthritis, or other immunologic arthritis. These decreased joint complement levels are caused by consumption of the complement induced by the antigen–antibody immune complexes within the joint cavity.

One of the most important tests routinely performed on synovial fluid is the microscopic examination for crystals. For example, urate crystals indicate gouty arthritis. Calcium pyrophosphate crystals are found in pseudogout. Cholesterol crystals occur in rheumatoid arthritis.

Contraindications

- Patients with skin or wound infections in the area of the needle puncture because of the risk of sepsis

Potential complications

- Joint infection
- Hemorrhage in the joint area

Procedure and patient care

Before

PT Explain the procedure to the patient.
- Obtain an informed consent if indicated.
- The physician may request that the patient be kept NPO after midnight on the day of the test.

During

- Have the patient lie on his or her back with the joint fully extended.
- Note the following procedural steps:
  1. The skin is locally anesthetized to minimize pain.
  2. The area is aseptically cleansed, and a needle is inserted through the skin and into the joint space.
  3. Fluid is obtained for analysis. The joint area sometimes may be wrapped with an elastic bandage to compress free fluid within a certain area, thereby ensuring maximal collection of fluid.
  4. If a corticosteroid or other medications (e.g., antibiotics) are to be administered, a syringe containing the steroid preparation is attached to the needle, and the drug is injected.
  5. The needle is removed, and a pressure dressing may be applied to the site.

6. Sometimes a peripheral venous blood sample is taken to compare chemical tests on the blood with chemical studies on the synovial fluid.

- Note that a physician performs this procedure in an office or at the patient's bedside in approximately 10 minutes.

PT Tell the patient that the only discomfort associated with this test is the injection of the local anesthetic.

- Be aware that joint-space pain may worsen after fluid aspiration, especially in patients with acute arthritis.

After

PT Assess the joint for any pain, fever, or swelling. Teach the patient to look for signs of infection at home.

PT Apply ice to decrease pain and swelling, and instruct the patient to continue this at home.

- Keep a pressure dressing on the joint to avoid re-collection of joint fluid or development of a hematoma.

PT Tell the patient to avoid strenuous use of the joint for the next several days.

PT Teach the patient to walk on crutches if indicated.

PT Instruct the patient to look for signs of bleeding into the joint (significant swelling, increasing pain, or joint weakness).

PT Educate the patient to look for signs of phlebitis. The involved leg may become swollen, painful, and edematous.

PT Instruct the patient not to drive until it is approved by the physician.

Abnormal findings

Infection
Osteoarthritis
Synovitis
Neoplasm
Joint effusion
Septic arthritis
Systemic lupus erythematosus
Rheumatoid arthritis
Gout
Pseudogout

notes

arthroscopy

Type of test Endoscopy

Normal findings Normal ligaments, menisci, and articular surfaces of the joint

Test explanation and related physiology

Arthroscopy is an endoscopic procedure that allows examination of a joint interior with a specially designed endoscope. Arthroscopy is a highly accurate test because it allows direct visualization of an anatomic site (Figure 4). Although this technique can visualize many joints of the body, it is most often used to evaluate the knee for meniscus cartilage or ligament injury. It is also used in the differential diagnosis of acute and chronic disorders of the knee (e.g., arthritic inflammation vs. injury).

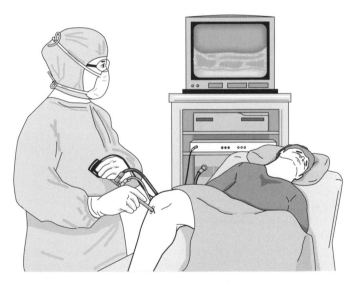

FIGURE 4 Arthroscopy. The arthroscope is placed in the joint space of the knee. Video arthroscopy requires a water source to distend the joint space, a light source to see the contents of the joint, and a television monitor to project the image. Other trocars are used for access of the joint space for other operative instruments.

Physicians can perform corrective surgery on the knee through the endoscope. Meniscus removal, spur removal, ligamentous repair, and biopsy are but a few of the procedures that are done through the arthroscope. Arthroscopy provides a safe, convenient alternative to open surgery (arthrotomy) because surgery is done through small trocars that are placed into the joint. Surgical maneuvers are carried out under direct vision of the camera, which is attached to the arthroscope. Because a large incision is avoided, recovery is faster and more comfortable.

Arthroscopy is also used to monitor the progression of disease and the effectiveness of therapy. Visual findings may be recorded by attaching a video camera to the arthroscope. Joints that can be evaluated by the arthroscope include the tarsal, ankle, knee, hip, carpal, wrist, shoulder, and temporomandibular joints. Synovial fluid can be obtained for fluid analysis through arthroscopy. See arthrocentesis, p. 121.

Contraindications

- Patients with ankylosis
- Patients with local skin or wound infections
- Patients who have recently had an arthrogram

Potential complications

- Infection
- Hemarthrosis
- Swelling
- Thrombophlebitis
- Joint injury
- Synovial rupture

Procedure and patient care

Before

PT Explain the procedure to the patient.
- Ensure that the physician has obtained written consent for this procedure.
- Follow the routine preoperative procedure of the institution.
- Keep the patient NPO after midnight on the day of the test.
PT Instruct the patient who will use crutches after the procedure regarding the appropriate crutch gait. The patient should use crutches after arthroscopy until able to walk without limping.
- Shave the hair in the area 6 inches above and below the joint before the test (as ordered).

During

- Place the patient on his or her back on an operating room table.
- Note the following procedural steps:
    1. Local or general anesthesia is used.
    2. The leg is carefully scrubbed, elevated, and wrapped with an elastic bandage from the toes to the lower thigh to drain as much blood from the leg as possible.
    3. A tourniquet is placed on the patient's leg. If the tourniquet is not used, a fluid solution may be instilled into the patient's knee immediately before insertion of the arthroscope to distend the knee and help reduce bleeding.
    4. The foot of the table is lowered so that the patient's knee is at a 45-degree angle.
    5. A small incision is made in the skin around the knee.
    6. The arthroscope (a lighted instrument) is inserted into the joint space to visualize the inside of the knee joint. In the past, the surgeon looked directly into the scope. More recently, a video camera has been attached to the scope in order for the image to be projected onto a TV monitor.
    7. Although the entire joint can be viewed from one puncture site, additional punctures for better visualization are often necessary.
    8. After the area is examined, biopsy or appropriate surgery can be performed.
    9. Before removal of the arthroscope, the joint is irrigated. Pressure is then applied to the knee to remove the irrigating solution.
    10. After a few stitches are placed into the skin, a pressure dressing is applied over the incision site.
- Note that this procedure is performed in the operating room by an orthopedic surgeon in approximately 15 to 30 minutes.
- **PT** Tell the patient receiving local anesthesia that there may be transient discomfort from the injection of the local anesthetic and from the pressure of the tourniquet on the leg.
- **PT** Inform the patient that a thumping sensation may be felt as the arthroscope is inserted into the joint and that the joint may be painful for several days.

After

- Assess the patient's neurologic and circulatory status.
- Assess vital signs and observe the patient for signs of infection, including fever, swelling, increased pain, and redness or drainage at the incision site.

PT Instruct the patient to elevate the knee when sitting and to avoid overbending the knee, so that swelling is minimized.

PT Inform the patient that he or she can usually walk with the assistance of crutches; however, this depends on the extent of the procedure and the physician's protocol.

PT Tell the patient to minimize use of the joint for several days.

• Examine the incision site for bleeding.

PT Educate the patient to look for signs of bleeding into the joint (significant swelling, increasing pain, or joint weakness).

• Apply ice to reduce pain and swelling, and instruct the patient to continue this at home.

PT Educate the patient to look for signs of phlebitis. This is not uncommon in a person immobilized by joint pain. The involved leg may become swollen, painful, and edematous.

PT Instruct the patient not to drive until it is approved by the physician.

PT Inform the patient that the sutures will be removed in approximately 7 to 10 days.

Abnormal findings

Torn cartilage
Torn ligament
Patellar disease
Patellar fracture
Chondromalacia
Osteochondritis dissecans
Cyst (e.g., Baker)
Synovitis
Rheumatoid arthritis
Degenerative arthritis
Meniscal disease
Osteochondromatosis
Trapped synovium

notes

aspartate aminotransferase (AST; Formerly called serum glutamic-oxaloacetic transaminase [SGOT])

Type of test   Blood

Normal findings

Adult: 0-35 units/L or 0-0.58 µKat/L (SI units); females tend to have slightly lower values than males
Elderly: values slightly higher than adult values
Children:
    0-5 days: 35-140 units/L
    <3 years: 15-60 units/L
    3-6 years: 15-50 units/L
    6-12 years: 10-50 units/L
    12-18 years: 10-40 units/L

Test explanation and related physiology

This test is used in the evaluation of suspected hepatocellular diseases. When disease or injury affects the cells of these tissues, the cells lyse. The AST is released and picked up by the blood, and the serum level rises. The amount of AST elevation is directly related to the number of cells affected by the disease or injury. Furthermore, the elevation depends on the time after the injury that the blood is drawn. AST is cleared from the blood in a few days. Serum AST levels become elevated 8 hours after cell injury, peak at 24 to 36 hours, and return to normal in 3 to 7 days. If the cellular injury is chronic, levels will be persistently elevated.

Because AST exists within the liver cells, diseases that affect the hepatocytes cause elevated levels of this enzyme. In acute hepatitis, AST levels can rise to 20 times the normal value. In acute extrahepatic obstruction (e.g., gallstones), AST levels quickly rise to 10 times the normal value and fall swiftly. In cirrhotic patients, the level of AST depends on the amount of active inflammation.

Serum AST levels are often compared with alanine aminotransferase (ALT, see p. 21) levels. The AST/ALT ratio is usually greater than 1.0 in patients with alcoholic cirrhosis, liver congestion, or metastatic tumor of the liver. Ratios less than 1.0 may be seen in patients with acute hepatitis, viral hepatitis, or infectious mononucleosis. The ratio is less accurate if AST levels exceed 10 times the normal value.

Patients with acute pancreatitis, acute renal diseases, musculoskeletal diseases, or trauma may have a transient rise in serum AST. Patients with red blood cell abnormalities, such as acute hemolytic anemia and severe burns, also can have elevations of this enzyme.

Interfering factors

- Exercise may cause increased levels.
- Pyridoxine deficiency (beriberi or pregnancy), severe long-standing liver disease, uremia, or diabetic ketoacidosis may cause decreased levels.
- ✄ Drugs that may cause *increased* levels include antihypertensives, cholinergic agents, coumarin-type anticoagulants, digitalis preparations, erythromycin, hepatotoxic medications, isoniazid, methyldopa, opiates, oral contraceptives, salicylates, statins, and verapamil.

Procedure and patient care

- See inside front cover for Routine Blood Testing.
- Fasting: no
- Blood tube commonly used: red
- If possible, avoid giving the patient any IM injection because increased enzyme levels may result.
- Record the time and date of any IM injection given.
- Record the exact time and date when the blood test is performed. This aids in the interpretation of the temporal pattern of enzyme elevations.

Abnormal findings

▲ **Increased levels**

Liver diseases

Hepatitis

Hepatic cirrhosis

Drug-induced liver injury

Hepatic metastasis

Hepatic necrosis (initial stages
only)

Hepatic surgery

Infectious mononucleosis with
hepatitis

Hepatic infiltrative process
(e.g., tumor)

Skeletal muscle diseases

Skeletal muscle trauma

Recent noncardiac surgery

Multiple traumas

Severe, deep burns

Progressive muscular
dystrophy

Recent convulsions

Heat stroke

Primary muscle diseases
(e.g., myopathy, myositis)

Other diseases

Acute hemolytic anemia

Acute pancreatitis

▼ **Decreased levels**

Acute renal disease

Beriberi

Diabetic ketoacidosis

Pregnancy

Chronic renal dialysis

notes

barium enema (BE, Lower GI series)

Type of test X-ray with contrast dye

Normal findings

Normal filling, contour, patency, and positioning of barium in the colon

Normal filling of the appendix and terminal ileum

Test explanation and related physiology

The BE study consists of a series of x-rays visualizing the colon. It is used to demonstrate the presence and location of polyps, tumors, and diverticula. Anatomic abnormalities (e.g., malrotation) also can be detected. Therapeutically, the BE may be used to reduce nonstrangulated ileocolic intussusception in children. Bleeding from diverticula can cease with a BE.

The BE is occasionally used to assess filling of the appendix. When the clinical picture suggests possible appendicitis, failure of the appendix to fill with barium may support the diagnosis. Although the colon is the main organ evaluated by a BE, reflux of barium into the terminal ileum also allows adequate visualization of the distal part of the small intestine. Diseases that affect the terminal ileum, especially Crohn disease (regional enteritis), can be identified. Inflammatory bowel disease involving the colon can be detected with a BE. Fistulas involving the colon can be demonstrated by a BE.

In many instances, air is insufflated into the colon after the instillation of barium. This provides an air contrast to the barium. With air contrast, the colonic mucosa can be much more accurately visualized. This is called an *air-contrast BE*. It is used especially when small polyps are suspected. The accuracy of the regular BE in detecting small colonic tumors is approximately 60%; however, the accuracy of an air-contrast BE in detecting small colonic tumors exceeds 85%.

Contraindications

- Patients suspected of a perforation of the colon
  In these patients, diatrizoate (Gastrografin), a water-soluble contrast medium, is used.
- Patients who are unable to cooperate
  This test requires the patient to hold the barium in the rectum and colon. This is especially difficult for elderly patients.
- Patients with megacolon
  Barium may worsen the disease.

Potential complications
- Colonic perforation, especially when the colon is weakened by inflammation, tumor, or infection
- Barium fecal impaction

Interfering factors
- Barium within the abdomen from previous barium tests
- Significant residual stool within the colon precludes adequate visualization of the entire bowel wall. Stool may be confused with polyps.
- Spasm of the colon can mimic the radiographic signs of a cancer.

Procedure and patient care

Before
PT Explain the procedure to the patient. Encourage the patient to verbalize questions and fears.
- Assist the patient with the bowel preparation, which varies among institutions. In elderly patients, this preparation can be exhausting and may even cause severe dehydration. A typical preparation for most adults would include the following actions:

Day before examination
- Give the patient clear liquids for lunch and supper (no dairy products).
PT Instruct the patient to drink one glass of water or clear fluid every hour for 8 to 10 hours.
- Administer a cathartic (10 ounces of magnesium citrate) or X-Prep (extract of senna fruit) at 2 PM. In children, lesser volumes may be used.
- Administer three 5-mg bisacodyl (Dulcolax) tablets at 7 PM.
- A pediatric Fleet enema the night before testing and repeated 3 hours before testing may be adequate prep for an infant.
- Keep the patient NPO after midnight the day of the test.

Day of examination
- Keep the patient NPO.
- Administer a bisacodyl suppository at 6 AM and/or a cleansing enema.
- Note that pediatric patients will have individualized bowel preparations.
- Note that special preparations will be ordered for patients with an ileostomy or colostomy.
- Determine whether the bowel is adequately cleansed. When the fecal return is similar to clear water, preparation is

adequate; if large, solid fecal waste is still being evacuated, preparation is inadequate. Notify the radiologist, who may want to extend the bowel preparation.

PT Suggest that the patient take reading material to the x-ray department to occupy the time while expelling the barium.

During

- Note the following procedural steps:
    1. The test begins with placement of a rectal balloon catheter.
    2. The balloon on the catheter is inflated tightly against the anal sphincter to hold the barium within the colon.
    3. The patient is asked to roll into the lateral, supine, and prone positions.
    4. The barium is dripped into the rectum by gravity. The colon of the young child is not able to tolerate the volume and pressure of instillation of barium that an adult's can. Both volume and pressure should be reduced.
    5. The barium flow is monitored fluoroscopically.
    6. The colon is thoroughly examined as the barium flow progresses through the large colon and into the terminal ileum.
    7. The barium is drained out.
    8. If an air-contrast BE has been ordered, air is insufflated into the large bowel.
    9. The patient is asked to expel the barium, and a postevacuation x-ray image is taken.
- The standard procedure for administering the barium through a *colostomy* is to instill the contrast medium through an irrigation cone placed in the stoma. When the x-ray series is completed, the barium is allowed to be expelled from the stoma. A gentle stream of clean water for irrigation is helpful in expelling residual barium.
- Note that this test is usually performed in the radiology department by a radiologist in approximately 45 minutes.

PT Inform the patient that abdominal bloating and rectal pressure will occur during instillation of barium.

After

- Ensure that the patient defecates as much barium as possible.
PT Suggest the use of soothing ointments on the anal area to minimize any anorectal pain that may result from the test preparation.
PT Encourage ingestion of fluids to avoid dehydration caused by the cathartics.
PT Encourage rest after the procedure. The cleansing regimen and BE procedure may be exhausting.

PT Be aware of dehydration and electrolyte abnormalities. Instruct parents to hydrate the child well with electrolyte-containing fluids after the BE.

PT Inform the patient that bowel movements will be white. When all the barium has been expelled, the stool will return to a normal color.

- Note that laxatives may be ordered to facilitate evacuation of barium.

Abnormal findings

Malignant tumor

Polyps

Diverticula

Inflammatory bowel diseases (e.g., ulcerative colitis, Crohn disease)

Colonic stenosis secondary to ischemia, infection, or previous surgery

Perforated colon

Colonic fistula

Appendicitis

Extrinsic compression of the colon from extracolonic tumors (e.g., ovarian)

Extrinsic compression of the colon from an abscess

Malrotation of the gut

Colon volvulus

Intussusception

Hernia

notes

barium swallow

Type of test X-ray with contrast dye

Normal findings Normal size, contour, filling, patency, and positioning of the esophagus

Test explanation and related physiology

This barium contrast study provides a more thorough examination of the esophagus than most upper GI series (see p. 941). As in most barium contrast studies, defects in normal filling and narrowing of the barium column indicate tumor, strictures, or extrinsic compression from extraesophageal tumors or an abnormally enlarged heart and great vessels. Varices also can be seen as serpiginous, linear-filling defects. Such anatomic abnormalities as hiatal hernia, Schatzki rings, and diverticula (Zenker or epiphrenic) can be seen as well.

In patients with esophageal reflux, the radiologist may identify reflux of the barium from the stomach back into the esophagus. Muscular abnormalities (e.g., achalasia, diffuse esophageal spasm) can be detected easily by a barium swallow. If perforations or rupture of the esophagus are suspected, it is best not to use barium; rather, water-soluble x-ray contrast should be used. If swallowing function is to be evaluated and there is a concern for the potential of aspiration during the test, barium should be used instead of Gastrografin, which can cause a chemical pneumonitis.

Contraindications

- Patients with evidence of bowel obstruction
  Barium may create a stonelike impaction.
- Patients with a perforated viscus
  If barium were to leak, the degree and duration of infection would be much worse. Usually, when perforation is suspected, diatrizoate (Gastrografin), a water-soluble contrast medium, is used.
- Patients who are unable to cooperate for the test

Potential complications

- Barium-induced fecal impaction

Interfering factors

- Food within the esophagus prevents adequate visualization.

Procedure and patient care

Before

PT Explain the procedure to the patient.

PT Instruct the patient not to take anything by mouth for at least 8 hours before testing. Usually the patient is kept NPO after midnight on the day of the test.

• Assess the patient's ability to swallow. If the patient tends to aspirate, inform the radiologist.

• Accompany the hospitalized patient to the x-ray department if vital signs are not stable and the test still needs to be performed.

During

• Note the following procedural steps:

1. The fasting patient is asked to swallow the contrast medium. Usually this is barium sulfate in a milkshake-like substance; however, if a perforated viscus is possible, Gastrografin is used.

2. As the patient drinks the contrast through a straw, the x-ray table is tilted to the near-erect position.

3. The patient is asked to roll into various positions so that the entire esophagus can be adequately visualized.

4. With fluoroscopy, the radiologist follows the barium column through the entire esophagus.

• Note that this procedure is usually performed in the radiology department by a radiologist in approximately 15 to 20 minutes.

PT Tell the patient that no discomfort is associated with this test.

After

PT Inform the patient of the need to evacuate all the barium. Cathartics are recommended. Initially stools are white but should return to a normal color with complete evacuation.

Abnormal findings

Total or partial esophageal obstruction
Cancer
Scarred strictures
Lower esophageal rings
Peptic esophageal ulcers
Varices
Peptic or corrosive esophagitis
Achalasia
Esophageal motility disorders (e.g., presbyesophagus, diffuse
  esophageal spasm)
Diverticula
Chalasia
Extrinsic compression from extraesophageal tumors,
  cardiomegaly, or aortic aneurysm

notes

Bence Jones protein (Free kappa and lambda light chains)

Type of test   Urine

Normal findings

Kappa total light chain: <0.68 mg/dL
Lambda total light chain: <0.40 mg/dL
Kappa/lambda ratio: 0.7-6.2

Test explanation and related physiology

The detection of Bence Jones protein in the urine most commonly indicates multiple myeloma (especially when the urine levels are high). The test is used to detect and monitor the treatment and clinical course of multiple myeloma and other similar diseases.

Bence Jones proteins are monoclonal light-chain portions of immunoglobulins found in 75% of patients with multiple myeloma. These proteins are made most notably by the plasma cells in these patients. They also may be associated with tumor metastases to the bone, chronic lymphocytic leukemias, lymphoma, macroglobulinemia, and amyloidosis.

Immunoglobulin light chains are usually cleared from the blood through the renal glomeruli and are reabsorbed in the proximal tubules; thus, urine light-chain concentrations are very low or undetectable. The production of large amounts of monoclonal light chains, however, can overwhelm this reabsorption mechanism. Because the Bence Jones protein is rapidly cleared from the blood by the kidneys, it may be very difficult to detect in the blood; therefore, urine is used for this study. Normally urine should contain no Bence Jones proteins.

Routine urine testing for proteins using reagent strips often does not reflect the type or amount of proteins in the urine. In fact, the strip may show a completely negative result despite large amounts of Bence Jones globulins in the urine. Proteins in the urine are best identified by *protein electrophoresis* of the urine. With this method, the proteins are separated based on size and electrical charge in an electric field when the urine specimen is applied to a gel plate. After the various proteins are separated, antisera to specific proteins can be added to the gel and specific precipitin arcs can be identified and quantified *(immunofixation)*. Monitoring the urine M-spike (a spike on electrophoresis indicating multiple myeloma) is especially useful in patients with light-chain multiple myeloma in whom the serum M-spike may be very small or absent, but in whom the urine M-spike is large.

Interfering factors

- Dilute urine may yield a false-negative result.
- ✘ High doses of aspirin or penicillin can cause false-positive results.

Procedure and patient care

- See inside front cover for Routine Urine Testing.
- **PT** Instruct the patient to collect an early morning specimen of at least 50 mL of uncontaminated urine in a container. It may be helpful to know the amount of these proteins excreted over 24 hours. If so, a 24-hour collection is ordered.
- Immediately transport the specimen to the laboratory. If it cannot be taken to the laboratory immediately, refrigerate it. Heat-coagulable proteins can decompose, causing a false-positive test.

Abnormal findings

▲ **Increased levels**
  Multiple myeloma (plasmacytoma)
  Various metastatic tumors
  Chronic lymphocytic leukemia
  Amyloidosis
  Lymphoma
  Waldenström macroglobulinemia
  Osteogenic sarcoma
  Cryoglobulinemia
  Rheumatoid diseases

notes

B

11 beta-prostaglandin F(2) alpha

Type of test Urine

Normal findings >1000 ng/24 hours

Test explanation and related physiology

Measurement of 11 beta-prostaglandin F(2) alpha in urine is useful in the evaluation of patients suspected of having systemic mastocytosis (systemic mast cell disease [SMCD]). SMCD is characterized by mast cell infiltration of extracutaneous organs (usually the bone marrow). Focal mast cell lesions in the bone marrow are found in approximately 90% of adult patients with SMCD.

Prostaglandin D(2) (PGD[2]) is generated by human mast cells, activated alveolar macrophages, and platelets. Although the most definitive test for SMCD is bone marrow biopsy (p. 166), measurement of mast cell mediators like beta prostaglandin in urine is advised for the initial evaluation of suspected cases. Elevated levels of 11 beta-prostaglandin F(2) alpha in urine are not specific for SMCD and may be found in patients with angioedema, diffuse urticaria, or myeloproliferative diseases in the absence of diffuse mast cell proliferation.

Procedure and patient care

• See inside front cover for Routine Urine Testing.

Abnormal findings

▲ **Increased levels**
   Systemic mast cell disease (SMCD)

notes

bilirubin

Type of test Blood

Normal findings

Adult/elderly/child:
  Total bilirubin: 0.3-1.0 mg/dL or 5.1-17 μmol/L (SI units)
    Indirect bilirubin: 0.2-0.8 mg/dL or 3.4-12.0 μmol/L (SI units)
    Direct bilirubin: 0.1-0.3 mg/dL or 1.7-5.1 μmol/L (SI units)
Newborn:
  Total bilirubin: 1.0-12.0 mg/dL or 17.1-205 μmol/L (SI units)

Possible critical values

Total bilirubin

Adult: >12 mg/dL
Newborn: >15 mg/dL

Test explanation and related physiology

Bile, which is formed in the liver, has many constituents, including bile salts, phospholipids, cholesterol, bicarbonate, water, and bilirubin. Bilirubin metabolism begins with the breakdown of red blood cells (RBCs) in the reticuloendothelial system (Figure 5). Hemoglobin is released from RBCs and broken down to heme and globin molecules. Heme is then catabolized to form biliverdin, which is transformed into bilirubin. This form of bilirubin is called *unconjugated (indirect) bilirubin*. In the liver, indirect bilirubin is conjugated with a glucuronide, resulting in *conjugated (direct) bilirubin*. The conjugated bilirubin is then excreted from the liver cells and into the intrahepatic canaliculi, which eventually lead to the hepatic ducts, the common bile duct, and the bowel.

Jaundice is the discoloration of body tissues caused by abnormally high blood levels of bilirubin. This yellow discoloration is recognized when the total serum bilirubin exceeds 2.5 mg/dL.

Physiologic jaundice of the newborn occurs if the newborn's liver is immature and does not have enough conjugating enzymes. This results in a high circulating blood level of unconjugated bilirubin, which can pass through the blood-brain barrier and be deposited in the brain cells of the newborn. This can cause encephalopathy *(kernicterus)*.

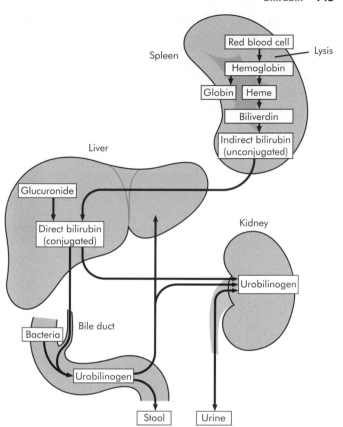

FIGURE 5 Bilirubin metabolism and excretion. The spleen, liver, kidneys, and gastrointestinal tract contribute to this process.

When the jaundice is recognized either clinically or chemically, it is important (for therapy) to differentiate whether it is predominantly caused by unconjugated or conjugated bilirubin. This in turn will help differentiate the etiology of the defect. In general, jaundice caused by hepatocellular dysfunction (e.g., hepatitis) results in elevated levels of unconjugated bilirubin. Jaundice resulting from extrahepatic obstruction of the bile ducts (e.g., gallstones or tumor blocking the bile ducts) results in elevated conjugated bilirubin levels; this type of jaundice usually can be resolved surgically or endoscopically.

The total serum bilirubin level is the sum of the conjugated (direct) and unconjugated (indirect) bilirubin. These are separated out when *fractionation* or *differentiation* of the total bilirubin to its direct and indirect parts is requested from the laboratory. Normally the unconjugated bilirubin makes up 70% to 85% of the total bilirubin. In patients with jaundice, when more than 50% of the bilirubin is conjugated, it is considered a conjugated hyperbilirubinemia from gallstones, tumors, inflammation, scarring, or obstruction of the extrahepatic ducts. Unconjugated hyperbilirubinemia exists when less than 15% to 20% of the total bilirubin is conjugated. Diseases that typically cause this form of jaundice include accelerated erythrocyte (RBC) hemolysis or hepatitis.

Interfering factors

- Blood hemolysis and lipemia can produce erroneous results.
- ☒ Drugs that may cause *increased* levels of total bilirubin include allopurinol, anabolic steroids, antibiotics, antimalarials, ascorbic acid, azathioprine, chlorpropamide, cholinergics, codeine, dextran, diuretics, epinephrine, meperidine, methotrexate, methyldopa, monoamine oxidase inhibitors, morphine, nicotinic acid (large doses), oral contraceptives, phenothiazines, quinidine, rifampin, salicylates, steroids, sulfonamides, theophylline, and vitamin A.
- ☒ Drugs that may cause *decreased* levels of total bilirubin include barbiturates, caffeine, penicillin, and salicylates (large doses).

Procedure and patient care

- See inside front cover for Routine Blood Testing.
- Fasting: verify with lab
- Blood tube commonly used: red
- Note that fasting requirements vary among different laboratories. Some require keeping the patient NPO after midnight the day of the test except for water.
- Use a heel puncture for blood collection in infants.
- Prevent hemolysis of blood during phlebotomy.
- Do *not* shake the tube; inaccurate test results may occur.
- Protect the blood sample from bright light. Prolonged exposure (longer than 1 hour) to sunlight or artificial light can reduce bilirubin content.

Abnormal findings

▲ **Increased levels of conjugated (direct) bilirubin**
Gallstones
Extrahepatic duct obstruction (tumor, inflammation,
 gallstone, scarring, or surgical trauma)
Extensive liver metastasis
Cholestasis from drugs
Dubin-Johnson syndrome
Rotor syndrome

▲ **Increased levels of unconjugated (indirect) bilirubin**
Hemolytic disease of the newborn
Hemolytic jaundice
Large-volume blood transfusion
Resolution of a large hematoma
Hepatitis
Sepsis
Neonatal hyperbilirubinemia
Hemolytic anemia
Crigler-Najjar syndrome
Gilbert syndrome
Pernicious anemia
Cirrhosis
Transfusion reaction
Sickle cell anemia

notes

bioterrorism infectious agents testing

Type of test Various (e.g., blood, urine, stool, tissue culture, sputum, lymph node biopsy, skin)

Normal findings Negative for evidence of infectious agent

Test explanation and related physiology

There are many infectious agents used in bioterrorism, and it would be difficult to discuss each possible agent. In this test, those agents to which humans are most likely to be exposed, either in war or a civilian terrorist attack, are discussed. Refer to Table 4 for specific information on each agent. All documented cases must be reported to the Department of Public Health.

Botulism infection

The botulinum toxin produced by *Clostridium botulinum* causes this disease. The GI tract usually absorbs this organism after eating undercooked meat or sauces exposed to room temperature for prolonged periods. The organism also can be inhaled by handling these items or by open wound contamination of soil that contains *C. botulinum*.

Blurred vision, dysphagia, and muscle weakness progressing to flaccid paralysis are symptoms of the disease. Symptoms begin 6 to 12 hours after ingestion of the contaminated food or approximately 1 week after wound contamination.

The test used to diagnose this disease involves the identification of the toxin in the blood, stool, or vomitus of the affected individual. The food itself can also be tested.

Treatment involves the use of botulinum antitoxin, which can be obtained from the Centers for Disease Control and Prevention (CDC). However, this antitoxin presents a risk of *serum sickness* in nearly one fourth of the patients who receive it.

Anthrax

Anthrax is caused by *Bacillus anthracis*, which is a spore-forming gram-positive rod. Gastrointestinal anthrax is contracted by eating undercooked meat. Pulmonary anthrax results from inhalation of spores or tissues from infected animals. Once inhaled, it is always fatal without treatment. Cutaneous anthrax occurs after contact with contaminated meat, wool, hides, or leather from infected animals.

The three forms of the disease are cutaneous, GI, and pulmonary. Symptoms include fever, malaise, and fatigue progressing to cutaneous lesions, or pulmonary failure. Symptoms occur about 2 to 6 days after exposure.

TABLE 4 Bioterrorism infectious agents testing

Infection/Infectious agent	Site of entry	Sources	Specimen	Tests
Botulism/ *Clostridium botulinum*	GI mucosal surfaces, lung, wound contamination	Undercooked meats, soil, dust	Blood, stool, vomitus, food	Botulinum toxin, mouse bioassay
Anthrax/ *Bacillus anthracis*	Lung, GI	Undercooked meats, inhalation of spores from animal products, skin	Sputum, blood, stool, skin vesicle, food, spores	Culture, Gram stain
Yellow fever/ Hantavirus, Ebola virus, multiple other viruses	Skin bite	Rodent or mosquito bites	Blood, sputum, tissue	Culture, serology for viral antigens
Plague infections/ *Yersinia pestis*	Skin bite	Infected fleas	Blood, sputum, lymph node aspirate	Culture of organism

(Continued)

TABLE 4 Bioterrorism infectious agents testing—cont'd

Brucellosis/ *Brucella abortus, canis,* etc.	GI, lung, wound	Infected meat and milk products	Blood, sputum, food	Culture of organism
Smallpox/ Variola virus	Lungs	Respiratory droplets, direct contact, contaminated clothing	Vesicle	Viral culture or viral identification with electron microscopy
Tularemia/ *Francisella tularensis*	Skin, GI tract, lungs	Ingestion of contaminated plants or water	Blood, sputum, stool	Culture of organism

Culturing the organism in sheep blood agar makes the diagnosis. Appropriate specimens for culture would be stool, blood, sputum, and the cutaneous vesicle. Treatment for this disease is early institution of antibiotics and supportive care.

Hemorrhagic fever (yellow fever)

This disease complex has many causative viruses, including arenavirus, bunyavirus (including hantavirus), filovirus (including Ebola), and flavivirus. Symptoms include fever, thrombocytopenia, shock, multiorgan failure, lung edema, and jaundice. Symptoms develop 4 to 21 days after a mosquito or rodent bite (depending on the disease). This disease is contagious, and patients with suspicious symptoms should be quarantined.

The diagnosis is determined by clinical evaluation. However, viral cultures with polymerase chain reaction identification, serology, and immunohistochemistry of tissue specimens are possible. There is no specific treatment other than aggressive medical therapy and support of organ failure.

Plague

This disease is caused by *Yersinia pestis* and has three forms: bubonic (enlarged lymph nodes), septicemic (blood-borne), and pneumonic (aerosol). Pneumonic is by far the deadliest form of the infection. Symptoms may include fever, chills, weakness, enlarged lymph nodes, or pneumonia and respiratory failure.

The diagnosis is made by culture of the blood, sputum, or lymph node aspirate. This disease complex can be treated with antibiotics when started early in the course of the disease. The risk for bioterrorism is attack or spread by aerosol transmission.

Brucellosis

This disease is caused by *Brucella abortus, suis, melitensis,* or *canis.* It is contracted by ingestion of contaminated milk products, direct puncture of the skin (in butchers and farmers), or by inhalation. The illness is characterized by acute or insidious onset of fever, night sweats, undue fatigue, anorexia, weight loss, headache, and arthralgia. *Brucella* can be cultured from a blood, sputum, or food specimen. Serology testing is also possible. Diagnosis is confirmed by a fourfold or greater rise in *Brucella* agglutination titer between acute- and convalescent-phase serum specimens obtained 2 weeks or more apart and studied at the same laboratory. Demonstration by immunofluorescence of a *Brucella* organism in a clinical specimen is another method of diagnosis.

Smallpox

Smallpox is a serious, contagious, and sometimes fatal infectious disease caused by the variola virus (a DNA virus). There is no specific treatment for smallpox disease, and the only prevention is vaccination. There are two clinical forms of smallpox. Variola major is the severe and most common form of smallpox, with a more extensive rash and higher fever. Variola minor is a less common presentation of smallpox and a much less severe disease. The disease was eradicated after a successful worldwide vaccination program. It is very easily spread and is therefore considered a potential bioterrorism weapon.

The first symptoms of smallpox include fever, malaise, head and body aches, and sometimes vomiting. Next a rash occurs in the mouth and then on the skin. This rash proceeds to become pustular. As the pustules dry up and scab, the patient is no longer contagious.

Viral culture, serology, immunohistochemistry, or electron microscopy can make the diagnosis. The best specimen is the vesicular rash. There is no treatment for the disease, but vaccination is available and is offered to all those at risk for bioterrorism.

Tularemia

This disease is caused by a bacterium called *Francisella tularensis*. It is contracted by drinking contaminated water or eating vegetation contaminated by infected animals. When it enters through the skin, tularemia can be recognized by the presence of a lesion and swollen glands. Ingestion of the organism may produce a throat infection, intestinal pain, diarrhea, and vomiting. Symptoms generally appear from 2 to 10 days—but usually 3 days—after exposure.

Inhalation of the organism may produce fever only or combined with a pneumonia-like illness. Diagnosis is made by culture of the blood, sputum, or stool.

Procedure and patient care

Before

- Maintain strict adherence to all procedures to avoid violations in isolation or contamination.
- Biohazard precautions are to be taken with each specimen.
- Laboratory personnel must strictly adhere to all universal standard precautions.

During

- If an enema is used to obtain a botulinum stool specimen, use sterile water. Saline can negate results.
- Send enough blood for adequate testing. Usually two red-top tubes are adequate. It is best to send it on ice.

- If food is sent for testing, it should be sent in its original container.
- For anthrax or smallpox testing of a cutaneous lesion, soak one or two culture swabs with fluid from a previously unopened lesion.

After

- Identify all potential sources of contamination.
- Isolate individuals who are suspected of having a contagious disease.

Abnormal findings

See Table 4.

notes

> **bladder cancer markers** (Bladder tumor antigen [BTA], Nuclear matrix protein 22 [NMP22])

Type of test Urine

Normal findings

BTA: <14 units/mL
NMP22: <10 units/mL
FISH: No chromosomal amplification or deletions noted

Test explanation and related physiology

The recurrence rate for superficial bladder cancers that have been resected by transurethral cystoscopy is high. Surveillance testing requires frequent urine testing for cytology and frequent cystoscopic evaluations. The use of bladder tumor markers may provide an easier, cheaper, and more accurate method of diagnosing recurrent bladder cancer.

Bladder tumor antigen (BTA) and nuclear matrix protein 22 (NMP22) are proteins produced by bladder tumor cells and deposited into the urine. Normally, none or very low levels of these proteins are found in the urine. When levels of bladder cancer tumor markers are normal, cystoscopy rarely yields positive results. When these markers are elevated, bladder tumor recurrence is strongly suspected and cystoscopy is indicated to confirm bladder cancer recurrence.

NMP22 may also be a good screening test for patients at increased risk for developing bladder cancer. However, these markers can be elevated in other circumstances (i.e., recent urologic surgery, urinary tract infection, calculi). Cancers involving the ureters and renal pelvis may also be associated with increased BTA and NMP22.

Bladder cancer cells have been found to exhibit aneuploidy (gene amplifications on chromosomes 3, 7, and 17, and the loss of the 9p21 locus on chromosome 9). Using DNA probes, through *fluorescence in situ hybridization (FISH)*, these chromosomal abnormalities can be identified with great accuracy. FISH can be performed on cells isolated in a fresh urine specimen or cells available on a ThinPrep slide (similar to Pap smears [see p. 681]). When these chromosomal abnormalities are present, fluorescent staining will be obvious using a fluorescence microscope.

Although not actually a tumor marker, a cytology test is available that can be used in the early detection of bladder cancer recurrence. It is an immunocytofluorescence technique based on a patented cocktail of three monoclonal antibodies labeled with fluorescence markers. These antibodies bind to two antigens: a mucin glycoprotein and a carcinoembryonic antigen (CEA). These antigens are expressed by tumor cells found in bladder cancer patients and are exfoliated in the urine.

Interfering factors

- These proteins are very unstable. If the urine is not immediately stabilized, false negatives may occur.
- Active infection (including sexually transmitted diseases) of the lower urologic tract can cause false elevations.
- Kidney or bladder calculi can cause false elevations.

Procedure and patient care

- See inside front cover for Routine Urine Testing.
- **PT** Tell the patient that no fasting is required.
- A urine specimen should be collected, preferably from the first void of the day.
- The specimen should be transported to the lab immediately to avoid deterioration of the cells.
- If a time delay is required, the specimen should be refrigerated.

Abnormal findings

Bladder cancer
Non-bladder urologic cancer (ureters, renal pelvis, etc.)

notes

blood culture and sensitivity

Type of test Blood

Normal findings Negative

Test explanation and related physiology

Blood cultures are obtained to detect the presence of bacteria in the blood. Bacteremia (the presence of bacteria in the blood) can be intermittent and transient, except in endocarditis or suppurative thrombophlebitis. An episode of bacteremia is usually accompanied by chills and fever; thus, the blood culture should be drawn when the patient manifests these signs to increase the chances of growing bacteria on the cultures. It is important that at least two culture specimens be obtained from two different sites. If one produces bacteria and the other does not, it is safe to assume that the bacteria in the first culture may be a contaminant and not the infecting agent. When both cultures grow the infecting agent, bacteremia exists and is caused by the organism that is growing in the culture.

If the patient is receiving antibiotics during the time that the cultures are drawn, the laboratory should be notified. Resin can be added to the culture medium to negate the antibiotic effect in inhibiting growth of the offending bacteria in the culture. If cultures are to be performed while the patient is on antibiotics, the blood culture specimen should be taken shortly before the next dose of the antibiotic is administered. All cultures preferably should be performed before antibiotic therapy is initiated.

Culture specimens drawn through an IV catheter are frequently contaminated, and tests using them should not be performed unless catheter sepsis is suspected. In these situations, blood culture specimens drawn through the catheter help identify the causative agent more accurately than a culture specimen from the catheter tip.

Most organisms require approximately 24 hours to grow in the laboratory, and a preliminary report can be given at that time. Often, 48 to 72 hours are required for growth and identification of the organism. Anaerobic organisms may take longer to grow.

Interfering factors

- Contamination of the blood specimen, especially by skin bacteria, may occur.

Procedure and patient care
Before
PT Explain the procedure to the patient.
PT Tell the patient that no fasting is required.

During
- Carefully prepare the venipuncture site with povidone-iodine (Betadine). Allow the skin to dry.
- Clean the tops of the Vacutainer tubes or culture bottles with povidone-iodine and allow them to dry. Some laboratories suggest cleaning with 70% alcohol after cleaning with povidone-iodine and air drying.
- Collect approximately 10 to 15 mL of venous blood by venipuncture from each site in a 20-mL syringe.
- Discard the needle on the syringe and replace it with a second sterile needle before injecting the blood sample into the culture bottle.
- Inoculate the anaerobic bottle first if both anaerobic and aerobic cultures are needed.
- Mix gently after inoculation.
- Label the specimen with the patient's name, date, time, and tentative diagnosis.
- Indicate on the laboratory slip any medications that may affect test results.

After
- Transport the culture bottles immediately to the laboratory (or at least within 30 minutes).
- Notify the physician of any positive results so that appropriate antibiotic therapy can be initiated.

Abnormal findings
Bacteremia

notes

blood smear (Peripheral blood smear, Red blood cell [RBC] morphology, RBC smear)

Type of test Blood

Normal findings

Normal quantity of red and white blood cells (RBCs, WBCs) and platelets
Normal size, shape, and color of RBCs
Normal WBC differential count
Normal size and granulation of platelets

Test explanation and related physiology

Examination of the peripheral blood smear can provide a significant amount of information concerning drugs and diseases that affect erythrocytes (RBCs), leukocytes (WBCs), or platelets. Furthermore, other congenital and acquired diseases can be diagnosed. When special stains are applied to the blood smear, leukemia, infection, infestation, and other diseases can be identified.

When adequately prepared and examined microscopically by an experienced technologist or pathologist, a smear of peripheral blood is the most informative of all hematologic tests. All three hematologic cell lines—RBCs, platelets, and WBCs—can be examined. In the peripheral blood, five different types of WBCs can routinely be identified: neutrophils, eosinophils, basophils, lymphocytes, and monocytes. The first three are also referred to as *granulocytes*. Please see the discussion in bone marrow biopsy (p. 166) for more information concerning the various elements of blood.

Microscopic examination of the RBCs can reveal variations in RBC size (anisocytosis), shape (poikilocytosis), color, or intracellular content (Box 3). Classification of RBCs according to these

---

BOX 3 Microscopic examination of RBCs

RBC size abnormalities
  Microcytes (small RBCs)
    Iron deficiency
    Thalassemia
    Hemoglobinopathies
  Macrocytes (larger size)
    Vitamin B_{12} or folic acid deficiency

BOX 3   Microscopic examination of RBCs—cont'd

B

    Reticulocytosis secondary to increased erythropoiesis
      (RBC production)
    Occasional liver disorder

RBC shape abnormalities
    Spherocytes (small and round)
      Hereditary spherocytosis
      Acquired immunohemolytic anemia
    Elliptocytes (crescent)
      Iron deficiency
      Hereditary elliptocytosis
    Codocytes or target cells (thin cells with less
      hemoglobin)
      Hemoglobinopathies
      Thalassemia
    Echinocytes (Burr cells)
      Uremia
      Liver disease

RBC color abnormalities
    Hypochromic (pale)
      Iron deficiency
      Thalassemia
    Hyperchromasia (more colored)
      Concentrated hemoglobin, usually caused by dehydration

RBC intracellular structure
    Nucleated (normoblasts) (Mature RBCs are round with a small
      central pallor without any intracellular structures. They do not
      have a nucleus. Immature RBCs (reticulocytes) do contain
      intracellular RNA. Immature nucleated cells are not normally
      found in the peripheral blood and indicate increased RBC
      synthesis.)
      Anemia
      Chronic hypoxemia
      Normal for an infant
      Marrow-occupying neoplasm or fibrotic tissue
    Basophilic stippling (refers to bodies enclosed or included in the
      cytoplasm of the RBCs)
      Lead poisoning
      Reticulocytosis
    Howell-Jolly bodies (small, round remnants of nuclear material
      remaining within the RBC)
      After a surgical splenectomy
      Hemolytic anemia
      Megaloblastic anemia
      Functional asplenia (after splenic infarction)

variables is most helpful in identifying the causes of anemia and the presence of other diseases.

The WBCs are examined for total quantity, differential count, and degree of maturity. An increased number of immature WBCs may indicate leukemia or infection. A decreased WBC count indicates a failure of marrow to produce WBCs (due to drugs, chronic disease, neoplasia, or fibrosis), peripheral destruction, or sequestration.

Platelet examination

Finally, an experienced laboratory technologist also can estimate platelet number. Platelets are small cell fragments that do not contain a nucleus. The contents of the granules in a platelet are released to promote clotting.

Procedure and patient care

Before

PT Explain the procedure to the patient.

PT Tell the patient that no fasting is required.

During

- Collect a drop of blood from a finger stick or heel stick and place it on a slide.
- If necessary, perform a venipuncture and collect the blood in a lavender-top tube.
- Note that a blood smear is first studied with an automated cytometer programmed to recognize abnormal blood cell shapes and other variations. An evaluation smear is performed by a technologist. Low counts may be hand counted to ensure accuracy. The most accurate smear requires review by a pathologist.

After

- Apply pressure to the venipuncture site.

Abnormal findings

See Box 3 in the Test explanation and related physiology section.

notes

blood typing (Blood group microarray testing)

Type of test Blood

Normal findings Compatibility

Test explanation and related physiology

With blood typing, ABO and Rh antigens can be detected in the blood of prospective blood donors and potential blood recipients. This test is also used to determine the blood type of expectant mothers and newborns. A description of the ABO system, Rh factors, and blood crossmatching is reviewed here.

ABO system

Human blood is grouped according to the presence or absence of A or B antigens. The surface membranes of group A red blood cells (RBCs) contain A antigens; group B RBCs contain B antigens on their surface; group AB RBCs have both A and B antigens; and group O RBCs have neither A nor B antigens. In general, a person's serum does not contain antibodies to match the surface antigen on their RBCs. That is, persons with group A antigens (type A blood) will not have anti-A antibodies; however, they will have anti-B antibodies. The converse is true for persons with group B antigens. Group O blood will have both anti-A and anti-B antibodies (Table 5). These antibodies against A and B blood group antigens are formed in the first 3 months of life after exposure to similar antigens on the surface of naturally occurring bacteria in the intestine.

TABLE 5 Blood typing

Blood type (ABO, Rh)	Antigens present	Antibodies possibly present	Percent of general population
O, +	Rh	A, B	35
O, –*	None	A, B, Rh	7
A, +	A, Rh	B	35
A, –	A	B, Rh	7
B, +	B, Rh	A	8
B, –	B	A, Rh	2
AB, +†	A, B, Rh	None	4
AB, –	A, B	Rh	2

* Universal donor; † Universal recipient

Blood transfusions are actually transplantations of tissue (blood) from one person to another. It is important that the recipient not have antibodies to the donor's RBCs. If this were to occur, there could be a hypersensitivity reaction, which can vary from mild fever to anaphylaxis with severe intravascular hemolysis. If donor ABO antibodies are present against the recipient antigens, usually only minimal reactions occur.

Persons with group O blood are considered *universal donors* because they do not have antigens on their RBCs. People with group AB blood are considered *universal recipients* because they have no antibodies to react to the transfused blood. Group O blood is usually transfused in emergent situations in which rapid, life-threatening blood loss occurs and immediate transfusion is required. The chance of a transfusion reaction is least when type O is used. Women of childbearing potential should receive group O negative blood, and men generally receive group O positive blood when emergency transfusion prior to type-specific or crossmatched blood is required.

ABO typing is not required for autotransfusions (blood donated by a patient several weeks prior to a major operation and then transfused post-operatively). However, in most hospitals, ABO typing is performed on those patients in the event that further blood transfusion of banked blood is required.

Rh factors

The presence or absence of Rh antigens on the RBC's surface determines the classification of Rh positive or Rh negative. After ABO compatibility, Rh factor is the next most important antigen affecting the success of a blood transfusion. The major Rh factor is $Rh_o(D)$. There are several minor Rh factors. If $Rh_o(D)$ is absent, the minor Rh antigens are tested. If negative, the patient is considered *Rh negative (Rh–)*.

Rh– persons may develop antibodies to Rh antigens if exposed to Rh-positive (Rh+) blood by transfusions or fetal–maternal blood mixing. All women who are pregnant should have a blood typing and Rh factor determination. If the mother's blood is Rh–, the father's blood should also be typed. If his blood is Rh+, the woman's blood should be examined for the presence of Rh antibodies (by the indirect Coombs test; see page 299). Hemolytic disease of the newborn can be prevented by Rh typing during pregnancy. If the mother is Rh–, she should be advised that she is a candidate for RhoGAM (Rh immunoglobulin that "neutralizes" the Rh antigen) after the delivery. RhoGAM can reduce the chance of fetal hemolytic problems during subsequent pregnancies.

B

Other blood typing systems

There are nine different gene codes for blood groups assayed. Most are minor and not clinically significant. However in certain clinical circumstances, these minor blood group antigens and acquired antigens can become significant. This may occur with frequent blood transfusions or in patients with leukemia or lymphoma. Multiplex PCR microarray analysis provides identification of the many variants involving these blood group systems and is particularly helpful in the described patients.

Blood crossmatching

Although typing for the major ABO and Rh antigens is no guarantee that a reaction will not occur, it does greatly reduce the possibility of such a reaction. Many potential minor antigens are not routinely detected during blood typing. If allowed to go unrecognized, these minor antigens also can initiate a blood transfusion reaction. Therefore, blood is not only typed but also crossmatched to identify a mismatch of blood caused by minor antigens. Crossmatching always includes an indirect Coombs test. Only blood products containing RBCs need to be crossmatched. Plasma products do not need to be crossmatched but should be ABO compatible because other cells (WBCs and platelets) have ABO antigens.

Homologous (donor and recipient are different people) and directed (recipient chooses the donor) blood for donation must be rigorously tested before transfusion. Autologous (recipient and donor is the same person) blood for transfusions, however, is not subject to that same testing.

Finally, one must be aware of graft-versus-host disease (GVHD) in which donor lymphocytes included in the blood transfusion may engraft and multiply in the recipient.

Procedure and patient care

- See inside front cover for Routine Blood Testing.
- Fasting: yes
- Blood tube commonly used: red. Verify with lab.

Abnormal findings

See Test explanation and related physiology section (p. 159).

notes

bone densitometry (Bone mineral content [BMC], Bone mineral density [BMD], DEXA scan)

Type of test X-ray

Normal findings

Normal: <1 standard deviation below normal (>–1)
Osteopenia: 1-2.5 standard deviations below normal (–1 to –2.5)
Osteoporosis: >2.5 standard deviations below normal (<–2.5)

Test explanation and related physiology

Bone densitometry is used to determine bone mineral content (BMC) and density (BMD) to diagnose osteoporosis as early as possible. It is also used to monitor patients who are undergoing treatment for osteoporosis. *Osteoporosis* and *low bone mass (osteopenia)* are terms used for bones that become weakened and fracture easily. This most commonly occurs in postmenopausal women. However, other diseases are associated with osteoporosis, such as malnourishment and osteopenic endocrinopathies (e.g., hyperparathyroidism).

The earlier that osteoporosis is recognized, the more effective the treatment and the milder the clinical course. If the diagnosis of osteoporosis is delayed until fractures occur or even until plain film images identify *thin* bones, successful treatment is less likely. Because therapy can be expensive and is not without risks, the diagnosis of osteoporosis must be made on the basis of accurate data. Bone densitometry can provide early and accurate measurements of bone strength based on BMD.

Several groups of bones are routinely evaluated. The lumbar spine is one of the best representatives of cancellous bone. The radius is the most frequently studied cortical bone. The proximal hip (neck of the femur) is the best representative of mixed (cancellous and cortical) bone. However, specific bone sites can be evaluated if they are particularly symptomatic.

Dual-energy x-ray absorptiometry (DEXA) is the method most commonly used. Because DEXA uses two photons, more energy is produced so that bones (spine and hip [femoral neck]) surrounded by a lot of soft tissue can be more easily penetrated. The source of the photon is placed on one side of the bone to be studied. The gamma detector is placed on the other side. Increased bone density is associated with increased bone photon absorption and, therefore, less photon recognition at the site of the gamma detector.

Several other methods are available to measure BMD. *Quantitative computed tomography (QCT)* uses CT technology to measure central bones, especially the spine. *Ultrasound absorption (quantitative ultrasound)* can be used to measure peripheral bones (heel [calcaneus], patella, or midtibia).

BMD is usually reported in terms of standard deviation (SD) from mean values. T scores compare the patient's results to a group of young healthy adults. Z scores compare the patient's results to a group of age-matched controls. The World Health Organization has defined *low bone mass* as a BMD value greater than 1 SD below peak bone mass levels in young women, and *osteoporosis* as a value greater than 2.5 SD below that same measurement scale. Positive T scores indicate a normal BMD. Negative T scores indicate reduced BMD.

Based on the BMD of the femoral neck, and upon other clinical criteria, the risk of a major osteoporotic fracture and the risk of a hip fracture can be calculated (see www.shef.ac.uk/FRAX/index.htm). This is called *Fracture Risk Assessment.* Furthermore, the identification of vertebral fracture is important in the diagnosis of osteoporosis because the presence of one or more of these fractures is a strong indicator of a patient's future fracture risk at the spine, hip, and other sites. *Vertebral Fracture Assessment (VFA)* can be performed utilizing the images generated by the DEXA scan. Images of the lower thoracic and lumbar spine are examined. If a vertebral fracture is identified, bone mineral strengthening medications are recommended despite T score. Presence of a vertebral fracture indicates a substantial risk for a subsequent vertebral or nonvertebral fracture independent of the bone mineral density or other osteoporosis risk factors. VFA is commonly recommended on postmenopausal women with reduced BMD and the following:

- Age >70
- Height loss >1.6 inches
- Prior vertebral fracture
- Chronic disease with increased risk for vertebral fracture (e.g., COPD, rheumatoid arthritis, Crohn disease)
- Women with osteoporosis
- Postmenopausal women chronically receiving glucocorticoid therapy

BMD testing is an important part of routine screening testing for postmenopausal women. In general, BMD is recommended every 2 years to screen for osteoporosis. Women and men with known osteoporotic fractures, hyperparathyroidism, or administration of long-term steroid therapy may benefit from annual BMD testing.

Interfering factors

- Barium may falsely increase the density of the lumbar spine. BMD measurements should not be performed for about 10 days after barium studies.
- Calcified abdominal aortic aneurysm may falsely increase BMD of the spine.
- Internal fixation devices of the hip or radius will falsely increase BMD of those bones.
- Overlying metal jewelry or other objects may falsely increase BMD.
- Previous fractures or severe arthritis changes of the bone can falsely increase BMD.
- Metallic clips placed in the vertebrae of patients who have had previous abdominal surgery can falsely increase BMD.
- Prior bone scans can falsely decrease BMD because the photons generated from the bone (as a result of the previously administered bone scan radionuclide) will be detected by the scintillator detector.

Procedure and patient care

Before

PT Explain the procedure to the patient.

PT Tell the patient that no fasting or sedation is required.

PT Instruct the patient to remove all metallic objects (e.g., belt buckles, zippers, coins, keys) that might be in the scanning path.

During

- Note the following procedural steps:
  1. The patient lies supine on an imaging table, with his or her legs supported and placed on a padded box to flatten the pelvis and lumbar spine.
  2. Under the table, a photon generator is slowly and successively passed under the lumbar spine.
  3. A scintillator (gamma or x-ray) detector/camera is passed over the patient in a manner parallel to that of the generator. An image of the lumbar spine and hip bone is obtained by the scintillator camera and projected onto a computer monitor.
  4. Next, the appropriate foot is applied to a brace that internally rotates the nondominant hip, and the procedure is

repeated over the hip. A similar procedure is performed for radius evaluation.

5. When the radius is examined, the nondominant arm is preferred unless there is a history of fracture to that bone.

- Note that the data are interpreted and reported by a radiologist or a physician trained in nuclear medicine.
- Note that BMD studies take about 15 minutes to perform and are free of any discomfort. Only minimal radiation is used for this procedure.
- Note that there are numerous types of bone densitometry machines. Peripheral units that quickly scan the finger, heel, or forearm are often used to identify patients at risk for osteoporosis. Abnormal results are followed up with the more comprehensive table procedure previously described.

After

- On the computer screen, a small window of the lumbar spine, femoral neck, or distal radius is drawn. The computer calculates the amount of photons not absorbed by the bone. This is the BMC. BMD is computed as follows:

$$BMD = \frac{BMC\left(g/cm^2\right)}{Surface\ area\ of\ the\ bone}$$

Abnormal findings

Low bone mass
Osteoporosis

notes

bone marrow biopsy (Bone marrow examination, Bone marrow aspiration)

Type of test Microscopic examination of tissue

Normal findings

Active erythroid cell line, myeloid and lymphoid cell lines, and megakaryocyte (platelet) production. See range of cell types below.

Cell type	Range (%)
Neutrophilic series	49.2-65.0
Myeloblasts	0.2-1.5
Promyelocytes	2.1-4.1
Myelocytes	8.2-15.7
Eosinophilic series	1.2-5.3
Myelocytes	0.2-1.3
Metamyelocytes	0.4-2.2
Bands	0.2-2.4
Segmented	0-1.3
Basophilic and mast cells	0-0.2
Erythrocyte series	18.4-33.8
Pronormoblasts	0.2-1.3
Basophilic	0.5-2.4
Polychromatophilic	17.9-29.2
Orthochromatic	0.4-4.6
Monocytes	0-0.8
Lymphocytes	11.1-23.2
Plasma cells	0.4-3.9
Megakaryocytes	0-0.4
Reticulum cells	0-0.9
Monocyte to erythrocyte (M/E) ratio	1.5-3.3

Normal iron content is demonstrated by staining with Prussian blue.

Test explanation and related physiology

Bone marrow examination is an important part of the evaluation of patients with hematologic diseases. Indications for bone marrow examination include the following:

- To evaluate anemias, leukopenia, or thrombocytopenia
- To diagnose leukemia, myelodysplastic syndromes, myeloproliferative neoplasms, and plasma cell dyscrasia
- To document abnormal iron stores

- To document bone marrow infiltrative diseases (e.g., neoplasm, infection, or fibrosis)
- To stage lymphomas or other cancers

The bone marrow is located in the central fatty core of cancellous bone (particularly sternum, rib, and pelvis). There, the blood-forming cells produce blood cells and release them into the circulation.

By examining a bone marrow specimen, a hematologist can fully evaluate hematopoiesis. Examination of bone marrow reveals the number, size, and shape of the RBCs, WBCs, and megakaryocytes (platelet precursors) as these cells evolve through their various stages of development in the bone marrow. Samples of bone marrow can be obtained by aspiration, bone marrow biopsy, or surgical removal. An aspiration is obtained for cell morphology, immunophenotyping, cytogenetics, or microbiology cultures. Microscopic examination of the marrow biopsy includes estimation of cellularity, identification of disordered hematopoiesis, and determination of the presence of infiltrative diseases (fibrosis or neoplasms, both primary and metastatic). Estimation of iron storage is performed on bone marrow aspirates or non-decalcified clot sections.

For the estimation of cellularity, the specimen is examined and the relative quantity of each cell type is determined. Leukemias or leukemoid drug reactions are suspected when increased numbers of leukocyte precursors are present. Physiologic marrow leukemoid compensation is also seen with infection. Decreased numbers of marrow leukocyte precursors occur in patients with myelofibrosis, metastatic neoplasia, or agranulocytosis/aplastic anemia; in elderly patients; and following radiation therapy or chemotherapy. Some drugs or infections can diminish leukocyte production.

Increased numbers of marrow RBC precursors occur with polycythemia vera or as physiologic compensation to blood loss (hemorrhage or hemolysis). Decreased numbers of marrow RBC precursors occur with erythroid hypoplasia following chemotherapy, infection (parvovirus), aplastic anemia, radiation therapy, administration of other toxic drugs, iron administration, or marrow replacement by fibrotic tissue or neoplasms.

Increased numbers of platelet precursors (megakaryocytes) can be the result of compensation to platelet loss from a recent hemorrhage. They are also seen in some forms of acute and chronic myeloid leukemias. This increase also may be compensatory in patients with platelet sequestration (secondary hypersplenism associated with portal hypertension) or platelet destruction (idiopathic thrombocytopenic purpura). Platelet counts decrease, and the marrow compensates by increasing production. Decreased numbers of megakaryocytes occur in patients who have had radiation therapy, chemotherapy, or other drug therapy and in patients with neoplastic or fibrotic marrow infiltrative diseases. Patients with aplastic anemia also have decreased numbers of megakaryocytes.

Increased numbers of lymphocyte precursors occur in chronic, viral, or mycoplasmal infections (e.g., mononucleosis), lymphocytic leukemia, and lymphoma. Plasma cells and lymphocytes are increased in patients with plasma cell dyscrasia, lymphomas, hypersensitivity states, autoimmune disease, chronic infections, and other chronic inflammatory diseases.

Estimation of cellularity also can be expressed as a ratio of myeloid (WBC) to erythroid (RBC) cells (M/E ratio). The normal M/E ratio is approximately 3:1. The M/E ratio is greater than normal in those diseases in which leukocyte precursors are increased or erythroid precursors are decreased. The M/E ratio is below normal when either leukocyte precursors are decreased or erythroid precursors are increased.

Drug-induced myelofibrosis or myelofibrosis associated with hematologic, myeloproliferative, or other neoplasms can be detected by examination of the bone marrow using reticulin or collagen stains. Using special stains, iron stores can be estimated with a marrow aspirate or decalcified clot sections (biopsies are decalcified leading to artificial decrease in iron staining).

Bone marrow aspiration and biopsy are performed by a physician or mid-level health care provider. The duration of these procedures is approximately 20 minutes. The patient may have some apprehension when pressure is applied to puncture the outer table of the bone during biopsy-specimen removal or aspiration. The patient probably will feel pain during lidocaine infiltration and pressure when the syringe plunger is withdrawn for aspiration.

Contraindications

- Patients with acute coagulation disorders, because of the risk of excessive bleeding
- Patients who cannot cooperate or remain still during the procedure

Potential complications

- Hemorrhage, especially if the patient has a coagulopathy
- Infection, especially if the patient is leukopenic

Procedure and patient care
Before
PT Explain the procedure to the patient.
- Obtain a written informed consent for this procedure.
- Encourage the patient to verbalize fears because many patients are anxious concerning this study. Conscious sedation may be required.
- Assess the results of the coagulation studies. Report any evidence of coagulopathy to the physician. Platelets should be >20,000 and INR should be <1.5.
- Obtain an order for sedatives if the patient appears extremely apprehensive.

PT Instruct the patient to remain very still throughout the procedure.

During
PT Inform the patient that during bone marrow aspiration, most patients feel pain or a burning sensation during lidocaine infiltration and pressure when the syringe plunger is withdrawn for aspiration.
- Conscious sedation may be provided for this procedure.
- Note the following procedural steps for *bone marrow aspiration*:
  1. The procedure is usually begun as described in step 1 below for bone marrow biopsy.
  2. For aspiration, an Illinois or Jamshedi type large-bore needle is used.
  3. When inside the marrow, a syringe is used to aspirate marrow contents (Figure **6**).

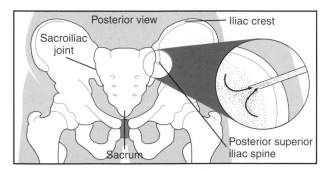

FIGURE 6 Bone marrow aspiration. Samples of the bone marrow are taken from along the posterior superior iliac spine.

4. Several small-volume (0.5- to 2-mL) samples of bone marrow are aspirated.
5. The aspirate is placed in an appropriate blood specimen
   collecting test tube depending on the test requested.
- Note the following procedural steps for *bone marrow biopsy*:
  1. The skin and soft tissues overlying the posterior superior
     spine of the iliac bone are prepped and draped. A small
     skin incision is made in that area after local anesthesia is
     provided.
  2. A Jamshedi needle is positioned into the bone.
  3. The aspiration specimen is obtained first. With reposition-
     ing of the needle (to avoid aspiration artifact), the biopsy
     specimen is obtained and placed in a formalin fixative. It is
     then sent to the pathology laboratory for analysis.
  4. Bilateral bone marrow biopsies may be performed for stag-
     ing of lymphoma or other neoplasms.

After

- Apply pressure to the puncture site to arrest any bleeding.
- Apply an adhesive bandage.
- Observe the puncture site for bleeding. Ice packs may be used
  to minimize bleeding.
- Assess for tenderness and erythema, which may indicate infection. Report this to the physician.
- Normally, place the patient in the supine position at bed rest
  for 30 to 60 minutes after the test. This provides pressure on
  the biopsy site.
- Note that some patients complain of tenderness at the puncture site for several days after this study. Mild analgesics may
  be ordered.

Abnormal findings

Metastatic neoplasm
Myeloproliferative neoplasms
Infection (e.g., viral, bacterial,
   fungal)
Agranulocytosis
Red cell aplasia
Plasma cell dyscrasia
Hodgkin lymphoma
Non-Hodgkin lymphoma

Lymphoblastic leukemia
Myeloid leukemia
Myelodysplastic syndromes
Anemia
Chronic inflammatory disease
Acquired immunodeficiency
   syndrome (AIDS)
Bone marrow aplasia

notes

bone scan

Type of test Nuclear scan

Normal findings No evidence of abnormality

Test explanation and related physiology

The bone scan permits examination of the skeleton by a scanning camera after IV injection of a radionuclide material. After injection, the radiopharmaceutical is taken up by the bone. Gamma rays are emitted from the radionuclide through the body and detected by a scintillator. The scintillator emits light with each photon it receives from the gamma ray. When these light patterns are arranged in a spatial order, a realistic image of the bones is apparent.

The degree of radionuclide uptake is related to the metabolism of the bone. Normally a uniform concentration should be seen throughout the bones of the body. There is symmetrical distribution of activity throughout the skeletal system in healthy adults. Urinary bladder activity, faint renal activity, and minimal soft tissue activity are also normally present. An increased uptake of radionuclide is abnormal and may represent tumor, arthritis, fracture, degenerative bone and joint changes, osteomyelitis, bone necrosis, osteodystrophy, and Paget disease. These areas of concentrated radionuclide uptake are often called *hot spots* and are detectable months before an ordinary x-ray image can reveal the pathology. Hot spots occur because new bone growth is usually stimulated around areas of pathology. If pathology exists and there is no new bone formation around the lesion, the scan will not pick up the abnormality. Increased uptake of radionuclide is also seen in the normal physiologic active epiphyses of children.

The major reason a bone scan is performed is to detect metastatic cancer to the bone. All malignancies capable of metastasis may reach the bone, especially those of the prostate, breast, lung, kidney, urinary bladder, and thyroid gland. Bone scans are also useful in staging primary bone tumors, such as osteogenic sarcomas and Ewing sarcoma. Bone scans may be serially repeated to monitor tumor response to antineoplastic therapy.

Bone scans also provide valuable information in the evaluation of patients with trauma or unexplained pain. Bone scanning is much more sensitive than routine x-ray images in detecting small and difficult-to-find fractures, especially in the spine, ribs, face, and small bones of the extremities. Bone scans are used to determine the age of a fracture as well. If a fracture line is seen on a plain x-ray image and the uptake around that fracture is not increased on a bone scan, the injury is said to be an *old* fracture, exceeding several months in age.

Although the bone scan is extremely sensitive, unfortunately it is not very specific. Fractures, infections, tumors, and arthritic changes all appear similar in this scan. A three-phase bone scan may be performed if inflammation (arthritis) or infection (osteomyelitis, septic arthritis) is suspected. In a three-phase bone scan, imaging is performed at three different times after injection of the radionuclide. Early uptake of the radionuclide would indicate infection or inflammation rather than neoplasm. Uptake of the radionuclide on delayed imaging that is not present on early imaging would indicate neoplasm.

When the metastatic process is diffuse, virtually all of the radionuclide is concentrated in the skeleton, with little or no activity in the soft tissues or urinary tract. The resulting pattern, which is characterized by excellent bone detail, is frequently referred to as a *superscan*. A superscan may also be associated with metabolic bone diseases (e.g., Paget disease, renal osteodystrophy, or osteomalacia). Unlike in metastatic disease, however, the uptake in metabolic bone disease is more uniform in appearance and extends into the distal appendicular skeleton.

Contraindications

- Patients who are pregnant, unless the benefits outweigh the risk of fetal damage
- Patients who are lactating

Procedure and patient care

Before

PT Explain the procedure to the patient.

PT Assure patients they will not be exposed to large amounts of radioactivity because only tracer doses of the isotope are used.

PT Tell the patient that no fasting or sedation is required.

PT Inform the patient that the injection of the radionuclide may cause slight discomfort, nausea, or vomiting.

During

- Note the following procedural steps:
    1. The patient receives an IV injection of radionuclide, usually ^{99m}Tc-MDP (technetium-99 m-methylene diphosphonate) or ^{99m}Tc-HDP 99 m (hydroxymethane diphosphonate), into a peripheral vein in the arm.

2. The patient is encouraged to drink several glasses of water between the time of radionuclide injection and the scanning. This facilitates renal clearance of the circulating tracer not picked up by the bone. The waiting period before scanning is approximately 2 to 3 hours.
3. The patient is instructed to urinate.
4. The patient is situated in the supine position on the scanning table in nuclear medicine.
5. A radionuclide detector is placed over the patient's body and records the radiation emitted by the skeleton.
6. This information is translated into a two- or three-dimensional view of the skeleton.
7. The patient may be repositioned in the prone and lateral positions during the test.

- Note that this scan is performed by a nuclear medicine technician in 30 to 60 minutes. It is interpreted by a physician trained in nuclear medicine imaging.

PT Inform patients in significant pain that lying on the hard scanning table can be uncomfortable.

After

- Because only tracer doses of radionuclide are used, no radiation precautions need to be taken.

PT Assure the patient that the radioactive substance is usually excreted from the body within 6 to 24 hours.

PT Encourage the patient to drink fluids to aid in the excretion of the radioactive substance.

Abnormal findings

Primary or metastatic tumor of the bone
Fracture
Degenerative arthritis
Rheumatoid arthritis
Osteomyelitis
Bone necrosis
Renal osteodystrophy
Paget disease of bone

notes

> **bone turnover markers** (BTMs, N-telopeptide [NTx], Bone collagen equivalents (BCEs), Osteocalcin [bone G1 a protein, BGP, osteocalc], Pyridinium [PYD] crosslinks, Bone-specific alkaline phosphatase [BSAP], Amino-terminal propeptide of type I procollagen [P1NP], C-telopeptide [CTx])

Type of test Blood; urine

Normal findings (Results vary greatly with age)

N-telopeptide

    Urine (nm BCE*/mm creatinine)

        Male: 21-83

        Female, premenopausal: 17-94

        Female, postmenopausal: 26-124

    Serum (nm BCE*)

        Male: 5.4-24.2

        Female: 6.2-19.0

    (*BCE = bone collagen equivalents)

C-telopeptide

    Urine (ng/mL)

        Adults: 1.03 ± 0.41

        Children: 8.00 ± 3.37

    Serum (pg/mL)

        Female, premenopausal: 40-465

        Female, postmenopausal: 104-1008

        Male: 60-700

Amino-terminal propeptide of type I procollagen, serum (µg/L)

    Male: 22-105

    Female, premenopausal: 19-101

    Female, postmenopausal: 16-96

Osteocalcin, serum (ng/mL)

    Adult (>22 years)

        Male: 5.8-14.0

        Female: 3.1-14.4

Pyridium, urine (nm/mm)

    Male: 10.3-33.6

    Female: 15.3-33.6

Bone-specific alkaline phosphatase, serum (µg/L)

    Male: 6.5-20.1

    Female, premenopausal: 4.5-16.9

    Female, postmenopausal: 7.0-22.4

Test explanation and related physiology

With the increased use of bone density scans (see p. 162), osteoporosis can now be diagnosed and treated more easily. This has prompted an interest in biochemical markers of bone metabolism. Bone is continuously turned over: bone resorption by osteoclasts and bone formation by osteoblasts. Osteoporosis is a common disease of postmenopausal women and is associated with increased bone resorption and decreased bone formation. The result is thin and weak bones that are prone to fracture. The same process is now becoming increasingly recognized in elderly men as well. Early diagnosis allows therapeutic intervention to prevent bone fracture.

Bone mineral density studies (p. 162) are valuable tools in the identification of osteoporosis; however, they cannot recognize small changes in bone metabolism. Although bone density studies can be used to monitor the effectiveness of therapy, it takes years to detect measurable changes in bone density. Bone turnover markers (BTMs), however, can identify significant improvement in a few months after instituting successful therapy. Furthermore, the cost of bone density studies limits the feasibility of performing this test as frequently as may be required to monitor treatment.

Because the levels of BTMs vary according to the time of day and bone volume, these studies are not widely used or helpful in screening for detection of osteoporosis. Their use is in determining the effect of treatment by comparing BTMs with pretreatment levels. Levels will decline with the use of antiresorption drugs (e.g., estrogen, bisphosphonates, calcitonin, raloxifene). BTMs have been shown to be accurately predictive of early improvement in bone mineral density and antifracture treatment efficacy. BTMs are also useful in documenting treatment compliance.

N- and *C-telopeptides (NTx and CTx)* are protein fragments used in type 1 collagen that make up nearly 90% of the bone matrix. The *C* and *N* terminals of these proteins are crosslinked to provide tensile strength to the bone. When bone breaks down, CTx and NTx are released into the bloodstream and excreted in the urine. Serum levels of these fragments have been shown to correlate well with urine measurements normalized to creatinine. Measurements of these fragments show early response to antiresorptive therapy (within 3 to 6 months) and are good indicators of bone resorption. Normal levels may vary with the method of testing.

Amino-terminal propeptide of type 1 procollagen (P1NP), like NTx, is directly proportional to the amount of new collagen produced by osteoblasts. Concentrations are increased in patients with various bone diseases that are characterized by increased osteoblastic activity. P1NP is the most effective marker of bone formation and is particularly useful for monitoring bone formation therapies and antiresorptive therapies.

Osteocalcin, or *bone G1a protein (BGP)*, is a noncollagenous protein in the bone and is made by osteoblasts. It enters the circulation during bone resorption and bone formation; it is a good indicator of bone metabolism. Serum levels of BGP correlate with bone formation and destruction (turnover). Increased levels are associated with increased bone mineral density loss. BGP is a vitamin K–dependent protein. A reduced vitamin K intake is associated with reduced BGP levels. This probably explains the pathophysiology of vitamin K–dependent deficiency osteoporosis.

Pyridinium (PYD) crosslinks are formed during maturation of the type 1 collagen during bone formation. During bone resorption, these PYD crosslinks are released into the circulation.

Bone-specific alkaline phosphatase (BSAP) is an isoenzyme of alkaline phosphatase (p. 29) and is found in the cell membrane of the osteoblast. It is, therefore, an indicator of the metabolic status of osteoblasts and bone formation.

These BTMs cannot indicate the risk of bone fracture nearly as well as a bone density measurement scan. These markers can be used to monitor the activity and treatment of Paget disease, hyperparathyroidism, and bone metastasis.

BTMs are normally high in children because of increased bone resorption associated with growth and remodeling of the ends of the long bones. The levels reach a peak at about age 14 and then gradually decline to adult values. Because estrogen is a strong inhibitor of osteoclastic (bone resorption) activity, loss of bone density begins soon after menopause begins. Marker levels therefore rise after menopause. Most urinary assays are correlated with creatinine excretion for normalization.

Interfering factors

- Measurements of these urinary markers can differ by as much as 30% in one person, even on the same day. Collecting double-voided specimens in the morning can minimize variability.
- Bodybuilding treatments, such as testosterone, can cause reduced levels of NTx.

Procedure and patient care

- See inside front cover for Routine Blood Testing.
- Fasting: yes

- Blood tube commonly used: verify with lab
- It is important to obtain baseline levels before instituting therapy.
- See inside front cover for Routine Urine Testing.

Urine
- Preferably, obtain a double-voided specimen.
- Collect the urine specimen 30 to 40 minutes before the time the specimen is needed.
- Discard this first specimen.
- Give the patient a glass of water to drink.
- At the requested time, obtain a second specimen.

Blood
- Collect a venous blood sample in a red-top tube for NTx and/or a lavender- or green-top tube for osteocalcin. Check with the laboratory for guidelines with other markers.

Abnormal findings

▲ **Increased levels**
  Osteoporosis
  Paget disease of bone
  Advanced bone tumors
    (primary or metastatic)
  Acromegaly
  Hyperparathyroidism
  Hyperthyroidism

▼ **Decreased levels**
  Hypoparathyroidism
  Hypothyroidism
  Cortisol therapy
  Effective antiresorptive
    therapy

notes

bone x-ray

Type of test X-ray

Normal findings No evidence of fracture, tumor, infection, or congenital abnormalities

Test explanation and related physiology

X-ray images of the long bones are usually taken when the patient has complaints about a particular body area. Fractures or tumors are readily detectable by x-ray studies. In patients who have a severe or chronic infection overlying a bone (osteomyelitis), an x-ray image may detect the infection involving that bone. X-ray studies of the long bones also can detect joint destruction and bone spurring as a result of persistent arthritis. Growth patterns can be followed by serial x-ray studies of a long bone, usually the wrists and hands. Healing of a fracture can be documented and followed. X-ray images of the joints reveal the presence of joint effusions and soft tissue swelling as well. Calcifications in the soft tissue indicate chronic inflammatory changes of the nearby bursa or tendons. Soft tissue swelling also can be seen on these bone x-rays. Because the cartilage and tendons are not directly visualized, cartilage fractures, sprains, or ligamentous injuries cannot be seen.

At least two x-rays at 90-degree angles are required so that the bone region being studied can be visualized from two different angles (usually anterior to posterior and lateral). Some bone studies (e.g., skull, spine, hip) require oblique views to visualize all the parts that need to be seen.

Interfering factors

- Jewelry or clothing can obstruct radiographic visualization of part of the bone to be evaluated.
- Prior barium studies can diminish the full radiographic visualization of some of the bones surrounding the abdomen (e.g., spine and pelvis).

Procedure and patient care

Before

PT Explain the procedure to the patient.

- Handle carefully any injured parts of the patient's body.

PT Instruct the patient that he or she will need to keep the extremity still while the x-ray image is being taken. This can sometimes be difficult, especially when the patient has severe pain associated with a recent injury.

- Shield the patient's testes, ovaries, or pregnant abdomen to avoid exposure from scattered radiation.
- **PT** Tell the patient that no fasting or sedation is required.

During

- Note that, in the x-ray department, the patient is asked to place the involved extremity in several positions. An x-ray image is taken of each position.
- Note that this test is routinely performed by a radiologic technologist within several minutes.
- **PT** Tell the patient that no discomfort is associated with this test, except possibly from moving an injured extremity.

After

- Administer an analgesic for relief of pain if indicated.

Abnormal findings

Fractures
Congenital bone disorders (e.g., achondroplasia, dysplasia, dysostosis)
Tumors (osteogenic sarcoma, Paget disease, myeloma, or metastatic)
Infection/osteomyelitis
Osteoporosis/osteopenia
Joint destruction (arthritis)
Bone spurring
Abnormal growth pattern
Joint effusion
Foreign bodies

notes

brain scan (Cisternogram, Cerebral blood flow, DaT scan)

Type of test Nuclear scan

Normal findings No areas of altered radionuclide uptake within the brain.

Test explanation and related physiology

The usefulness of a nuclear brain scan is narrow when compared with computed tomography (CT), magnetic resonance imaging (MRI), and positron emission tomography (PET) scans of the brain. Primarily, a nuclear brain scan is used to indicate complete and irreversible cessation of brain function (brain death). This determination, when combined with appropriate clinical data, allows for cessation of medical therapy and opportunity for the harvest of potential donor organs. With brain death, there is complete absence of blood perfusion to the brain.

The brain scan can also be used to indicate cerebral vascular occlusion or stenosis. With the use of Diamox (acetazolamide), an accurate assessment of local cerebral blood flow can be determined. Diamox is a carbonic anhydrase inhibitor that results in the elevation of Pco_2 in the bloodstream. Normally, this causes dilatation of the cerebral blood vessels. If asymmetric blood flow is noted after Diamox injection, cerebral vascular occlusion or stenosis can be suspected.

Brain scans are also used to investigate the ventricular system (cisternogram) of the central nervous system. Normal pressure hydrocephalus and ventricular shunt dysfunction can be identified and located.

Contraindications

- Patients who are pregnant unless the benefits outweigh the risk of fetal damage
- Patients who cannot cooperate during the testing

Interfering factors

⚑ Many sedative drugs can affect brain nuclear imaging.
⚑ Angiotensin-converting enzyme (ACE) inhibitors, vasoconstrictors, and vasodilators can alter blood flow distribution in nuclear brain imaging.

Procedure and patient care

Before

PT Explain the procedure to the patient.
- Administer blocking agents as ordered before scanning.
- Consider having a sedative ordered for agitated patients.

During

- Note the following procedural steps:
  1. After administration of the radioisotope, the patient is placed in the supine position while planar and single-photon emission computed tomography (SPECT) images are obtained.
  2. When cerebral flow studies are performed, the counter is immediately placed over the head.
  3. The counts are anatomically recorded in timed sequence to follow the isotope during its first flow through the brain.
- Note that this study is performed by a technologist in the nuclear medicine department in approximately 35 to 45 minutes.

After

Because only tracer doses of radioisotopes are used, inform the patient that no precautions need to be taken to prevent radioactive exposure to other personnel or family present.

Encourage the patient to drink fluids to aid in the excretion of the isotope from the body.

Abnormal findings

Cerebral death
Cerebral vascular stenosis/occlusion
Cerebral neoplasm
CSF leakage
Hydrocephalus

notes

breast cancer genomics (Oncotype DX, Genotyping, MammaPrint)

Type of test Microscopic examination

Normal findings Recurrence score <18

Test explanation and related physiology

Genomic testing using either Oncotype DX or MammaPrint is a clinically validated, multigene assay that provides a quantitative assessment of the likelihood of distant breast cancer recurrence; it also assesses the benefit from certain types of chemotherapy in newly diagnosed breast cancer patients. In early stage invasive breast cancer, the evaluation of the likelihood of distant recurrence is usually based on multiple pathologic factors, such as nodal status, tumor size, tumor grade, estrogen and progesterone receptors, and *HER-2* status (see p. 184). However, these factors are often inaccurate and cannot quantify the recurrence risk sufficiently to provide significant insight into the risks and benefits of adjuvant chemotherapy. Genomic testing is designed to provide quantitative data to assist in clinical decision making regarding the use of adjuvant systemic therapies.

The Oncotype DX rtPCR assay—performed using formalin-fixed, paraffin-embedded tumor tissue—analyzes the expression of a panel of 21 genes (16 tumor-related genes and 5 reference genes) and provides the results as a recurrence score (0 to 100). The gene panel was selected and the recurrence score calculation derived through extensive laboratory testing followed by appropriate corroboration with multiple clinical studies in which Oncotype DX predictability was validated. The MammaPrint, using microarray assay on fresh-frozen breast cancer tissue, analyzes the expression of 70 prognostic genes. A 5-gene IHC assay, the Mammostrat, uses monoclonal antibody biomarkers and a diagnostic algorithm with fresh-frozen cancer tissue. Molecular genomics is sensitive, specific, and highly reproducible, and has a wide dynamic range.

Patients whose tumor genomics have low recurrence scores have only a slight chance of recurrence and derive minimal or no benefit from chemotherapy. Patients with tumors that have high recurrence scores have a significant chance of recurrence and can experience considerable benefit from chemotherapy. At present, genomic testing is intended for newly diagnosed patients whose breast cancer is stage I or II, node negative, *HER-2/neu* negative, and estrogen receptor positive. Clinical studies in other populations are currently underway.

Procedure and patient care

Before

PT Explain the significance of the prognostic data available for the patient's tumor.

PT Explain the benefits of genomics in helping the physician and the patient make appropriate decisions regarding the use of adjuvant chemotherapy.

• Provide the patient with emotional support through the postoperative period.

• Ensure that the patient's insurance will cover this expensive testing.

During

• The pathologist will send paraffin-embedded tissue to the centralized laboratory.

• Results will be available in about 2 weeks.

After

PT Provide education and support to patients as they evaluate their results.

Abnormal findings

Aggressive breast cancer

notes

breast cancer tumor analysis (DNA ploidy status, S-phase fraction, Cathepsin D, HER-2 [c erbB2, neu] protein, p53 protein, Ki67 protein)

Type of test Microscopic examination

Normal findings

DNA ploidy
>Aneuploid is unfavorable.
>Diploid is favorable.

S-phase fraction
>>5.5% is unfavorable.
><5.5% is favorable.

HER-2 protein
>IHC method: 0 to 1+
>FISH method: <2 copies/cell
>Oncotype DX method: <10.7 units

Cathepsin D
>>10% is unfavorable.
><10% is favorable.

p53 protein
>>10% is unfavorable.
><10% is favorable.

Ki67 protein
>>20% is unfavorable.
>10% to 20% is borderline.
><20% is favorable.

Test explanation and related physiology

The most important predictor of recurrent breast cancer is stage of disease, including lymph node status. Patients with positive lymph node metastasis are more likely to develop recurrence. However, nearly 30% of the patients whose tumors have been completely removed and who have no evidence of lymph node metastasis will also develop recurrence. Conventional predictors such as tumor size, grade, histologic type, and hormone receptors (see p. 408) are able to identify some of those patients who are at increased risk for recurrence. However, it is important to accurately predict the patients who are destined for recurrence so they can be selected for systemic therapy; patients who will not have a recurrence can be spared the morbidity of a treatment that is not needed.

DNA ploidy status and S-phase fraction

Measurement of the rapidity with which the cells in a breast cancer grow includes ploidy status and S-phase analysis. Normally, cells are diploid (one set of paired chromosomes) and have a small number of cells in the S phase of cell division. During the mitotic phase of cell division, the amount of DNA doubles (two sets of paired chromosomes) in preparation for cell division. Because the more aggressive cancer cells divide more rapidly, many cells are in various stages of the mitotic phase. These cells may have a variable number of chromosome sets (aneuploid).

It has been noted that the more aggressive cancer cells are more often in S phase (a time of DNA replication where the amount of DNA in the cell doubles while ploidy remains unchanged). This is usually reported as S-phase fraction (SPF), which is the number of cells in S phase divided by the total number of cancer cells in the particular specimen.

Cathepsin D

This protein catabolic enzyme was found to be absent in resting breast tissue but significantly elevated in malignant tissue. This protein exists on tumor cell membrane and is correlated with worse clinical outcomes. The exact cutoff point between a favorable prognosis and unfavorable prognosis has yet to be standardized.

HER-2 (c erbB2, neu) protein

HER-2/neu, which stands for *human epidermal growth factor receptor 2*, is a protein associated with worse clinical outcomes. The *HER-2/neu* oncogene encodes a transmembrane tyrosine kinase receptor with extensive similarity to other epidermal growth factor receptors. It is normally involved in the pathways leading to cell growth and survival. Approximately 15% to 20% of breast cancers have an amplification of the *HER-2/neu* gene or overexpression of its protein product.

There are two commonly used methods to measure *HER-2/neu* protein, *immunohistochemistry (IHC)* and *fluorescence in situ hybridization (FISH)*. *HER-2* testing is also helpful in making treatment decisions. The *HER-2* gene can act as a target for an antineoplastic monoclonal antibody drug such as trastuzumab (Herceptin).

p53 protein

The p53 gene is a tumor suppressor gene that is overexpressed in more aggressive breast cancer cells. Mutation of the gene causes overexpression and a buildup of mutant proteins on the surface of the cancer cells.

Ki67 protein

The Ki67 gene encodes the synthesis for Ki67 protein that is associated with worse clinical outcomes.

Interfering factors

- Delay in tissue fixation may cause deterioration of marker proteins and may produce lower values.
- ☑ Preoperative use of some chemotherapy agents may cause *decreased* levels of some marker proteins.

Procedure and patient care

Before

PT Inform the patient that an examination for these tumor predictor markers may be performed on their breast cancer tissue.

PT Provide psychological and emotional support to the breast cancer patient.

During

- The surgeon obtains tumor tissue.
- This tissue should be placed on ice or in formalin.
- Part of the tissue is used for routine histology. A portion of the paraffin block is sent to a reference laboratory.

After

PT Explain to the patient that results are usually available in 1 week.

Abnormal findings

Unfavorable test results indicating a risk of cancer reoccurrence

notes

breast ductal lavage

Type of test Fluid analysis

Normal findings No atypical cells in the effluent

Possible critical values Cancer cells in the effluent

Test explanation and related physiology

The theory behind ductal lavage is that by washing out exfoliated cells from a few breast ducts, the risk of breast cancer developing in the near future can be assessed. If atypical cells are obtained, the risk of breast cancer developing in the next decade may be as high as 4 to 10 times normal. Once that risk is identified, the patient may choose to attempt to alter that risk by using chemopreventative medications (e.g., selective estrogen receptor modulators) or surgery.

Initially, it was hoped that ductal lavage would be able to identify ductal carcinoma of the breast at its earliest stages. The results of several large studies did not support that fact. Its use has now been limited to women who have been found to be at a statistically higher risk for breast cancer by *Gail or Claus breast cancer risk models.* These statistical models are based on age at menarche, age at first pregnancy, prior breast surgery, family history, and history of atypical changes in previous breast biopsies. Many women found to be at increased risk would like more data before they decide to take a medication designed to reduce those risks. If these women were found to have atypical cells in the lavage, most would choose to take the medication. If no atypical cells were found, they might choose close observation only.

There are still no data to confirm that the findings do accurately reflect a true risk for breast cancer. Furthermore, there are no data to indicate what a negative lavage means.

Contraindications

- Patients with prior breast cancer surgery, because their risks are already known to be high

Potential complications

- Infection

Procedure and patient care

Before

PT Explain the procedure to the patient. Often these women have already received extensive counseling regarding their risk of breast cancer.

- Be sure the breast exam and mammogram are normal.
- Apply a topical anesthetic to the nipple area about ½ hour before the test.

During

- Note the following procedural steps:
  1. A suction apparatus is applied to the nipple area. Ducts that reveal fluid with the suction are then chosen for cannulation.
  2. A tiny catheter is gently placed into the nipple duct, and the duct is lavaged with 1 to 3 mL of saline.
  3. The effluent is collected in a small tube and sent for cytology.
  4. The procedure is then repeated for the other ducts that produced fluid with nipple suction.
- This procedure is performed by a surgeon in the office. There is minimal to moderate discomfort associated with the nipple suction, duct cannulation, and lavage.

After

PT Inform the patient of the possibility of mild breast discomfort.

- Arrange for follow-up to discuss test results.

PT Provide counseling if results indicate atypical or malignant cells.

Abnormal findings

Atypical cells

Ductal cancer cells

notes

breast ultrasonography (Ultrasound mammography, Breast sonogram)

Type of test Ultrasound

Normal findings No evidence of cyst or tumor

Test explanation and related physiology

Ultrasound examination of the breast is diagnostically performed to determine if a mammographic abnormality or a palpable lump is a cyst (fluid-filled) or a solid tumor (benign or malignant). It is also used in screening for breast cancer in women whose breasts are dense on mammography.

In diagnostic real-time ultrasonography, harmless high-frequency sound waves are emitted and penetrate the breast. The sound waves are reflected back to the sensor and are arranged in a pictorial image by electronic conversion. Ultrasonography of the breast is used to:

- Differentiate cystic from solid breast lesions.
- Identify masses in women with breast tissue too dense for accurate mammography.
- Monitor a cyst to determine whether it enlarges or disappears.
- Measure the size of a tumor.
- Evaluate the axilla in women who are newly diagnosed with breast cancer.

Ultrasonography is also useful for examination of symptomatic breasts in women in whom the radiation of mammography is potentially harmful. These include:

- Pregnant women. Radiation may be harmful to the fetus.
- Women younger than age 25, who may be at greater oncologic risk from the radiation of mammography.
- Women who refuse mammography because of unreasonable fear of diagnostic radiation.

With high-quality diagnostic ultrasonography, the characteristics of an abnormality can be evaluated and a reasonable prediction can be made whether it is malignant. Diagnostic accuracy is improved when breast ultrasonography is combined with mammography (see p. 624). Ultrasound is especially useful in patients with an abnormal mass identified on a mammogram, because the nature (cystic or solid) of the mass can be determined. Most cysts are benign.

Ultrasound can be used to locate and accurately direct percutaneous biopsy probes to a nonpalpable breast abnormality for biopsy or aspiration. Ultrasound is painless, harmless, and with-out any radiation effects on the breast tissue.

Procedure and patient care

Before

PT Explain the procedure to the patient.

PT Assure the patient that no discomfort is associated with this study.

PT Inform the patient that no fasting or sedation is required before the tests. Instruct the patient not to apply any lotions or powders to the breasts on the examination day.

During

- The patient is placed in the supine position, and the trans-ducer is directly applied to the breast using contact gel to improve sound transmission.
- Note that this test is performed by an ultrasound technician in approximately 15 minutes.
- There is no discomfort associated with this procedure.

After

- After the test is completed, the breasts are dried and the con-ductive paste is removed.

Abnormal findings

Cyst
Hematoma
Cancer
Fibroadenoma
Fibrocystic disease
Abscess

notes

bronchoscopy

Type of test Endoscopy

Normal findings Normal larynx, trachea, bronchi, and alveoli

Test explanation and related physiology

Bronchoscopy permits endoscopic visualization of the larynx, trachea, and bronchi by either a flexible fiberoptic bronchoscope or a rigid bronchoscope. There are many diagnostic and therapeutic uses for bronchoscopy.

Diagnostic uses of bronchoscopy include:
- Direct visualization of the tracheobronchial tree for abnormalities (e.g., tumors, inflammation, strictures)
- Biopsy of tissue from observed lesions
- Aspiration of deep sputum for culture, sensitivity, and cytology determinations
- Direct visualization of the larynx for identification of vocal cord paralysis if present

Therapeutic uses of bronchoscopy include:
- Aspiration of retained secretions in patients with airway obstruction or postoperative atelectasis
- Control of bleeding within the bronchus
- Removal of foreign bodies that have been aspirated
- Brachytherapy, which is endobronchial radiation therapy using an iridium wire placed via the bronchoscope
- Palliative laser obliteration of bronchial neoplastic obstruction

The *flexible fiberoptic bronchoscope* has accessory lumens through which cable-activated instruments can be used for removing biopsy specimens of pathologic lesions. Also, the collection of bronchial washings (obtained by flushing the airways with saline solution), pulmonary toilet, and the instillation of anesthetic agents can be carried out through these extra lumens. Double-sheathed, plugged-protected brushes also can be passed through this accessory lumen. Specimens for cytology and bacteriology can be obtained with these brushes. This allows more accurate determination of pulmonary infectious agents. Needles can be placed through the scope to obtain biopsies from tissue immediately adjacent to the bronchi. Laser therapy to burn out endotracheal lesions can now be performed through the bronchoscope.

Laryngoscopy is often performed through a short bronchoscope to allow inspection of the larynx and paralaryngeal structures. This is most commonly performed by an ENT surgeon. Cancers, polyps, inflammation, and infections of those structures can be identified. The vocal cord motion can be evaluated also. Anesthesiologists use laryngoscopy to visualize the vocal cord structures on patients who are difficult to intubate for general anesthesia. In this instance, the laryngoscope is shaped very much like a rigid scope routinely used to see the vocal cords under direct visualization using retraction of the anterior neck during intubation. This endoscopic laryngoscope, however, is attached to a camera that projects the image of the vocal cords onto a monitor.

Contraindications

- Patients with hypercapnia and severe shortness of breath who cannot tolerate interruption of high-flow oxygen. However, bronchoscopy can be performed through a special oxygen mask or an endotracheal tube so that the patient can receive oxygen if required.
- Severe tracheal stenosis may make it difficult to pass the scope.

Potential complications

- Fever
- Hypoxemia
- Laryngospasm
- Bronchospasm
- Pneumothorax
- Aspiration
- Hemorrhage (after biopsy)

Procedure and patient care

Before

PT Explain the procedure to the patient. Allay any fears and allow the patient to verbalize any concerns.
- Obtain informed consent for this procedure.
- Keep the patient NPO for 4 to 8 hours before the test to reduce the risk of aspiration.
PT Instruct the patient to perform good mouth care to minimize the risk of introducing bacteria into the lungs during the procedure.
- Remove and safely store the patient's dentures, glasses, or contact lenses before administering the preprocedure medications.
- Administer the preprocedure medications as ordered.
PT Reassure the patient that he or she will be able to breathe during this procedure.

PT Instruct the patient not to swallow the local anesthetic sprayed into the throat. Provide a basin for expectoration of the lidocaine.

- Have emergency resuscitation equipment available.

During

- Note the following procedural steps for *fiberoptic bronchoscopy*:
  1. This test is performed by a pulmonary specialist or a surgeon at the bedside or in an appropriately equipped room.
  2. The patient's nasopharynx and oropharynx are anesthetized topically with lidocaine spray before insertion of the bronchoscope.
  3. The patient is placed in a sitting or supine position, and the tube is inserted through the nose or mouth and into the pharynx (Figure 7).
  4. After the tube is passed into the larynx and through the glottis, more lidocaine is sprayed into the trachea to prevent the cough reflex.
  5. The tube is passed farther, well into the trachea, bronchi, and first- and second-generation bronchioles, for systematic examination of the bronchial tree.
  6. Biopsy specimens and washings are taken if pathology is suspected.
  7. If bronchoscopy is performed for pulmonary toilet (removal of mucus), each bronchus is aspirated until it is clear.
- Note that this procedure is performed by a physician in approximately 30 to 45 minutes.

PT Tell the patient that because of sedation, no discomfort is usually felt.

After

PT Instruct the patient not to eat or drink anything until the tracheobronchial anesthesia has worn off and the gag reflex has returned, usually in approximately 2 hours.

- Observe the patient's sputum for hemorrhage if biopsy specimens were removed. A small amount of blood streaking may be expected and is normal for several hours after the procedure. Large amounts of bleeding can cause a chemical pneumonitis.
- Observe the patient closely for evidence of impaired respiration or laryngospasm. The vocal cords may go into spasms after intubation.

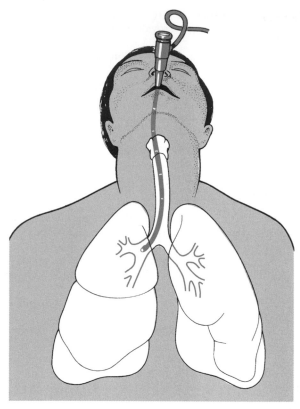

FIGURE 7 Bronchoscopy. A bronchoscope is inserted through the trachea and into the bronchus.

- **PT** Inform the patient that postbronchoscopy fever often develops within the first 24 hours. High, persistent fever should be reported immediately.
- If a tumor is suspected, collect a postbronchoscopy sputum sample for a cytology determination.
- **PT** Inform the patient that warm saline gargles and lozenges may be helpful if a sore throat develops.
- **PT** Inform the patient that biopsy or culture reports will be available in 2 to 7 days.

Abnormal findings

Inflammation
Strictures
Tuberculosis
Cancer
Hemorrhage
Foreign body
Abscess
Infection

notes

CA 15-3 and CA 27.29 tumor markers (Cancer antigen 15-3, Cancer antigen 27.29)

Type of test Blood

Normal findings

CA 15-3: <31 units/mL or <31 kU/L (SI units)
CA 27.29: <38 units/mL or <38 kU/L (SI units)

Test explanation and related physiology

CA 15-3 and CA 27.29 are tumor-associated serum markers available for staging breast cancer and monitoring its treatment. CA 15-3 or CA 27.29 levels are high in less than 50% of patients who have a localized breast cancer or a small tumor burden. Of patients with metastatic breast cancer, however, 80% do have elevated CA 15-3 levels, and 65% have elevated CA 27.29 levels. Therefore, the usefulness of these antigen tests as a screening technique in early breast cancers is quite limited. Benign breast disease and nonbreast malignancies also can cause elevation of these antigen levels.

Interfering factors

• Other benign and malignant diseases associated with elevations include cancer of the lung, ovary, pancreas, prostate, and colon; fibrocystic disease of the breast; cirrhosis; and hepatitis.

Procedure and patient care

• See inside front cover for Routine Blood Testing.
• Fasting: no.
• Blood tube commonly used: red.
• The blood sample may be sent to a central diagnostic laboratory. The results may not be available for 7 to 10 days.

Abnormal findings

▲ **Increased levels**
Metastatic breast cancer

notes

CA 19-9 tumor marker (Cancer antigen 19-9)

Type of test Blood

Normal findings <37 units/mL or <37 kU/L (SI units)

Test explanation and related physiology

CA 19-9 is a tumor marker used in diagnosis, evaluation of a patient's response to treatment, and surveillance of patients with pancreatic or hepatobiliary cancer. CA 19-9 is a carbohydrate antigen that exists on the surface of cancer cells. In the diagnosis of pancreatic carcinoma, the presence of a pancreatic mass or biliary obstruction and greatly elevated CA 19-9 levels would support pancreatic cancer as the diagnosis over benign pancreatitis. Likewise, patients whose symptoms are ascites, jaundice, and elevated CA 19-9 levels would be suspected of having hepatobiliary cancer. Approximately 70% of patients with pancreatic carcinoma and 65% of patients with hepatobiliary cancer have elevated levels.

CA 19-9 levels are used in the posttreatment surveillance of those who have had pancreatic or hepatobiliary cancers. In the few patients with pancreatic or biliary cancers who have a positive response to surgery, chemotherapy, or radiation therapy, a decline in serum levels of CA 19-9 will confirm this response. A rapid rise in CA 19-9 levels may be associated with a recurrent or progressive tumor growth. Mildly elevated levels may exist in patients with gastric cancer, colorectal cancer, or hepatoma and even in 6% to 7% of patients with nongastrointestinal malignancies. Patients who have pancreatitis, gallstones, cirrhosis, inflammatory bowel disease, or cystic fibrosis also can have minimally elevated levels of CA 19-9.

Because of its lack of sensitivity and specificity, CA 19-9 is not effective in screening for pancreaticobiliary tumors in the general population.

Procedure and patient care

- See inside front cover for Routine Blood Testing.
- Fasting: no.
- Blood tube commonly used: red.
- The blood may be sent to a central diagnostic laboratory for CA 19-9 determinations. The results may not be available for 7 to 10 days.

Abnormal findings

▲ **Increased levels**
   Pancreatic carcinoma
   Hepatobiliary carcinoma
   Pancreatitis
   Cholecystitis
   Cirrhosis
   Gastric cancer
   Colorectal cancer
   Gallstones
   Cystic fibrosis
   Lung cancer
   Inflammatory bowel disease
   Rheumatoid diseases

notes

CA-125 tumor marker (Cancer antigen-125)

Type of test Blood

Normal findings 0-35 units/mL or <35 kU/L (SI units)

Test explanation and related physiology

CA-125 is an extremely accurate marker for nonmucinous epithelial tumors of the ovary. It is elevated in more than 80% of women with ovarian cancer. This tumor marker has a high degree of sensitivity and specificity for ovarian cancer and has been of great benefit to clinicians.

The CA-125 serum tumor marker is also used to determine a patient's response to therapy. Serial comparative testing will show a progressive decline in CA-125 levels for patients responding to treatment. Also, CA-125 tumor markers can predict whether a second-look (repeat) diagnostic laparotomy will be positive. A second-look laparotomy will detect a residual tumor in 97% of patients whose CA-125 level is greater than 35 units/mL, whereas only 56% of patients with ovarian cancer whose CA-125 level is less than 35 units/mL will have a positive second-look laparotomy. A precipitous fall in CA-125 after two courses of chemotherapy is an accurate predictor of a complete response to chemotherapy and is used as a good prognostic sign.

Finally, CA-125 determinations can be used in posttreatment surveillance of patients with ovarian cancer. In a patient who has had a complete response as a result of radiation therapy, chemotherapy, or surgery, a delayed rise in the CA-125 level is an early predictor of a recurrent tumor in 93% of patients. Abnormal levels can antedate the appearance of obvious recurrent ovarian cancer by 2 to 7 months.

CA-125 is not an effective screening test for the asymptomatic general public because of its lack of specificity. It is used in a high-risk population of women who have a strong family history of ovarian cancer. Elevated levels in the general population indicate that either benign or malignant disease is present in 95% of patients.

Other tumors and benign processes can cause elevated CA-125 levels as well. Diseases that affect the peritoneum, such as cirrhosis, pancreatitis, peritonitis, endometriosis, and pelvic inflammatory disease, can create elevated levels of CA-125. Other malignancies occurring in the female genital tract, pancreas, colon, lung, and breast can also be associated with elevated levels of this protein. Of the normal population, 1% to 2% have CA-125 levels in excess of 35 units/mL.

Interfering factors

- The first trimester of pregnancy and normal menstruation may be associated with mild elevations of CA-125 levels.
- Patients with benign peritoneal diseases (e.g., cirrhosis, endometriosis) have mildly increased levels.
- Smoking can falsely increase CA-125 values.
- Patients who have had recent abdominal surgery may have elevated levels for as long as 3 weeks after surgery.

Procedure and patient care

- See inside front cover for Routine Blood Testing.
- Fasting: no.
- Blood tube commonly used: red.
- The blood may be sent to a central diagnostic laboratory for determination of the CA-125 level. The results are usually available in 3 to 7 days.

Abnormal findings

▲ Increased levels

Malignant disorders
Cancer of the ovary
Cancer of the pancreas
Cancer of the nonovarian female genital tract
Cancer of the breast
Cancer of the colon
Cancer of the lung
Lymphoma
Peritoneal carcinomatosis
Benign disorders
Cirrhosis
Peritonitis
Pregnancy
Endometriosis
Pancreatitis
Pelvic inflammatory disease

notes

calcitonin (Human calcitonin [HCT], Thyrocalcitonin)

Type of test Blood

Normal findings

Basal (plasma)
  Males: ≤19 pg/mL or ≤19 ng/L (SI units)
  Females: ≤14 pg/mL or ≤14 ng/L (SI units)
Calcium infusion (2.4 mg/kg)
  Males: ≤190 pg/mL or ≤190 ng/L
  Females: ≤130 pg/mL or ≤130 ng/L
Pentagastrin injection (0.5 mcg/kg)
  Males: ≤110 pg/mL or ≤110 ng/L
  Females: ≤30 pg/mL or ≤30 ng/L

Test explanation and related physiology

Calcitonin is a hormone secreted by the parafollicular or C cells of the thyroid gland. Its secretion is stimulated by elevated serum calcium levels. The purpose of calcitonin is to contribute to calcium homeostasis.

This test is usually used in the evaluation of patients with or suspected to have medullary carcinoma of the thyroid. Calcitonin is also useful in monitoring response to therapy for and predicting recurrences of medullary thyroid cancer and as a screening test for those with a family history of medullary cancer (who are therefore at high risk for medullary cancer). This is a cancer of the thyroid with a familial tendency; if it is found late, it has a poor prognosis. Routine screening for elevated calcitonin levels can detect medullary cancer early and can improve chances for cure. C-cell hyperplasia, a benign calcitonin-producing disease that also has a familial tendency, is also associated with elevated calcitonin levels.

Equivocal elevations in calcitonin levels should be followed with further provocative testing using pentagastrin or calcium to stimulate calcitonin secretion. *Pentagastrin stimulation* involves an IV infusion with blood samples drawn before the injection and at 90 seconds, 2 minutes, and 5 minutes after the infusion. The *calcium infusion test* can be performed in a variety of ways but is most commonly administered with baseline and 5- and 10-minute postinfusion blood levels.

Elevated levels of calcitonin also may be seen in people with cancer of the lung, breast, or pancreas. This is probably a form of paraneoplastic syndrome in which there is an ectopic production of calcitonin by the nonthyroid cancer cells.

Interfering factors

- Levels are often elevated in pregnancy and in newborns.
- ✘ Drugs that may cause *increased* levels include calcium, cholecystokinin, epinephrine, glucagon, pentagastrin, and oral contraceptives.

Procedure and patient care

- See inside front cover for Routine Blood Testing.
- Fasting: yes.
- Blood tube commonly used: green or red.
- Collect a venous sample of blood in a heparinized green-top tube or a chilled red-top tube according to the laboratory's protocol.
- The specimen should be placed on ice immediately. The blood may be frozen and sent to a reference laboratory.
- PT Tell the patient that results may not be available for several days.

Abnormal findings

▲ Increased levels
  Medullary carcinoma of the thyroid
  C-cell hyperplasia
  Oat cell carcinoma of the lung
  Breast carcinoma
  Pancreatic cancer
  Primary hyperparathyroidism
  Secondary hyperparathyroidism because of chronic renal
    failure
  Pernicious anemia
  Zollinger-Ellison syndrome
  Alcoholic cirrhosis
  Thyroiditis

notes

calcium (Total/ionized calcium, Ca, Serum calcium)

Type of test Blood; urine

Normal findings

Age	mg/dL	mmol/L
Total calcium		
<10 days	7.6–10.4	1.9–2.6
Umbilical	9.0–11.5	2.25–2.88
10 days-2 years	9.0–10.6	2.3–2.65
Child	8.8–10.8	2.2–2.7
Adult*	9.0–10.5	2.25–2.62
Ionized calcium		
Newborn	4.20–5.58	1.05–1.37
2 months-18 years	4.80–5.52	1.20–1.38
Adult	4.5–5.6	1.05–1.3

*In elderly individuals, values tend to decrease.

Possible critical values

Total calcium: <6 or >13 mg/dL
Ionized calcium: <2.2 or >7 mg/dL

Test explanation and related physiology

The serum calcium test is used to evaluate parathyroid function and calcium metabolism by directly measuring the total amount of calcium in the blood. Determination of serum calcium is used to monitor patients with renal failure, renal transplantation, hyperparathyroidism, and various malignancies. It is also used to monitor calcium levels during and after large-volume blood transfusions.

About half the total calcium in the blood exists in its free (ionized) form, and about half exists in its protein-bound form (mostly with albumin). The serum calcium level is a measure of both. As a result, when the serum albumin level is low (as in malnourished patients), the serum calcium level will also be low and vice versa. As a rule of thumb, the total serum calcium level decreases by approximately 0.8 mg for every 1-g decrease in the serum albumin level. Serum albumin should be measured with serum calcium. An advantage of measuring only the ionized form is that it is unaffected by changes in serum albumin levels.

When the serum calcium level is elevated on at least three separate determinations, the patient is said to have *hypercalcemia*. The most common cause of hypercalcemia is hyperparathyroidism.

Parathyroid hormone (see p. 689) causes elevated calcium levels by increasing gastrointestinal absorption, decreasing urinary excretion, and increasing bone resorption. Malignancy, the second most common cause of hypercalcemia, can cause elevated calcium levels in two main ways. First, tumor metastasis (myeloma, lung, breast, renal cell) to the bone can destroy the bone, causing resorption and pushing calcium into the blood. Second, the cancer (lung, breast, renal cell) can produce a parathyroid hormone–like substance that drives the serum calcium up (ectopic PTH). Excess vitamin D ingestion can increase serum calcium by increasing renal and gastrointestinal absorption. Granulomatous infections, such as sarcoidosis and tuberculosis, are associated with hypercalcemia.

Hypocalcemia occurs in patients with hypoalbuminemia. The most common causes of hypoalbuminemia are malnutrition (especially in alcoholics) and large-volume IV infusions. Large blood transfusions are associated with low serum calcium levels because the citrate additives used in banked blood for anticoagulation bind the free calcium in the recipient's bloodstream. Intestinal malabsorption, renal failure, rhabdomyolysis, alkalosis, and acute pancreatitis (caused by saponification of fat) are also known to be associated with low serum calcium levels. Hypomagnesemia can be associated with refractory hypocalcemia.

Urinary calcium can also be measured. Excretion of calcium in the urine is increased in all patients with hypercalcemia. Urinary calcium levels are decreased in patients with hypocalcemia. The test is helpful in determining the cause of recurrent nephrolithiasis.

Interfering factors

- Vitamin D intoxication may cause increased calcium levels.
- Excessive ingestion of milk may cause increased levels.
- Serum pH can affect calcium values. A decrease in pH causes increased calcium levels.
- Prolonged tourniquet time will lower pH and falsely increase calcium levels.
- There is normally a small diurnal variation in calcium, with peak levels occurring around 9 PM.
- Hypoalbuminemia is artifactually associated with decreased levels of total calcium.
- Drugs that may cause *increased* serum levels include alkaline antacids, androgens, calcium salts, ergocalciferol, hydralazine, lithium, parathyroid hormone (PTH), thiazide diuretics, thyroid hormone, and vitamin D.

❧ Drugs that may cause *decreased* serum levels include acetazolamide, albuterol, anticonvulsants, asparaginase, aspirin, calcitonin, cisplatin, corticosteroids, diuretics, estrogens, heparin, laxatives, loop diuretics, magnesium salts, and oral contraceptives.

C

Procedure and patient care

- See inside front cover for Routine Blood Testing.
- Fasting: verify with lab.
- Blood tube commonly used: red.

Abnormal findings

▲ **Increased levels (hypercalcemia)**
Hyperparathyroidism
Nonparathyroid PTH-
  producing tumor
  (e.g., lung or renal
  carcinoma)
Metastatic tumor to the
  bone
Paget disease of bone
Prolonged immobilization
Milk-alkali syndrome
Vitamin D intoxication
Lymphoma
Granulomatous infections
  (e.g., sarcoidosis and
  tuberculosis)
Addison disease
Acromegaly
Hyperthyroidism

▼ **Decreased levels (hypocalcemia)**
Hypoparathyroidism
Renal failure
Hyperphosphatemia
  secondary to renal failure
Rickets
Vitamin D deficiency
Osteomalacia
Malabsorption
Pancreatitis
Fat embolism
Alkalosis
Hypoalbuminemia

notes

caloric study (Oculovestibular reflex study)

Type of test   Electrodiagnostic

Normal findings   Nystagmus with irrigation

Test explanation and related physiology

Caloric studies are used to evaluate the vestibular portion of the eighth cranial nerve (CN VIII) by irrigating the external auditory canal with hot or cold water. This is considered a part of a complete neurological exam. Normally stimulation with cold water causes rotary nystagmus (involuntary rapid eye movement) away from the ear being irrigated; hot water induces nystagmus toward the side of the ear being irrigated. If the labyrinth is diseased or CN VIII is not functioning (e.g., from tumor compression), no nystagmus is induced. This study aids in the differential diagnosis of abnormalities that may occur in the vestibular system, brainstem, or cerebellum.

Contraindications

- Patients with a perforated eardrum
  Cold air may be substituted for the fluid, although this method is much less reliable.
- Patients with an acute disease of the labyrinth (e.g., Ménière syndrome)
  The test can be performed when the acute attack subsides.

Interfering factors

☑ Drugs such as sedatives and antivertigo agents can alter test results.

Procedure and patient care

Before

PT Explain the procedure to the patient.

PT Instruct the patient to avoid solid foods before the test to reduce the incidence of vomiting.

During

- Although the exact procedures for caloric studies vary, note the following steps in a typical test:
  1. Before the test, the patient is examined for the presence of nystagmus, postural deviation (Romberg sign), and past-pointing. This examination provides the baseline values for comparison during the test.

2. The ear canal should be examined and cleaned before testing to ensure that the water will freely flow to the middle ear area.

3. The ear on the suspected side is irrigated first because the patient's response may be minimal.

4. After an emesis basin is placed under the ear, the irrigation solution is directed into the external auditory canal until the patient complains of nausea and dizziness or nystagmus is seen. Usually this occurs in 20 to 30 seconds.

5. If after 3 minutes no symptoms occur, the irrigation is stopped.

6. The patient is tested again for nystagmus, past-pointing, and Romberg sign.

7. After approximately 5 minutes, the procedure is repeated on the other side.

- Note that this procedure is usually performed by a physician or technician in approximately 15 minutes.

PT Tell the patient that he or she will probably experience nausea and dizziness during the test.

After

- Usually place the patient on bed rest for approximately 30 to 60 minutes until nausea or vomiting subsides.
- Ensure patient safety related to dizziness.

Abnormal findings

Brainstem inflammation, infarction, or tumor
Cerebellar inflammation, infarction, or tumor
Vestibular or cochlear inflammation or tumor
Acoustic neuroma
Eighth nerve neuritis/neuropathy

notes

carbon dioxide content (CO$_2$ content, CO$_2$ combining power)

Type of test Blood

Normal findings

Adult/elderly: 23-30 mEq/L or 23-30 mmol/L (SI units)
Child: 20-28 mEq/L
Infant: 20-28 mEq/L
Newborn: 13-22 mEq/L

Possible critical values <6 mEq/L

Test explanation and related physiology

The CO$_2$ content is a measure of CO$_2$ in the blood. In the peripheral venous blood, this assists in evaluation of the pH status of the patient and in evaluation of electrolytes. The serum CO$_2$ test is usually included with other assessments of electrolytes. It is usually done with a multiphasic testing machine that also measures sodium, potassium, chloride, BUN, and creatinine.

It is important not to get this test confused with Pco_2. This CO$_2$ content measures the H$_2$CO$_3$, the dissolved CO$_2$, and the bicarbonate ion (HCO$_3$) that exists in the serum. Because the amounts of H$_2$CO$_3$ and dissolved CO$_2$ in the blood are so small, CO$_2$ content is an indirect measure of the HCO$_3$ anion. The HCO$_3$ anion is second in importance to the chloride ion in electrical neutrality (negative charge) of extracellular and intracellular fluid; its major role is in acid-base balance.

Levels of HCO$_3$ are regulated by the kidneys. Increases cause alkalosis, and decreases cause acidosis. See further discussion of this test as it is performed on arterial blood (p. 109). When CO$_2$ content is measured in the laboratory with other serum electrolytes, air affects the specimen and the CO$_2$ partial pressure can be altered. Therefore, venous blood specimens are not very accurate for true CO$_2$ content or HCO$_3$ determination. This test is used mostly as a rough guide to the patient's acid-base balance.

Interfering factors

- Underfilling the tube with blood allows CO$_2$ to escape from the serum specimen and may significantly decrease HCO$_3$ values.
- ✄ Drugs that may cause *increased* serum CO$_2$ and HCO$_3$ levels include aldosterone, barbiturates, bicarbonates, ethacrynic acid, hydrocortisone, loop diuretics, mercurial diuretics, and steroids.

✠ Drugs that may cause *decreased* levels include methicillin, nitrofurantoin (Furadantin), paraldehyde, phenformin hydrochloride, tetracycline, thiazide diuretics, and triamterene.

Procedure and patient care

- See inside front cover for Routine Blood Testing.
- Fasting: no.
- Blood tube commonly used: red or green.

Abnormal findings

▲ **Increased levels**
  Severe diarrhea
  Starvation
  Severe vomiting
  Aldosteronism
  Emphysema
  Metabolic alkalosis
  Gastric suction

▼ **Decreased levels**
  Renal failure
  Salicylate toxicity
  Diabetic ketoacidosis
  Metabolic acidosis
  Shock
  Starvation

notes

carboxyhemoglobin (COHb, Carbon monoxide)

Type of test Blood

Normal findings

Saturation of hemoglobin

Nonsmoker: <3%

Smoker: ≤12%

Newborn: ≥12%

Possible critical values >20%

Test explanation and related physiology

This test is used to detect carbon monoxide poisoning. It measures the amount of serum COHb, which is formed by the combination of carbon monoxide (CO) and hemoglobin (Hb). CO combines with Hb 200 times more readily than oxygen (O_2) can combine with Hb; thus fewer Hb bonds are available to combine with O_2. Furthermore, when CO occupies the O_2 binding sites, Hb is changed to bind the remaining O_2 more tightly. This greater affinity of CO for Hb and this change in O_2 binding strength do not allow O_2 to pass readily from RBCs to tissue. Less O_2 is therefore available for tissue cell respiration. This results in hypoxemia.

CO poisoning is documented by Hb analysis for COHb. A specimen should be drawn as soon as possible after exposure because CO is rapidly cleared from Hb by breathing normal air. O_2 saturation studies and oximetry are inaccurate in CO-exposed patients because they measure all forms of oxygen-saturated Hb, including COHb. In these circumstances, the patient's oximetry will be good, yet the patient will be hypoxemic.

This test can also be used to evaluate patients with complaints of headache, irritability, nausea, vomiting, and vertigo, who unknowingly may have been exposed to CO. Its greatest use, however, is in patients exposed to smoke inhalation, exhaust fumes, and fires. Other sources of CO include tobacco smoke, petroleum and natural gas fuel fumes, automobile exhaust, unvented natural gas heaters, and defective gas stoves. The treatment of CO toxicity is administration of high concentrations of O_2 to displace the COHb.

Procedure and patient care

- See inside front cover for Routine Blood Testing.
- Fasting: no.
- Blood tube commonly used: lavender or green.

- Obtain the patient's history for possible sources of CO.
- Assess the patient for signs and symptoms of mild CO toxicity (e.g., headache, weakness, dizziness, malaise, dyspnea) and moderate to severe CO toxicity (e.g., severe headache, bright red mucous membranes, cherry-red blood). Maintain patient safety precautions if confusion is present.
- Treat the patient as indicated by the physician. Usually the patient receives high concentrations of O_2.
- **PT** Encourage respirations to allow the patient to clear CO from the Hb.

Abnormal findings

Carbon monoxide poisoning

notes

carcinoembryonic antigen (CEA)

Type of test Blood

Normal findings <5 ng/mL or <5 mcg/L (SI units)

Test explanation and related physiology

The CEA is a protein that normally occurs in fetal gut tissue. By the time of birth, detectable serum levels disappear. In the early 1960s, CEA was found to exist in the bloodstream of adults who had colorectal tumors. Thus, the antigen was thought to be a specific indicator of the presence of colorectal cancer. Subsequently, however, this protein has been found in patients who have a variety of carcinomas (e.g., breast, pancreatic, gastric, hepatobiliary), sarcomas, and even many benign diseases (e.g., ulcerative colitis, diverticulitis, cirrhosis). Chronic smokers also have elevated CEA levels.

Because the CEA level can be elevated in both benign and malignant diseases, it is not considered to be a specific test for colorectal cancer. As a result, CEA is not a reliable screening test for the detection of colorectal cancer in the general population. Its use is limited to determining the prognosis and monitoring the response of tumor to antineoplastic therapy in a patient with cancer. This is especially helpful in patients with breast and gastrointestinal cancers. The CEA level on the initial test is an indicator of tumor burden and prognosis. Smaller and earlier-staged tumors are likely to have minimal CEA elevations, if not normal CEA levels. A drastic reduction of normal CEA levels is expected with complete eradication of tumor. Therefore, this test is used to determine the adequacy of treatment.

This test also is used in the surveillance of patients with cancer. A steadily rising CEA level is occasionally the first sign of tumor recurrence. This makes CEA testing very valuable in the follow-up of patients who have had potentially curative therapy. It is important to note that many patients with advanced breast or gastrointestinal tumors may not have elevated CEA levels.

CEA can also be detected in bodily fluids other than blood. Its presence in those bodily fluids indicates metastasis. This antigen is commonly measured in peritoneal fluid or chest effusions. An elevated CEA in these fluids indicates metastasis to the peritoneum or pleurae, respectively. Likewise, elevated CEA levels in the CSF would indicate central nervous system metastasis.

Interfering factors

- Smokers tend to have higher CEA levels than nonsmokers.
- Benign diseases (e.g., cholecystitis, colitis, diverticulitis) are associated with elevated CEA levels.
- Liver diseases (e.g., hepatitis, cirrhosis) are associated with elevated CEA levels.
- Results may vary considerably depending on the method used for quantification. Because of this, results from different laboratories cannot be compared or interchangeably interpreted.

Procedure and patient care

- See inside front cover for Routine Blood Testing.
- Fasting: no.
- Blood tube commonly used: verify with lab.
- Indicate on the laboratory slip if the patient smokes or has diseases that can affect test results.

Abnormal findings

▲ **Increased levels**

Cancer (gastrointestinal, breast, lung, pancreatic, hepatobiliary)

Inflammation (colitis, cholecystitis, pancreatitis, diverticulitis)

Cirrhosis

Peptic ulcer

Crohn disease

notes

cardiac catheterization (Coronary angiography, Ventriculography)

Type of test X-ray with contrast dye

Normal findings Normal heart-muscle motion, normal coronary arteries, normal great vessels, and normal intracardiac pressures and volumes

Test explanation and related physiology

Cardiac catheterization is used to visualize the heart chambers, arteries, and great vessels. It is used most often to evaluate patients with chest pain. Patients with a positive stress test are also studied to locate the region of coronary occlusion. This test is also used to determine the effects of valvular heart disease. Right heart catheterization is performed to calculate cardiac output and to measure right heart pressures. This is the most accurate method to determine cardiac output. Right heart catheterization is also used to identify pulmonary emboli (see pulmonary angiography, p. 771).

For cardiac catheterization, a catheter is passed into the heart through a peripheral vein or artery, depending on whether catheterization of the right or left side of the heart is being performed. Pressures are recorded through the catheter, and radiographic dyes are injected. With the assistance of a computer, cardiac output and other measures of cardiac functions can be determined. Cardiac catheterization is indicated for the following reasons:

- To identify, locate, and quantitate the severity of atherosclerotic, occlusive coronary artery disease
- To evaluate the severity of acquired and congenital cardiac valvular or septal defects
- To detect congenital cardiac abnormalities, such as transposition of great vessels, patent ductus arteriosus, and anomalous venous return to the heart
- To evaluate the success of previous cardiac surgery or balloon angioplasty
- To evaluate cardiac muscle function
- To identify and quantify ventricular aneurysms
- To detect disease of the great vessels, such as atherosclerotic occlusion or aneurysms within the aortic arch
- To evaluate and treat patients with acute myocardial infarction
- To insert a catheter to monitor right-sided heart pressures, such as pulmonary artery and pulmonary wedge pressures (Table 6 provides pressures and volumes used in cardiac monitoring.)

TABLE 6 Pressures and volumes used in cardiac monitoring

Pressures/Volumes	Description	Normal values
Pressures		
Routine blood pressure	Routine brachial artery pressure	90-140/60-90 mm Hg
Systolic left ventricular pressure	Peak pressure in the left ventricle during systole	90-140 mm Hg
End-diastolic left ventricular pressure	Pressure in the left ventricle at the end of diastole	4-12 mm Hg
Central venous pressure	Pressure in the superior vena cava	2-14 cm H_2O
Pulmonary wedge pressure	Pressure in the pulmonary venules, an indirect measurement of left atrial pressure and left ventricular end-diastolic pressure	Left atrial: 6-15 mm Hg
Pulmonary artery pressure	Pressure in the pulmonary artery	15-28/5-16 mm Hg
Aortic artery pressure	Same as routine blood pressure	
Volumes		
End-diastolic volume (EDV)	Amount of blood present in the left ventricle at the end of diastole	50-90 mL/m²
End-systolic volume (ESV)	Amount of blood present in the left ventricle at the end of systole	25 mL/m²
Stroke volume (SV)	Amount of blood ejected from the heart in one contraction (SV = EDV − ESV)	45 ± 12 mL/m²
Ejection fraction (EF)	Proportion (fraction) of EDV ejected from the left ventricle during systole (EF = SV/EDV)	0.67 ± 0.07
Cardiac output (CO)	Amount of blood ejected by the heart in 1 minute	3-6 L/min
Cardiac index (CI)	Amount of blood ejected by the heart in 1 minute per square meter of body surface area (CI = CO/body surface area)	2.8-4.2 L/min/m² for a patient with 1.5 m² of body surface area

C

- To perform dilation of stenotic coronary arteries (angioplasty), place coronary artery stents, or perform laser atherectomy

Cardiac catheterization is performed under sterile conditions. In right-sided heart catheterization, usually the jugular, subclavian, brachial, or femoral vein is used for vascular access. In left-sided heart catheterization, usually the right femoral artery is cannulated; alternatively, however, the radial or brachial artery may be chosen (Figure 8). As the catheter is placed into the great vessels of the heart chamber, pressures are monitored and recorded. Blood samples for analysis of O_2 content are also obtained. The catheter is advanced with appropriate guidance into the desired position. After pressures are obtained, angiographic visualization of the heart chambers, valves, and coronary arteries is achieved with the injection of radiographic dye.

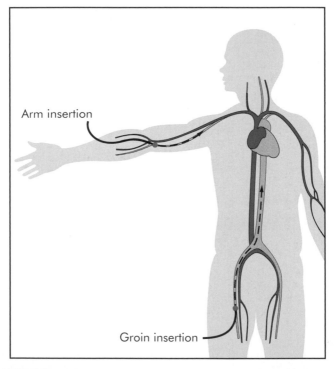

Arm insertion

Groin insertion

FIGURE 8 Cardiac catheterization. Brachial (arm) or femoral (groin) arterial insertion for cardiac catheterization.

Percutaneous transluminal coronary angioplasty and *intra-coronary stents* are therapeutic procedures that can be performed during cardiac catheterization in medical centers where open heart surgery is available. During this procedure, a specially designed balloon catheter is introduced into the coronary arteries and placed across the stenotic area of the coronary artery. This area can then be dilated by controlled inflation of the balloon and subsequently stented. The coronary arteriogram is then repeated to document the effects of the forceful dilation of the stenotic area. Coronary arterial stents can be placed at the site of previous stenosis after angioplasty to maintain patency for longer periods of time.

Likewise, *atherectomy* of coronary arterial plaques can be performed to more permanently open some of the hard, atheromatous plaques. There are certain occlusive lesions with characteristics unfavorable for balloon angioplasty that appear to be ideally suited for atherectomy. Rotational atherectomy is most commonly used. A tiny, rotating knife inside a catheter is moved to the arterial obstruction. A balloon is inflated to position the knife precisely on the fatty deposit, and the fatty deposit is then shaved off the wall of the artery. The shavings are collected in the catheter and removed.

Contraindications

- Patients who are unable to cooperate during the test
- Patients with an iodine dye allergy who have not received preventive medication for allergy
- Patients who are pregnant because of radiation exposure to the fetus
- Patients with renal disorders because iodinated contrast is nephrotoxic
- Patients with a bleeding propensity

Potential complications

- Cardiac arrhythmias (dysrhythmias)
- Perforation of the heart myocardium
- Catheter-induced embolic stroke (cerebrovascular accident) or myocardial infarction
- Complications associated with the catheter insertion site (e.g., arterial thrombosis, embolism, or pseudoaneurysm)
- Infection at the catheter insertion site
- Pneumothorax following subclavian vein catheterization of the right side of the heart

- Lactic acidosis in patients who are taking metformin and receiving iodine contrast. Metformin should be held the day of the test to prevent this complication.

Procedure and patient care

Before

PT Explain the procedure to the patient.

- Obtain written permission from the fully informed patient.
- Allay the patient's fears and anxieties regarding this test. Although this test creates tremendous fear in a patient, it is performed often and complications are rare.

PT Instruct the patient to abstain from oral intake for at least 4 to 8 hours before the test.

- Prepare the catheter insertion site as per protocol.
- Mark the patient's peripheral pulses with a pen before catheterization. This will facilitate postcatheterization assessment of the pulses at the affected and nonaffected extremities.
- Provide appropriate precatheterization sedation as ordered by the physician.

PT Instruct the patient to void before going to the catheterization laboratory.

- Remove all valuables and dental prostheses before transporting the patient to the catheterization laboratory.
- Obtain IV access for delivery of IV fluids and cardiac drugs if necessary.

During

- Take the patient to the cardiac catheterization laboratory.
- Note the following procedural steps:
    1. The chosen catheter insertion site is prepared and draped in a sterile manner.
    2. The desired vessel is punctured with a needle.
    3. A wire is placed through the needle and a sheath is placed over the wire and into the vessel.
    4. The angiographic catheter is threaded through the sheath over a guidewire.
    5. When the catheter is in the desired location, the appropriate cardiac pressures and volumes are measured.
    6. Cardiac ventriculography is performed with controlled injection of contrast.
    7. Each coronary artery is catheterized. Cardiac angiography is then carried out with a controlled injection of contrast material.
    8. During the injection, x-ray images are rapidly made.

9. The patient's vital signs must be monitored constantly during this procedure.
10. If *angioplasty* is performed, the cardiologist appropriately places the catheter and balloon at the stenotic area. Note the following procedural steps:
   a. As the ECG tracing is observed, the balloon is inflated and the stenotic areas are forcefully dilated.
   b. If signs of myocardial ischemia develop, the balloon is immediately deflated.
   c. Usually inflation of the balloon is continued only for 10 seconds.
11. After obtaining all the required information, the catheter is removed and a vascular closure device may be placed.
12. A chemical vascular closure device designed to seal the arterial puncture is often placed.

- Note that this test is usually performed by a cardiologist in approximately 1 hour.
- **PT** Tell the patient that during the injection he or she may experience a severe hot flush. This is uncomfortable but lasts only 10 to 15 seconds.
- Note that some patients have a tendency to cough as the catheter is placed into the pulmonary artery.
- Verbally support the patient as the x-ray images are taken because the loud noises may be frightening.

After

- Monitor the patient's vital signs to check for bleeding.
- Apply pressure to the site of vascular access.
- Keep the patient on bed rest for 4 to 8 hours to allow for complete sealing of the arterial puncture.
- Keep the affected extremity extended and immobilized with sandbags to decrease bleeding.
- Assess the puncture site for signs of bleeding, hematoma, or absence of pulse.
- Assess the patient's pulses for both extremities. Compare with preprocedure baseline values.
- **PT** Encourage the patient to drink fluids to maintain adequate hydration. Dehydration may be caused by the diuretic action of the dye. Monitor urinary output.
- **PT** Instruct the patient to report any signs of numbness, tingling, pain, or loss of function in the involved extremity.
- See p. xviii for appropriate interventions concerning care of patients with iodine allergy.

PT Instruct the patient that the test will be reviewed by the cardiologist and the results will be available in 1 or 2 days.

Abnormal findings

Anatomic variation of the cardiac chambers and great vessels
Coronary artery occlusive disease
Coronary aneurysm
Coronary fistula
Cardiomyopathy
Ventricular aneurysm
Ventricular mural thrombi
Intracardiac tumor
Aortic root arteriosclerotic or aneurysmal disease
Anomalies in pulmonary venous return
Acquired or congenital septal defects and valvular abnormalities
Pulmonary emboli
Pulmonary hypertension

notes

> **cardiac nuclear scan** (Myocardial perfusion scan, Myocardial perfusion imaging, Myocardial scan, Cardiac scan, Heart scan, Thallium scan, MUGA scan, Isonitrile scan, Sestamibi cardiac scan, Cardiac flow studies, and Nuclear stress test)

C

Type of test Nuclear scan

Normal Findings

Heterogeneous uptake of radionuclide throughout the myocardium of the left ventricle

Left ventricular end-diastolic volume ≤70 mL

Left ventricular end-systolic volume ≤25 mL

Left ventricular ejection fraction >50%

Right ventricular ejection fraction >40%

Normal cardiac wall motion

No muscle wall thickening

Test explanation and related physiology

A cardiac perfusion scan measures the coronary blood flow at rest and during exercise. It is often used to evaluate the cause of chest pain. It may be done after a coronary ischemic event to evaluate coronary patency or heart muscle function.

In this test, a radionuclide is injected intravenously into the patient. Myocardial perfusion images are then obtained while the patient is lying down under a single-photon emission computed tomography (SPECT) camera that generates a picture of the radioactivity coming from the heart. This scan can be performed at rest or with exercise such as treadmill or bicycling (*myocardial nuclear stress testing*). Medications may be administered that duplicate exercise stress testing. Vasodilators (dipyridamole, adenosine, and regadenoson) or chronotropic agents (dobutamine) are commonly used. Regadenoson is the most recent A_{2A} adenosine receptor agonist that instigates coronary vasodilatation. It is associated with fewer side effects (e.g., heart block, bronchospasm) and can be injected more quickly.

The initial radioisotope used was thallium (thus the name *thallium scan*). Technetium agents such as tetrofosmin and sestamibi (isonitrile) are now more commonly used. The uptake of these agents is proportional to the myocardial coronary flow. At rest, a coronary stenosis must exceed 90% of the normal diameter before blood flow is impaired enough to see it on the perfusion scan. With exercise stress testing, however, stenosis of 50% becomes obvious. Often, stenosis or coronary obstruction is noted by a normal resting perfusion scan followed by stress perfusion scan that demonstrates cold spots compatible with decreased coronary perfusion. Myocardial perfusion scans can be synchronized by gating the images with the cardiac cycle and thereby allowing the visualization and evaluation of cardiac muscle function. The contractility of the muscle wall can be evaluated at the same time. Prior muscle injury is demonstrated by reduced muscle wall motion. Most times, nuclear myocardial scans include both perfusion and gated wall motion images. Cardiac ejection fraction, the end-systolic volume of the left ventricle, can be calculated.

Cardiac nuclear imaging when gated to the cardiac cycle (*multigated acquisition scan [MUGA], gated blood pool scan*) can provide an accurate measure of ventricular function through the calculation of the *ventricular ejection fraction.* In this scan, the patient's red blood cells are tagged with technetium. Ventricular volumes can be calculated and used to accurately calculate the amount of blood that is ejected from the ventricle with each contraction (ejection fraction). This is used in the initial assessment of cardiac function and subsequently to monitor therapy designed to improve cardiac function. Patients with cardiomyopathies (ischemic, infiltrative, inflammatory), cardiac transplant, or drug-induced cardiac muscle toxicity (from doxorubicin or Herceptin) require frequent evaluation of ventricular ejection fraction.

Contraindications

- Patients who are uncooperative or medically unstable
- Patients with severe cardiac arrhythmia.
- Patients who are pregnant, (unless the benefits outweigh the risks) because of fetal exposure to radionuclide material (unless the benefits outweigh the risks)

Interfering factors

- Myocardial trauma
- Cardiac flow studies can be altered by excessive alterations in chest pressure (as exists with excessive crying in children).
- Recent nuclear scans (e.g., thyroid or bone scan)
- ✗ Drugs, such as long-acting nitrates, may only temporarily improve coronary perfusion and cardiac function.

Procedure and patient care

Before

PT Explain the procedure to the patient.
PT Instruct the patient that a short fasting period may be required, especially when using sestamibi or tetrofosmin.

PT Tell the patient that the only discomfort associated with this test is the venipuncture required for injection of the radioisotope.

- Be sure all jewelry is removed from the chest wall.
- Obtain a consent form if stress testing is to be performed.

During

- Take the patient to the nuclear medicine department. Depending on the type of nuclear myocardial scan, each scanning protocol is different.
- Note the following general procedural steps:
  1. One or more intravenous (IV) injection of radionuclide material is performed.
  2. Electrocardiographic (EKG) leads may be applied.
  3. Depending on the radionuclide used, scanning is performed 15 minutes to 4 hours later.
  4. SPECT camera is placed at the level of the precordium.
  5. If a single gamma camera is used, the patient is placed in a supine position, then may be repositioned to the lateral position or in the right and left oblique positions. In some departments, the detector can be rotated around the patient, who remains in the supine position.
  6. The gamma ray scanner records the image of the heart, and an image is immediately developed.
  7. For an *exercise stress test*, additional radionuclide is injected during exercise when the patient reaches a maximum heart rate. The patient then lies on a table, and scanning is done. A repeat scan may be done 3 to 4 hours later.
  8. If an *isonitrile stress test* is needed, the radionuclide material is injected and a scan performed 30 to 60 minutes later for the resting phase. Four hours later, cardiac stress testing is done. After a second injection, scanning is repeated.
- Note that myocardial scans are usually performed in less than 30 minutes by a nuclear medicine technician.
- If nuclear cardiac stress testing is performed, follow routine protocol described on page 225.

After

PT Inform the patient that because only tracer doses of radioisotopes are used, no precautions need to be taken against radioactive exposure to personnel or family.

PT Instruct the patient to drink fluids to aid in the excretion of the radioactive substance.

- Apply pressure or a pressure dressing to the venipuncture site.
- Assess the venipuncture site for bleeding.

- If stress testing was performed, evaluate the patient's vital signs at frequent intervals (as indicated).
- Remove any applied EKG leads.

Abnormal findings

Coronary artery occlusive disease

Decreased myocardial function associated with ischemia, myocarditis, cardiomyopathy, or congestive heart failure

Decreased cardiac output

notes

cardiac stress testing (Exercise stress testing; Nuclear stress testing; Echo stress testing)

Type of test Electrodiagnostic; nuclear

Normal findings Patient able to obtain and maintain maximal heart rate of 85% for predicted age and gender with no cardiac symptoms or ECG change. No cardiac muscle wall dysfunction present.

Test explanation and related physiology

Stress testing is used in the following situations:
- To evaluate chest pain in a patient suspected of having coronary disease
- To determine the limits of safe exercise during a cardiac rehabilitation program or to assist patients with cardiac disease in maintaining good physical fitness
- To detect labile or exercise-related hypertension
- To detect intermittent claudication in patients with suspected vascular occlusive disease in the extremities
- To evaluate the effectiveness of treatment in patients who take antianginal or antiarrhythmic medications
- To evaluate the effectiveness of cardiac intervention (e.g., bypass grafting or angioplasty)

Stress testing is a noninvasive study that provides information about the patient's cardiac function. In stress testing, the heart is stressed in some way and then evaluated during the stress. Changes indicating ischemia suggest coronary occlusive disease. By far the most commonly used method is *exercise stress testing*. *Chemical stress testing* methods are becoming more commonly used because of their safety and increased accuracy. A third method, less commonly used, is *pacer stress testing*.

During *exercise stress testing*, the ECG, heart rate, and blood pressure are monitored while the patient engages in some type of physical activity (stress). The treadmill test is the most frequently used because it is the most easily standardized and reproducible.

The usual goal of exercise stress testing is to increase the heart rate to just below maximal levels or to the *target heart rate*. Usually this target heart rate is 80% to 90% of the maximal heart rate. The test is usually discontinued if the patient reaches that target heart rate or develops any symptoms or ECG changes. The maximal heart rate is determined by a chart that takes into account the patient's age and gender. (Target rate is about 220 minus the patient's age.) Patients taking calcium channel blockers and sympathetic blockers have a lower-than-expected maximal heart rate.

Exercise stress testing is based on the principle that occluded arteries will be unable to meet the heart's increased demand for blood during the testing. This may become obvious with symptoms (e.g., chest pain, fatigue, dyspnea, tachycardia, cardiac arrhythmias [dysrhythmias], fall in blood pressure) or ECG changes (e.g., ST-segment variance >1 mm, increasing premature ventricular contractions, or other rhythm disturbances). Besides the electrodiagnostic method of cardiac evaluation, the stressed heart can also be evaluated by nuclear scanning or echocardiography (which are more sensitive and accurate).

When exercise testing is not advisable or the patient is unable to exercise at a level adequate to stress the heart (e.g., patients with an orthopedic, arthritic, neurologic, vascular, or pulmonary limitation), *chemical stress testing* is recommended. Although chemical stress testing is less physiologic than exercise testing, it is safer and more controllable. *Dipyridamole (Persantine)* is a coronary vasodilator. If one coronary artery is significantly occluded, the coronary blood flow is diverted to the opened vessels. *Adenosine* works similarly to dipyridamole. *Dobutamine* is another chemical that can stress the heart. Dobutamine stimulates the heart muscle function. The normal heart muscle increases (augments) its contractility (wall motion). Ischemic muscle has no augmentation. In fact, in time the ischemic area becomes hypokinetic. Infarcted tissue is akinetic. In chemical stress testing, the stressed heart is evaluated by nuclear scanning or echocardiography.

Pacing is another method of stress testing. In patients with permanent pacemakers, the rate of capture can be increased to a rate that would be considered a cardiac stress. The heart is then evaluated electrodiagnostically or with nuclear scanning or echocardiography.

The methods of evaluation of the heart are electrophysiologic parameters (e.g., ECG, blood pressure, and heart rate), cardiac nuclear scanning, and echocardiography. These other tests are discussed separately (see pp. 221 and 356). Echocardiography is fast becoming the method of choice for urgent and elective cardiac evaluation with or without stress testing.

Contraindications

- Patients with unstable angina
- Patients with severe aortic valvular heart disease

- Patients who have recently had a myocardial infarction (however, limited stress testing can be done)
- Patients with severe congestive heart failure
- Patients with severe left main coronary artery disease

Potential complications

- Fatal cardiac arrhythmias
- Severe angina
- Myocardial infarction
- Fainting

Interfering factors

- Heavy meals before testing can divert blood to the gastrointestinal tract.
- Nicotine from smoking can cause coronary artery spasm.
- Caffeine blocks the effect of dipyridamole.
- Medical problems, such as left ventricular hypertrophy, hypertension, valvular heart disease, left bundle-branch block, severe anemia, hypoxemia, and chronic pulmonary disease, can affect results.
- ✘ Drugs that can affect test results include beta-blockers, calcium channel blockers, digoxin, and nitroglycerin.

Procedure and patient care

Before

- **PT** Explain the procedure to the patient.
- **PT** Instruct the patient to abstain from eating, drinking, and smoking for 4 hours prior to testing.
- **PT** Inform the patient about the risks of the test and obtain informed consent.
- **PT** Instruct the patient to bring comfortable clothing and athletic shoes for exercise. Slippers are not acceptable.
- **PT** Inform the patient if any medications should be discontinued for a time period before testing.
- Obtain a pretest ECG.
- Record the patient's vital signs for baseline values.
- Apply and secure appropriate ECG electrodes.

During

- Note that a physician usually is present during stress testing.
- After the patient begins to exercise, adjust the treadmill machine settings to apply increasing levels of stress. Encourage and support the patient at each level of increased stress.
- **PT** Encourage patients to verbalize any symptoms.

- Note that during the test the ECG tracing and vital signs are monitored continuously.
- Terminate the test if the patient complains of chest pain, exhaustion, dyspnea, fatigue, or dizziness.
- Note that testing usually takes approximately 45 minutes.
- **PT** Inform the patient that the physician in attendance usually interprets and explains the results.

After

- Place the patient in the supine position to rest after the test.
- Monitor the ECG tracing and record vital signs at poststress intervals until recordings and values return to pretest levels.
- Remove electrodes and paste.
- **PT** Tell the patient when the test results will be available.

Abnormal findings

Coronary artery occlusive disease
Exercise-related hypertension or hypotension
Intermittent claudication
Abnormal cardiac rhythms: stress induced
Arrhythmias (e.g., ventricular tachycardia or supraventricular tachycardia)

notes

carotid artery duplex scanning (Carotid ultrasound)

Type of test Ultrasound

Normal findings Carotid artery free of plaques and stenosis

Test explanation and related physiology

Carotid duplex scanning is a noninvasive ultrasound test used on the vertebral and extracranial carotid artery to detect occlusive disease directly. It is recommended for patients with peripheral vascular disease, headaches, and neurologic symptoms (e.g., transient ischemic attacks [TIAs], hemiparesis, paresthesia, and acute speech or visual deficits).

This scan is called *duplex* because it combines the benefits of two methods of ultrasonography—Doppler and B-mode. With the use of the transducer, a B-mode ultrasound grayscale image of the carotid vessel is obtained. A pulsed Doppler probe within the transducer is used to evaluate blood flow velocity and direction in the artery and to measure the amplitude and waveform of the carotid arterial pulse. A computer combines that information and provides a two-dimensional image of the carotid artery along with an image of blood flow. With this technique, one is able to directly visualize areas of stenotic or occluded arteries and arterial flow disruption. The degree of occlusion is measured in the percentage of the entire lumen that is occluded.

Color Doppler ultrasound (CDU) can be added to duplex scanning. CDU assigns color for direction of blood flow within the vessel, and the intensity of that color is dependent on the mean computed velocity of blood traveling in the vessel. This allows visualization of stenotic areas by seeing slowing or reversal of direction of blood flow at a particular area of the artery. Reversal of blood flow is sometimes associated with contralateral arterial occlusion, which can be easily demonstrated by using this technique.

Measurement of the thickness of the wall of the carotid artery (*carotid intima–media thickness [CIMT]*) is used as a measurement of cerebrovascular atherosclerosis specifically and is a predictor of coronary atherosclerosis in general. CIMT is also used to monitor progression of atherosclerosis (particularly in diabetics). It is used to monitor atherosclerotic regression in patients who are undergoing a treatment for atherosclerosis.

Procedure and patient care

Before
PT Explain the procedure to the patient.
PT Tell the patient that no special preparation is required.
PT Assure the patient that the test is painless.

During
- Place the patient in the supine position with the head supported to prevent lateral motion.
- Note the following procedural steps:
  1. A water-soluble gel is used to couple the sound from the transducer to the skin surface.
  2. Images of the carotid artery and pulse waveform are obtained.
- Note that this test is performed by an ultrasound technologist in the ultrasound or radiology department in approximately 15 to 30 minutes.

PT Tell the patient that no discomfort is associated with this test.

After
- Remove the water-soluble gel from the patient.

Abnormal findings
Carotid artery occlusive disease
Carotid artery aneurysm

notes

cell culture drug resistance testing (CCDRT, Chemosensitivity assay, Drug response assay)

Type of test Miscellaneous

Normal findings Cells sensitive to planned therapeutic drugs

Test explanation and related physiology

Cell culture drug resistance testing (CCDRT) refers to testing the reaction of a patient's own cancer cells in the laboratory to drugs that may be used to treat the patient's cancer. The idea is to identify which drugs are more likely to work and which drugs are less likely to work. By avoiding the latter and choosing from among the former, the patient's probability of benefiting from the chemotherapy may be improved. This testing is still considered experimental because there is no extensive clinical experience to support its accuracy. However, a growing number of studies have shown a superior survival rate for patients treated with drugs targeting their tumor cells.

There are multiple tests available for drug sensitivity testing, but all have four common steps. Cancer cells from the patient's tumor must be obtained and isolated. The cells are then isolated with various potentially therapeutic drugs. Assessment of cell survival is then performed and the results are provided. Based on those results, the clinician can recommend more appropriate chemotherapy for a particular cancer. In most cases, this testing is used for patients with refractory or recurrent epithelial tumors (usually breast or ovarian cancer).

Procedure and patient care

Before

PT Explain the process to the patient. (Tumor cells are usually obtained by a surgical procedure.)

During

- Tumor cells are sent to a reference laboratory. The method of tissue preservation varies among laboratories.

After

- After the results are obtained, appropriate chemotherapy targeted to the patient's tumor cells is administered.

Abnormal findings

Epithelial cancer

notes

cell-free maternal DNA testing (Noninvasive prenatal testing [NIPT, cell-free DNA in maternal blood])

Type of test Blood

Normal findings Low risk of chromosomal abnormality

Test explanation and related physiology

Trisomy 21 (Down syndrome), trisomy 18 (Edwards syndrome), and trisomy 13 (Patau syndrome) are the three most common chromosomal abnormalities affecting live births. Although one in 450 live births has one of these aneuploidy abnormalities, trisomy 21 is the most common. Abnormal findings on pelvic ultrasonography of the fetus, including fetal nuchal translucency or thickness (page 697) along with biochemical markers (e.g., hCG, page 530; PAAP-A, page 742), can identify pregnancies at high risk for these chromosomal defects. The definitive diagnosis requires chorionic villus sampling (CVS; page 254) and amniocentesis (page 49), which are invasive and increase the risk for miscarriage.

Cell-free (cf) DNA from the placental fetal cells circulate in maternal blood. This DNA can be extracted and, through advanced laboratory techniques of targeting genomic sequencing, allows 99% of the cases of trisomy to be detected. False-positive rates instigating unnecessary invasive testing are less than 1%. This testing can be performed as early as 10 weeks' gestation but is typically done between 10 and 22 weeks. Because of newer laboratory techniques of multiplexing, results can be available in about 1 week.

In 2012, the American College of Obstetricians and Gynecologists (ACOG) and the Society for Maternal-Fetal Medicine (SMFM) issued a joint committee opinion that supported noninvasive prenatal testing that uses cell-free fetal DNA for women at increased risk for having a baby with a chromosomal abnormality. See Box 4.

BOX 4 Women at high risk for having children with chromosomal abnormalities

- Maternal age 35 years or older at delivery
- Fetal ultrasonographic findings indicating an increased risk for trisomy
- History of prior pregnancy with trisomy
- Positive maternal screen result
- Other translocation abnormalities with increased risk of trisomy

Testing of high-risk pregnant women may be done in several ways:

- Cell-free DNA test done in the first trimester along with ultrasonography
- Cell-free DNA test done in the second trimester without ultrasonography
- A combination of both

If the results of these screening tests are positive, more invasive testing such as CVS or amniocentesis is required to make definitive diagnosis of trisomy.

Procedure and patient care

- See inside front cover for Routine Blood Testing.
- Fasting: no.
- Blood tube commonly used: red.
- **PT** Encourage all women undergoing cell-free (cf) DNA to have genetic counseling.
- **PT** Results should be reviewed with the patient, and the risks, benefits, and alternatives to further testing should be explained.

Abnormal findings

Trisomy 21 (Down syndrome)
Trisomy 18 (Edwards syndrome)
Trisomy 13 (Patau syndrome)

notes

cell surface immunophenotyping (Flow cytometry cell surface immunophenotyping, Lymphocyte immunophenotyping, AIDS T-lymphocyte cell markers, CD4 marker, CD4/CD8 ratio, CD4 percentage)

Type of test Blood

Normal findings

Cells	Percent	No. of cells/μL
T-cells	60-95	800-2500
T-helper (CD4) cells	60-75	600-1500
CD8 T-cells	25-30	300-1000
B-cells	4-25	100-450
Natural killer cells	4-30	75-500

CD4/CD8 ratio: >1

Test explanation and related physiology

This test is used to detect the progressive depletion of CD4 T-lymphocytes, which is associated with an increased likelihood of clinical complications from acquired immunodeficiency syndrome (AIDS). Test results can indicate if a patient with AIDS is at risk for developing opportunistic infections. It is also used to confirm the diagnosis of acute myelocytic leukemia (AML) and to differentiate AML from acute lymphocytic leukemia (ALL).

All lymphocytes originate from reticulum cells in the bone marrow. Normal hematopoietic cells undergo changes in expression of cell surface markers as they mature from stem cells into cells of a committed lineage. Monoclonal antibodies have been developed that react with lymphoid and myeloid glycoprotein antigens on the cell surface of peripheral blood cells. One kind of lymphocyte that matures in the bone marrow is called a B-lymphocyte. B-lymphocytes provide humoral immunity (i.e., produce antibodies). A second type of lymphocyte matures in the thymus and is called a T-lymphocyte. T-lymphocytes are responsible for cellular immunity. Finally, there is a group of lymphocytes that have neither T nor B markers. These are called *natural killer cells* because they chemically attack foreign or cancer cells without prior sensitization. Monoclonal antibodies against cell-surface markers are used to identify the various forms of lymphocytes. The absolute numbers and percentages are then counted using *flow cytometry*. This can be performed on blood or on cell suspensions of tissue. Flow cytometry is able to analyze thousands of cells in less than a minute.

CD4 (T-helper cells) and CD8 (T-suppressor cells) are examples of T-lymphocytes. T-lymphocytes, and especially CD4 counts, when combined with HIV viral load testing (p. 517) are used to determine the time to initiate antiviral therapy. They also can be used to monitor antiviral therapy. Successful antiviral therapy is associated with an increase in CD4 counts. Worsening of disease or unsuccessful therapy is associated with decreasing T-lymphocyte counts.

There are three related measurements of CD4 T-lymphocytes. The first measurement is the *total CD4 count*. This is measured in whole blood and is the product of the WBC count, the lymphocyte differential count, and the percentage of lymphocytes that are CD4 T-cells. The second measurement, the *CD4 percentage*, is a more accurate prognostic marker. It measures the percentage of CD4 lymphocytes in the whole blood sample by combining immunophenotyping with flow cytometry. This procedure relies on detecting specific antigenic determinants on the surface of the CD4 lymphocyte by antigen-specific monoclonal antibodies labeled with a fluorescent dye. The third prognostic marker, which is also more reliable than the total CD4 count, is the *CD4 to CD8 ratio*.

Of the three T-cell measurements, the total CD4 count is the most variable. There is substantial diurnal variation in this count. Because it is a calculated measurement, the combination of possible laboratory error and personal fluctuation can result in wide variations in test results. With the CD4 percentage and the CD4 to CD8 ratio, very little diurnal variation and laboratory error exist. The Multicenter AIDS Cohort Study suggests that the latter two measurements are more accurate than the total CD4 count. However, because the total CD4 count was originally thought to be the best marker, this test was used in many of the studies that now form the basis for practice recommendations.

The pathogenesis of AIDS is largely attributed to a decrease in the T-lymphocyte that bears the CD4 receptor. Progressive depletion of CD4 T-lymphocytes is associated with an increased likelihood of clinical complications from AIDS. Therefore, CD4 measurement is a prognostic marker that can indicate whether a patient infected with HIV is at risk for developing opportunistic infections. The measurement of CD4 levels is used to decide whether to initiate *Pneumocystis jirovecii* pneumonia prophylaxis and antiviral therapy, and for determining the prognosis of patients with HIV.

Both immunodeficiency and the dosage of immunosuppressive medications used after organ transplant are also monitored with the use of this cell surface immunophenotyping. Lymphomas and other lymphoproliferative diseases are now classified and treated according to the predominant lymphocyte type identified. In some instances, the prognosis of these diseases depends on this lymphocyte phenotyping.

Contraindications

- Patients who are not emotionally prepared for the prognosis that the results may indicate

Interfering factors

- Diurnal variation occurs.
- A recent viral illness can decrease total T-lymphocyte counts.
- Nicotine and very strenuous exercise have been shown to decrease lymphocyte counts.
- ✶ Steroids can *increase* lymphocyte counts.
- ✶ Immunosuppressive drugs will *decrease* lymphocyte counts.

Procedure and patient care

- See inside front cover for Routine Blood Testing.
- Fasting: no.
- Blood tube commonly used: green or purple.
- Never recap needles. Dispose of needles and syringes in a puncture-proof container.
- Keep the specimen at room temperature. Do not refrigerate.
- The specimen must be evaluated within 24 hours.
- **PT** Instruct the patient to observe the venipuncture site for infection. Patients with leukemia or AIDS are immunocompromised and susceptible to infection.
- **PT** Encourage the patient to discuss his or her concerns regarding the prognostic information that may be obtained by these results.
- Do not give test results over the phone. Decreasing CD4 counts can have devastating consequences.

Abnormal findings

▲ Increased counts
Leukemias
Lymphoma

▼ Decreased counts
Organ transplant patients
Immunodeficiency diseases

notes

cervical biopsy (LEEP procedure, Cone biopsy)

Type of test Microscopic examination

Normal findings Normal squamous cells

Possible critical values Cancer cells

Test explanation and related physiology

When a PAP smear reveals an *epithelial cell abnormality* or when a pelvic exam reveals a possible abnormality in the cervix, a biopsy of that structure is performed. There are several different methods of biopsy, all of which obtain an increasing amount of tissue. Cervical biopsy procedures include:

- A *simple cervical biopsy*, sometimes called a *punch biopsy*, removes a small piece of tissue from the surface of the cervix. This is often performed during colposcopy, see p. 274.
- An *endocervical biopsy (endocervical curettage)* removes tissue from high in the cervical canal by scraping with a sharp instrument.
- *Loop electrosurgical excision procedure (LEEP)* uses a thin, low-voltage electrified wire loop to cut out abnormal tissue on the cervix and high in the endocervical canal (sometimes called a *large loop excision of the transformation zone [LLETZ]*).
- A *cone biopsy (conization)* is a more extensive form of a cervical biopsy. It is called a cone biopsy because a cone-shaped wedge of tissue is removed from the cervix. Both normal and abnormal cervical tissues are removed. This can be performed by LEEP, surgical knife (scalpel), or carbon dioxide laser.

After colposcopy and a cervical biopsy, LEEP may be used to treat abnormal, precancerous cells found on biopsy. It can also be used to assess the extent of and sometimes to treat noninvasive cervical cancers.

Contraindications

- Patients with active menstrual bleeding
- Patients who are pregnant

Potential complications

- After the surgery, a small number of women (less than 10%) may have significant bleeding that requires vaginal packing or a blood transfusion.
- Infection of the cervix or uterus may occur. (This is rare.)

- Narrowing of the cervix (cervical stenosis) may occur, which can cause infertility. (This is rare.)

Procedure and patient care

Before

PT Explain the procedure to the patient.

- Obtain informed consent if required by the institution.

During

- Note the following procedural steps:
  1. The patient is placed in the lithotomy position and a vaginal speculum is used to expose the vagina and cervix.
  2. The cervix is cleansed with a 3% acetic acid solution or antiseptic to remove excess mucus and cellular debris and to accentuate the difference between normal and abnormal epithelial tissues.
  3. Medication is injected to numb the cervix *(cervical block)*.
  4. With the instrument chosen by the doctor, a punch biopsy, endocervical biopsy, LEEP, or cone biopsy is performed.
- Note that the physician performs the procedure in approximately 5 to 10 minutes.
- Whereas cone biopsy is done in the operating room, the other procedures can be performed in the doctor's office.
PT Tell the patient that some women complain of pressure pains from the vaginal speculum and that discomfort may be felt if biopsy specimens are obtained.
- Most women can return to normal activities immediately after a simple cervical biopsy or an endocervical biopsy.
- Most women will be able to return to normal activities within 2 to 4 days after LEEP or cone biopsies. This can vary, depending on the amount of tissue removed.

After

PT Inform the patient that it is normal to experience the following:
  o Vaginal bleeding if biopsy specimens were taken. Suggest that she wear a sanitary pad.
  o Mild cramping for several hours after the procedure
  o Brownish-black vaginal discharge during the first week
  o Vaginal discharge or spotting for about 1 to 3 weeks
PT Instruct the patient to use sanitary napkins instead of tampons for 1 to 3 weeks.
PT Tell the patient to avoid sexual intercourse for 3 to 4 weeks.
PT Inform the patient not to douche for 3 to 4 weeks.
PT Tell the patient how to obtain the test results.

PT Instruct the patient to call the doctor for any of the following symptoms:
- Fever
- Spotting or bleeding that lasts longer than 1 week
- Bleeding that is heavier than a normal menstrual period and contains blood clots
- Increasing pelvic pain
- Bad-smelling, yellowish vaginal discharge, which may indicate an infection

Abnormal findings

Chronic cervical infection
Cervical intraepithelial neoplasia
Cervical carcinoma in situ
Invasive cervical carcinoma
Endocervical adenocarcinoma

notes

chest x-ray (CXR)

Type of test X-ray

Normal findings Normal lungs and surrounding structures

Test explanation and related physiology

The chest x-ray image is important in a complete evaluation of the pulmonary and cardiac systems. Much information can be provided by the chest x-ray image. One can identify or follow (by repeated chest x-ray images) the following:

- Tumors of the lung (primary and metastatic), heart (myxoma), chest wall (soft tissue sarcomas), and bony thorax (osteogenic sarcoma)
- Inflammation of the lung (pneumonia), pleura (pleuritis), and pericardium (pericarditis)
- Fluid accumulation in the pleura (pleural effusion), pericardium (pericardial effusion), and lung (pulmonary edema)
- Air accumulation in the lung (chronic obstructive pulmonary disease) and pleura (pneumothorax)
- Fractures of the bones of the thorax or vertebrae
- Diaphragmatic hernia
- Heart size, which may vary depending on cardiac function
- Calcification, which may indicate large-vessel deterioration or old lung granulomas
- Location of centrally placed intravenous access devices

Most chest x-rays are taken with the patient standing. The sitting or supine position also can be used, but x-ray images taken with the patient in the supine position will not demonstrate fluid levels. A *posteroanterior (PA)* view, with the x-rays passing through the back of the body (posterior) to the front of the body (anterior), is taken first. Then a *lateral* view, with the x-rays passing through the patient's side, is taken.

Oblique views may be taken with the patient turned at different angles as the x-rays pass through the body. *Lordotic* views provide visualization of the apices (rounded upper portions) of the lungs and are usually used for detection of tuberculosis. *Decubitus* images are taken with the patient in the recumbent lateral position to localize fluid, which becomes dependent within the pleural space (pleural effusion).

Chest x-ray studies are best performed in the radiology department. Studies using a portable x-ray machine may be done at the bedside and are often performed on critically ill patients who cannot leave the nursing unit.

Contraindications

- Patients who are pregnant, unless the benefits outweigh the risks

Interfering factors

- Conditions (e.g., severe pain) that prevent the patient from taking and holding a deep breath
- Scarring from previous lung surgery, which makes interpretation difficult
- Obesity, which requires more x-rays to penetrate the body to provide a readable picture

Procedure and patient care

Before

PT Explain the procedure to the patient.

PT Tell the patient that no fasting is required.

PT Instruct the patient to remove clothing to the waist and to put on an x-ray gown.

PT Inform the patient to remove all metal objects (e.g., necklaces, pins) so that they do not block visualization of part of the chest.

PT Tell the patient that he or she will be asked to take a deep breath and hold it while the x-ray images are taken.

PT Instruct men to ensure that their testicles are covered and women to have their ovaries covered, using a lead shield to prevent radiation-induced abnormalities.

During

PT After the patient is correctly positioned, tell him or her to take a deep breath and hold it until the images are taken.

- Note that x-ray images are taken by a radiologic technologist in several minutes.

PT Inform the patient that no discomfort is associated with chest radiography.

After

- Note that no special care is required following the procedure.

Abnormal findings

Lung

Lung tumor (primary or metastatic)
Pneumonia
Pulmonary edema
Pleural effusion
Chronic obstructive pulmonary disease
Pneumothorax
Atelectasis
Tuberculosis
Lung abscess
Congenital lung diseases (hypoplasia)
Pleuritis
Foreign bodies (chest, bronchus, or esophagus)

Heart

Cardiac enlargement
Pericarditis
Pericardial effusion

Chest wall

Soft tissue sarcoma
Osteogenic sarcoma
Fracture (ribs or thoracic spine)
Thoracic spine scoliosis
Metastatic tumor to the bony thorax

Diaphragm

Diaphragmatic/hiatal hernia

Mediastinum

Aortic calcinosis
Enlarged lymph nodes
Dilated aorta
Thymoma
Lymphoma
Substernal thyroid
Widened mediastinum

notes

Chlamydia

Type of test Blood; microscopic examination

Normal findings

Negative culture
Antibodies:
Chlamydophila pneumoniae
 IgG: <1:64
 IgM: <1:10
Chlamydophila psittaci
 IgG: <1:64
 IgM: <1:10
Chlamydia trachomatis
 IgG: <1:64
 IgM: <1:10
Nucleic Acid Detection: negative

Test explanation and related physiology

There are many *Chlamydia* species that cause various diseases within the human body. *Chlamydophila psittaci* causes respiratory tract infections, headache, altered mentation, and hepatosplenomegaly. It occurs as a result of close contact with infected birds. *C. pneumoniae*, another species, causes pneumonia. *C. trachomatis* infection is probably the most frequently occurring sexually transmitted disease in developed countries. Infections of the genitalia, pelvic inflammatory disease, urethritis, cervicitis, salpingitis, and endometritis are most common. *C. trachomatis* may also infect the conjunctiva, pharynx, urethra, and rectum and cause lymphogranuloma venereum. The second serotype of *C. trachomatis* causes the eye disease *trachoma*, which is the most common form of preventable blindness. A third serotype produces genital and urethral infections different from lymphogranuloma. Most women colonized with *Chlamydia* are asymptomatic. *Chlamydia* infection is thought to be the most prevalent sexually transmitted disease in the United States.

Chlamydia infection can be diagnosed by identification and quantification of antibodies to the organism. Cytologic detection and culture testing is also available. Molecular testing through nucleic acid amplification/PCR represents the most sensitive diagnostic techniques. Tests can be performed on the blood of infected patients or swabs from the conjunctiva, nasopharynx, urethra, rectum, vagina, or cervix. Urine, seminal fluid, or pelvic washing can be used in culture and in direct identification of *Chlamydia*. Early identification of infection enables sexual partners to seek testing and/or treatment as soon as possible and reduces the risk of disease spread. Prompt treatment reduces the risk of infertility in women.

Interfering factors

- Women presently having routine menses
- Patients undergoing antibiotic therapy

Procedure and patient care

Before

PT Explain the procedure to the patient.

During

- For *Chlamydia* antibody testing, collect venous blood in a red-top tube. Acute and convalescent serum should be drawn 2 to 3 weeks apart.
- Sputum cultures (see p. 858) are used to check for *C. psittaci* respiratory infections.
- *Chlamydia* can be tested by direct nucleic acid identification or culture. A conjunctival smear is obtained by swabbing the eye lesion with a cotton-tipped applicator or scraping with a sterile ophthalmic spatula and smearing on a clean glass slide.
- Note the following procedural steps for *cervical culture*:
  1. The patient should refrain from douching and bathing in a tub before the cervical culture is performed.
  2. The patient is placed in the lithotomy position.
  3. A nonlubricated vaginal speculum is inserted to expose the cervix.
  4. Excess mucus is removed from the cervix using a cleaning swab.
  5. A second sterile, cotton-tipped swab is inserted into the endocervical canal and moved from side to side for 30 seconds to obtain the culture.
  6. The swab is then placed into an appropriate transport tube for testing.
- Note the following procedural steps for *urethral culture*:
  1. The urethral specimen should be obtained from the man before voiding within the previous hour.
  2. A culture is taken by inserting a thin sterile swab with rotating movement about 3 to 4 cm into the urethra.
- Note the following procedural steps for a *urine specimen:*
  1. The patient should not have urinated for at least 1 hour before specimen collection.

2. The patient should collect the first portion (first part of stream) of a random voided urine into a sterile, plastic, preservative-free container.

3. Transfer 2 mL of urine into the urine specimen collection tube using the disposable pipette provided. (The correct volume of urine has been added when the fluid level is between the black fill lines on the urine tube.)

- Note that these tests are performed by a physician, nurse, or other health care provider in several minutes.

PT Tell the patient that these procedures cause minimal discomfort.

After

- Treat patients who have positive smears with antibiotics.

PT Tell affected patients to have their sexual partners examined.

Abnormal findings

Chlamydia infection

notes

chloride, blood (Cl)

Type of test   Blood

Normal findings

Adult/elderly: 98-106 mEq/L or 98-106 mmol/L (SI units)
Child: 90-110 mEq/L
Newborn: 96-106 mEq/L
Premature infant: 95-110 mEq/L

Possible critical values   <80 or >115 mEq/L

Test explanation and related physiology

This test is performed as a part of *multiphasic testing* in what is usually called *electrolytes*. By itself, not much information is obtained. However, with interpretation of the other electrolytes, chloride can give an indication of acid-base balance and hydrational status.

Chloride is the major extracellular anion. Its main purpose is to maintain electrical neutrality, mostly as a salt with sodium. It follows sodium (cation) losses and accompanies sodium excesses to maintain electrical neutrality. For example, when aldosterone encourages sodium resorption, chloride follows to maintain electrical neutrality. Because water moves with sodium and chloride, chloride also affects water balance. Finally, chloride also serves as a buffer to assist in acid-base balance. As carbon dioxide (and H^+ cations) increases, bicarbonate must move from the intracellular space to the extracellular space. To maintain electrical neutrality, chloride will shift back into the cell.

Hypochloremia and hyperchloremia rarely occur alone and are usually part of parallel shifts in sodium or bicarbonate levels. Signs and symptoms of hypochloremia include hyperexcitability of the nervous system and muscles, shallow breathing, hypotension, and tetany. Signs and symptoms of hyperchloremia include lethargy, weakness, and deep breathing.

Interfering factors

• Excessive infusions of saline can result in increased chloride levels.

✘ Drugs that may cause *increased* serum chloride levels include acetazolamide, ammonium chloride, androgens, chlorothiazide, cortisone preparations, estrogens, guanethidine, hydrochlorothiazide, methyldopa, and nonsteroidal antiinflammatory drugs.

✠ Drugs that may cause *decreased* levels include aldosterone, bicarbonates, corticosteroids, cortisone, hydrocortisone, loop diuretics, thiazide diuretics, and triamterene.

Procedure and patient care

- See inside front cover for Routine Blood Testing.
- Fasting: no.
- Blood tube commonly used: red or green.

Abnormal findings

▲ Increased levels
(hyperchloremia)
Dehydration
Renal tubular acidosis
Excessive infusion of normal saline
Cushing syndrome
Eclampsia
Multiple myeloma
Kidney dysfunction
Metabolic acidosis
Hyperventilation
Anemia
Respiratory alkalosis
Hyperparathyroidism

▼ Decreased levels
(hypochloremia)
Overhydration
Congestive heart failure
Syndrome of inappropriate antidiuretic hormone
Vomiting
Chronic gastric suction
Chronic respiratory acidosis
Salt-losing nephritis
Addison disease
Burns
Metabolic alkalosis
Diuretic therapy
Hypokalemia
Aldosteronism
Respiratory acidosis

notes

cholesterol

Type of test Blood

Normal findings

Adult/elderly: <200 mg/dL or <5.20 mmol/L (SI units)
Child: 120-200 mg/dL
Infant: 70-175 mg/dL
Newborn: 53-135 mg/dL

Test explanation and related physiology

Cholesterol is the main lipid associated with arteriosclerotic vascular disease. However, cholesterol is required for the production of steroids, sex hormones, bile acids, and cellular membranes. Most of the cholesterol we eat comes from foods of animal origin. The liver metabolizes the cholesterol to its free form, and cholesterol is transported in the bloodstream by lipoproteins. Nearly 75% of the cholesterol is bound to low-density lipoproteins (LDLs) and 25% is bound to high-density lipoproteins (HDLs). Therefore, cholesterol is the main component of LDLs and only a minimal component of HDLs and very low-density lipoproteins. LDLs are most directly associated with increased risk of coronary heart disease (CHD).

The purpose of cholesterol testing is to identify patients at risk for arteriosclerotic heart disease. Cholesterol testing is usually done as a part of *lipid profile* testing, which also evaluates lipoproteins (see p. 587) and triglycerides (see p. 927), because by itself cholesterol is not a totally accurate predictor of heart disease.

Elevated results should be corroborated by repeating the study. The two results should be averaged to obtain an accurate cholesterol for risk assessment.

Because the liver is required to make cholesterol, low serum cholesterol levels are indicative of severe liver diseases. Furthermore, because our main source of cholesterol is our diet, malnutrition is also associated with low cholesterol levels. Certain illnesses can affect cholesterol levels. For example, patients with an acute myocardial infarction may have as much as a 50% reduction in cholesterol level for as many as 6 to 8 weeks.

The Adult Treatment Panel III (ATP III) of the National Cholesterol Education Program issued an evidence-based set of guidelines on cholesterol management. The goal for high-risk patients (those with known coronary artery disease or more than two risk factors) is LDL <70 mg/dL. All ATP reports have identified low-density lipoprotein cholesterol (LDL-C) as the primary target of cholesterol lowering therapy. Many prospective studies have shown that high serum concentrations of LDL-C are a major risk factor for CHD. Moreover, lowering of LDL-C levels will reduce the risk for major coronary events. The cholesterol-to-HDL ratio has been used to assess the risk of CHD (Table 7). Familial hyperlipidemias and hyperlipoproteinemias are often associated with high cholesterol.

Interfering factors

- Pregnancy is usually associated with elevated cholesterol levels.
- Oophorectomy increases levels.
- Drugs that may cause *increased* levels include adrenocorticotropic hormone, anabolic steroids, beta-adrenergic blocking agents, corticosteroids, cyclosporine, epinephrine, oral contraceptives, phenytoin (Dilantin), sulfonamides, thiazide diuretics, and vitamin D.
- Drugs that may cause *decreased* levels include allopurinol, androgens, bile salt-binding agents, captopril, chlorpropamide, clofibrate, colchicine, colestipol, erythromycin, isoniazid, liothyronine (Cytomel), monoamine oxidase inhibitors, neomycin (oral), niacin, nitrates, and statins.

Procedure and patient care

- See inside front cover for Routine Blood Testing.
- Fasting: yes.
- Blood tube commonly used: red.
- PT Instruct the patient to fast 12 to 14 hours after eating a low-fat diet before testing. Only water is permitted. Food can elevate triglyceride levels.
- PT Inform the patient that dietary intake at least 2 weeks before testing will affect results.

TABLE 7 Cholesterol-to-HDL ratio as an indicator of risk of CHD

Risk	Ratio	
	Male	Female
½ Average	3.4	3.3
Average	5.0	4.4
2× Average	10.0	7.0
3 × Average	24.0	11.0

^{PT} Tell the patient that no alcohol should be consumed 24 hours before the test.

• The fingerstick method is often used in mass screening.

^{PT} Instruct patients with high levels regarding a low-cholesterol diet, exercise, and appropriate body weight.

Abnormal findings

▲ **Increased levels**
Hypercholesterolemia
Hyperlipidemia
Hypothyroidism
Uncontrolled diabetes
  mellitus
Nephrotic syndrome
Pregnancy
High-cholesterol diet
Xanthomatosis
Hypertension
Myocardial infarction
Atherosclerosis
Biliary cirrhosis
Stress
Nephrosis

▼ **Decreased levels**
Malabsorption
Malnutrition
Hyperthyroidism
Cholesterol-lowering
  medication
Pernicious anemia
Hemolytic anemia
Sepsis
Stress
Liver disease
Acute myocardial infarction

notes

cholinesterase (CHS, Pseudocholinesterase [PChE], Cholinesterase RBC, Red blood cell cholinesterase, Acetylcholinesterase)

Type of test Blood

Normal findings

Serum cholinesterase: 8-18 units/mL or 8-18 units/L (SI units)

RBC cholinesterase: 5-10 units/mL or 5-10 units/L (SI units)

Dibucaine inhibition: 79% to 84%

(Values vary with laboratory test methods.)

Test explanation and related physiology

This test is done to identify patients with pseudocholinesterase deficiency before anesthesia or to identify patients who may have been exposed to phosphate poisoning. Cholinesterases hydrolyze acetylcholine and other choline esters and thereby regulate nerve impulse transmission at the nerve synapse and neuromuscular junction. There are two types of cholinesterases: *acetylcholinesterase*, also known as *true cholinesterase*, and pseudocholinesterase. True cholinesterase exists primarily in the red blood cells and nerve tissue. It is not in the serum. *Pseudocholinesterase*, on the other hand, exists in the serum. Deficiencies in either of these enzymes can be acquired or congenital.

Because succinylcholine (the most commonly used muscle relaxant during anesthesia induction) is inactivated by pseudocholinesterase, people with an inherited pseudocholinesterase enzyme deficiency exhibit increased and/or prolonged effects of succinylcholine. Patients with a genetic variant of pseudocholinesterase may have a nonfunctioning form of pseudocholinesterase and will also experience prolonged effects of succinylcholine administration. Prolonged muscle paralysis and apnea will occur after anesthesia in these patients. This situation can be avoided by measuring serum cholinesterase (pseudocholinesterase) in all patients with a family history of prolonged apnea after surgery.

Because patients with a nonfunctioning variant of pseudocholinesterase will have normal total quantitative pseudocholinesterase levels yet still have prolonged paralytic effects of succinylcholine, a second test (dibucaine inhibition) usually is also performed. Dibucaine is a known local anesthetic that inhibits the function of normal pseudocholinesterase. The *dibucaine inhibition number* is the percent of pseudocholinesterase activity that is inhibited when dibucaine is added to the patient's serum sample. If total pseudocholinesterase is normal and dibucaine numbers are low, the presence of a nonfunctioning pseudocholinesterase variant is suspected and the patient will be at risk for succinylcholine-induced prolonged paralysis.

A common form of acquired cholinesterase deficiency, either true or pseudocholinesterase, is caused by overexposure to pesticides, organophosphates, or nerve gas. The half-life of the pseudo-enzyme in serum is about 8 days, and the true cholinesterase (AChE) of red cells is more than 3 months (determined by erythropoietic activity). Recent exposure up to several weeks is determined by assay of the pseudo-enzyme and months after exposure by measurement of the red cell enzyme. Persons with jobs associated with chronic exposure to these chemicals are often monitored by the frequent testing of RBC cholinesterase activity. Other potential causes of reduced cholinesterase activity include chronic liver diseases, malnutrition, and hypoalbuminemia.

Increased cholinesterase activity, when found in the amniotic fluid, represents strong evidence for a *neural tube defect (NTD)*. When an NTD is suspected based upon maternal serum alpha-fetoprotein (AFP) screening results or diagnosed via ultrasound, analysis of AFP and acetylcholinesterase (AChE) in amniotic fluid are useful diagnostic tools.

Interfering factors

- Pregnancy decreases test values.
- ✘ Drugs that may cause *decreased* values include atropine, caffeine, codeine, estrogens, morphine sulfate, neostigmine, oral contraceptives, phenothiazines, quinidine, theophylline, and vitamin K.

Procedure and patient care

- See inside front cover for Routine Blood Testing.
- Fasting: no.
- Blood tube commonly used: red.
- If the test is done to identify the presurgical patient who may be at risk for cholinesterase deficiency, be sure the test is completed several days before the planned surgery.
- It may be recommended to withhold medications that could alter test results for 12 to 24 hours before the test.

Abnormal findings

▲ **Increased serum levels**
Hyperlipidemia
Nephrosis
Diabetes mellitus

▼ **Decreased serum levels**
Poisoning from
organophosphate
insecticides
Hepatocellular disease
Persons with congenital
pseudocholinesterase
enzyme deficiency
Malnutrition

▲ **Increased RBC levels**
Reticulocytosis
Sickle cell disease

▼ **Decreased RBC levels**
Congenital
cholinesterase
deficiency
Poisoning from
organophosphate
insecticides

notes

chorionic villus sampling (CVS, Chorionic villus biopsy [CVB])

Type of test Cell analysis

Normal findings No genetic or biochemical disorders

Test explanation and related physiology

CVS is performed on women whose unborn children may be at risk for life-threatening or significant life-altering genetic defects. This would include women who:

- Are older than age 35 years at the time of pregnancy
- Have had frequent spontaneous abortions
- Have had previous pregnancies with fetuses or infants with chromosomal or genetic defects (e.g., Down syndrome)
- Have a genetic defect themselves (e.g., hemoglobinopathies)

CVS can be performed between 8 and 12 weeks of gestation for the early detection of genetic and biochemical disorders. Because CVS detects congenital defects early, first-trimester therapeutic abortions can be performed if indicated.

For this study, a sample of chorionic villi from the chorion frondosum, which is the trophoblastic origin of the placenta, is obtained for analysis. These villi are present from 8 to 12 weeks on and reflect fetal chromosome, enzyme, and deoxyribonucleic acid content, thus permitting a much earlier diagnosis of prenatal problems than amniocentesis (see p. 49), which cannot be done before 14 to 16 weeks. Furthermore, the cells derived by CVS are more easily grown in tissue culture for *karyotyping* (determination of chromosomal/genetic abnormalities). The cells obtained with amniocentesis take a longer time to grow in culture, further adding to the delay in obtaining results.

Potential complications

- Accidental abortion
- Infection
- Bleeding
- Fetal limb deformities

Procedure and patient care

Before

PT Explain the procedure to the patient.
- Be certain that the physician has obtained a signed consent.
PT Tell the patient that no food or fluid restrictions are necessary.
PT Encourage the patient to drink at least 1 to 2 glasses of fluid before testing.

PT Instruct the patient not to urinate for several hours before testing. A full bladder is an excellent reference point for pelvic ultrasound.

- Assess the vital signs of the mother and the fetal heart rate of the fetus before testing. These are baseline studies that should be repeated during and on completion of the test.

During

- Note the following procedural steps:
  1. The patient is placed in the lithotomy position.
  2. Samples of vaginal mucus may be obtained to rule out preprocedural infections (such as *Chlamydia*).
  3. A cannula from the endoscope is inserted into the cervix and uterine cavity (Figure 9).
  4. Under ultrasound guidance, the cannula is rotated to the site of the developing placenta.
  5. A syringe is attached, and suction is applied to obtain several samples of villi.
  6. As many as three or more samples may be obtained to get sufficient tissue for accurate sampling.

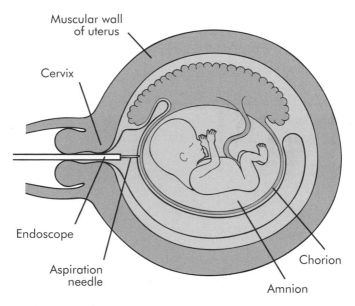

FIGURE 9 Chorionic villus sampling. Diagram of an 8-week pregnancy showing endoscopic aspiration of extraplacental villi.

7. If ultrasound indicates that the trophoblastic tissue is remote from the cervix, a transabdominal approach similar to that described for amniocentesis (see p. 49) may be used.

- Note that this procedure is performed by an obstetrician in approximately 30 minutes.

PT Inform the patient that discomfort associated with this test is similar to that of a Pap smear.

After

- Note that Rh-negative women (who have not been sensitized to Rh incompatability) receive RhoGAM. This procedure may be contraindicated for women with known pre-existing Rh sensitization.
- Monitor the vital signs and check for signs of bleeding.
- Schedule the patient for an ultrasound in 2 to 4 days to confirm the continued viability of the fetus.
- Assess the vaginal area for discharge and drainage; note the color and amount.

PT Assess and educate the patient for signs of spontaneous abortion (e.g., cramps, bleeding).

PT Inform the patient how she can obtain the results from her physician. Make sure she understands that the results usually will not be available for several weeks. (Results may be available much sooner at major medical centers that perform this test.)

PT Educate the patient about how to identify and report signs of endometrial infection (vaginal discharge, fever, crampy abdominal pain).

PT Inform the patient about genetic counseling services if needed.

Abnormal findings

Genetic and biochemical disorders

notes

chromosome karyotype (Blood chromosome analysis, Chromosome studies, Cytogenetics, Karyotype)

Type of test Blood

Normal findings

Female: 44 autosomes+2 X chromosomes; karyotype: 46,XX
Male: 44 autosomes+1 X, 1 Y chromosome; karyotype: 46,XY

Test explanation and related physiology

This test is used to study an individual's chromosomal makeup to determine chromosomal defects associated with disease or the risk of developing disease. The term *karyotyping* refers to the arrangement and pairing of cell chromosomes in order from the largest to the smallest to analyze their number and structure. Variations in either can produce numerous developmental abnormalities and diseases. A normal karyotype of chromosomes consists of a pattern of 22 pairs of autosomal chromosomes and a pair of sex chromosomes (XY for the male and XX for the female). Chromosomal karyotype abnormalities can be congenital or acquired. These karyotype abnormalities can occur because of duplication, deletion, translocation, reciprocation, or genetic rearrangement.

Chromosomal karyotyping is useful in evaluating congenital anomalies, mental retardation, growth retardation, delayed puberty, infertility, hypogonadism, primary amenorrhea, ambiguous genitalia, chronic myelogenous leukemia, neoplasm, recurrent miscarriage, prenatal diagnosis of serious congenital diseases (especially in situations of advanced maternal age), Turner syndrome, Klinefelter syndrome, Down syndrome, and other suspected genetic disorders. The products of conception also can be studied to determine the cause of stillbirth or miscarriage.

Procedure and patient care

Before

PT Explain the procedure to the patient.

- Determine how the specimen will be collected. Obtain preparation guidelines from the laboratory if indicated.
- Many patients are fearful of the test results and require considerable emotional support.
- In some states, informed consent is required.

During

- Specimens for chromosome analysis can be obtained from numerous sources. Leukocytes from a peripheral venipuncture are most easily and most often used for this study.
- Bone marrow biopsies and surgical specimens also can be used sometimes as sources for analysis.
- During pregnancy, specimens can be collected by amniocentesis (see p. 49) and chorionic villus sampling (see p. 254).
- Fetal tissue or products of conception can be studied to determine the reason for loss of a pregnancy.
- Smears and stains of buccal mucosal cells are less costly but not as accurate as other tissue for karyotyping.

After

- Aftercare depends on how the specimen was collected.
- **PT** Inform the patient that test results generally will not be available for several months.
- If an abnormality is identified, often the entire family line must be tested. This can be exhaustive and expensive.
- **PT** If the test results show an abnormality, encourage the patient to verbalize his or her feelings. Provide emotional support.

Abnormal findings

Congenital anomalies
Mental retardation
Growth retardation
Delayed puberty
Infertility
Hypogonadism
Primary amenorrhea
Ambiguous genitalia
Chronic myelogenous leukemia
Neoplasm
Recurrent miscarriage
Trisomy 21 (Down syndrome)
Tay-Sachs disease
Sickle cell anemia
Turner syndrome
Klinefelter syndrome

notes

Clostridium difficile (*C. diff*, Clostridial toxin assay)

Type of test Stool

Normal findings Negative (no *Clostridium* toxin identified)

Test explanation and related physiology

Clostridium difficile–associated disease (CDAD) bacterial infections usually affect the intestine (pseudomembranous colitis) and occur in patients who are immunocompromised or taking broad-spectrum antibiotics (e.g., clindamycin, ampicillin, cephalosporins). The disease severity can range from mild nuisance diarrhea to severe pseudomembranous colitis and bowel perforation. The overwhelming predisposing factor is ongoing antibiotic therapy. Patient age, length of hospital stay, acuity of illness, and comorbidities are risk factors.

The infection possibly results from depression of the normal flora of the bowel caused by the administration of antibiotics. The clostridial bacterium produces two toxins (A and B) that cause inflammation and necrosis of the colonic epithelium. The standard for laboratory detection of *C. difficile* toxins is the cytotoxicity assay in cell cultures. Toxin detection by enzyme immunoassay (EIA) is insensitive. *C. difficile* can also be diagnosed by obtaining colonic-rectal tissue for this toxin. Stool cultures (p. 862) for *C. difficile* can be performed but are also labor intensive and take longer to get results.

A polymerase chain reaction (PCR) assay for the qualitative in vitro rapid detection of *C. difficile* toxin B gene (tcdB) in human liquid or soft stool specimens is available. This method rapidly provides a definitive diagnosis of *C. difficile*. Quickly reaching a definitive diagnosis allows CDAD patients to get the proper treatment without delay and reduce hospital stays for inpatients with CDAD. At the same time, they can be placed in isolation sooner to reduce transmission and prevent outbreaks. Definitive results can reduce inappropriate antimicrobial use in negative patients.

A positive PCR result for the presence of the gene-regulating toxin C production (tcdC) indicates the presence of *C. difficile* and toxin A and/or B. A negative result indicates the absence of detectable *C. difficile* tcdC DNA in the specimen but does not rule out *C. difficile* infection.

Procedure and patient care

Before

PT Explain the method of stool collection to the patient. Be matter-of-fact to avoid embarrassment to the patient.

PT Instruct the patient not to mix urine or toilet paper with the stool specimen.

- Handle the specimen carefully, as though it were capable of causing infection.

During

PT Instruct the patient to defecate into a clean container. A rectal swab cannot be used because it collects inadequate amounts of stool. The stool cannot be retrieved from the toilet.

- Stool can be obtained from incontinence pads.
- A stool specimen also can be collected by proctoscopy.
- Place the specimen in a closed container and transport it to the laboratory to prevent deterioration of the toxin.
- If the specimen cannot be processed immediately, refrigerate it (depending on laboratory protocol).

After

- Maintain enteric isolation precautions on all patients until appropriate therapy is completed.

Abnormal findings

▲ **Increased levels**

Antibiotic-related pseudomembranous colitis

C. difficile colitis

notes

coagulating factors concentration (Coagulating factors, Blood-clotting factors)

Type of test Blood

C

Normal findings

Factor	Normal value (% of "normal")
II	80-120
V	50-150
VII	65-140
VIII	55-145
IX	60-140
X	45-155
XI	65-135
XII	50-150

Test explanation and related physiology

These tests measure the quantity of each specific factor thought to be responsible for suspected defects in hemostasis. Testing is available to measure the quantity of the factors listed in the normal findings section. When these factors exist in concentrations below their *minimal hemostatic levels*, clotting is impaired.

Deficiencies of these factors may be a result of inherited genetic defects, acquired diseases, or drug therapy. Common medical conditions associated with abnormal factor concentrations are listed in Table 8. It is important to identify the exact factor or factors involved in the coagulating defect so that appropriate blood component replacement can be administered.

The hemostasis and coagulation system is a homeostatic balance between factors encouraging clotting and those encouraging clot dissolution (Figure 10). See Table 9 for a list of factor names and routine coagulation test abnormalities associated with factor deficiency.

Fibrinogen (or factor I, see p. 439), like many of the coagulation proteins, is considered an acute reactant protein and is elevated in many severe illnesses. It is also considered a risk factor for coronary heart disease and stroke.

Prothrombin is a vitamin K–dependent clotting factor. Its production in the liver requires vitamin K. This vitamin is fat soluble and is dependent on bile for absorption. Bile duct obstruction or malabsorption causes a vitamin K–deficiency and

TABLE 8 Conditions that may result in coagulation factor excess or deficiency

Factor	Increased (excess)	Decreased (deficiency)
I (Fibrinogen)	Acute inflammatory reactions Trauma Coronary heart disease Cigarette smoking	Liver disease (hepatitis or cirrhosis) DIC Congenital deficiency
II (Prothrombin)	ND	Vitamin K deficiency Liver disease Congenital deficiency Warfarin ingestion
V (Proaccelerin)	ND	Liver disease DIC Fibrinolysis
VII (Proconvertin [stable factor])	ND	Congenital deficiency Vitamin K deficiency Liver disease Warfarin ingestion
VIII (Anti-hemophilic factor)	Acute inflammatory reactions Trauma/stress Pregnancy Birth control pills	Congenital deficiency (e.g., hemophilia A) DIC
von Willebrand factor	ND	Congenital deficiency (e.g., von Willebrand disease) Some myeloproliferative disorders
IX (Christmas factor)	ND	Congenital deficiency (e.g., hemophilia B) Liver disease Nephrotic syndrome Warfarin ingestion DIC Vitamin K deficiency

TABLE 8   Conditions that may result in coagulation factor excess
or deficiency—cont'd

Factor	Increased (excess)	Decreased (deficiency)
X (Stuart factor)	ND	Congenital deficiency Liver disease Warfarin ingestion Vitamin K deficiency
XII (Hageman factor)	ND	Congenital deficiency Liver disease DIC

ND, There is no common disease state known to be associated with an
excess of this factor; *DIC*, disseminated intravascular coagulation.

results in reduced quantity of prothrombin and other vitamin
K–dependent factors (e.g., VII, IX, X).

Factor VIII is actually a complex molecule with two components. The first component is related to hemophilia A and is
involved in the hemostatic mechanism. The second component
is von Willebrand factor and is related to von Willebrand disease. This second component is involved in platelet adhesion and
aggregation. Factor XII deficiency is a common cause of prolonged activated partial thromboplastin time (APTT) in a non-
bleeding patient.

Coagulation factor inhibitors arise in patients who are congenitally deficient in a specific factor in response to factor replacement therapy. They can also occur spontaneously without known
cause or in response to a variety of medical conditions, including
the postpartum state, immunologic disorders, certain antibiotic
therapies, some malignancies, and old age.

Interfering factors

- Many of these proteins are heat sensitive, and levels are
  decreased if the specimen is kept at room temperature.
- Pregnancy or the use of contraceptive medication can increase
  levels of several of these factors, especially VIII and IX.
- Many of these protein coagulation factors are *acute reactant*
  proteins. Acute illness, stress, exercise, or inflammation can
  raise levels.

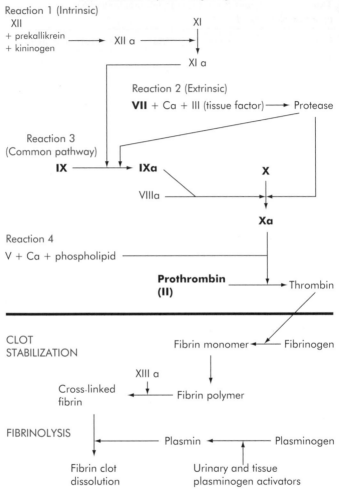

Hemostasis and Fibrinolysis

Bold = Vitamin K–dependent coagulating factors

Reaction 1 (Intrinsic)

XII
+ prekallikrein
+ kininogen → XII a → XI

XI → XI a

Reaction 2 (Extrinsic)

VII + Ca + III (tissue factor) → Protease

Reaction 3
(Common pathway)

IX → **IXa**   **X**

VIIIa → **Xa**

Reaction 4

V + Ca + phospholipid

**Prothrombin
(II)** → Thrombin

CLOT
STABILIZATION

Fibrin monomer ← Fibrinogen

XIII a

Cross-linked
fibrin ← Fibrin polymer

FIBRINOLYSIS

Fibrin clot
dissolution ← Plasmin ← Plasminogen

Urinary and tissue
plasminogen activators

FIGURE 10 Secondary hemostasis (fibrin clot formation) and fibrinolysis (fibrin clot dissolution). Primary hemostasis involves platelet plugging of the injured blood vessel. Secondary hemostasis, as described here, takes place most rapidly on the platelet surface after attachment to the fractured endothelium. Four different reactions result in the formation of fibrin. As seen beneath the dark line in the figure, the fibrin clot supports the platelet clump so that the clot does not get swept away by the tremendous shear forces of the fast-moving blood cells. Fibrinolysis follows formation of the fibrin clot in order to prevent complete occlusion of the injured blood vessel.

TABLE 9 List of minimum concentration of coagulation factors required for fibrin production

Factor	Name	Quantitation of minimum hemostatic level (mg/dL)	Abnormal coagulation tests associated with deficiency	Blood components to provide specific factor
I	Fibrinogen	60-100	PT, APTT	C, FFP, FWB
II	Prothrombin	10-15	PT	P, WB, FFP, FWB
III	Tissue factor or thromboplastin	Not applicable	PT	
IV	Calcium	See calcium, p. 203		
V	Proaccelerin	5-10	PT, APTT	FFP, FWB
VII	Stable factor	5-20	PT	P, WB, FFP, FWB
VIII	Antihemophilic factor	30	APTT	C, FFP, VIII CONC
IX	Christmas factor	30	APTT	FFP, FWB
X	Stuart factor	8-10	PT, APTT	P, WB, FFP, FWB
XI	Plasma thromboplastin antecedent	25	APTT	P, WB, FFP, FWB
XII	Hageman factor	Yes	APTT	
XIII	Fibrin stabilizing factor	No		P, C, XIII CONC

APTT, Activated partial thromboplastin time; *PT*, prothrombin time; *C*, cryoprecipitate; *FFP*, fresh frozen plasma; *FWB*, fresh whole blood (less than 24 hours old); *P*, unfrozen banked plasma; *WB*, banked whole blood; *VIII CONC*, factor VIII concentrate; *XIII CONC*, factor XIII concentrate. Note: Recombinant factors are now available for factor VII, VIII, IX, and XIII. Concentrates are also now available for II, VII, VIII, IX, and XIII.

Procedure and patient care
- See inside front cover for Routine Blood Testing.
- Fasting: no.
- Blood tube commonly used: blue.

Abnormal findings
See Table 8 on p. 262.

notes

cold agglutinins

Type of test Blood

Normal findings No agglutination in titers ≤1:64

Test explanation and related physiology

Cold agglutinins are antibodies (usually IgM) to erythrocytes. All individuals have circulating antibodies directed against red blood cells (RBCs), but their concentrations are often too low to trigger disease (titers under 1:64). In individuals with *cold agglutinin disease*, these antibodies are in much higher concentrations. At body temperatures of 28° C to 31° C, such as those encountered during winter months, these antibodies can cause a variety of symptoms, from chronic anemia due to intravascular hemolysis or extravascular sequestration of affected RBCs to acrocyanosis of the ears, fingers, or toes due to local blood stasis in the skin capillaries.

There are two forms of cold agglutinin disease: primary and secondary. The primary form has no precipitating cause. Secondary cold agglutinin disease is a result of an underlying condition, notably *Mycoplasma pneumoniae*. Other possible underlying conditions include influenza, mononucleosis, rheumatoid arthritis, lymphomas, HIV, Epstein Barr virus, and cytomegalovirus. Temperature regulation is important for the performance of these tests. Under no circumstance should the cold agglutinin specimen be refrigerated.

The cold agglutinin screen is performed on all specimens first to identify most of those with titer values in the normal range. If the screen is negative, no titration is required. If the screen is positive, a titer with serial saline dilutions is performed.

Interfering factors

✂ Some antibiotics (penicillin and cephalosporins) can interfere with the development of cold agglutinins.

Procedure and patient care

- See inside front cover for Routine Blood Testing.
- Fasting: no.
- Blood tube commonly used: red.

Abnormal findings

▲ **Increased levels**
Mycoplasma pneumoniae infection
Viral illness
Infectious mononucleosis
Multiple myeloma
Scleroderma
Cirrhosis
Staphylococcemia
Thymic tumor
Influenza
Rheumatoid arthritis
Lymphoma
Systemic lupus erythematosus
Primary cold agglutinin disease

notes

> **colon cancer tumor analysis** (Microsatellite instability [MSI] testing, DNA mismatch repair [MMR] genetic testing, BRAF mutation analysis, Oncotype DX colon cancer assay)

C

Type of test Microscopic examination

Normal findings

Recurrence score <10
No mismatch repair gene
No microsatellite instability

Test explanation and related physiology

Patients with stage I colon cancer have a high cure rate with surgery alone. Patients with stage III colon cancer benefit from the use of adjuvant chemotherapy. Patients with stage II colon cancer may or may not benefit from adjuvant chemotherapy. Colon cancer tumor analysis can help differentiate the stage II patients who may benefit from adjuvant chemotherapy. These tests are used to indicate the risk of recurrent colon cancer in the years succeeding surgical treatment.

Deficiencies in DNA mismatch repair (MMR) gene function, either due to decreased gene expression or mutation, result in the accumulation of DNA alterations that can manifest as abnormal shortening or lengthening of microsatellite DNA sequences in the colon cancer cell. This causes microsatellite instability (MSI). Patients with MMR-deficient (MMR-D) colon tumors have high MSI and have been shown to have significantly lower colon cancer recurrence risk. Therefore, testing the colon tumor for MMR and MSI can help determine the likelihood of recurrence after surgery and quantify any benefit from adjuvant chemotherapy.

Furthermore, hereditary colon cancers frequently are positive for MSI as compared to sporadic colon cancers. Lynch syndrome (a hereditary form of colon cancer) can be suspected if the tumor is MSI positive. MSI is performed by immunohistochemical identification of specific nucleic acid. MMR genetic testing is most frequently performed by PCR testing.

BRAF is another important gene that is used to indicate the likelihood that a colon tumor is hereditary. BRAF is a kinase-encoding gene in the RAS/RAF/MAPK pathway. The presence of a BRAF V600E mutation in a microsatellite unstable tumor indicates that the tumor is probably sporadic and not associated with hereditary non-polyposis colorectal cancer (HNPCC). The lack of this mutation indicates that a tumor may either be sporadic or HNPCC-associated.

The Oncotype DX colon cancer assay evaluates 12 genes and provides an individualized score reflective of the risk of colon cancer recurrence for individual patients with stage II colon cancer. The assay uses RT-PCR platform to quantitate the level of expression of each of the 12 genes in the panel using the patient's colon tumor. For each patient, the assay produces a Recurrence Score that is closely associated with the patient's risk of recurrent colon cancer 3 years after surgery (the peak time of recurrence). MMR and MSI testing can complement the information provided by the Oncotype DX colon cancer assay.

Procedure and patient care

Before

PT Inform the patient that an examination for these tumor predictor markers may be performed on their colon cancer tissue.

PT Provide psychological and emotional support to the colon cancer patient.

During

- The surgeon obtains tumor tissue.
- This tissue should be placed on ice or in formalin.
- Part of the tissue is used for routine histology. A portion of the paraffin block is sent to a reference laboratory.

After

PT Explain to the patient that results are usually available in 1 week.

Abnormal findings

Unfavorable test results indicating a high risk of cancer reoccurrence.

notes

colonoscopy

Type of test Endoscopy

Normal findings Normal colon

Test explanation and related physiology

With fiberoptic colonoscopy, the entire colon from anus to cecum can be examined in most patients. As with sigmoidoscopy, benign and malignant neoplasms, polyps, mucosal inflammation, ulceration, and sites of active hemorrhage can be visualized. Such diseases as cancer, polyps, ulcers, and arteriovenous (AV) malformations also can be visualized. Cancers, polyps, and inflammatory bowel diseases can be biopsied through the colonoscope with cable-activated instruments; sites of active bleeding can be coagulated with the use of laser, electrocoagulation, and injection of sclerosing agents.

This test is recommended for patients who have Hemoccult-positive stools, abnormal sigmoidoscopy, lower GI tract bleeding, or a change in bowel habits. This test is also recommended for patients who are at high risk for colon cancer. They include patients with a strong personal or family history of colon cancer, polyps, or ulcerative colitis. For asymptomatic individuals over 50 with no colorectal cancer risk factors, the American Cancer Society has recommended colonoscopy screening every 10 years. Virtual colonoscopy is now an option (see p. 282).

Contraindications

- Patients whose medical condition is not stable
- Patients who are bleeding profusely from the rectum
  The viewing lens will become covered with blood clots.
- Patients with a suspected perforation of the colon
- Patients with toxic megacolon
  These patients may worsen with the test preparation.
- Patients with a recent colon anastomosis (within the last 14 to 21 days)
  The anastomosis may break down with significant insufflation of CO_2.

Potential complications

- Bowel perforation
- Persistent bleeding from a biopsy site
- Oversedation, resulting in respiratory depression

Interfering factors

- Poor bowel preparation may result in stool obstructing the lens and precluding adequate visualization of the colon.
- Active bleeding obstructs the lens system and precludes adequate visualization of the colon.

Procedure and patient care

Before

PT Explain the procedure to the patient.

PT Fully inform the patient about the risks of the procedure and obtain an informed consent.

PT Assure patients that they will be appropriately draped to avoid unnecessary embarrassment.

PT Instruct the patient on appropriate bowel preparation. One type is the *2-day bowel preparation*, which uses clear liquids for 2 days, along with a strong cathartic such as magnesium citrate and bisacodyl (Dulcolax). On the day of examination, an enema is given. A *1-day preparation* using a glycol (CoLyte) bowel preparation is more widely used. After the patient ingests a gallon of CoLyte, enemas are not usually needed. The 1 gallon should be consumed within 4 hours if possible. Lemonade powder may be added to the glycol cathartic.

- Avoid an oral bowel preparation in patients with upper gastrointestinal obstruction, suspected acute diverticulitis, or recent bowel resectional surgery.
- Administer appropriate preendoscopy sedation.

During

- Note the following procedural steps:
  1. IV access is obtained for sedation.
  2. After a rectal examination indicates adequate bowel preparation, the patient is sedated.
  3. The patient is placed in the lateral decubitus position, and the colonoscope is placed into the rectum.
  4. Under direct visualization, the colonoscope is directed to the cecum. Often a significant amount of manipulation is required to obtain this position.
  5. As in all endoscopies, air is insufflated to distend the bowel for better visualization.
  6. Complete examination of the large bowel is carried out.
  7. Polypectomy, biopsy, and other endoscopic surgery is performed after appropriate visualization.

- Note that this test is performed by a physician trained in gastrointestinal endoscopy in approximately 30 to 60 minutes.
- **PT** Tell the patient that minimal discomfort is associated with the test.

After

PT Explain to patients that air has been insufflated into the bowel. They may experience flatulence or gas pains.
- Examine the abdomen for evidence of colon perforation (abdominal distention, tenderness, fever, and chills).
- Monitor vital signs for a decrease in blood pressure and an increase in pulse as an indication of hemorrhage.
- Inspect the stool for gross blood.
- Notify the physician if the patient develops increased pain or significant gastrointestinal bleeding.
- Allow the patient to eat when fully alert if no evidence of bowel perforation exists.
- **PT** Encourage the patient to drink a lot of fluids when intake is allowed. This will make up for the dehydration associated with the bowel preparation.
- **PT** Inform the patient that frequent, bloody bowel movements may indicate poor hemostasis after biopsy or polypectomy.
- **PT** Educate the patient to report abdominal bloating and inability to pass flatus, which may indicate colon obstruction if a neoplasm was identified.
- **PT** Assess the patient for and educate to report weakness and dizziness, which may indicate orthostasis and hypovolemia due to dehydration.

Abnormal findings

Colorectal cancer
Colon polyps
Inflammatory bowel disease (e.g., ulcerative or Crohn colitis)
Arteriovenous malformations
Hemorrhoids
Ischemic or postinflammatory strictures
Diverticulosis

notes

colposcopy

Type of test Endoscopy

Normal findings Normal vagina and cervix

Test explanation and related physiology

Colposcopy provides an *in situ* macroscopic examination of the vagina and cervix with a *colposcope*, which is a macroscope with a light source and a magnifying lens (Figure 11). With this procedure, tiny areas of dysplasia, carcinoma *in situ*, and invasive cancer that would be missed by the naked eye can be visualized, and biopsy specimens can be obtained. The study is performed on patients with abnormal vaginal epithelial patterns, cervical lesions, abnormal Pap smears, or positive HPV results and on those exposed to diethylstilbestrol in utero. This procedure is

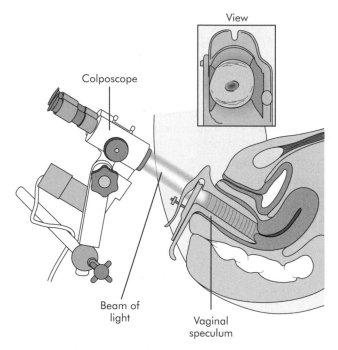

View

Colposcope

Beam of
light

Vaginal
speculum

FIGURE 11 Colposcopy. A colposcope is used to evaluate patients with an abnormal Pap smear and a grossly normal cervix.

used to determine the need for cone biopsy (removal and examination of a cone of tissue from the cervix) in evaluating the cause of abnormal cervical cytologic findings.

It is important to realize that colposcopy is useful only in identifying a suspicious lesion. Definitive diagnosis requires biopsy of the tissue. One of the major advantages of this procedure is the capability of directing the biopsy to the area most likely to be truly representative of the lesion. A biopsy performed without colposcopy may not necessarily be representative of the lesion's true pathological condition, resulting in a significant risk of missing a serious lesion.

The patient will need to have diagnostic conization if:

- Colposcopy and endocervical curettage do not explain the problem or match the cytologic findings of the Pap smear within one grade.
- The entire transformation zone is not seen.
- The lesion extends up the cervical canal beyond the vision of the colposcope.

The need for up to 90% of cone biopsies is eliminated by an experienced colposcopist. Endocervical curettage may accompany colposcopy to detect unknown lesions in the endocervical canal.

Contraindications

- Patients with heavy menstrual flow

Interfering factors

- Failure to cleanse the cervix of foreign materials (e.g., creams, medications) may impair visualization.

Procedure and patient care

Before

PT Explain the procedure to the patient.
- Obtain informed consent if required by the institution.

During

- Note the following procedural steps:
  1. The patient is placed in the lithotomy position, and a vaginal speculum is used to expose the vagina and cervix.
  2. The cervix is cleansed with a 3% acetic acid solution to remove excess mucus and cellular debris. The acetic acid also accentuates the difference between normal and abnormal epithelial tissues. Abnormal epithelium becomes white with application of dilute acetic acid.

3. An aggressive ecto-endocervical Pap smear using curettage is then performed.
4. The colposcope is focused on the cervix, which is then carefully examined.
5. Usually the entire lesion can be outlined and the most atypical areas selected for biopsy specimen removal.

- Note that colposcopy is performed by a physician, nurse practitioner, or physician's assistant in approximately 5 to 10 minutes.

PT Tell the patient that some women complain of pressure pains from the vaginal speculum and that momentary discomfort may be felt if biopsy specimens are obtained.

After

PT Inform the patient that she may have vaginal bleeding if biopsy specimens were taken. Suggest that she wear a sanitary pad.

PT Instruct the patient to abstain from intercourse and to not insert anything (except a tampon) into the vagina until healing of a biopsy is confirmed.

PT Inform the patient about when and how to obtain results of this study.

Abnormal findings

Dysplasia
Carcinoma *in situ*
Invasive cancer
Cervical lesions

notes

complement assay (Total, C3 and C4 complement)

Type of test Blood

Normal findings

Total complement: 30-75 units/mL
C3: 75-175 mg/dL
C4: 22-45 units/mL

Test explanation and related physiology

Measurements of complement are used primarily to diagnose hereditary and acquired deficiencies of complement peptides and to monitor the activity of infectious or autoimmune diseases (e.g., systemic lupus erythematosus, nephritis, membranoproliferative nephritis, poststreptococcal nephritis).

Serum complement is a group of 31 proteins that act as enzymes, cofactors, inhibitors, and membrane-integrated proteins. These effect a cascade-like series of reactions that lead to the synthesis of a group of proteins that facilitate the immunologic and inflammatory responses. The total complement, sometimes labeled *CH 50*, is made up of a series of reactions involving proteins C1 through C9 (classic cascade reactions). Besides these major components, subcomponents are involved in the system. When activated, total complement (and some precursor proteins) acts to increase vascular permeability, allowing antibodies and white blood cells (WBCs) to be delivered to the area of the immune/antigen complex. Complement also acts to increase chemotaxis (attracting WBCs to the area), phagocytosis, and immune adherence of the antibody to antigen. These processes are vitally important in the normal inflammatory or immunologic response.

Reduced complement levels can be congenital or acquired. As the complement system is activated, the complement components are consumed or used up. If the system is persistently or overly activated, serum levels can fall. The complement system is instigated by the presence of antibody/antigen complexes. As in hereditary angioedema, complement components are used up, and serum levels fall. Diseases associated with these immune complexes include serum sickness, lupus erythematosus, infectious endocarditis, renal transplant rejection, vasculitis, some forms of glomerulonephritis, and infections. As these diseases are successfully treated, complement levels can be expected to return to normal. Complement components can be increased after the onset of various acute inflammatory diseases (e.g., thyroiditis, periarteritis nodosum, rheumatoid arthritis) or acute tissue damage (e.g., acute myocardial infarction). This is very similar to an acute reaction protein.

The total complement assay should be used as a screen for suspected complement related diseases before ordering individual complement component assays. A deficiency of an individual component of the complement cascade will result in an undetectable total complement level. For a list of common diseases associated with complement abnormalities, see Table 10. Note, however, that this list is not complete. Complement abnormalities may occur in the face of normal blood levels when particular complement proteins are not functioning properly. Complement testing may include quantification of complement/subunit proteins, qualitative evaluation of complement/subunit function, and identification of genetic mutations affecting complement synthesis.

Complement levels can also be measured in other bodily fluids such as pleural, pericardial, and synovial fluids. Low fluid complement levels are characteristic of effusions from patients with rheumatoid arthritis (despite elevated serum levels), systemic lupus erythematosus, and bacterial infections.

TABLE 10   Diseases associated with complement deficiencies

Complement deficiency	Associated disease
C1q	Recurrent bacterial infection
C1r	Discoid lupus, glomerulonephritis
C1s	Systemic lupus
C1–INH	Hereditary angioedema
C1	Autoimmune diseases, hypogammaglobulinemia
C2	Lupus, glomerulonephritis, recurrent bacterial infections
C3	Recurrent bacterial infections
C4	Systemic lupus
C5	Systemic lupus, recurrent infections, *Neisseria* infection
C6	*Neisseria* infections
C7	Scleroderma, *Neisseria* infections, rheumatoid arthritis
C8	*Neisseria* infections
C9	*Neisseria* infections

Interfering factors

- C3 is very unstable at room temperature.

Procedure and patient care

- See inside front cover for Routine Blood Testing.
- Fasting: no.
- Blood tube commonly used: red.

Abnormal findings

▲ **Increased levels**
Rheumatic fever (acute)
Myocardial infarction (acute)
Ulcerative colitis
Cancer

▼ **Decreased levels**
Cirrhosis
Autoimmune disease
(e.g., systemic lupus
erythematosus)
Serum sickness (immune
complex disease)
Glomerulonephritis
Lupus nephritis
Renal transplant
rejection (acute)
Protein malnutrition
Anemia
Malnutrition
Hepatitis
Rheumatoid arthritis
Sjögren syndrome
Severe sepsis

notes

complete blood count and differential count
(CBC and diff)

The CBC and differential count are a series of tests of the peripheral blood; they provide a tremendous amount of information about the hematologic system and many other organ systems. These tests are inexpensively, easily, and rapidly performed as a screening test. The CBC and differential count include automated measurement of the following studies, which are discussed separately:

Red blood cell count (RBC, see p. 785)

Hemoglobin (Hgb, see p. 500)

Hematocrit (Hct, see p. 497)

Red blood cell indices (RBC indices, see p. 788)

  Mean corpuscular volume (MCV)

  Mean corpuscular hemoglobin (MCH)

  Mean corpuscular hemoglobin concentration (MCHC)

  Red blood cell distribution width (RDW)

White blood cell count (WBC) and differential count (see p. 991)

  Neutrophils (polymorphonuclear leukocytes or *polys*, segmented cells or *segs*, band cells, stab cells)

  Lymphocytes

  Monocytes

  Eosinophils

  Basophils

Blood smear (see p. 156)

Platelet count (see p. 718)

Platelet volume, mean (MPV) (see p. 724)

notes

computed tomography of the abdomen and pelvis
(CT scan of the abdomen and pelvis, Helical/spiral CT scan of the abdomen and pelvis)

C

Type of test X-ray with contrast dye

Normal findings No evidence of abnormality

Test explanation and related physiology

The CT scan of the abdomen is a noninvasive, yet very accurate, x-ray procedure used to diagnose pathologic conditions, such as tumors, cysts, abscesses, inflammation, perforation, bleeding, obstruction, aneurysms, and calculi of the abdominal and retroperitoneal organs. The CT scan image results from passing x-rays through the abdominal organs at many angles. The variation in density of each tissue allows for a variable penetration of the x-rays. Each density is given a numeric value, called a *density coefficient*, which is digitally computed into shades of gray. This is then interpolated to an accurate image on a computer monitor. Repeating the CT scan after IV or oral administration of an iodine-containing contrast dye can enhance the image. These images can be recorded as x-ray images or captured digitally.

Liver tumors, abscesses, trauma, cysts, and anatomic abnormalities can be seen; pancreatic tumors, pseudocysts, inflammation, calcification, bleeding, and trauma can also be detected. The kidneys and urinary outflow tract are well visualized.

Renal tumors and cysts, ureteral obstruction, stones, and congenital renal and ureteral abnormalities are easily seen with the use of IV contrast injection. Calculi can be seen without IV contrast. Extravasation of urine secondary to trauma or obstruction can also be demonstrated easily. Adrenal tumors and hyperplasia are best diagnosed with this technique.

Large tumors, perforations of the bowel, and appendicitis can be identified with the CT scan, especially when oral contrast is ingested. The spleen can be well visualized for hematoma, laceration, fracture, tumor infiltration, and splenic vein thrombosis with CT scanning. The retroperitoneal lymph nodes can be evaluated. These are usually present, but all nodes with a diameter greater than 2 cm are considered abnormal. The abdominal aorta and its major branches can be evaluated for aneurysmal dilation and intramural thrombi. The pelvic structures (including the uterus, ovaries, fallopian tubes, prostate, and rectum) and musculature can be evaluated for tumors, abscesses, infection, or hypertrophy. Ascites and hemoperitoneum can easily be demonstrated with the CT scan. Tumors, abscesses, or perforation of the pelvic organs can be seen when the CT scan is directed to the pelvis. Perineal CT scanning can demonstrate perianal abscesses or perirectal tumors or infection.

Helical (also called *spiral*, or *volume-averaging*) *CT scanning*, with the development in multidetector CT (MDCT) technology, continuously obtains data as the patient is passed through the gantry. With the use of multiple collimators (and multiple banks of detectors), large data images (called *slices*) can be obtained in a very short period of time. The entire abdomen can be scanned in slightly more than a few seconds with one breath hold. The slices are very thin (1 to 5 mm). With thin slices and rapid accession, breathing and motion distortion are minimized. This produces faster and more accurate images.

With this CT technique, 200 to 500 individual images can be obtained. Volume imaging with 3D real-time display of the data allows the interpreter to visualize and analyze the data in three dimensions. With these advances in software, 2D and 3D reconstructions of data can provide very accurate images of the intraabdominal organs and especially the mesenteric vessels in a few seconds. This allows radiologists to see these structures from multiple directions.

A three-dimensional perspective can be added to the abdominal and pelvic organs or tumors that are imaged. This provides data for virtual colonoscopy and virtual angiography.

Virtual colonoscopy (or *CT colonography*) uses a CT scanner and virtual reality software to look inside the body without inserting a colonoscope (for conventional colonoscopy, see p. 271). Virtual colonoscopy is an appropriate alternative to a screening endoscopic colonoscopy. No sedation is required and no discomfort is experienced. Patients need a cleansing bowel preparation prior to the test. The virtual colonoscopy procedure takes place in the radiology department. It begins with the insertion of a small, flexible rubber tube in the rectum. Air is inserted through this tube to inflate the colon for better visualization. The air acts as a contrast medium. The test is completed in 10 to 20 minutes. Because no sedation is required, patients are free to leave the CT suite without the need for observation and recovery. Patients can resume normal activities after the procedure, and they can eat, work, or drive without a delay. Unlike endoscopic colonoscopy, polypectomy and/or biopsy cannot be performed with virtual testing. If abnormalities are found with virtual colonoscopy, conventional colonoscopy is needed.

Increasingly, *fusion CT/PET* scans are now being used to provide both anatomic and physiologic information that can be fused onto one image. This allows the image to locate pathology and to indicate whether it is benign or malignant. Fusion CT/PET scans can provide an accurate image of the entire colon and indicate whether any abnormality that is seen is malignant.

CT arteriography or angiography is performed through the use of multichannel helical CT scanning. After IV injection of contrast, CT imaging can demonstrate the arteries in any given organ. With computerized subtraction of the surrounding tissue, the arteries can be even better displayed. Three-dimensional re-creations of the aorta and other abdominal vessels are possible. This is particularly helpful in identifying renal artery stenosis and hepatic vasculature for cancer-related resections. Renal helical arteriography can be used to demonstrate and evaluate each functional phase of urinary excretion. This procedure is also called *dynamic CT scanning*.

CT nephrotomography can be done by computerized re-creation of a 3D image of the kidneys, renal pelvis, and ureters. This is particularly helpful in identifying ureteral stones and small tumors of the kidney or collecting system. Using different protocols and radiopaque contrast, kidney function can be evaluated. This does require significant radiation exposure. A different protocol designed to identify ureteral stones can be performed with very little radiation exposure. This is called *CT urography*.

With the increasing use and development of 3D volumetric imaging, radiologists have expanded CT scanning to assist pathologists, coroners, and medical examiners to investigate a cadaver for clues as to the cause of death. This is now being termed *virtual autopsy*. This includes CT or MRI whole-body, post-mortem imaging. With these techniques, image-directed biopsies can be performed to obtain tissue for the pathologists to review. Post-mortem angiograms can be performed to more accurately indicate occlusive disease that may have contributed to death.

The CT scan can be used as a guide to aspirate fluid from the abdomen or one of the abdominal organs. This fluid can be sent for cultures and other studies. The CT scan can also be used to guide biopsy needles into areas of abdominal tumors to obtain tissue for study. Catheters for drainage of intraabdominal abscess can be placed with CT guidance.

The CT scan is an important part of staging and monitoring of many tumors before and after therapy. Tumors of the colon, rectum, liver, breast, lung, prostate, ovary, uterus, kidney, lymph, and adrenal gland commonly recur in the abdomen. Recurrence can be detected early with the CT scan.

Contraindications

- Patients who are allergic to iodinated dye or shellfish
- Patients who are pregnant, unless the benefits outweigh the risks
- Patients whose vital signs are unstable
- Patients who are very obese, usually more than 300 lb
- Patients who are claustrophobic

Potential complications

- Allergic reaction to iodinated dye
  See p. xviii for appropriate interventions concerning the care of patients with iodine allergy.
- Acute renal failure from dye infusion
  Adequate hydration before the infusion may reduce this likelihood.
- Lactic acidosis may occur in patients who are taking metformin and receiving iodine contrast. The metformin should be held the day of the test to prevent this complication.

Interfering factors

- Presence of metallic objects (e.g., hemostasis clips)
- Retained barium from previous studies
- Large amounts of fecal material or gas in the bowel

Procedure and patient care

Before

PT Explain the procedure to the patient. The patient's cooperation is necessary, because he or she must lie still during the procedure.
- Obtain informed consent if required by the institution.
- Assess the patient for allergies to iodinated dye or shellfish.
PT Show the patient a picture of the CT machine. Encourage the patient to verbalize his or her concerns because some patients may have claustrophobia. Most patients who are mildly claustrophobic can be scanned after appropriate premedication with antianxiety drugs.
- Keep the patient NPO for at least 4 hours before the test if oral contrast is to be administered; however, this test can be performed on an emergency basis on patients who have recently eaten.
- Note that this procedure is usually performed by a radiologist in less than 30 minutes. If dye is administered, the procedure

time may be doubled, because the CT scan is done both with and without contrast dye.

PT Tell the patient that the discomforts associated with this study include lying still on a hard table and the peripheral venipuncture. Mild nausea is a common sensation when contrast dye is used. An emesis basin should be readily available. Some patients may experience a salty taste, flushing, and warmth during the dye injection.

During

- Note the following procedural steps for an abdominal CT scan:
  1. The patient is taken to the radiology department and placed on the CT scan table.
  2. The patient then is placed in an encircling body scanner (gantry). The x-ray tube travels around the gantry and takes pictures of the various levels of the abdomen and pelvis. Any motion causes blurring and streaking of the final picture. Therefore, the patient is asked to remain motionless during x-ray exposure. Computer monitoring equipment allows for immediate display of the CT scan image, which is then recorded digitally. In a separate room, the technicians manipulate the CT scan table to change the level of the abdomen that is scanned.
  3. Through audio communication, the patient is instructed to hold his or her breath during x-ray exposure.
- Remember that oral and IV iodinated x-ray contrast dye provides better results for this test. One can accurately differentiate the gastrointestinal organs from the other abdominal organs with oral contrast. Likewise, the vessels and ureters are contrasted with the surrounding structures with use of IV dye. Sometimes contrast is given rectally to visualize the pelvic organs.

After

PT Encourage the patient to drink fluids to avoid dye-induced renal failure and to promote dye excretion.

PT Inform the patient that diarrhea may occur after ingestion of the oral contrast.

- Evaluate the patient for delayed reaction to dye.

Abnormal findings

Liver
Tumor
Abscess
Bile duct dilation

Pancreas
Tumor
Pseudocyst
Inflammation
Bleeding

Spleen
Hematoma
Fracture
Laceration
Tumor
Venous thrombosis

Gallbladder/biliary system
Gallstones
Tumor
Bile duct dilation

Kidneys
Tumor
Cyst
Ureteral obstruction
Calculi
Congenital abnormalities
Renal artery stenosis

Adrenal gland
Adenoma
Cancer
Pheochromocytoma
Hemorrhage
Myelolipoma hyperplasia

GI tract
Perforation
Tumor
Inflammatory bowel disease
Diverticulitis
Appendicitis

Uterus, tubes, ovaries
Tumor
Abscess
Infection
Hydrosalpinx
Cyst
Fibroid

Prostate
Hypertrophy
Tumor

Retroperitoneum
Tumor
Lymphadenopathy

Other
Abdominal aneurysm
Ascites, hemoperitoneum
Abscess

notes

computed tomography of the brain (CT scan of the brain, Helical/spiral CT scan of the brain)

Type of test X-ray with contrast dye

Normal findings No evidence of pathologic conditions

Test explanation and related physiology

Computed tomography of the brain consists of a computerized analysis of multiple tomographic x-rays taken of the brain tissue at successive layers, providing a 3D view of the cranial contents. The CT image provides a view of the head as if one were looking down through its top. The variation in density of each tissue allows for variable penetration of the x-ray beam. An attached computer calculates the amount of x-ray penetration of each tissue and displays this as shades of gray. This is then displayed digitally on a computer monitor as a series of actual anatomic pictures of coronal sections of the brain.

The CT scan is used in the differential diagnosis of intracranial neoplasms, cerebral infarctions, ventricular displacement or enlargement, cortical atrophy, cerebral aneurysms, intracranial hemorrhage and hematoma, and arteriovenous (AV) malformation. Information about the ventricular system can be obtained by CT scanning. Multiple sclerosis and other degenerative abnormalities can be identified also.

Visualization of a neoplasm, previous infarction, or any pathologic process that destroys the blood-brain barrier may be enhanced by IV injection of an iodinated contrast dye. CT scans may be repeated frequently to monitor the progress of any disease or to monitor the healing process. In most cases, CT scanning has eliminated the need for more invasive procedures, such as cerebral arteriography and pneumoencephalography. MRI brain scanning can provide more and different information in some instances and may be used in place of CT scanning of the brain.

CT arteriography is performed immediately after venous contrast injection. Three-dimensional re-creations of the carotid artery and its branches are also extremely helpful in the evaluation of cerebral vascular disease.

Helical (also called *spiral*, or *volume-averaging*) *CT scanning* represents a significant improvement over standard CT scanning. The helical CT scan continuously obtains images as the patient is passed through the gantry. This produces faster and more accurate images. Because the helical CT scan images the selected area in less than 30 seconds, the entire study can be performed with one breath hold. Therefore, breathing and motion misrepresentations are eliminated. Images are improved and scan time is reduced. This is particularly helpful in scanning uncooperative adults or children. Through volume averaging, 3D images can be re-created. Furthermore, when contrast material is used, contrast imaging is markedly improved.

Contraindications

- Patients who are allergic to iodinated dye or shellfish
- Patients who are claustrophobic
- Patients who are pregnant, unless benefits outweigh risks
- Patients whose vital signs are unstable
- Patients who are very obese, usually more than 300 lb

Potential complications

- Allergic reaction to iodinated dye
  See p. xviii for appropriate interventions concerning the care of patients with iodine allergy
- Acute renal failure from dye infusion
  Adequate hydration beforehand may reduce this likelihood.
- Lactic acidosis may occur in patients who are taking metformin and receiving iodine contrast.
  The metformin should be held the day of the test to prevent this complication.
- Apnea if xenon is used because it is an anesthetic gas

Procedure and patient care

Before

PT Explain the procedure to the patient. The patient's cooperation is necessary, because he or she must lie still during the procedure.
- Obtain informed consent if required by the institution.
PT Show the patient a picture of the CT machine and encourage the patient to verbalize his or her concerns, because some patients may have claustrophobia. Most patients who are mildly claustrophobic can be scanned after appropriate premedication with antianxiety drugs.
- Keep the patient NPO for 4 hours before the study, if oral contrast is to be used.
PT Instruct the patient that wigs, hairpins, clips, or partial dental plates cannot be worn during the procedure because they hamper visualization of the brain.
- Assess the patient for allergies to iodinated dye or shellfish.
PT Tell the patient that he or she may hear a clicking noise as the scanning machine moves around the head.

During

- Note the following procedural steps for the brain CT scan:
  1. The patient lies in the supine position on an examining table with the head resting on a platform. The face is not covered, and the patient can see out of the machine at all times. Sponges are placed along the side of the head to ensure that the patient's head does not move during the study.
  2. The scanner passes an x-ray beam through the brain from multiple angles.
  3. If an iodinated dye will be used, a peripheral IV line is started and the iodinated dye is administered through it. The entire scanning process is repeated.
- Note that this procedure is performed by a radiologist in less than 1 hour. If dye is administered, the procedure time is doubled, because the CT scan is done with and without the contrast dye.

PT Tell the patient that discomfort associated with this study includes lying still on a hard table and peripheral venipuncture. Mild nausea is a common sensation when contrast dye is used. An emesis basin should be readily available. Some patients may experience a salty taste, flushing, and warmth during the dye injection.

After

PT Encourage the patient to drink fluids, because dye is excreted by the kidneys and causes diuresis.

Abnormal findings

Intracranial neoplasm
Cerebral infarction
Ventricular displacement
Ventricular enlargement
Cortical atrophy
Cerebral aneurysm
Intracranial hemorrhage
Hematoma
Arteriovenous malformation
Meningioma
Multiple sclerosis
Hydrocephalus
Abscess

notes

computed tomography of the chest (Chest CT scan, Helical/spiral CT scan of the chest)

Type of test X-ray with contrast dye

Normal findings No evidence of pathologic conditions

Test explanation and related physiology

Computed tomography of the chest is a noninvasive yet very accurate x-ray procedure for diagnosing and evaluating pathologic conditions such as tumors, nodules, hematomas, parenchymal coin lesions, cysts, abscesses, pleural effusion, and enlarged lymph nodes affecting the lungs and mediastinum. Tumors, cysts, and fractures of the chest wall and pleura can also be seen. When IV contrast material is given, vascular structures can be identified, and a diagnosis of aortic or other vascular abnormality can be made. With oral contrast, the esophagus and upper structures can be evaluated for tumor and other conditions. This procedure provides a cross-sectional view of the chest and is especially useful in detecting small differences in tissue densities, demonstrating lesions that cannot be seen with conventional radiology and tomography.

The x-ray image results from using a body scanner (an x-ray tube held in a circular gantry) to deliver x-rays through the patient's chest at many different angles. The variation in density of each tissue allows for a variable penetration of the x-rays. Each density is given a numeric value called a *coefficient*, which is digitally computed into shades of gray. These data are then saved, collated, and reproduced to provide 2D or 3D images of the organ being evaluated.

Helical (also called *spiral*, or *volume-averaging*) *CT scanning* uses the developments in multidetector CT (MDCT) technology to continuously obtain data as the patient is passed through the gantry. With the use of multiple collimators (and multiple banks of detectors), large data images (called *slices*) can be obtained in a very short period of time. The entire chest can be scanned in slightly more than a few seconds with one breath hold. The slices are very thin (1 to 5 mm). With thin slices and rapid accession, breathing and motion distortion are minimized. This produces faster and more accurate images.

With this new CT study, 200 to 500 individual images can be obtained. Volume imaging with 3D real-time display of the data allows the interpreter to visualize and analyze the data in three dimensions. With these advances in software, 2D and 3D reconstructions of data can provide very accurate images of the heart (see p. 293), lungs, chest wall, pleura, esophagus, great vessels, and soft tissue in a few seconds, allowing radiologists to see these structures from multiple directions. With this new technology, *virtual bronchoscopy* and *virtual esophagoscopy* may increasingly be used in place of their invasive counterparts.

Contraindications

- Patients who are pregnant, unless benefits outweigh risks
- Patients who are allergic to iodinated dye or shellfish
- Patients who are claustrophobic
- Patients who are very obese, usually more than 300 lb
- Patients whose vital signs are unstable

Potential complications

- Allergic reaction to iodinated dye
  See p. xviii for appropriate interventions concerning the care of patients with iodine allergy.
- Acute renal failure from dye infusion
  Adequate hydration beforehand may reduce this likelihood.
- Lactic acidosis may occur in patients who are taking metformin and receiving iodine contrast.
  The metformin should be held the day of the test to prevent this complication.

Procedure and patient care

Before

PT Explain the procedure to the patient. The patient's cooperation is necessary because he or she must lie still during the procedure.

- Obtain informed consent if required by the institution.
- Assess the patient for allergies to iodinated dye or shellfish.

PT Show the patient a picture of the CT machine and encourage the patient to verbalize concerns regarding claustrophobia. Most patients who are mildly claustrophobic can tolerate this study after appropriate premedication with antianxiety drugs.

- Keep the patient NPO for 4 hours before the test in the event that contrast dye is administered.

During

- Note the following procedural steps for the chest CT scan:
  1. The patient is taken to the radiology department and asked to remain motionless in a supine position because any motion will cause blurring and streaking of the final picture.

2. An encircling x-ray camera (body scanner) takes pictures at varying intervals and levels over the chest area. Often IV dye is administered to enhance the chest image, and the x-ray studies are repeated.

- Note that this procedure is performed by a radiologist in less than 30 minutes.

PT Tell the patient that the discomforts associated with this study include lying still on a hard table and peripheral venipuncture. Mild nausea is a common sensation when contrast dye is used. An emesis basin should be readily available. Some patients may experience a salty taste, flushing, and warmth during the dye injection.

After

PT Encourage patients who received dye injection to increase their fluid intake, because the dye is excreted by the kidneys and causes diuresis.

Abnormal findings

Pulmonary tumor
Inflammatory nodules
Granuloma
Cyst
Pulmonary emboli
Pleural effusion
Enlarged lymph nodes
Aortic aneurysm
Postpneumonic scanning
Pneumonitis
Esophageal tumor
Hiatal hernia
Mediastinal tumor (e.g., lymphoma, thymoma)
Primary or metastatic chest wall tumor

notes

computed tomography of the heart (Coronary CT angiography, Coronary calcium score)

Type of test X-ray with contrast dye

Normal findings No evidence of coronary stenosis; calcium score average for age and gender

Test explanation and related physiology

With the developments in *multidetector CT (MDCT)* technology, much data can be obtained about the heart and coronary vessels. This test is now increasingly being used to help stratify patients according to risks of future cardiac events, to instigate preventative medicinal interventions (e.g., statin drugs), to monitor progression of coronary vascular disease and effects of statin drugs, to evaluate chest pain, and to indicate the need for stress testing or coronary angiography.

MDCT produces fast and accurate images of the heart. With the use of multiple collimators (and multiple banks of detectors—usually 4 to 64), large data images (called *slices*) can be obtained in a very short period of time. The entire heart can be scanned in 10 seconds with one breath hold. The slices are very thin (1 to 5 mm). With thin slices and rapid accession, breathing and motion distortion are minimized.

With advances in software technology, 2D and 3D reconstructions of data can provide very accurate images of the heart and coronary vessels in a few seconds, allowing radiologists to see these structures from multiple directions. Furthermore, with shorter scanning times, intravenous contrast effect can be greater while using less contrast volume. The newest MDCT scanners allow routine cardiac gating that synchronizes the scanning with each heartbeat, thereby eliminating further motion distortion.

MDCT is now considered the preferred study for the myocardium, cardiac chambers, cardiac valves, coronary arteries, and great vessels, and for detection of pulmonary emboli. Calcified atheromatous plaques can be seen and quantified (calcium score) with the use of MDCT. Coronary calcium is a surrogate marker for coronary atherosclerotic plaque. In the coronary arteries, calcifications occur almost exclusively in the context of atherosclerotic changes. Within a coronary vessel or larger segment of the vessel, the amount of coronary calcium correlates moderately closely with the extent of atherosclerotic plaque burden. On the other hand, not every serious atherosclerotic coronary plaque is calcified. However, in the vast majority of patients with acute coronary syndromes, coronary calcium can be detected, and the amount of calcium in these patients is substantially greater than in matched control subjects without coronary artery disease.

The *Agatston score* has most frequently been used to quantify the amount of coronary calcium in CT. Men develop calcifications about 10 to 15 years earlier than women. In the majority of asymptomatic men over 55 years of age and women over 65 years of age, calcification can be detected. See Table 11 for categorizing absolute Agatston scores. It is well established that individuals with Agatston scores above 400 have an increased occurrence of coronary procedures (bypass, stent placement, angioplasty) and events (myocardial infarction and cardiac death) within 2 to 5 years after the test. Individuals with very high Agatston scores (over 1000) have a 20% chance of suffering a myocardial infarction or cardiac death within a year.

Variability of the Agatston score can be high for patients with small amounts of calcium but is lower for higher calcium scores. There is a variability of about 20%. Excessively high calcium scores can inhibit the visualization of the coronary arteries. Therefore, when calcium scores are excessively high, injection of radiopaque dye is not performed and coronary CT cannot be carried out.

MDCT can directly and accurately visualize coronary artery lumen after intravenous injection of a contrast agent *(coronary CT angiography)*. Regular and low heart rates are a prerequisite for reliable visualization of the coronary arteries. Hence, most centers have proposed the administration of a short-acting beta-blocker or a calcium channel blocker prior to scanning if the heart rate exceeds 60 to 70 beats/minute. The use of sublingual nitroglycerin is also recommended to achieve coronary vasodilatation and to maximize image quality.

Contraindications

- Patients who are pregnant
- Patients who are allergic to iodinated dye or shellfish
- Patients who are very obese, usually more than 300 lb
- Patients whose vital signs are unstable

TABLE 11 Agatston score categories for coronary calcium quantification

	Minimal	Moderate	Increased	Severe
Agatston score	<10	11-99	100-400	>400

Potential complications

- Allergic reaction to iodinated dye
  See p. xviii for appropriate interventions concerning the care of patients with iodine allergies.
- Acute renal failure from dye infusion
  Adequate hydration beforehand may reduce this likelihood.
- Lactic acidosis may occur in patients who are taking metformin and receiving iodine contrast.
  The metformin should be held the day of the test to prevent this complication.

Procedure and patient care

Before

PT Explain the procedure to the patient. The patient's cooperation is necessary because he or she must lie still during the procedure.
- Obtain informed consent if required by the institution.
- Assess the patient for allergies to iodinated dye or shellfish.
- Assess the patient's vital signs. If the heart rate exceeds protocol levels, administer a rapid-acting beta-blocker or ACE inhibitor per protocol orders.

PT Show the patient a picture of the CT machine and encourage the patient to verbalize concerns regarding claustrophobia.
- Keep the patient NPO for 4 hours before the test.

During

- Note the following procedural steps for the cardiac CT scan:
  1. The patient is taken to the CT department and asked to remain motionless in a supine position.
  2. EKG leads are applied to synchronize the EKG signal to the image data (gating).
  3. An encircling x-ray camera (body scanner) takes pictures at varying intervals and levels over the heart while the patient holds his or her breath (for about 10 seconds).
  4. A nonenhanced scan is performed first for calcium scoring.
  5. If the calcium scoring is below threshold levels of the protocol, IV dye is rapidly administered through a large-bore intravenous catheter and the scan is repeated.
  6. A fast acting nitrate (usually nitroglycerin) is administered to maximize coronary dilatation.
- Note that a radiologist or cardiologist performs this procedure in about 20 minutes.

PT Tell the patient that discomfort associated with this study includes lying still on a hard table and peripheral venipuncture. Nausea is a common sensation when contrast dye is used. An emesis basin should be readily available. Some patients may experience a salty taste, flushing, and warmth during the dye injection.

After

PT Encourage patients to increase their fluid intake because the dye is excreted by the kidneys and causes diuresis.

PT Tell the patient that a headache from the nitroglycerin is not uncommon.

Abnormal findings

Coronary vascular disease
Coronary vascular congenital anomalies
Ventricular aneurysm
Aortic aneurysm or dissection
Pulmonary emboli
Cardiac tumors
Myocardial scarring
Cardiac valvular disease

notes

Coombs test, direct (Direct antiglobulin test [DAT])

Type of test Blood

Normal findings Negative; no agglutination

Test explanation and related physiology

This test is performed to identify immune hemolysis (lysis of RBCs) or to investigate hemolytic transfusion reactions. Most of the antibodies to RBCs are directed against the ABO/Rh blood grouping antigens, such as those that occur in hemolytic anemia of the newborn or transfusion of incompatible blood. When a transfusion reaction occurs, the Coombs test can detect the patient's antibodies or complement components coating the transfused RBCs. Therefore, the Coombs test is very helpful in evaluating suspected transfusion reactions.

Non–blood grouping antigens can develop on the RBC membrane and stimulate formation of antibodies. Such drugs as levodopa or penicillin cause this. Also, in autoimmune diseases, antibodies not originally directed against the patient's RBCs can attach to the RBCs and cause hemolysis that is detected by the direct Coombs test. Frequently the inciting factor for the production of these autoantibodies against RBCs is not associated with any identifiable disease, and the resulting hemolytic anemia is called *idiopathic*.

The direct Coombs test demonstrates if the patient's RBCs have been attacked by antibodies in the patient's own bloodstream. Coombs serum is a solution containing antibodies to human globulin (antibodies). Coombs serum is mixed with the patient's RBCs. If the RBCs have antibodies on them, agglutination of the patient's RBCs will occur. The greater the quantity of antibodies against RBCs, the more clumping occurs. This test is read as *positive*, with clumping on a scale of micropositive to +4. If the RBCs are not coated with autoantibodies against RBCs (immunoglobulins), agglutination will not occur; this is a *negative* test.

Interfering factors

- Antiphospholipid antibodies (see p. 64, anticardiolipin antibodies) can cause a false-positive DAT.
- Drugs that may cause false-positive results include ampicillin, captopril, cephalosporins, chlorpromazine, chlorpropamide, hydralazine, indomethacin, insulin, isoniazid, levodopa, methyldopa, penicillin, phenytoin, procainamide, quinidine, quinine, rifampin, streptomycin, sulfonamides, and tetracyclines.

Procedure and patient care

- See inside front cover for Routine Blood Testing.
- Fasting: no.
- Blood tube commonly used: red or lavender.
- Use venous blood from the umbilical cord to detect the presence of antibodies in the newborn.
- List on the laboratory slip all medications and any transfusions that the patient has had in the last few days.

Abnormal findings

Autoimmune hemolytic anemia
Transfusion reaction
Hemolytic disease of the newborn
Lymphoma
Systemic lupus erythematosus
Mycoplasmal infection
Infectious mononucleosis

notes

Coombs test, indirect (Blood antibody screening, Indirect antiglobulin test [IAT])

Type of test Blood

Normal findings Negative; no agglutination

Test explanation and related physiology

The indirect Coombs test detects circulating antibodies against RBCs. The major purpose of this test is to determine if the patient has minor serum antibodies (other than the major ABO/Rh system) to RBCs that he or she is about to receive by blood transfusion. Therefore, this test is the *screening* part of the *type and screen* routinely performed for blood compatibility testing (cross-matching in the blood bank). This test is also used to detect other agglutinins, such as cold agglutinins, which are associated with *Mycoplasma* infections.

Unlike the direct Coombs test that is performed on the patient's RBCs, this test is performed on the patient's serum. In this test, a small amount of the recipient's serum is added to donor RBCs containing known antigens on their surfaces. This is the first stage. In the second stage of the test, Coombs serum is added. Coombs serum is a solution containing antibodies to human globulin (antibodies). If antibodies exist in the patient's serum, agglutination occurs. In blood transfusion screening, visible agglutination indicates that the recipient has antibodies to the donor's RBCs. If the recipient has no antibodies against the donor's RBCs, agglutination will not occur; transfusion should then proceed safely and without any transfusion reaction. Circulating antibodies against RBCs also may occur in an Rh-negative pregnant woman who is carrying an Rh-positive fetus.

Interfering factors

☛ Drugs that may cause false-positive results include antiarrhythmics, antituberculins, cephalosporins, chlorpromazine, insulin, levodopa, methyldopa, penicillin, phenytoin, quinidine, sulfonamides, and tetracyclines.

Procedure and patient care

- See inside front cover for Routine Blood Testing.
- Fasting: no.
- Blood tube commonly used: red.
- Remember that if this antibody screening test is positive, antibody identification is then done.

Abnormal findings

Incompatible cross-matched blood
Maternal anti-Rh antibodies
Hemolytic disease of the newborn
Acquired immune hemolytic anemia
Presence of specific cold agglutinin antibody

notes

cortisol, blood, urine, saliva (Hydrocortisone, Serum cortisol, Salivary cortisol)

Type of test   Blood; urine; saliva

Normal findings

Serum

Adult/elderly
  8 AM: 5-23 mcg/dL or 138-635 nmol/L (SI units)
  4 PM: 3-13 mcg/dL or 83-359 nmol/L (SI units)
Child 1-16 years
  8 AM: 3-21 mcg/dL
  4 PM: 3-10 mcg/dL
Newborn: 1-24 mcg/dL

Urine (24-hour)

Adult/elderly: <100 mcg/24 hr or <276 nmol/day (SI units)
Adolescent: 5-55 mcg/24 hr
Child: 2-27 mcg/24 hr

Saliva

7 AM-9 AM: 100-750 ng/dL
3 PM-5 PM: <401 ng/dL
11 PM-midnight: <100 ng/dL

Test explanation and related physiology

An elaborate feedback mechanism for cortisol coordinates the function of the hypothalamus, pituitary gland, and adrenal glands. Corticotropin-releasing hormone (CRH) is made in the hypothalamus. This stimulates adrenocorticotropic hormone (ACTH) production in the anterior pituitary gland. ACTH stimulates the adrenal cortex to produce cortisol. The rising levels of cortisol act as a negative feedback to curtail further production of CRH and ACTH. Cortisol is a potent glucocorticoid released from the adrenal cortex. This hormone affects the metabolism of carbohydrates, proteins, and fats. It has a profound effect on glucose serum levels. Cortisol tends to increase glucose by stimulating gluconeogenesis from glucose stores. It also inhibits the effect of insulin and thereby inhibits glucose transport into the cells.

The best method of evaluating adrenal activity is by directly measuring plasma cortisol levels. Normally cortisol levels rise and fall during the day; this is called the diurnal variation. Cortisol levels are highest around 6 AM to 8 AM and gradually fall during the day, reaching their lowest point around midnight. Sometimes the earliest sign of adrenal hyperfunction is only the loss of this diurnal variation, even though the cortisol levels are not yet elevated. For example, individuals with Cushing syndrome often have upper normal plasma cortisol levels in the morning and do not exhibit a decline as the day proceeds. High levels of cortisol indicate Cushing syndrome, and low levels of plasma cortisol are suggestive of Addison disease.

For this test, blood is usually collected at 8 AM and again at around 4 PM. The 4 PM value is anticipated to be one third to two thirds of the 8 AM value. Normal values may be transposed in individuals who have worked during the night and slept during the day for long periods of time.

The measurement of late-night *salivary cortisol* is another effective test for Cushing syndrome. It seems to be more convenient and superior to plasma and urine for detecting cortisol in patients with mild Cushing syndrome. Salivary cortisol assay cannot be used to diagnose hypocortisolism or Addison disease because laboratory methods are not sensitive enough at low levels. If late-night salivary cortisol levels are elevated, the results should be confirmed with a repeat salivary cortisol measurement, a midnight blood sampling for cortisol, or a 24-hour urinary collection of free cortisol. A dexamethasone suppression test (p. 339) is another confirmation test that can be used.

Interfering factors

- Pregnancy is associated with increased levels.
- Physical and emotional stress can elevate cortisol levels. Stress stimulates the pituitary-cortical mechanism and thereby stimulates cortisol production.
- Drugs that may cause *increased* levels include amphetamines, cortisone, estrogen, oral contraceptives, and spironolactone (Aldactone).
- Drugs that may cause *decreased* levels include androgens, aminoglutethimide, betamethasone and other exogenous steroid medications, danazol, lithium, levodopa, metyrapone, and phenytoin (Dilantin).

Procedure and patient care

Before

PT Explain the procedure to the patient to minimize anxiety.

- Assess the patient for signs of physical stress (e.g., infection, acute illness) or emotional stress and report these to the physician.

During

Blood

- Collect a venous blood sample in a red-top or green-top tube in the morning after the patient has had a good night's sleep.
- Collect another blood sample at about 4 PM.
- Indicate the time of the venipuncture on the laboratory slip.

Saliva

1. Do not brush teeth before specimen collection.
2. Do not eat or drink for 15 minutes before specimen collection.
3. Collect the specimen between 11 PM and midnight, and record the collection time.
4. Collect at least 1.5 mL of saliva in a Salivette as follows:
   a. Place swab directly into mouth by tipping container so swab falls into mouth. Do not touch swab with fingers.
   b. Keep swab in mouth for approximately 2 minutes. Roll swab in mouth; do not chew swab.
   c. Place swab back into its container without touching and replace the cap.

Urine

PT Instruct the patient how to collect a 24-hour urine. See inside front cover for Routine Urine Testing.

- Keep the collection on ice and use a preservative.

After

- Apply pressure or a pressure dressing to the venipuncture site.

Abnormal findings

▲ **Increased levels**
Cushing syndrome
Adrenal adenoma or
   carcinoma
Ectopic ACTH-producing
   tumors
Hyperthyroidism
Obesity
Stress

▼ **Decreased levels**
Congenital adrenal
   hyperplasia
Addison disease
Hypopituitarism
Hypothyroidism
Liver disease

notes

C-peptide (Connecting peptide insulin, Insulin C-peptide, Proinsulin C-peptide)

Type of test Blood

Normal findings
Fasting: 0.78-1.89 ng/mL or 0.26-0.62 nmol/L (SI units)
1 hour after glucose load: 5-12 ng/mL

Test explanation and related physiology
In the islet of Langerhans of the pancreas, proinsulin chains are broken down to form insulin and C-peptide. Because C-peptide has a longer half-life than insulin, more C-peptide exists in the peripheral circulation. In general, C-peptide levels correlate with insulin levels in the blood. The capacity of the pancreatic beta cells to secrete insulin can be evaluated by directly measuring either insulin or C-peptide. In most cases, direct measurement of insulin is more accurate. C-peptide levels, however, more accurately reflect islet cell function in the following situations:

- Patients with diabetes who are treated with exogenous insulin and who have antiinsulin antibodies.
- Patients who secretly administer insulin to themselves (factitious hypoglycemia). Insulin levels will be elevated. Direct insulin measurement in these patients tends to be high because the insulin measured is the self-administered exogenous insulin. But C-peptide levels in that same specimen will be low because exogenously administered insulin suppresses endogenous insulin (and C-peptide) production.
- Diabetic patients who are taking insulin. This is done to see if the diabetic patient is in remission and may not need exogenous insulin.
- Distinguishing type I from type II diabetes. This is particularly helpful in newly diagnosed diabetics. A person whose pancreas does not make any insulin (type I diabetes) has low levels of insulin and C-peptide. A person with type II diabetes has a normal or high level of C-peptide.

Furthermore, C-peptide is used in evaluating patients who are suspected of having an insulinoma. In patients with an autonomous secreting insulinoma, C-peptide levels are high. C-peptide can also be used to monitor treatment for insulinoma. A rise in C-peptide levels indicates a recurrence or progression of the insulinoma. Likewise, some clinicians use C-peptide testing as an indicator of the adequacy of therapeutic surgical pancreatectomy in patients with pancreatic tumors. C-peptide also can be used to diagnose insulin resistance syndrome.

Interfering factors

- Because the majority of C-peptide is degraded in the kidney, renal failure can cause increased levels.
- ✗ Drugs that may cause *increased* levels of C-peptide include oral hypoglycemic agents (e.g., sulfonylureas).

Procedure and patient care

- See inside front cover for Routine Blood Testing.
- Fasting: yes.
- Blood tube commonly used: red.

Abnormal findings

▲ **Increased levels**
  Insulinoma
  Renal failure
  Pancreas transplant
  Type II diabetes mellitus

▼ **Decreased levels**
  Factitious hypoglycemia
  Radical pancreatectomy
  Type I diabetes mellitus

notes

C-reactive protein test (CRP, High-sensitivity C-reactive protein [hs-CRP])

Type of test Blood

Normal findings <1.0 mg/dL or <10.0 mg/L (SI units)

Cardiac risk:
  Low: <1.0 mg/dL
  Average: 1.0-3.0 mg/dL
  High: >3.0 mg/dL

Test explanation and related physiology

C-reactive protein (CRP) is a nonspecific, acute-phase reactant used to diagnose bacterial infectious disease and inflammatory disorders, such as acute rheumatic fever and rheumatoid arthritis. CRP levels do not consistently rise with viral infections. CRP is a protein produced primarily by the liver during an acute inflammatory process and other diseases. A positive test result indicates the presence but not the cause of the disease. The synthesis of CRP is initiated by antigen-immune complexes, bacteria, fungi, and trauma.

The CRP test is a more sensitive and rapidly responding indicator than the erythrocyte sedimentation rate (ESR, see p. 393). In an acute inflammatory change, CRP shows an earlier and more intense increase than ESR; with recovery, the disappearance of CRP precedes the return of ESR to normal. CRP also disappears when the inflammatory process is suppressed by salicylates or steroids.

The level of CRP correlates with peak levels of the MB isoenzyme of creatine kinase (see p. 308), but CRP peaks occur 1 to 3 days later. Failure of CRP to normalize may indicate ongoing damage to the heart tissue. Multiple prospective studies also have demonstrated that baseline CRP is a good marker of future cardiovascular events. The level of CRP is a stronger predictor of cardiovascular events than the low-density lipoprotein (LDL) cholesterol level. However, when used together with the lipid profile (in cholesterol, see p. 248), it adds prognostic information to that conveyed by the Framingham risk score.

The recent development of an assay for *high-sensitivity CRP (hs-CRP)* has enabled accurate assays at even low levels. Because of the individual variability in hs-CRP, two separate measurements are required to classify a person's risk level. In patients with stable coronary disease or acute coronary syndromes, hs-CRP measurement may be useful as an independent marker for assessing the likelihood of harmful events, including death, myocardial infarction, or restenosis after percutaneous coronary intervention. hs-CRP is most commonly used when other causes of systemic inflammation have been eliminated.

Interfering factors

- Elevated test results can occur in patients with hypertension, elevated body mass index, metabolic syndrome/diabetes mellitus, chronic infection (e.g., gingivitis, bronchitis), chronic inflammation (e.g., rheumatoid arthritis), and low HDL/high triglycerides.
- Cigarette smoking can cause increased levels.
- Decreased test levels can result from moderate alcohol consumption, weight loss, and increased activity/exercise.
- Drugs that may cause *increased* test results include estrogens and progesterones.
- Drugs that may cause *decreased* test results include fibrates, niacin, and statins.

Procedure and patient care

- See inside front cover for Routine Blood Testing.
- Fasting: verify with lab.
- Blood tube commonly used: red.

Abnormal findings

▲ **Increased levels**
Arthritis
Acute rheumatic fever
Reiter syndrome
Crohn disease
Vasculitis syndrome
Systemic lupus erythematosus
Tissue infarction or damage
Acute myocardial infarction
Pulmonary infarction
Kidney transplant rejection
Bone marrow transplant rejection
Soft tissue trauma
Bacterial infection
Postoperative wound infection
Urinary tract infection
Tuberculosis
Malignant disease
Bacterial meningitis

notes

creatine kinase (CK, Creatine phosphokinase [CPK])

Type of test Blood

Normal findings

Total CPK

Adult/elderly

Male: 55-170 units/L or 55-170 units/L (SI units)

Female: 30-135 units/L or 30-135 units/L (SI units)

(Values are higher after exercise.)

Newborn: 68-580 units/L (SI units)

Isoenzymes

CK-MM: 100%

CK-MB: 0%

CK-BB: 0%

Test explanation and related physiology

This test is used to support the diagnosis of myocardial muscle injury (infarction). It can also indicate neurologic or skeletal muscle diseases. Creatine kinase is found predominantly in the heart muscle, skeletal muscle, and brain. Serum CK levels are elevated when these muscle or nerve cells are injured. CK levels can rise within 6 hours after damage. If damage is not persistent, the levels peak at 18 hours after injury and return to normal in 2 to 3 days (Figure 12).

To test specifically for myocardial muscle injury, three CK isoenzymes are measured: CK-BB (CK1), CK-MB (CK2), and CK-MM (CK3). CK-MB appears to be specific for myocardial cells. CK-MB levels rise 3 to 6 hours after infarction occurs. If there is no further myocardial damage, the levels peak at 12 to 24 hours and return to normal 12 to 48 hours after infarction. CK-MB levels do not usually rise with transient chest pain caused by angina, pulmonary embolism, or congestive heart failure. One can expect to see a rise in CK-MB in patients with shock, malignant hyperthermia, myopathies, or myocarditis. Mild elevation of CK-MB (below the threshold of positive) can occur in patients with unstable angina and will signify an increased risk for an occlusive event. Very small amounts of CK-MB also exist in skeletal muscle. Severe injury to, or diseases of, the skeletal muscle can also raise the CK-MB above normal.

The CK-MB level is helpful in both quantifying the degree of myocardial infarction (MI) and timing the onset of infarction. The CK-MB level is often used to determine appropriateness of thrombolytic therapy, which is used for MI. High

C

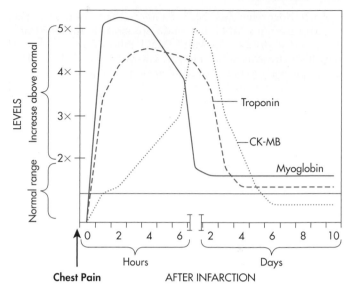

FIGURE 12 Blood studies useful in the diagnosis of myocardial infarction.

CK-MB levels suggest that significant infarction has already occurred, thereby precluding the benefit of thrombolytic therapy.

Because CK-BB is found predominantly in the brain and lung, injury to either of these organs (e.g., cerebrovascular accident, pulmonary infarction) will be associated with elevated levels of this isoenzyme.

CK-MM normally makes up almost all of the circulatory total CK enzymes in healthy people. When the total CK level is elevated as a result of increases in CK-MM, injury to or disease of the skeletal muscle is present. Examples of this include myopathies, vigorous exercise, multiple intramuscular injections, electroconvulsive therapy, cardioversion, chronic alcoholism, or surgery. Because CK is made only in the skeletal muscle, the normal value of total CK (and therefore CK-MM) varies according to a person's muscle mass. Large, muscular people may normally have a CK level in the high range of normal. Likewise, people of small stature or those with low muscle mass will be expected to have low CK levels. This is important because high normal CK levels in these patients can mask an MI.

Each isoenzyme has been found to have isoforms. The CK-MM isoforms MM1 and MM3 are most useful for identifying cardiac disease. An MM3/MM1 ratio of greater than 1 suggests acute myocardial injury. A CK-MB ratio of MB2/MB1 greater than 1 also indicates acute myocardial injury.

CK is the main cardiac enzyme studied in patients with heart disease. Because its blood clearance and metabolism are well known, its frequent determination (on admission, at 12 hours, and at 24 hours) can accurately reflect timing, quantity, and resolution of an MI. Troponin (p. 931) and myoglobin (p. 650) are also serum markers used to confirm an MI (see Figure 12). A new assay is ischemia-modified albumin (see p. 565).

Interfering factors

- IM injections may cause elevated CPK levels.
- Strenuous exercise and recent surgery may cause increased levels.
- Early pregnancy may cause decreased levels.
- ✗ Drugs that may cause *increased* levels include alcohol, amphotericin B, ampicillin, some anesthetics, anticoagulants, aspirin, captopril, colchicine, dexamethasone, fibrates, furosemide, lidocaine, lithium, morphine, propranolol, statins, and succinylcholine.

Procedure and patient care

- See inside front cover for Routine Blood Testing.
- Fasting: no.
- Blood tube commonly used: red.
- PT Discuss with the patient the need and reason for frequent venipuncture in diagnosing myocardial infarction.
- Avoid IM injections in patients with cardiac disease. These injections may falsely elevate the total CPK level.
- Blood collection is usually done daily for 3 days and then at 1 week.
- Record the exact time and date of venipuncture on each laboratory slip. This aids in the interpretation of the temporal pattern of enzyme elevations.

Abnormal findings

▲ **Increased levels of total CK**
Disease or injury affecting the heart muscle, skeletal
    muscle, or brain

▲ **Increased levels of CK-BB isoenzyme**
Disease affecting the central nervous system
Adenocarcinoma (especially breast and lung)
Pulmonary infarction

▲ **Increased levels of CK-MB isoenzyme**
Acute myocardial infarction
Cardiac aneurysm surgery
Cardiac defibrillation
Myocarditis
Ventricular arrhythmias
Cardiac ischemia

▲ **Increased levels of CK-MM isoenzyme**
Rhabdomyolysis
Muscular dystrophy
Myositis
Recent surgery
Electromyography
IM injections
Crush injuries
Delirium tremens
Malignant hyperthermia
Recent convulsions
Electroconvulsive therapy
Shock
Hypokalemia
Hypothyroidism
Trauma

notes

creatinine, blood (Serum creatinine)

Type of test Blood

Normal findings

Adult:

Female: 0.5-1.1 mg/dL or 44-97 μmol/L (SI units)

Male: 0.6-1.2 mg/dL or 53-106 μmol/L (SI units)

Elderly: decrease in muscle mass may cause decreased values

Adolescent: 0.5-1.0 mg/dL

Child: 0.3-0.7 mg/dL

Infant: 0.2-0.4 mg/dL

Newborn: 0.3-1.2 mg/dL

Possible critical values >4 mg/dL (indicates serious impairment in renal function)

Test explanation and related physiology

This test measures the amount of creatinine in the blood. Creatinine is a catabolic product of creatine phosphate, which is used in skeletal muscle contraction. The daily production of creatine, and subsequently creatinine, depends on muscle mass, which fluctuates very little. Creatinine, as with blood urea nitrogen (BUN, see p. 946), is excreted entirely by the kidneys and therefore is directly proportional to renal excretory function. Thus, with normal renal excretory function, the serum creatinine level should remain constant and normal. Besides dehydration, only such renal disorders as glomerulonephritis, pyelonephritis, acute tubular necrosis, and urinary obstruction will cause abnormal elevations in creatinine. There are slight increases in creatinine levels after meals, especially after ingestion of large quantities of meat. Furthermore, there may be some diurnal variation in creatinine—nadir at 7 AM and peak at 7 PM.

The serum creatinine test, as with BUN, is used to diagnose impaired renal function. Unlike BUN, however, the creatinine level is affected very little by hepatic function. The creatinine test is used as an approximation of *glomerular filtration rate (GFR)*. The serum creatinine level has much the same significance as the BUN level but tends to rise later. Therefore, elevations in creatinine suggest chronicity of the disease process. In general, a doubling of creatinine suggests a 50% reduction in GFR. The creatinine level is interpreted in conjunction with the BUN test. These tests are referred to as *renal function studies*. The BUN/creatinine ratio is a good measurement of kidney and liver function. The normal adult range is 6 to 25, with 15.5 being the optimal adult value for this ratio.

Although serum creatinine is the most commonly used biochemical parameter to estimate GFR in routine practice, there are some shortcomings. Such factors as muscle mass and protein intake can influence serum creatinine, leading to an inaccurate estimation of GFR. Moreover, in unstable, critically ill patients, acute changes in renal function can make real-time evaluation of GFR using serum creatinine difficult. On the other hand, *cystatin C*, a protein that is produced at a constant rate by all nucleated cells, is probably a better indicator of GFR. Because of its constant rate of production, its serum concentration is determined only by glomerular filtration. Its level is not influenced by those factors that affect creatinine and BUN.

Cystatin C might predict the risk for developing *chronic kidney disease*, thereby signaling a state of preclinical kidney dysfunction. Several studies have found that increased levels of cystatin C are associated with the risk of death and several types of cardiovascular disease (including MI, stroke, heart failure, peripheral arterial disease, and metabolic syndrome). For women, the average reference interval is 0.52 to 0.90 mg/L with a mean of 0.71 mg/L. For men, the average reference interval is 0.56 to 0.98 mg/L with a mean of 0.77 mg/L.

Interfering factors

☑ Drugs that may *increase* creatinine values include ACE inhibitors, aminoglycosides (e.g., gentamicin), cimetidine, heavy-metal chemotherapeutic agents (e.g., cisplatin), and other nephrotoxic drugs, such as cephalosporins (e.g., cefoxitin).

Procedure and patient care

- See inside front cover for Routine Blood Testing.
- Fasting: no.
- Blood tube commonly used: red.
- For pediatric patients, blood is usually drawn from a heel stick.

Abnormal findings

▲ **Increased levels**
  Glomerulonephritis
  Pyelonephritis
  Acute tubular necrosis
  Urinary tract obstruction
  Reduced renal blood flow
    (e.g., shock, dehydration,
    congestive heart failure,
    atherosclerosis)
  Diabetic nephropathy
  Nephritis
  Rhabdomyolysis
  Acromegaly
  Gigantism

▼ **Decreased levels**
  Debilitation
  Decreased muscle mass
    (e.g., muscular dystrophy,
    myasthenia gravis)

notes

creatinine clearance (CC, Estimated glomerular filtration rate [eGFR])

Type of test Urine (24-hour); blood

Normal findings

Adult (<40 years)
    Male: 107-139 mL/min or 1.78-2.32 mL/s (SI units)
    Female: 87-107 mL/min or 1.45-1.78 mL/s (SI units)
Newborn: 40-65 mL/min
Values decrease 6.5 mL/min/decade of life because of decline in GFR.
eGFR: >60 mL/min/$1.73 m^2$

Test explanation and related physiology

    Creatinine is a catabolic product of creatine phosphate, which is used in skeletal muscle contraction. The daily production of creatinine depends on muscle mass, which fluctuates very little. Creatinine is entirely excreted by the kidneys and therefore is directly proportional to the glomerular filtration rate (GFR; i.e., the number of milliliters filtered by all the nephrons in the kidneys per minute). The creatinine clearance (CC) is a measure of the GFR.

    The CC depends on the amount of blood present to be filtered and the ability of the nephron to act as a filter. The amount of blood present for filtration is decreased in renal artery atherosclerosis, dehydration, or shock. The ability of the nephron to act as a filter is decreased by such diseases as glomerulonephritis, acute tubular necrosis, and most other primary renal diseases. Significant bilateral obstruction to urinary outflow affects glomerular filtration only after it is long-standing.

    When one kidney becomes diseased, the opposite kidney, if normal, has the ability to compensate by increasing its filtration rate. Therefore, with unilateral kidney disease or nephrectomy, a decrease in CC is not expected if the other kidney is normal.

    Several nonrenal factors may influence CC. With each decade of age, the CC decreases 6.5 mL/min because of a decrease in the GFR. Urine collections are timed, and incomplete collections will falsely decrease CC. Muscle mass varies among people. Decreased muscle mass will give lower CC values.

The CC test requires a 24-hour urine collection and a serum creatinine level. The *uncorrected* CC is then computed using the following formula:

$$\text{Creatinine clearance} = \frac{UV}{P}$$

where

U = Number of milligrams per deciliter of creatinine excreted in the urine over 24 hours

V = Volume of urine in milliliters per minute

P = Serum creatinine in milligrams per deciliter

The *corrected* CC calculation takes into account the average body surface area.

A 24-hour urine collection for creatinine is often measured along with other urine collections to assess the completeness of other 24-hour collections. In patients with normal creatinine, the CC should indicate whether all the urine has been collected for the 24 hours.

The 24-hour urine collections used to measure CC are too time-consuming and expensive for routine clinical use. The GFR can be estimated *(estimated GFR [eGFR])* using the Modification of Diet in Renal Disease (MDRD) Study equation. This is an equation that uses the serum creatinine, age, and numbers that vary depending upon sex and ethnicity to calculate the GFR with very good accuracy. The prediction equation for GFR is as follows, with Pcr being serum or plasma creatinine in mg/dL:

$$\text{GFR (mL/min/1.73 m}^2) = 186 \times (Pcr)^{-1.154} \times (age)^{-0.203} \times (0.742 \text{ if female})$$
$$\times (1.210 \text{ if African American})$$

The GFR is expressed in mL / min/ 1.73 m^2.

More and more, institutions across the country are beginning to report an eGFR on patients 18 years and older with every serum creatinine ordered. The eGFR calculation can be programmed into most laboratory information systems. As a result, chronic renal disease is being recognized more frequently in its early stages. Chronic kidney disease can be treated and progression to renal failure slowed or prevented. For example, if a patient with diabetes is found to have a reduced GFR of 49 at an annual examination, that patient's primary care physician can and should take steps to treat the early chronic kidney disease. This may include the use of ACE inhibitors, more aggressive treatment of high blood pressure, glycemic dietary control, and treatment of high cardiac risk factors. The eGFR can also be used to calculate medication dosage in patients with decreased renal function.

TABLE 12   Mean estimated glomerular filtration rates (eGFRs)

Age (years)	Mean eGFR
20-29	$116\,mL/min/1.73\,m^2$
30-39	$107\,mL/min/1.73\,m^2$
40-49	$99\,mL/min/1.73\,m^2$
50-59	$93\,mL/min/1.73\,m^2$
60-69	$85\,mL/min/1.73\,m^2$
70+	$75\,mL/min/1.73\,m^2$

Table 12 shows population estimates for mean (average) eGFR by age. There is no difference between races or sexes when eGFRs are expressed per meter squared body surface area. For diagnostic purposes, most laboratories report eGFR values above 60 as $>60\,mL/min/1.73\,m^2$, not as an exact number.

Cystatin C is a cysteine proteinase inhibitor that is produced by all nucleated cells and found in serum. Because it is formed at a constant rate and freely filtered by the kidneys, its serum concentration (like creatinine) is another accurate test that can estimate GFR.

Interfering factors

- Exercise may cause increased creatinine values.
- Incomplete urine collection may give a falsely lowered value.
- Pregnancy increases CC.
- A diet high in meat can transiently elevate CC.
- The eGFR may be inaccurate in extremes of age and in patients with obesity, severe malnutrition, paraplegia, quadriplegia, or pregnancy.
- Drugs that may cause *increased* levels include aminoglycosides (e.g., gentamicin), cimetidine, heavy-metal chemotherapeutic agents (e.g., cisplatin), and nephrotoxic drugs such as cephalosporins (e.g., cefoxitin).
- Drugs that may cause *decreased* eGFR are drugs that interfere with creatinine secretion (e.g., cimetidine or trimethoprim) or creatinine assay (cephalosporins). In these cases, a 24-hour CC may be necessary to accurately estimate kidney function.

Procedure and patient care

- See inside front cover for Routine Urine Testing.
- **PT** Note that some laboratories instruct the patient to avoid cooked meat, tea, coffee, or drugs on the day of the test.

- Make sure a venous blood sample is drawn in a red-top tube during the 24-hour collection.
- Mark the patient's age, weight, and height on the requisition sheet.

Abnormal findings

▲ **Increased levels**
Exercise
Pregnancy
High cardiac output
syndromes

▼ **Decreased levels**
Impaired kidney
function (e.g., renal
artery atherosclerosis,
glomerulonephritis,
acute tubular
necrosis)
Conditions causing
decreased GFR
(e.g., congestive
heart failure, cirrhosis
with ascites, shock,
dehydration)

notes

cryoglobulin

Type of test Blood

Normal findings No cryoglobulins detected

Test explanation and related physiology

Cryoglobulins are abnormal globulin protein complexes that exist in the blood of patients with various diseases. These proteins precipitate reversibly at low temperatures and redissolve with rewarming. They can precipitate in the blood vessels of the fingers when exposed to cold temperatures. This precipitation causes sludging of the blood in those blood vessels. These patients may have symptoms of purpura, arthralgia, or Raynaud phenomenon (pain, cyanosis, coldness of the fingers).

These proteins exist in varying quantities, depending on the disease entity with which they are associated. The cryoglobulins can be classified, which helps determine the underlying disease state. Type I (monoclonal) cryoglobulinemia is associated with monoclonal gammopathy of undetermined significance, macroglobulinemia, or multiple myeloma. Type II (mixed, two or more immunoglobulins of which one is monoclonal) cryoglobulinemia is associated with autoimmune disorders, such as vasculitis, glomerulonephritis, systemic lupus erythematosus, rheumatoid arthritis, and Sjögren syndrome. It may also be seen in such infections as hepatitis, infectious mononucleosis, cytomegalovirus, and toxoplasmosis. Type II cryoglobulinemia may also be essential (i.e., occurring in the absence of underlying disease). Type III (polyclonal) cryoglobulinemia is associated with the same disease spectrum as type II cryoglobulinemia.

For this test, the blood sample is taken to the chemistry laboratory, where it is refrigerated for 72 hours. After that time, the specimen is evaluated for precipitation. If precipitation is identified, it is measured and recorded. The tube is then rewarmed, and the specimen is reexamined for dissolution of that precipitation. If precipitation of the refrigerated specimen is identified and dissolved on rewarming, cryoglobulins are present. If cryoglobulin qualitative is positive, then immunofixation electrophoresis typing and quantitative IgA, IgG, and IgM are performed to classify the type of cryoglobulin that exists.

Procedure and patient care

- See inside front cover for Routine Blood Testing.
- Fasting: verify with lab.
- Blood tube commonly used: red.

PT Inform the patient that an 8-hour fast may be required. This will minimize turbidity of the serum caused by ingestion of a recent (especially fatty) meal. Turbidity may make the detection of precipitation rather difficult.

PT If cryoglobulins are found to be present, warn the patient to avoid cold temperatures and contact with cold objects to minimize Raynaud symptoms. Tell the patient to wear gloves in cold weather.

Abnormal findings

Connective tissue disease (e.g., lupus erythematosus, Sjögren syndrome, rheumatoid arthritis)

Lymphoid malignancies (e.g., multiple myeloma, leukemia, Waldenström macroglobulinemia, lymphoma)

Acute and chronic infections (e.g., infectious mononucleosis, endocarditis, poststreptococcal glomerulonephritis)

Liver disease (e.g., hepatitis, cirrhosis)

notes

cystography (Cystourethrography, Voiding cystography, Voiding cystourethrography [VCUG])

Type of test X-ray with contrast dye

Normal findings Normal bladder structure and function

Test explanation and related physiology

Filling the bladder with radiopaque contrast material provides visualization of the bladder for radiographic study. Either fluoroscopic or x-ray images demonstrate bladder filling and collapse after emptying. Filling defects or shadows within the bladder indicate primary bladder tumors. Extrinsic compression or distortion of the bladder is seen with pelvic tumor (e.g., rectal, cervical) or hematoma (secondary to pelvic bone fractures). Extravasation of the dye is seen with traumatic rupture, perforation, and fistula of the bladder. Vesicoureteral reflux (abnormal backflow of urine from bladder to ureters), which can cause persistent or recurrent pyelonephritis, also may be demonstrated during cystography. Although the bladder is visualized during an intravenous pyelogram (see p. 778), primary pathologic bladder conditions are best studied by cystography.

Contraindications

• Patients with urethral or bladder infection or injury

Potential complications

• Urinary tract infection
  This may result from catheter placement or the instillation of contaminated contrast material.
• Allergic reaction to iodinated dye
  This rarely occurs because the dye is not administered intravenously.

Procedure and patient care

Before

PT Explain the procedure to the patient.
• Obtain informed consent if required by the institution.
• Give clear liquids for breakfast on the morning of the test.
PT Assure the patient that he or she will be draped to prevent unnecessary exposure.
• Insert a Foley catheter if ordered.

During

- Note the following procedural steps:
  1. The patient is taken to the radiology department and placed in a supine or lithotomy position.
  2. Unless the catheter is already present, one is placed.
  3. Through the catheter, approximately 300 mL of air or radiopaque dye (much less for children) is injected into the bladder.
  4. The catheter is clamped.
  5. X-ray images are taken.
  6. If the patient is able to void, the catheter is removed, and the patient is asked to urinate while images are taken of the bladder and urethra (voiding cystourethrogram).
- Ensure that males wear a lead shield over the testes to prevent irradiation of the gonads.
- Remember that female patients cannot be shielded without blocking bladder visualization.
- Note that a radiologist performs the study in approximately 15 to 30 minutes.
- **PT** Tell the patient that this test is moderately uncomfortable if bladder catheterization is required.

After

- Assess the patient for signs of urinary tract infection.
- **PT** Encourage the patient to drink fluids to eliminate the dye and to prevent accumulation of bacteria.

Abnormal findings

Bladder tumor
Pelvic tumor
Hematoma
Bladder trauma
Vesicoureteral reflux

notes

cystometry (Cystometrogram [CMG])

Type of test Manometric

Normal findings

Normal sensations of fullness and temperature
Normal pressures and volumes
Maximal cystometric capacity
    Male: 350-750 mL
    Female: 250-550 mL
Intravesical pressure when bladder is empty: usually <40 cm H_2O
Detrusor pressure: <10 cm H_2O
Maximal urethral pressures in normal patients (cm H_2O):

Age	Male	Female
<25 years	37-126	55-103
25-44 years	35-113	31-115
45-64 years	40-123	40-100
>64 years	35-105	35-75

Test explanation and related physiology

The purpose of cystometry is to evaluate the motor and sensory functions of the bladder when incontinence is present or neurologic bladder dysfunction is suspected. A graphic recording of pressure exerted at varying phases of the filling of the urinary bladder is produced. A pressure/volume relationship of the bladder is made. This urodynamic study assesses the neuromuscular function of the bladder by measuring the efficiency of the detrusor muscle; intravesical pressure and capacity; and the bladder's response to thermal stimulation.

Cystometry can determine whether bladder pathology is caused by neurologic, infectious, or obstructive diseases. Cystometry is indicated to elucidate the causes for frequency and urgency, especially before surgery on the urologic outflow tract. Cystometry is also part of the evaluation for incontinence, persistent residual urine, vesicoureteral reflux, neurologic disorders, sensory disorders, and the effects of certain drugs on bladder function.

A *urethral pressure profile (UPP)* is often performed during cystometry. The UPP indicates the intraluminal pressure along the length of the urethra with the bladder at rest.

Indications for cystometry include the following:
- Assessment of prostatic obstruction
- Assessment of stress incontinence in females

- Assessment of postprostatectomy sequelae of incontinence
- Assessment of the adequacy of external sphincterotomy
- Analysis of the effects of drugs on the urethra
- Analysis of the effects of stimulation on urethral flow
- Assessment of the adequacy of implanted artificial urethral sphincter devices

Contraindications

- Patients with urinary tract infections because of the possibility of false results and the potential for the spread of infection

Procedure and patient care

Before

PT Explain the purpose and the procedure to the patient.

PT Tell the patient that no fluid or food restrictions are needed.

- Assess the patient for signs and symptoms of urinary tract infection.

PT Instruct the patient not to strain while voiding, because the results can be skewed.

During

- Note the following procedural steps:
  1. Cystometry, usually performed in a urologist's office or a special procedure room, begins with the patient being asked to void.
  2. The amount of time required to initiate voiding and the size, force, and continuity of the urinary stream are recorded. The amount of urine, the time of voiding, and the presence of any straining, hesitancy, or terminal urine dribbling are also recorded.
  3. The patient is placed in a lithotomy or supine position.
  4. A retention catheter is inserted through the urethra and into the bladder.
  5. Residual urine volume is measured and recorded.
  6. Thermal sensation is evaluated by the instillation of approximately 30 mL of room-temperature saline solution into the bladder followed by an equal amount of warm water. The patient reports any sensations.
  7. This fluid is withdrawn from the bladder.
  8. The urethral catheter is connected to a cystometer (a tube used to monitor bladder pressure).
  9. Sterile water, normal saline solution, or carbon dioxide gas is slowly introduced into the bladder at a controlled rate, usually with the patient in a sitting position.

10. Patients are asked to indicate the first urge to void and then when they have the feeling that they must void.
11. The pressures and volumes are plotted on a graph.
12. The patient is asked to void, and the maximal intravesical voiding pressure is recorded.
13. The bladder is drained of any residual urine.
14. If no additional studies are to be done, the urethral catheter is removed.
15. For urethral pressures, fluid or gas is instilled through the catheter, which is withdrawn while pressures along the urethral wall are obtained.

PT Throughout the study, ask the patient to report any sensations of pain, flushing, sweating, nausea, bladder filling, or an urgency to void.

- Note that certain drugs may be administered during the cystometric examination to distinguish between underactivity of the bladder because of muscle failure and underactivity associated with denervation. Cholinergic drugs (e.g., bethanechol) may be given to enhance the tone of a flaccid bladder. Anticholinergic drugs (e.g., atropine) may be given to promote relaxation of a hyperactive bladder.
- Note that this test is performed by a urologist in approximately 45 minutes.

PT Explain to the patient that the only discomfort is that associated with the urethral catheterization.

After

- Observe the patient for any manifestations of infection (e.g., elevated temperature, chills).
- Examine the urine for hematuria. Notify the physician if the hematuria persists after several voidings.
- Offer a warm sitz bath or tub bath for the patient's comfort.

Abnormal findings

Neurogenic bladder
Bladder obstruction
Bladder infection
Bladder hypertonicity
Diminished bladder capacity
Prostatic obstruction secondary to benign prostatic hypertrophy or cancer
Urinary incontinence

notes

cystoscopy (Endourology)

Type of test Endoscopy

Normal findings Normal structure and function of the urethra, bladder, ureters, and prostate (in males)

Test explanation and related physiology

Cystoscopy provides direct visualization of the urethra and bladder through the transurethral insertion of a cystoscope into the bladder (Figure 13). Cystoscopy is used *diagnostically* to allow:

- Direct inspection and biopsy of the prostate, bladder, and urethra
- Collection of a separate urine specimen directly from each kidney by the placement of ureteral catheters

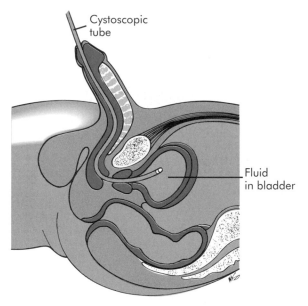

FIGURE 13 Cystoscopic examination of the male bladder. The cystoscope is passed through the urethra into the bladder. Although shown here as a flexible scope, usually the scope is rigid. Through the scope, fluid is instilled to maintain bladder distention.

- Measurement of bladder capacity and determination of ureteral reflux
- Identification of bladder and ureteral calculi
- Placement of ureteral catheters (Figure 14) for retrograde pyelography (see p. 778)
- Identification of the source of hematuria

Cystoscopy is used *therapeutically* to provide:

- Resection of small, superficial bladder tumors
- Removal of foreign bodies and stones
- Dilation of the urethra and ureters
- Placement of stents to drain urine from the renal pelvis
- Coagulation of bleeding areas
- Implantation of radium seeds into a tumor

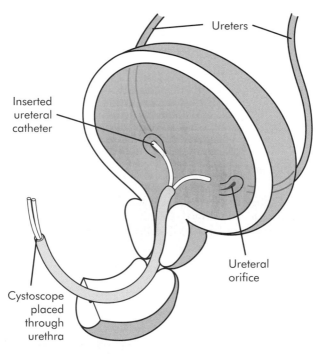

FIGURE 14 Ureteral catheterization through the cystoscope. Note the ureteral catheter inserted into the right orifice. The left ureteral catheter is ready to be inserted.

- Resection of hypertrophied or malignant prostate gland overgrowth
- Placement of ureteral stents for identification of ureters during pelvic surgery

The cystoscope consists primarily of an obturator and a telescope. The obturator is used to insert the cystoscope atraumatically. After the cystoscope is in the bladder, the obturator is removed and the telescope is passed through the cystoscope. The lens and lighting system of the telescope permit adequate visualization of the lower genitourinary tract. Transendoscopic instruments (e.g., forceps, scissors, needles, and electrodes) are used when appropriate. *Endourology* refers to endoscopic surgery performed on the bladder and urethra during cystoscopy.

Cystoscopy is important in the evaluation of hematuria, chronic infection, suspected stones, and radiographic filling defects. On inspection, the urethra may show inflammation or structural causes of obstruction (e.g., stricture, neoplasia, prostatic hypertrophy). If the obstruction is functional rather than structural (e.g., detrusor–bladder neck dyssynergia), no site of obstruction will be demonstrated by endoscopy.

Potential complications

- Perforation of the bladder
- Sepsis by seeding the bloodstream with bacteria from infected urine
- Hematuria
- Urinary retention

Procedure and patient care

Before

PT Explain the procedure to the patient.
- Ensure that an informed consent is obtained.
- If enemas are ordered to clear the bowel, assist the patient as needed and record the results.

PT Encourage the patient to drink fluids several hours before the procedure to maintain a continuous flow of urine for collection and to prevent multiplication of bacteria that may be introduced during this technique.
- If the procedure will be done with the patient under local anesthesia, allow a liquid breakfast.
- If the procedure will be performed with the patient under general anesthesia, follow routine precautions. Keep the patient NPO after midnight on the day of the test. Fluids may be given intravenously.

- Administer the preprocedure medications as ordered 1 hour before the study. Sedatives decrease the spasm of the bladder sphincter, decreasing the patient's discomfort.

During

- Note the following procedural steps:
  1. Cystoscopy is performed in the operating room or in the urologist's office.
  2. The patient is placed in the lithotomy position with his or her feet in stirrups.
  3. The external genitalia are cleansed with an antiseptic solution.
  4. A local anesthetic is instilled into the urethra if general anesthesia has not been used.
  5. The cystoscope is inserted, and the desired diagnostic or therapeutic studies are performed.
- **PT** Instruct the patient to lie very still during the entire procedure to prevent trauma to the urinary tract.
- **PT** Tell the patient that he or she will have the desire to void as the cystoscope passes the bladder neck.
- When the procedure is completed, keep the patient on bed rest for a short time.
- Note that if endourology is performed, the urethra will also be evaluated.
- Note that this procedure is performed by a urologist in approximately 25 minutes.
- **PT** When local anesthesia is used, inform the patient of the associated discomfort (much more than with urethral catheterization).

After

- **PT** Instruct the patient not to walk or stand alone immediately after his or her legs have been removed from the stirrups. The orthostasis that may result from standing erect may cause dizziness and fainting.
- Assess the patient's ability to void for at least 24 hours after the procedure. Urinary retention may be secondary to edema caused by instrumentation.
- **PT** Instruct the patient to note the urine color. Pink-tinged urine is common. The presence of bright red blood or clots should be reported to the physician.
- Monitor the patient for complaints of back pain, bladder spasms, urinary frequency, and burning on urination. Warm sitz baths and mild analgesics may be ordered and given. Sometimes belladonna and opium (B&O) suppositories are

given to relieve bladder spasms. Warm, moist heat to the lower abdomen may help relieve pain and promote muscle relaxation.

PT Encourage increased intake of fluids. A dilute urine decreases dysuria. Fluids also maintain a constant flow of urine to prevent stasis and the accumulation of bacteria in the bladder.

• Monitor the patient's vital signs for a decrease in blood pressure and an increase in pulse as an indication of hemorrhage.

• Observe for signs and symptoms of sepsis (elevated temperature, flush, chills, decreased blood pressure, increased pulse).

PT Note that antibiotics are occasionally ordered 1 day before and 3 days after the procedure to reduce the incidence of bacteremia that may occur with instrumentation of the urethra and bladder.

PT Instruct the patient to watch for fever, shaking chills, or prolonged dysuria as possible signs of a urinary tract infection.

PT Encourage the patient to use cathartics, especially after cystoscopic surgery. Increases in intraabdominal pressure caused by constipation may initiate urologic bleeding.

• If postprocedure irrigation is ordered, use an isotonic solution containing mannitol, glycine, or sorbitol to prevent fluid overhydration in the event any of the irrigation is absorbed through opened venous sinuses in the bladder.

PT If a catheter is left in after the procedure, provide catheter care instructions.

Abnormal findings

Lower urologic tract tumor
Stones in the ureter or bladder
Prostatic hypertrophy
Prostate cancer
Inflammation of the bladder and urethra
Urethral/ureteral stricture
Prostatitis
Vesical neck contracture

notes

cytokines

Type of test Blood

Normal findings Vary by laboratory and technique

Test explanation and related physiology

Cytokines are a group of proteins that have multiple functions. In general, they are produced by immune cells to communicate and orchestrate the immune response. The immune system has many different cells that must act together to effectively protect the body from infection, inflammation, or tumor. The cytokines are made by many different types of cells, including lymphocytes (T-cells, B-cells), monocytes, and eosinophils. Originally, cytokines were named by their function (T-cell growth factor, colony stimulating factor, etc.). As more was learned about this complex group of proteins, it became apparent that a single cytokine might act differently in different cells. Therefore, naming the cytokine by function was confusing and misleading. As more cytokines were identified, they were named *interleukins* and were numbered by the sequence of discovery. Interleukins, in general, are made by leukocytes. Lymphokines and monokines are made by lymphocytes and monocytes, respectively. Other cytokines include *interferon* and *growth factors*.

Cytokines have receptors in other cells to which they attach and instigate a series of intracellular activities that may be associated with secretion, motion, or cell division. Cytokines are used therapeutically to stimulate bone marrow production of blood cells in patients with suppression (by chemotherapy) or disease of the bone marrow. They are used as potent antiinflammatory or antineoplastic agents. Some cytokines are produced at increased levels in certain disease states and therefore become markers for disease extent, progression, and response to therapy. They can act as tumor markers in cancers associated with elevated cytokines. *Human interferon inducible protein 10* is a small cytokine belonging to the chemokine family that affects cellular chemotaxis, immune response, and bone marrow inhibition. This protein, when present in high quantities in an acutely ill patient, is an accurate predictor of multiple organ failure.

Any table created to list all the cytokines and their functions quickly becomes inaccurate. The discovery of new cytokines and new functions changes so frequently that any such table would be outdated in the delay to publication. Likewise, any listing of normal values would be just as quickly obsolete, as methods of testing change so frequently. It is suggested that reference to normal values be directed to the laboratory performing the assay.

At present, cytokine quantitative and qualitative assays are predominantly used for research. Clinically, cytokine assays may have the following uses:

- Measurement of AIDS progression
- Measurement of progression of inflammatory diseases, such as rheumatoid arthritis and other autoimmune diseases
- Tumor markers (e.g., breast cancer, lymphoma, and leukemia)
- Determination of disease risk (e.g., risk of developing Kaposi sarcoma in AIDS patients)
- Determination of treatment of disease (e.g., which patients with rheumatoid arthritis may benefit from cytokine therapy)
- Determination of immune function and response
- Monitoring of patients receiving cytokine therapy or anti-cytokine therapy

Usually, cytokine testing is performed on serum. However, joint fluid is often tested in the evaluation of the patient with arthritis. Likewise, if inflammatory encephalitis or meningitis is considered, cerebrospinal fluid may be the specimen.

Interfering factors

- Cells can still produce cytokines after specimen collection. It is best to freeze the specimen.
- Cytokines can degrade in the specimen container.
- Cytokines can stimulate or inhibit other cytokines while in the specimen container.

Procedure and patient care

- See inside front cover for Routine Blood Testing.
- Fasting: no.
- Blood tube commonly used: red.

Abnormal findings

Inflammatory disease
AIDS
Various malignancies

notes

cytomegalovirus (CMV)

Type of test   Blood

Normal findings   No virus isolated

Test explanation and related physiology

Cytomegalovirus (CMV) is part of the viral family that includes herpes simplex, Epstein-Barr, and varicella-zoster viruses. CMV infection is widespread and common. Infections usually occur in the fetus, during early childhood, and in the young adult. Certain populations are at increased risk. Male homosexuals, transplant patients, and AIDS patients are particularly susceptible. Infections are acquired by contact with body secretions or urine. Blood transfusions are a common form of spread for CMV. Most patients with acute disease have no or very few (mononucleosis-like) symptoms.

CMV is the most common congenital infection. Pregnant mothers can get the disease during their pregnancy, or a previous CMV infection can become reactivated. Approximately 10% of infected newborns exhibit permanent damage, usually mental retardation and auditory damage. Fetal infection can cause microcephaly, hydrocephaly, cerebral palsy, mental retardation, or death. The term TORCH (*t*oxoplasmosis, *o*ther, *r*ubella, *c*ytomegalovirus, *h*erpes) has been applied to infections with recognized detrimental effects on the fetus.

Virus culture is the most definitive method of diagnosis. However, a culture cannot differentiate a primary infection from a chronic, non-primary infection. Antibodies reveal much more information about the activity of the infection. CMV IgG antibody levels persist for years after infection. Identification of IgM antibodies, however, indicates a relatively recent primary infection. Three different CMV antigens can be detected immunologically. They are called *early*, *intermediate-early*, and *late* antigens and indicate onset of infection. A fourfold increase in CMV titer in paired sera drawn 10 to 14 days apart is usually indicative of an acute infection. PCR assays demonstrate sensitive and specific detection of CMV nucleic acid.

More recently, measurement of *CMV-specific IgG avidity* is able to distinguish primary from non-primary CMV infections. In this test, the strength with which the IgG attaches to the CMV antigen is measured. IgG avidity matures with the length of time after primary infection. Therefore, IgG produced in the first few months after primary CMV infection will exhibit "low avidity."

IgG produced more than 6 to 8 months after CMV infection will have "high avidity" and represent non-primary chronic CMV infection.

Procedure and patient care

- See inside front cover for Routine Blood Testing.
- Fasting: no.
- Blood tube commonly used: red or gold.
- For culture specimens, a urine, sputum, or mouth swab is the specimen of choice. Fresh specimens are essential.
- The specimens are cultured in a virus laboratory, which takes about 3 to 7 days.
- For antibody or antigen titer, collect a venous blood sample in a gold- or red-top tube.
- Collect a specimen from a mother with suspected acute infection as early as possible.
- Collect the convalescent specimen 2 to 4 weeks later.

Abnormal findings

Cytomegalovirus infection

notes

D-dimer (Fragment D-dimer, Fibrin degradation product [FDP], Fibrin split products)

Type of test Blood

Normal findings <250 ng/mL or <0.4 mcg/mL

Test explanation and related physiology

The fragment D-dimer test assesses both thrombin and plasmin activity. D-dimer is a fibrin degradation fragment that is made through lysis of cross-linked (D-dimerized) fibrin. As plasmin acts on the fibrin polymer clot, fibrin degradation products (FDPs) and D-dimer are produced. The D-dimer assay provides a highly specific measurement of the amount of fibrin degradation that occurs. Normal plasma does not have detectable amounts of fragment D-dimer. For discussion of other fibrin degradation products, see thrombosis indicators (p. 896)

This test provides a simple and confirmatory test for disseminated intravascular coagulation (DIC). Positive results of the D-dimer assay correlate with positive results of other thrombosis indicators. The D-dimer assay may be more specific than the FDP assay but is less sensitive. Therefore, combining the FDP and the D-dimer provides a highly sensitive and specific test for recognizing DIC.

Levels of D-dimer can increase when a fibrin clot is lysed by thrombolytic therapy. Thrombotic problems, such as deep vein thrombosis (DVT), pulmonary embolism (PE), sickle cell anemia, and thrombosis of malignancy, are also associated with high D-dimer levels. D-dimer is used as an effective screening test for DVT. It is able to accurately identify patients with DVT who are then sent for venous duplex scanning (p. 977). The D-dimer test, however, is often positive in patients who are already hospitalized. If the D-dimer test is negative, its high predictability indicates that the patient does not have PE/DVT; further testing may not be necessary.

Finally, the D-dimer test can be used to determine the duration of anticoagulation therapy in patients with DVT. Patients with an abnormal D-dimer level 1 month after the discontinuation of anticoagulant therapy have a significant incidence of recurrent DVT. This incidence can be reduced by restarting anticoagulation therapy.

Interfering factors

- D-dimer level may be decreased in lipemic patients.
- The presence of rheumatoid factor at a level >50 IU/mL may lead to increased D-dimer levels.

Procedure and patient care

- See inside front cover for Routine Blood Testing.
- Fasting: no.
- Blood tube commonly used: blue.
- Remember that if the patient is receiving anticoagulants or has coagulopathies, the bleeding time will be increased.

Abnormal findings

▲ **Increased levels**

Fibrinolysis

During thrombolytic or defibrination therapy with tissue plasminogen activator

Deep-vein thrombosis

Pulmonary embolism

Arterial thromboembolism

Disseminated intravascular coagulation

Sickle cell anemia with or without vasoocclusive crisis

Pregnancy

Malignancy

Surgery

notes

delta-aminolevulinic acid (Aminolevulinic acid [ALA], δ-ALA)

Type of test Urine (24-hour)

Normal findings 1.5-7.5 mg/24 hr or 11-57 µmol/24 hr (SI units)

Possible critical values >20 mg/24 hr

Test explanation and related physiology

As the basic precursor for the porphyrins (p. 729), δ-ALA is needed for the normal production of porphobilinogen, which ultimately leads to heme synthesis in erythroid cells. Heme is used in the synthesis of hemoglobin. Genetic disorders (porphyria) are associated with a lack of a particular enzyme vital to heme metabolism. These disorders are characterized by an accumulation of porphyrin products in the liver or red blood cells. The liver porphyrias are much more common. Symptoms of liver porphyrias include abdominal pain, neuromuscular signs and symptoms, constipation, and occasionally psychotic behavior. Acute intermittent porphyria (AIP) is the most common form of the liver porphyrias; this is caused by a deficiency in uroporphyrinogen-I-synthase (also called porphobilinogen deaminase).

Most patients with AIP have no symptoms (latent phase) until the acute phase is precipitated by medication or other factors (see uroporphyrinogen, p. 972). The acute phase is highlighted by symptoms of abdominal pain, muscular pain, nausea, vomiting, hypertension, mental symptoms (anxiety, insomnia, hallucinations, and paranoia), sensory loss, and urinary retention. Hemolytic anemia also may occur with these acute attacks. These acute symptoms are associated with increased serum and urine levels of porphyrin precursors (aminolevulinic acid, porphyrins, and porphobilinogens).

In lead intoxication, heme synthesis is similarly diminished by the inhibition of ALA dehydrase. This enzyme assists in the conversion of ALA to porphobilinogen. As a result of lead poisoning, ALA accumulates in the blood and urine.

Interfering factors

☝ Drugs that may cause *increased* ALA levels include barbiturates, griseofulvin, and penicillin.

Procedure and patient care

- See inside front cover for Routine Urine Testing.
- Keep the urine in a light-resistant container with a preservative.
- If the patient has a Foley catheter in place, cover the drainage bag to prevent exposure to light.

Abnormal findings

▲ **Increased levels**
Porphyria
Lead intoxication
Chronic alcoholic disorders
Diabetic ketoacidosis

notes

> **dexamethasone suppression test** (DST, Prolonged/rapid DST, Cortisol suppression test, ACTH suppression test)

Type of test Blood; urine (24-hour)

Normal findings

Prolonged method

Low dose: >50% reduction of plasma cortisol
High dose: >50% reduction of plasma cortisol
Urinary free cortisol: <20 µg/24 hr (<50 nmol/24 hr)

Rapid (overnight) method

Normal: plasma cortisol levels suppressed to <2 µg/dL

Test explanation and related physiology

An elaborate feedback mechanism for cortisol exists to coordinate the functions of the hypothalamus, pituitary gland, and adrenal glands. The DST is based on pituitary adrenocorticotropic hormone (ACTH) secretion being dependent on the plasma cortisol feedback mechanism. As plasma cortisol levels increase, ACTH secretion is suppressed; as cortisol levels decrease, ACTH secretion is stimulated. Dexamethasone is a synthetic steroid (similar to cortisol) that normally should suppress ACTH secretion. Under normal circumstances, this results in reduced stimulation to the adrenal glands and ultimately a drop of 50% or more in plasma cortisol and 17-OCHS levels. This important feedback system does not function properly in patients with hypercortisol states.

In Cushing syndrome caused by bilateral adrenal hyperplasia (Cushing disease), the pituitary gland is reset upward and responds only to high plasma levels of cortisol or its analogues. In Cushing syndrome caused by adrenal adenoma or cancer (which acts autonomously), cortisol secretion continues despite a decrease in ACTH. When Cushing syndrome is caused by an ectopic ACTH-producing tumor (as in lung cancer), that tumor is also considered autonomous and will continue to secrete ACTH despite high cortisol levels. Again, no decrease occurs in plasma cortisol. Knowledge of the following defects in the normal cortisol-ACTH feedback system is the basis for differentiating hypercortisol states using DST. ACTH and plasma cortisol levels are measured during this test.

When hypercortisol is caused by:
- Bilateral adrenal hyperplasia (Cushing disease)
  - Low dose: no change
  - High dose: >50% reduction of plasma cortisol and ACTH is elevated
- Adrenal adenoma or carcinoma (primary hypercortisolism)
  - Low dose: no change
  - High dose: no change
  - ACTH is undetectable or low
- Ectopic ACTH-producing tumor
  - Low dose: no change
  - High dose: no change
  - ACTH is normal to elevated

The DST also may identify depressed persons likely to respond to electroconvulsive therapy or antidepressants rather than to psychologic or social interventions. ACTH production will not be fully suppressed after administration of low-dose dexamethasone in these patients.

The *prolonged* DST can be performed over a 2-day period on an outpatient basis. The *rapid* DST is easily and quickly performed and is used primarily as a screening test to diagnose Cushing syndrome. It is less accurate and informative than the prolonged DST, but when its results are normal, the diagnosis of Cushing syndrome can be safely excluded.

Interfering factors
- Physical and emotional stress can elevate ACTH release.
- ✶ Drugs that can affect test results include barbiturates, estrogens, oral contraceptives, phenytoin, spironolactone, steroids, and tetracyclines.

Procedure and patient care
Before
Explain the procedure (prolonged or rapid test) to the patient.

During
There are several documented methods of performing this test by varying the dose and duration of testing.

Prolonged test
- Obtain a baseline 24-hour urine collection for urinary free cortisol (p. 301). See inside front cover for Routine Urine Testing.
- Collect blood for determination of baseline plasma cortisol levels (see p. 301) if indicated.

- Collect 24-hour urine specimens daily over a 2-day period. Because 2 continuous days of urine collections are needed, no urine specimens are discarded except for the first voided specimen on day 1, after which the collection begins.
- On days 1 and 2, administer a low dose (2 mg) of dexamethasone by mouth every 6 hours for 48 hours.
- Administer the dexamethasone with milk or an antacid to prevent gastric irritation.
- Note that the urine samples for free cortisol do not need a preservative.
- Note that creatinine is measured in all the 24-hour urine collections to demonstrate their accuracy and adequacy.
- Keep the urine specimens refrigerated or on ice during the collection period.

Rapid test
- Give the patient a low dose (0.5 mg) of dexamethasone by mouth at 11 PM.
- Administer the dexamethasone with milk or an antacid to prevent gastric irritation.
- Attempt to ensure a good night's sleep. However, use sedative-hypnotics only if absolutely necessary.
- At 8 AM the next morning, draw blood for determination of plasma cortisol level before the patient arises.
- If no cortisol suppression occurs after the dose of dexamethasone, at 11 PM administer a higher dose and obtain a cortisol level as described above. This is referred to as the *overnight dexamethasone suppression test*. Patients with adrenal hyperplasia will suppress. Patients with adrenal or ectopic tumors will not suppress.

After
- Assess the patient for steroid-induced side effects by monitoring glucose levels and potassium levels.

Abnormal findings

Cushing syndrome
Cushing disease
Ectopic ACTH-producing tumors
Adrenal adenoma or carcinoma
Bilateral adrenal hyperplasia
Mental depression
Hyperthyroidism

notes

diabetes mellitus autoantibody panel (Insulin autoantibody [IAA], Islet cell antibody [ICA], Glutamic acid decarboxylase antibody [GAD Ab])

Type of test Blood

Normal findings <1:4 titer; no antibody detected

Test explanation and related physiology

Type I diabetes mellitus (DM) is insulin-dependent (IDDM). It is becoming increasingly recognized that this disease is an *organ-specific* form of autoimmune disease that results in destruction of the pancreatic islet cells and their products. These antibodies are used to differentiate type I DM from type II non–insulin-dependent DM. Nearly 90% of type I diabetics have one or more of these autoantibodies at the time of their diagnosis. Type II diabetics have low or negative titers.

These antibodies often appear years before the onset of symptoms. The panel is useful to screen relatives of IDDM patients who are at risk of developing the disease. GAD Ab provides confirmatory evidence. The presence of these antibodies identifies which gestational diabetic will eventually require insulin permanently.

The presence of insulin antibodies is diagnostic of factitious hypoglycemia from surreptitious administration of insulin. This antibody panel is also used in surveillance of patients who have received pancreatic islet cell transplantation. Finally, these antibodies can be used to identify late onset type I diabetes in those patients previously thought to have type II diabetes.

Interfering factors

- Radioactive scans within 7 days before the test may interfere with the test result.

Procedure and patient care

- See inside front cover for Routine Blood Testing.
- Fasting: no.
- Blood tube commonly used: red or serum separator.

Abnormal findings

▲ Increased levels

Insulin-dependent diabetes mellitus
Insulin resistance
Allergies to insulin
Factitious hypoglycemia

notes

2,3-diphosphoglycerate (2,3-DPG in erythrocytes)

Type of test Blood

Normal findings

$12.3 \pm 1.87\,\mu mol/g$ of hemoglobin or $0.79 \pm 0.12\,mol/mol$ hemoglobin (SI units)

$4.2 \pm 0.64\,\mu mol/mL$ of erythrocytes or $4.2 \pm 0.64\,mmol/L$ erythrocytes (SI units)

(Levels are lower in newborns and even lower in premature infants.)

Test explanation and related physiology

This test is used in the evaluation of nonspherocytic hemolytic anemia. 2,3-DPG is a by-product of the glycolytic respiratory pathway of the RBC. A congenital enzyme deficiency in this vital pathway alters the RBC shape and survival significantly. Anemia is the result. Another result of the enzyme deficiency is reduced synthesis of 2,3-DPG. Because 2,3-DPG controls oxygen transport from RBCs to tissues, deficiencies of this enzyme result in alterations of the RBC-oxygen dissociation curve that controls release of oxygen to the tissues. Many anemias not due to 2,3-DPG deficiency are associated with increased levels of 2,3-DPG as a compensatory mechanism.

Usually 2,3-DPG levels increase in response to anemia or hypoxic conditions (e.g., obstructive lung disease, congenital cyanotic heart disease, after vigorous exercise). Increases in 2,3-DPG decrease the oxygen binding to hemoglobin so that oxygen is more easily released to the tissues when needed (lower arterial Po_2). Levels of 2,3-DPG are decreased as a result of inherited genetic defects. This genetic defect parallels that of sickle cell anemia and hemoglobin C diseases.

Interfering factors

- Vigorous exercise may cause increased levels.
- High altitudes may increase levels.
- Banked blood has decreased amounts of 2,3-DPG.
- Acidosis decreases levels.

Procedure and patient care

- See inside front cover for Routine Blood Testing.
- Fasting: no.
- Blood tube commonly used: red.

Abnormal findings

▲ Increased levels
Anemia
Hypoxic heart (e.g., cyanotic
  heart disease) or lung
  (e.g., chronic obstructive
  pulmonary disease) diseases
Hyperthyroidism
Chronic renal failure
Pyruvate kinase deficiency
Cystic fibrosis
Adjustment to higher altitudes

▼ Decreased levels
Polycythemia
Acidosis
Post–massive blood
  transfusion
2,3-DPG mutase
  deficiency
2,3-DPG phosphatase
  deficiency
Respiratory distress
  syndrome

notes

Type of test Blood

Normal findings No evidence of DIC

D

Test explanation and related physiology

This is a group of tests used to detect disseminated intravascular coagulation. Many pathologic conditions can instigate or are associated with DIC. The more common ones include bacterial septicemia, amniotic fluid embolism, retention of a dead fetus, malignant neoplasia, liver cirrhosis, extensive surgery (especially on the liver), postextracorporeal heart bypass, extensive trauma, severe burns, and transfusion reactions.

In DIC, the entire clotting mechanism is inappropriately triggered. This results in significant systemic or localized intravascular formation of fibrin clots. Consequences of this futile clotting are small blood vessel occlusion and excessive bleeding caused by consumption of the platelets and clotting factors that have been used in intravascular clotting. The fibrinolytic system is also activated to break down the clot formation and the fibrin involved in the intravascular coagulation. This fibrinolysis results in the formation of fibrin degradation products (FDPs), which by themselves act as anticoagulants; these FDPs serve only to enhance the bleeding tendency.

Organ injury can occur as a result of the intravascular clots, which cause microvascular occlusion in various organs. This may cause serious anoxic injury in affected organs. Also, red blood cells passing through partly plugged vessels are injured and subsequently hemolyzed. The result may be ongoing hemolytic anemia. Figure 15 summarizes DIC pathophysiology and effects.

When a patient with a bleeding tendency is suspected of having DIC, a series of readily performed laboratory tests should be done (Table 13). With these tests, a hematologist can make the appropriate diagnosis confidently. These tests as noted in Table 13 are discussed separately in this book.

Abnormal findings

Disseminated intravascular coagulation

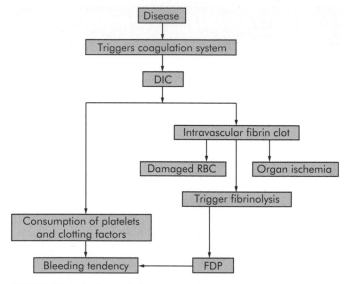

FIGURE 15 Pathology of disseminated intravascular coagulation *(DIC)*, which may result in bleeding tendency, organ ischemia, and hemolytic anemia. *RBC*, Red blood cell; *FDP*, fibrin degradation product.

TABLE 13   Disseminated intravascular coagulation screening tests

Test	Result
Platelet count (p. 718)	Decreased
Prothrombin time (p. 767)	Prolonged
Partial thromboplastin time (p. 693)	Prolonged
Coagulating factors (p. 261)	Decreased factors I, II, V, VIII, X, and XIII (more commonly used for diagnosis rather than for screening)
Fibrin degradation products (p. 896)	Increased
Fibrinogen (p. 439)	Decreased
D-dimer (p. 335)/in Δs	Increased
Fibrinopeptide A (p. 896)	Increased
Prothrombin fragment (p. 896)	Increased

drug monitoring (Therapeutic drug monitoring [TDM])

Type of test   Blood

Normal findings   See Table 14.

Test explanation and related physiology

TDM entails measuring blood drug levels to determine effective drug dosages and to prevent toxicity. Drug monitoring is helpful in patients who take other medicines that may affect drug levels or act in a synergistic or antagonistic manner with the drug to be tested. There are some medicines (e.g., antiarrhythmics, bronchodilators, antibiotics, anticonvulsants, cardiotonics) that have a very narrow therapeutic margin (i.e., the difference between therapeutic and toxic drug levels is small).

TDM is helpful if the desired therapeutic effect of the drug is not observed as expected. Dosages beyond normal may have to be prescribed. Likewise, if toxic symptoms appear with standard doses, TDM can be used to determine a more appropriate dosage.

Table 14 (p. 348) lists the therapeutic and toxic ranges for the average patient for some commonly tested drug levels. This list is far from complete. These ranges may not apply to all patients because clinical response is influenced by many factors. Also, note that different laboratories use different units for reporting test results and normal ranges. It is important that sufficient time pass between the administration of the medication and the collection of the blood sample to allow for adequate absorption and therapeutic levels to occur.

Blood is routinely used for TDM, because results indicate what is presently going on with the drug at any one particular time. Urine drug levels reflect the presence of the drug over the last several days. Therefore, if data concerning drug levels at a particular time are necessary, blood testing is required.

Blood samples can be taken at the drug's *peak level* (highest concentration) or at the *trough level* (lowest concentration). Peak levels are useful when testing for toxicity, and trough levels are useful for demonstrating a satisfactory therapeutic level. Trough levels are often referred to as residual levels. The time when the sample should be drawn after the last dose of the medication varies according to whether a peak or trough level is requested and according to the half-life (the time required for the body to decrease the drug blood level by 50%) of the drug. If peak levels

TABLE 14 Drug monitoring data

Drug	Use	Therapeutic level*	Toxic level*
Acetaminophen	Analgesic, antipyretic	Depends on use	>25 mcg/mL
Aminophylline	Bronchodilator	10-20 mcg/mL	>20 mcg/mL
Digoxin	Cardiac glycoside	0.8-2.0 ng/mL	>2.4 ng/mL
Gentamicin	Antibiotic	5-10 mcg/mL	>12 mcg/mL
Lidocaine	Antiarrhythmic	1.5-5.0 mcg/mL	>5 mcg/mL
Lithium	Manic episodes of bipolar psychosis	0.8-1.2 mEq/L	>2.0 mEq/L
Methotrexate	Antitumor agent	>0.01 μmol/24 hr	>10 μmol/24 hr
Phenobarbital	Anticonvulsant	10-30 mcg/mL	>40 mcg/mL
Phenytoin	Anticonvulsant	10-20 mcg/mL	>30 mcg/mL
Propranolol	Antiarrhythmic	50-100 ng/mL	>150 ng/mL
Salicylate	Antipyretic, antiinflammatory, analgesic	100-250 mcg/mL	>300 mcg/mL
Theophylline	Bronchodilator	10-20 mcg/mL	>20 mcg/mL
Tobramycin	Antibiotic	5-10 mcg/mL	>12 mcg/mL
Valproic acid	Anticonvulsant	50-100 mcg/mL	>100 mcg/mL
Vancomycin	Antibiotic	Peak: 20-40 mcg/mL Trough: 5-15 mcg/mL	>40 mcg/mL

* Levels vary according to the institution performing the test.

are higher than the therapeutic range, toxicity may be experienced. If trough levels are below the therapeutic range, drug therapy is inadequate.

Pharmacogenetics (genetic testing for drug monitoring)

TDM is used to alter the dosage of medications to maximize efficacy and minimize side effects. There are several factors that affect efficacy and toxicity: patient compliance, patient age and size, access to adequate care, optimal dosing, and drug pharmacology issues (e.g., absorption, elimination, and drug interactions). Drugs undergo metabolism by enzyme systems to activate a bound (proactive) drug or to deactivate an active drug. The effectiveness of these enzyme systems of metabolism are determined by the genetic makeup of the patient. With pharmacogenetics, four categories of drug metabolizers can be identified:

- Poor metabolizers (PMs)
- Intermediate metabolizers (IMs)
- Extensive metabolizers (EMs)
- Ultrametabolizers (UMs).

Overall, PMs and, to a lesser extent, IMs are prone to exaggerated side effects from active drugs, whereas normal doses of the same drugs tend to be ineffectual for UMs. If a proactive drug is administered and must be hydrolyzed to its active form, PMs will not benefit from normal doses whereas UMs will experience drug benefit from even small doses.

The cytochrome P450 (CYP450) system is a major family of drug-metabolizing enzymes. Several CYP450 enzymes are involved in the metabolism of a significant proportion of drugs (Table 15). *Cytochrome P450 genotype testing* is a pharmacogenetic method of evaluating the metabolic effectiveness of the CYP450 system.

Thiopurine methyltransferase (TPMT) is another metabolic enzyme system that is used in the metabolism of thiopurine drugs (e.g., azathioprine, 6-mercaptopurine [6MP], and 6-thioguanine). Defects in TPMT noted on *TPMT gene mutation testing* lead to decreased methylation and decreased inactivation of 6MP. This can lead to enhanced bone marrow toxicity which may cause myelosuppression, anemia, bleeding tendency, leukopenia, and infection.

Pharmacogenetics allows physicians to consider genetic information from patients in selecting medications and dosages of medications for a variety of common conditions (e.g., cardiac disease, psychiatric disease, and cancer).

TABLE 15   Enzymes involved in drug metabolism

Enzyme	Drugs
CYP2C9	Warfarin, phenytoin, nonsteroidal antiinflammatory drugs
CYP2C19	Omeprazole, proguanil, amitriptyline, diazepam, propranolol
CYP2D6	Codeine, tricyclic antidepressants, venlafaxine, procainamide, haloperidol, amiodarone
CYP2D6	Tricyclic antidepressants, dihydropyrimidine, dehydrogenase, fluorouracil, tamoxifen
Atypical pseudocholinesterase	Succinylcholine
NAT2 (slow acetylator)	Isoniazid, hydralazine
UGT1A1	Irinotecan
GST	D-penicillamine
TPMT	Azathioprine, mercaptopurine
CYP1A1	Polycyclic aromatic hydrocarbons
CYP1A2	Caffeine, theophylline, imipramine
CYP2 CYP2A6	Nicotine
CYP2E1	Ethanol
CYP3 CYP3A4	Amitriptyline, clarithromycin, cyclosporine, erythromycin, tacrolimus, lidocaine, nifedipine, tamoxifen

Procedure and patient care
Before
PT Explain the procedure to the patient.

PT Tell the patient that no food or fluid restrictions are needed.

- For patients suspected of having symptoms of drug toxicity, the best time to draw the blood specimen is when the symptoms are occurring.
- If there is a concern regarding whether an adequate dose of the drug is achieved, it is best to obtain trough levels.

During

- Collect a venous blood sample in a tube designated by the laboratory. Peak levels are usually obtained 1 to 2 hours after oral intake, approximately 1 hour after intramuscular (IM) administration, or approximately 30 minutes after intravenous (IV) administration. Residual (trough) levels are usually obtained shortly before (0 to 15 minutes) the next scheduled dose. Consult with the pharmacy for specific times.

After

- Apply pressure or a pressure dressing to the venipuncture site.
- Clearly mark all blood samples with the following information: patient's name, diagnosis, name of drug, time of last drug ingestion, time of sample, and any other medications the patient is currently taking.
- Promptly send the specimen to the laboratory.

Abnormal findings

Nontherapeutic levels of drugs
Toxic levels of drugs

notes

drug sensitivity genotype testing (AccuType)

Type of test Blood

Normal findings No abnormal genetic abnormalities

Test explanation and related physiology

The efficacy of therapeutic drugs can vary considerably among different patients. Factors that influence these variations include genetic aberrations, age, race, body weight/surface area, gender, tobacco use, concomitant medications, and comorbid medical conditions. It is extremely important to identify differences in drug metabolism to preclude the possibility of overdosing or underdosing.

Drug sensitivity genotype testing identifies genetic aberrations that encode various proteins required for drug metabolism. If the gene is abnormal, the protein may be deficient in quantity or character to properly metabolize the medication provided to the patient. Various laboratories have "trademarked" their testing methods. A common test is called *AccuType Testing*.

Drug sensitivity genotype testing is available for predicting a patient's response to warfarin, clopidogrel, interferon–ribavirin (and other retroviral medications), metformin, and anti–TB drugs (rifampin/isoniazid).

Procedure and patient care

- See inside front cover for Routine Blood Testing.
- Fasting: no.
- Blood tube commonly used: verify with lab.
- Alternatively 1 mL of saliva in an Oragene DNA self-collection kit can be submitted. The specimen should be maintained at room temperature.

Abnormal findings

Genetic aberrations that may vary drug metabolism

notes

ductoscopy (Mammary ductoscopy)

Type of test Endoscopy

Normal findings No tumor or premalignant changes

Test explanation and related physiology

Most breast cancers start in the cells that line the milk ducts within the breast. Mammary ductoscopy refers to a procedure where a miniaturized endoscope is used to get a closer look at the lining of the milk ducts and to provide access for biopsy or cell retrieval. Ductoscopy is used to visualize the breast ducts in women who have nipple discharge. Its accuracy and diagnostic potential depend upon the experience of the surgeon and the patient's anatomy.

The mammary ductoscope consists of an outer sheath with an external diameter that is barely larger than a piece of thread. The sheath has two channels; a camera light source is inserted in one channel, and water is injected into the other channel to dilate the ducts for better visibility. A video/endoscopic camera is attached, and the images are projected on a TV monitor through a video system (Figure 16). The scope is then advanced to the smallest branches of the milk ducts.

Breast diseases, including cancers, can be found at their very earliest stages with the use of this technique. Ductoscopy can identify cancers so small that mammography, ultrasound, and even MRI cannot see them. With this technique, premalignant changes can be identified and treated in an attempt to prevent breast cancer.

Breast ductal lavage (p. 187) is a technique used to obtain and identify premalignant, atypical cells from breast ducts in patients who are considered at high risk for cancer and who have no evidence of breast malignancy on a mammogram or ultrasound. Ductoscopy is used in the hopes of identifying the causes of those changes (e.g., intraductal papillomas and early cancers) and possibly delivering ablative therapies to eradicate them.

Interfering factors

• The inability to access the duct precludes performance of this endoscopic procedure.

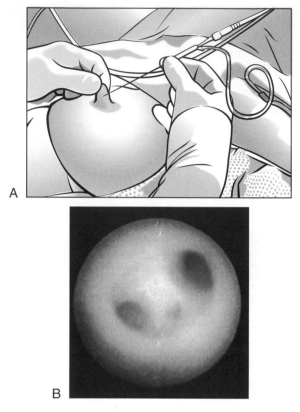

FIGURE 16 A, Ductoscope is passed into the breast nipple. **B,** Image of normal ducts in the breast.

Procedure and patient care
Before
PT Explain the procedure to the patient.
- Be sure the breast exam and mammogram are normal.
- Obtain informed consent.
PT If the procedure is to be performed under general anesthesia, instruct the patient to abstain from eating and drinking for at least 8 hours.

- If the procedure is to be performed under local anesthesia, apply a topical anesthetic to the nipple area about ½ hour to 1 hour prior to the test.

During
- Note the following procedural steps:
    1. The breast is massaged to promote the discharge of nipple fluid. This helps to visually identify the ductal orifice in the nipple for endoscopy.
    2. The ductal opening in the nipple is gently dilated with progressively larger dilators. The mammary sheath containing the ductoscope is inserted and advanced under direct visualization while saline is injected to dilate the branches of the duct.
    3. The ductoscopy findings can be recorded on videotape.
    4. If any disease is identified, the scope can pinpoint the area for directed surgical removal.
    5. Ductal washings can also be obtained by aspirating some of the fluid for microscopic analysis.
- This procedure is usually performed by a surgeon in the office in approximately 30 minutes.

After
PT Inform the patient to contact the physician if she develops any redness, breast pain, or elevated temperature, which may indicate mastitis.

Abnormal findings

Invasive ductal cancer
Noninvasive ductal cancer
Atypical ductal hyperplasia
Papilloma

notes

echocardiography (Cardiac echo, Heart sonogram, Transthoracic echocardiography [TTE])

Type of test Ultrasound

Normal findings

Normal position, size, and movement of the cardiac valves and heart muscle wall

Normal directional flow of blood within the heart chambers

Test explanation and related physiology

Echocardiography is a noninvasive ultrasound procedure used to evaluate the structure and function of the heart. In diagnostic ultrasonography, a harmless, high-frequency sound wave emitted from a transducer penetrates the heart. Sound waves are bounced off the heart structures and reflected back to the transducer as a series of echoes. These echoes are amplified and displayed on an oscilloscope. Tracings also can be recorded on moving graph paper or videotape. The study usually includes M-mode recordings, two-dimensional recordings, color Doppler studies, and real-time three-dimensional imaging.

M-mode echocardiography is a linear tracing of the motion of the heart structures over time. This allows the various cardiac structures to be located and studied regarding their movement during a cardiac cycle.

Two-dimensional echocardiography angles a beam within one sector of the heart. This produces a picture of the spatial anatomic relationships within the heart.

Three-dimensional echocardiography allows for improved images of the heart wall and valves. The addition of high temporal resolution further improves images.

Color Doppler echocardiography detects the pattern of the blood flow and measures changes in velocity of blood flow within the heart and great vessels. Turbulent blood or altered velocity and direction of blood flow can be identified by changes in color. This is seen in a photograph. In most Doppler ultrasound color flow imaging, blue and red represent the direction of a given stream of blood; the various hues from dull to bright represent varying blood velocities. The most useful application of the color flow imaging is in determining the direction and turbulence of blood flow across regurgitant or narrowed valves. Doppler color flow imaging also may be helpful in assessing proper functioning of prosthetic valves.

Echocardiography, in general, is used in the diagnosis of a pericardial effusion, valvular heart disease (e.g., mitral valve prolapse, stenosis, regurgitation), subaortic stenosis, myocardial wall abnormalities (e.g., cardiomyopathy), infarction, and aneurysm. Cardiac tumors (e.g., myxomas) are easily diagnosed with ultrasound. Atrial and ventricular septal defects and other congenital heart diseases are also recognized by ultrasound. Finally, postinfarction mural thrombi are readily apparent with this testing.

Echocardiography is also used in *cardiac stress testing*. It is fast becoming the method of choice in heart imaging for stress testing. During an exercise or chemical cardiac stress test, ischemic muscle areas are evident as hypokinetic areas within the myocardium. Echocardiography is being used with increasing frequency in emergent and urgent evaluations of patients with chest pains. If the myocardium is normal and without areas of hypokinesia, no coronary artery occlusive disease is suspected. If, however, a hypokinetic or akinetic area is noted, ischemia or infarction has occurred, and the chest pain is cardiac in origin.

Echocardiography can be performed via the esophagus with use of a probe mounted on an endoscope. This is referred to as *transesophageal echocardiography* or *TEE* (p. 921).

Contraindications

- Patients who are uncooperative

Interfering factors

- Chronic obstructive pulmonary disease (COPD)
  Patients who have severe COPD have a significant amount of air space between the heart and the chest cavity. Air space does not conduct ultrasound waves well.
- Obesity
  In obese patients the space between the heart and the transducer is greatly enlarged; therefore, accuracy of the test is decreased.

Procedure and patient care

Before

PT Assure the patient that this is a painless study.
- Complete the request for the echocardiogram, including the pertinent patient history.

During

- Note the following procedural steps:
  1. The patient is placed in the supine position.
  2. Electrocardiographic (ECG) leads are placed (p. 359).

3. A gel, which allows better transmission of sound waves, is placed on the chest wall immediately under the transducer.
4. Ultrasound is directed to the heart, and appropriate tracings are obtained.

- Note that this procedure usually takes approximately 45 minutes and is performed by an ultrasound technician in a darkened room within the cardiac laboratory or radiology department.
- **PT** Tell the patient that no discomfort is associated with this study but that the transmission gel is usually cooler than body temperature.

After

- Remove the gel from the patient's chest wall.
- **PT** Inform the patient that the physician must interpret the study and that the results will be available in a few hours.

Abnormal findings

Valvular stenosis
Valvular regurgitation
Mitral valve prolapse
Pericardial effusion
Ventricular or atrial mural thrombi
Myxoma
Poor ventricular muscle motion
Septal defects
Ventricular hypertrophy
Endocarditis

notes

electrocardiography (Electrocardiogram [ECG, EKG])

Type of test Electrodiagnostic

Normal findings Normal rhythm, wave deflections, and heart rate (60 to 100 beats/min)

Test explanation and related physiology

The ECG is a graphic representation of the electrical impulses that the heart generates during the cardiac cycle. These electrical impulses are conducted to the body's surface, where they are detected by electrodes placed on the patient's limbs and chest. The monitoring electrodes detect the electrical activity of the heart from a variety of spatial perspectives. The ECG lead system is composed of several electrodes that are placed on each of the four extremities and at varying sites on the chest. Each combination of electrodes is called a *lead*.

A *12-lead ECG* provides a comprehensive view of the flow of the heart's electrical currents in two different planes. There are six limb leads (combination of electrodes on the extremities) and six chest leads (corresponding to six sites on the chest). The limb leads provide a *frontal-plane view* that bisects the body, separating the front and back; the chest leads provide a *horizontal-plane view* that bisects the body, separating the top and bottom (Figure **17**).

Leads I, II, and III are considered the standard limb leads. Lead I records the difference in electrical potential between the left arm (LA) and the right arm (RA). Lead II records the electrical potential between the RA and the left leg (LL). Lead III reflects the difference between the LA and the LL. The right leg (RL) electrode is an inactive ground in all leads. There are three *augmented* limb leads: aV_R, aV_L, and aV_F (*a*, augmented; *V*, vector [unipolar]; *R*, right arm; *L*, left arm; *F*, left foot or leg). The augmented leads measure the electrode potential between a calculated center point and the right arm (aV_R), the left arm (aV_L), and the left leg (aV_F).

The six standard chest, or precordial, leads (V_1, V_2, V_3, V_4, V_5, V_6) are placed at six different positions on the chest, surrounding the heart.

In general, leads II, III, and aV_F look at the inferior part of the heart. Leads I and aV_L look at the lateral part of the heart, and leads V_2 through V_4 look at the anterior part of the heart.

The ECG is recorded on special paper with a graphic background of horizontal and vertical lines for rapid measurement of

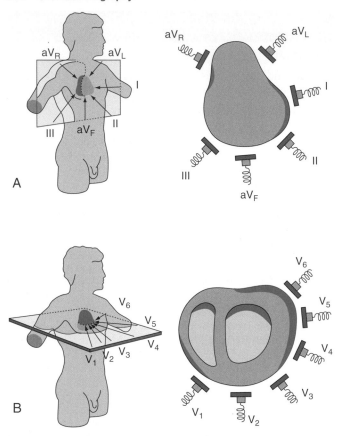

FIGURE 17 Planes of reference. **A,** The frontal plane. **B,** The horizontal plane.

time intervals (*X* coordinate) and voltages (*Y* coordinate). Time duration is measured by vertical lines 1 mm apart, each representing 0.04 second. Voltage is measured by horizontal lines 1 mm apart. Five 1-mm squares equals 0.5 mV.

The normal ECG pattern is composed of waves arbitrarily designated by the letters *P, Q, R, S, T,* and *U.* The Q, R, and S waves are grouped together and described as the QRS complex. The significance of the waves and time intervals is as follows (Figure 18):

- *P wave.* This represents atrial electrical depolarization associated with atrial contraction. It represents electrical activity

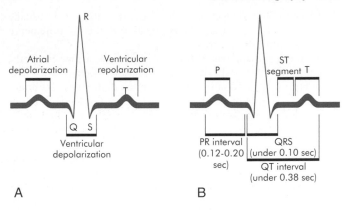

FIGURE 18 Electrocardiography. **A,** Normal ECG deflections during depolarization and repolarization of the atria and ventricles. **B,** Principal ECG intervals between P, QRS, and T waves.

associated with the spread of the original impulse from the sinoatrial (SA) node through the atria. If P waves are absent or altered, the cardiac impulse originates outside the SA node.

- *PR interval.* This represents the time required for the impulse to travel from the SA node to the atrioventricular (AV) node. If this interval is prolonged, a conduction delay exists in the AV node (e.g., a first-degree heart block). If the PR interval is shortened, the impulse must have reached the ventricle through a "shortcut" (e.g., Wolff-Parkinson-White syndrome).
- *QRS complex.* This represents ventricular electrical depolarization associated with ventricular contraction. This complex consists of an initial downward (negative) deflection (Q wave), a large upward (positive) deflection (R wave), and a small downward deflection (S wave). A widened QRS complex indicates abnormal or prolonged ventricular depolarization time (e.g., a bundle-branch block), Wolff-Parkinson-White syndrome, or pacemaker rhythms.
- *ST segment.* This represents the period between the completion of depolarization and the beginning of repolarization of the ventricular muscle. This segment may be elevated or depressed in transient muscle ischemia (e.g., angina) or in muscle injury (e.g., the early stages of myocardial infarction).
- *T wave.* This represents ventricular repolarization (i.e., return to the resting state).

- *U wave.* This deflection follows the T wave and is usually quite small. It represents repolarization of the Purkinje nerve fibers within the ventricles.

Through the analysis of these waveforms and time intervals, valuable information about the heart may be obtained. The ECG is used primarily to identify abnormal heart rhythms (arrhythmias [dysrhythmias]) and to diagnose acute myocardial infarction, conduction defects, and ventricular hypertrophy. It is important to note that the ECG may be normal, even in the presence of heart disease.

For some patients at high risk for malignant ventricular arrhythmias, a *signal-averaged ECG (SAECG)* can be performed. This test averages several hundred QRS waveforms to detect late potentials that are likely to lead to ventricular arrhythmias. SAECGs have been a useful precursor to electrophysiologic studies (p. 378) because they can identify patients with unexplained syncope who may have ventricular tachycardias induced by the electrophysiologic study. SAECGs can be performed at the bedside in 15 to 20 minutes and must be ordered separate from a standard ECG. This type of ECG uses a nonstandard ECG patch placement and is not performed like a standard ECG.

Microvolt T-wave alternans (MTWA) detects T-wave alternans (variations in the vector and amplitude of the T waves) on ECG signals as small as one-millionth of a volt. MTWA is defined as an alteration in the morphology of the T wave in an every-other-beat pattern. It has long been associated with ventricular arrhythmias and sudden death. MTWA is linked to the rapid onset of ventricular tachyarrhythmias.

MTWA is significant in the clinical context because it acts as a risk stratifier between patients who need implantable cardiac defibrillators (ICDs) and those who do not. Patients who test negative for MTWA have a very low risk of sudden cardiac death and are less likely to require ICDs than those who test positive.

In this test, high fidelity ECG leads are placed on the patient's chest during an exercise test. The goal is to get the patient walking fast enough to get the heart rate in the range of 105 to 110 beats per minute, but no higher. Minute changes in T waves are measured and recorded via computer analysis.

Interfering factors

- Inaccurate placement of the electrodes
- Electrolyte imbalances
- Poor contact between the skin and the electrodes
- Movement or muscle twitching during the test

☑ Drugs that can affect results include barbiturates, digitalis, and quinidine.

Procedure and patient care

Before

PT Explain the procedure to the patient.

PT Tell the patient that no food or fluid restriction is necessary.

PT Assure the patient that the flow of electric current is *from* the patient. He or she will feel nothing during this procedure.

• Expose only the patient's chest and arms. Keep the abdomen and thighs adequately covered.

During

• Note the following procedural steps:
   1. The skin areas designated for electrode placement are prepared by using alcohol swabs or sandpaper to remove skin oil or debris. Sometimes the skin is shaved if the patient has a large amount of hair.
   2. Pads with special gel are applied to ensure electrical conduction between the skin and the electrodes.
   3. Electrodes are applied to the four extremities. Many cardiologists recommend that arm electrodes be placed on the upper arm because fewer muscle tremors are detected there.
   4. The chest leads are applied one at a time, three at a time, or six at a time, depending on the type of ECG machine. These leads are positioned as follows:
       V_1: in the fourth intercostal space (4ICS) at the right sternal border
       V_2: in 4ICS at the left sternal border
       V_3: midway between V_2 and V_4
       V_4: in 5ICS at the midclavicular line
       V_5: at the left anterior axillary line at the level of V_4 horizontally
       V_6: at the left midaxillary line on the level of V_4 horizontally
• Note that cardiac technicians, nurses, or physicians perform this procedure in less than 5 minutes at the bedside or in the cardiology clinic.

PT Tell the patient that, although this procedure carries no discomfort, he or she must lie still in the supine position without talking while the ECG is recorded.

After

- Remove the electrodes from the patient's skin and wipe off the electrode gel.
- Indicate on the ECG strip or request slip if the patient was experiencing chest pain during the study. The pain may be correlated with an arrhythmia on the ECG.

Abnormal findings

Cardiac arrhythmias
Acute myocardial infarction
Myocardial ischemia
Old myocardial infarction
Conduction defects
Conduction system disease
Wolff-Parkinson-White syndrome
Ventricular hypertrophy
Cor pulmonale
Pulmonary embolus
Electrolyte imbalance
Pericarditis

notes

electroencephalography (Electroencephalogram [EEG])

Type of test Electrodiagnostic

Normal findings Normal frequency, amplitude, and characteristics of brain waves

Test explanation and related physiology

The EEG is a graphic recording of the electrical activity of the brain. EEG electrodes are placed on the scalp over multiple areas of the brain to detect and record electrical impulses within the brain. This study is invaluable in the investigation of epileptic states, in which the focus of seizure activity is characterized by rapid, spiking waves seen on the graph. Patients with cerebral lesions (e.g., tumors, infarctions) have abnormally slow EEG waves, depending on the size and location of the lesion. Because this study determines the overall activity of the brain, it can be used to evaluate trauma and drug intoxication and to determine cerebral death in comatose patients.

The EEG also can be used to monitor the electrophysiologic effects of cerebral blood flow. For example, during carotid endarterectomy, the carotid vessel must be temporarily occluded. When this surgery is performed with the patient under general anesthesia, the EEG can be used for early detection of cerebral tissue ischemia. Temporary shunting of the blood during the surgery is then required.

Electrocorticography (ECoG) is a form of EEG performed during craniotomy. Electrodes are placed directly on the exposed surface of the brain to record electrical activity from the cerebral cortex. ECoG is currently considered to be the standard for defining epileptogenic zones before attempts at surgical interruption are made. This procedure is invasive. The same information can be obtained by a noninvasive brain imaging technique called *magnetoencephalography (MEG)*.

MEG is a noninvasive imaging technique used to measure the magnetic fields produced by electrical activity in the brain with an extremely sensitive device called a *superconducting quantum interference device (SQID)*. The data obtained by MEG are commonly used to assist neurosurgeons in localizing pathology or defining sites of origin for epileptic seizures. MEG is also used in localizing important adjacent cortical areas for surgical planning in patients with brain tumors or intractable epilepsy.

Interfering factors

- Fasting may cause hypoglycemia, which could modify the EEG pattern.
- Drinks containing caffeine (e.g., coffee, tea, cocoa, cola) interfere with test results.
- Body and eye movements during the test can cause changes in brain wave patterns.
- ✘ Drugs that may affect test results include sedatives.

Procedure and patient care

Before

PT Explain the procedure to the patient.

PT Assure the patient that this test cannot read the mind or detect senility.

PT Assure the patient that the flow of electrical activity is *from* the patient. He or she will not feel anything.

PT Instruct the patient to wash his or her hair the night before the test. No oils, sprays, or lotion should be used.

- Check to see if the physician wants to discontinue any medications before the study.

PT Instruct the patient if sleeping time should be shortened the night before the test. Adults may not be allowed to sleep more than 4 or 5 hours and children not more than 5 to 7 hours if a sleep EEG will be done.

During

- Note the following procedural steps:
  1. The EEG is usually performed in a specially constructed room that is shielded from outside disturbances.
  2. The patient is placed in a supine position on a bed or reclining in a chair.
  3. Sixteen or more electrodes are applied to the scalp with electrode paste in a uniform pattern over both sides of the head, covering the prefrontal, frontal, temporal, parietal, and occipital areas.
  4. One electrode may be applied to each earlobe for grounding.
  5. After the electrodes are applied, the patient is instructed to lie still with eyes closed.
  6. The technician observes the patient during the EEG recording for movements that could alter results.
  7. Approximately every 5 minutes, the recording is interrupted to permit the patient to move if desired.

- In addition to the resting EEG, note that the following *activating procedures* can be performed:
    1. The patient is *hyperventilated* (asked to breathe deeply 20 times a minute for 3 minutes) to induce alkalosis and cerebral vasoconstriction, which can activate abnormalities.
    2. *Photostimulation* is performed by flashing a light over the patient's face with the eyes opened or closed. Seizure activity may be seen on the EEG.
    3. A *sleep EEG* may be performed to aid in the detection of some abnormal brain waves that are seen only if the patient is sleeping (e.g., frontal lobe epilepsy). The sleep EEG is performed after orally administering a sedative/hypnotic. A recording is performed while the patient is falling asleep, while the patient is sleeping, and while the patient is awakening.
- Note that this study is performed by an EEG technician in approximately 45 minutes to 2 hours.
- **PT** Tell the patient that no discomfort is associated with this study, other than possibly missing sleep.

After
- Help the patient remove the electrode paste.
- Ensure safety precautions until the effects of any sedatives have worn off. Keep the bed's siderails up.

Abnormal findings

Seizure disorders (e.g., epilepsy)
Brain tumor
Brain abscess
Head injury
Cerebral death
Encephalitis
Intracranial hemorrhage
Cerebral infarct
Narcolepsy
Alzheimer disease

notes

electromyography (EMG)

Type of test Electrodiagnostic

Normal findings No evidence of neuromuscular abnormalities

Test explanation and related physiology

By placing a recording electrode into a skeletal muscle, the electrical activity of a skeletal muscle can be monitored in a way very similar to electrocardiography (p. 359). The electrical activity is displayed on an oscilloscope as an electrical waveform. An audioelectrical amplifier can be added to the system so that the appearance and sound of electrical potentials can be analyzed and compared simultaneously. EMG is used to detect primary muscular disorders, along with muscular abnormalities caused by other system diseases (e.g., nerve dysfunction, sarcoidosis, paraneoplastic syndrome).

Spontaneous muscle movement, such as fibrillation and fasciculation, can be detected during EMG. When evident, these waveforms indicate injury or disease of the nerve or muscle being evaluated. A decrease in the number of muscle fibers able to contract is typically observed with peripheral nerve damage. This study is usually done in conjunction with nerve conduction studies (p. 373) and may also be called electromyoneurography.

Contraindications

- Patients receiving anticoagulant therapy
- Patients with extensive skin infection

Potential complications

- Rarely, hematoma at the needle insertion site

Interfering factors

- Edema, hemorrhage, or thick subcutaneous fat can interfere with test results.
- Patients with excessive pain may have false results.

Procedure and patient care

Before

PT Explain the procedure to the patient. Allay any fears and allow the patient to express concerns.
- Obtain informed consent if required by the institution.
PT Tell the patient that fasting is not usually required; however, some facilities may restrict stimulants (coffee, tea, cocoa, cola, cigarettes) for 2 to 3 hours before the test.

- If serum enzyme tests (e.g., AST, CPK, LDH) are ordered, the specimen should be drawn before EMG or 5 to 10 days after the test, because the EMG may cause misleading elevations of these enzymes.
- Premedication or sedation is usually avoided because of the need for patient cooperation.

During
- Note the following procedural steps:
  1. This study is usually done in an EMG laboratory.
  2. The patient's position depends on the muscle being studied.
  3. A tiny needle that acts as a recording electrode is inserted into the muscle being examined or overlying the nerve itself. In most circumstances, however, that reference electrode is in the needle itself.
  4. A reference electrode is placed nearby on the skin surface.
  5. The patient is asked to keep the muscle at rest.
  6. The oscilloscope display is viewed for any evidence of spontaneous electrical activity, such as fasciculation or fibrillation.
  7. The patient is asked to contract the muscle slowly and progressively.
  8. The electrical waves produced are examined for their number, form, and amplitude.
  9. A nerve innervating a particular muscle group is stimulated, and the resulting muscle contraction is evaluated as described if nerve conduction studies are performed concomitantly.
- Note that the EMG is performed by a physical therapist, physiatrist, or neurologist in approximately 20 minutes.
- **PT** Tell the patient that the small needle size makes this procedure nearly painless.

After
- Observe the needle site for hematoma or inflammation.
- Provide pain medication if needed.

Abnormal findings

Polymyositis
Muscular dystrophy
Myopathy
Traumatic injury
Hyperadrenalism
Hypothyroidism
Paraneoplastic syndrome (e.g., lung cancer)
Sarcoidosis
Guillain-Barré syndrome
Myasthenia gravis
Peripheral nerve injury, entrapment, or compression
Spinal cord injury or disease
Acetylcholine blockers (e.g., curare, snake venom)
Multiple sclerosis
Diabetic neuropathy
Anterior poliomyelitis
Muscle denervation
Amyotrophic lateral sclerosis

notes

electromyography of the pelvic floor sphincter
(Pelvic floor sphincter electromyography, Pelvic floor sphincter EMG, Rectal EMG procedure)

Type of test Electrodiagnostic

Normal findings

Increased EMG signal during bladder filling
Silent EMG signal on voluntary micturition
Increased EMG signal at the end of voiding
Increased EMG signal with voluntary contraction of the anal sphincter

Test explanation and related physiology

This test uses the placement of electrodes on or in the pelvic floor musculature to evaluate the neuromuscular function of the urinary or anal sphincter. It is performed most often in patients who have urinary or fecal incontinence. The pathology causing the muscle weakness can be muscular or neurologic. With pelvic floor sphincter EMG, these two causes can be separated.

The main benefit of this study is to evaluate the external sphincter (skeletal muscle) activity during voiding. This test is also used to evaluate the bulbocavernous reflex and voluntary control of external sphincter or pelvic floor muscles. The pelvic floor sphincter EMG also aids in the investigation of functional or psychological disturbances of voiding. Fecal incontinence caused by muscular dysfunction can also be evaluated by rectal sphincter EMG.

Recordings may be made from surface or needle electrodes within the muscle; surface electrodes are most often used. These electrodes allow for observation of and change in the muscle activity before and during voiding.

Contraindications

• Patients who cannot cooperate during the procedure

Procedure and patient care

Before

PT Explain the procedure to the patient.
PT Inform the patient that cooperation is essential.

During
- Note the following procedural steps:
  1. Electrodes are placed at the 2 o'clock and 10 o'clock positions on the perianal skin to monitor the pelvic floor musculature during voiding.
  2. A third electrode is usually placed on the thigh and serves as a ground.
  3. Electrical activity is recorded with the bladder empty and the patient relaxed.
  4. Reflex activity is evaluated by asking the patient to cough and by stimulating the urethra and trigone by gently tugging on an inserted Foley catheter (bulbocavernous reflex).
  5. Voluntary activity is evaluated by asking the patient to contract and relax the sphincter muscle.
  6. The bladder is filled with sterile water at room temperature at a rate of 100 mL/min.
  7. The EMG responses to filling and detrusor hyperreflexia (if present) are recorded.
  8. Finally, when the bladder is full and with the patient in a voiding position, the filling catheter is removed and the patient is asked to urinate. In the normal patient, the EMG signals build during bladder filling and cease promptly on voluntary micturition, remaining silent until the pelvic floor contracts at the end of voiding.
  9. The electrical waves produced are examined for their number and form.
- Note that a urologist performs this study in less than 30 minutes.
- **PT** Explain to the patient that this study is slightly more uncomfortable than urethral catheterization.

After
- If needle electrodes were used, observe the needle sites for hematoma or inflammation.

Abnormal findings

Neuromuscular dysfunction of lower urinary sphincter
Pelvic floor muscle dysfunction of anal sphincter

notes

electroneurography (ENG, Nerve conduction studies)

Type of test Electrodiagnostic

Normal findings

No evidence of peripheral nerve injury or disease
(Conduction velocity is usually decreased in the elderly.)

Test explanation and related physiology

Nerve conduction studies (NCS) evaluate the integrity of the nerves and allow for the detection and location of peripheral nerve injury or disease. By initiating an electrical impulse at one site (proximal when evaluating motor nerves or distal when evaluating sensory nerves) of a nerve and recording the time required for that impulse to travel to a second site (opposite above) of the same nerve, the conduction velocity of an impulse in that nerve can be determined. This study is usually done in conjunction with EMG (p. 368) and also may be called *electromyoneurography.*

Trauma or contusion of a nerve will usually cause slowing of conduction velocity in the affected side compared with the normal side. Neuropathies, both local and generalized, also will cause a slowing of conduction velocity. A velocity greater than normal does not indicate a pathologic condition. With complete nerve transection, no nerve conduction is noted.

Because conduction velocity may require contraction of a muscle as an indication of an impulse arriving at the recording electrode, significant primary muscular disorders may cause a falsely slow nerve conduction velocity. This "muscular" variable is eliminated if one evaluates the suspected pathologic muscle group before performing NCS. This muscular factor is evaluated by measuring distal latency (i.e., the time required for stimulation of the nerve to cause muscular contraction). As the distal latency is calculated, the motor NCS is performed normally by stimulating the nerve bundle. Conduction velocity can then be determined by the following equation:

$$\frac{\text{Conduction velocity}}{\text{(in meters per second)}} = \frac{\text{Distance (in meters)}}{\text{Total latency} - \text{Distal latency}}$$

NCS can also indicate diseases affecting either the motor or sensory nerves. Diseases affecting the neuromuscular junction, nerve axon loss, and variations in nerve recovery time can be evaluated.

Interfering factors

- Patients in severe pain may have false results.

Procedure and patient care

Before

PT Explain the procedure to the patient. Allay any fears.

- Obtain informed consent if required by the institution.

PT Tell the patient that no fasting or sedation is usually required.

During

- Note the following procedural steps:
  1. This test can be performed in a nerve conduction laboratory or at the patient's bedside.
  2. The patient's position depends on the area of suspected peripheral nerve injury or disease.
  3. A recording electrode is placed on the skin overlying a muscle innervated solely by the relevant nerve or overlying the nerve itself. All skin-to-electrode connections are ensured by using electrical gel.
  4. A reference electrode is placed nearby.
  5. The nerve is stimulated by a shock-emitting device at an adjacent location.
  6. The time between nerve impulse and muscular contraction (distal latency) is measured in milliseconds.
  7. The nerve is similarly stimulated at a location proximal to the area of suspected injury or disease.
  8. The time required for the impulse to travel from the site of initiation to muscle contraction (total latency) is recorded in milliseconds.
  9. The distance between the site of stimulation and the recording electrode is measured in centimeters.
  10. Conduction velocity is converted to meters per second and is computed as in the previous equation.
- Note that this test takes approximately 40 minutes and is performed by a physiatrist or a neurologist.

PT Tell the patient that this test may be uncomfortable because a mild shock is required for nerve impulse stimulation.

After

- Remove the electrode gel from the patient's skin.

Abnormal findings

Peripheral nerve injury or disease
Carpal tunnel syndrome
Herniated disc disease
Poliomyelitis
Diabetic neuropathy
Myasthenia gravis
Guillain-Barré syndrome

notes

electronystagmography (Electrooculography)

Type of test Electrodiagnostic

Normal findings Normal nystagmus response

Normal oculovestibular reflex

Test explanation and related physiology

Electronystagmography is used to evaluate nystagmus (involuntary rapid eye movement) and the muscles controlling eye movement. By measuring changes in the electrical field around the eye, this study can make a permanent recording of eye movement at rest, with a change in head position, and in response to various stimuli. The test delineates the presence or absence of nystagmus, which is caused by the initiation of the oculovestibular reflex. Nystagmus should occur when initiated by positional, visual, or caloric stimuli. Unlike caloric studies (p. 206), in which nystagmus is usually determined visually, electronystagmography electrically records the direction, velocity, and degree of nystagmus.

If nystagmus does not occur with stimulation, the vestibular cochlear apparatus, cerebral cortex (temporal lobe), auditory nerve, or brainstem is abnormal. Tumors, infection, ischemia, and degeneration can cause such abnormalities. When put together with the entire clinical picture, the pattern of nystagmus helps in the differentiation between central and peripheral vertigo. This test is used in the differential diagnosis of lesions in the vestibular system, brainstem, and cerebellum.

This study also may help evaluate unilateral hearing loss and vertigo. Unilateral hearing loss may be caused by middle ear problems or nerve injury. If the patient experiences nystagmus with stimulation, the auditory nerve is working and hearing loss can be blamed on the middle ear.

Contraindications

- Patients with perforated eardrums, who should not have water irrigation
- Patients with pacemakers

Interfering factors

- Blinking of the eyes can alter test results.
- ✶ Drugs that can alter results include antivertigo agents, sedatives, and stimulants.

Procedure and patient care

Before

PT Explain the procedure to the patient.

PT Instruct the patient not to apply facial makeup before the test because electrodes will be taped to the skin around the eyes.

PT Instruct the patient not to eat solid food before the test to reduce the likelihood of vomiting.

PT Instruct the patient not to drink caffeine or alcoholic beverages for approximately 24 to 48 hours (as ordered).

• Check with the physician regarding withholding any medications that could interfere with the test results.

During

• Note the following procedural steps:
  1. This procedure is usually performed in a darkened room with the patient seated or lying down.
  2. If there is any wax in the ear, it is removed.
  3. Electrodes are taped to the skin around the eyes.
  4. Various procedures are used to stimulate nystagmus, such as pendulum tracking, changing head position, changing gaze position, and caloric tests (p. 206).
  5. Several recordings are made with the patient at rest and to demonstrate patient response to various procedures (e.g., blowing air into the ear, irrigating the ear with water).
  6. Nystagmus response is compared with the expected ranges, and the results are recorded as normal, borderline, or abnormal.

• Note that this procedure is performed by a physician or audiologist in approximately 1 hour.

PT Tell the patient that nausea and vomiting may occur.

After

• Consider prescribing bed rest until nausea, vertigo, or weakness subsides.

Abnormal findings

Brainstem lesions
Cerebellum lesions
Auditory nerve damage

Vestibular system lesions
Congenital disorder
Demyelinating disease

notes

electrophysiologic study (EPS, Cardiac mapping)

Type of test Electrodiagnostic; manometric

Normal findings Normal conduction intervals, refractive periods, and recovery times

Tilt-table testing

<20 mm Hg decrease in systolic blood pressure
<10 mm Hg increase in diastolic blood pressure
Heart rate increase should be less than 10 beats/min

Test explanation and related physiology

In this invasive procedure, multiple electrode catheters are fluoroscopically placed through a peripheral vein and into the right atrium and/or ventricle or, less often, through an artery into the left atrium and/or ventricle. With close cardiac monitoring, the electrode catheters are used to pace the heart and potentially induce arrhythmias. Defects in the heart conduction system can then be identified; arrhythmias that are otherwise inapparent also can be induced, identified, and treated. The effectiveness of antiarrhythmic drugs (e.g., lidocaine, phenytoin, quinidine) can be assessed by determining the electrical threshold required to induce arrhythmias.

EPS can also be therapeutic. With the use of radiofrequency, sites with documented low thresholds for inducing arrhythmias can be obliterated to stop the arrhythmias.

The *tilt-table test* is sometimes performed with an electrophysiologic cardiac study and is a provocative test used to diagnose vasopressor syncope syndrome. Patients with this syndrome usually demonstrate symptomatic hypotension and syncope within a few to 30 minutes of being tilted upright by approximately 60 to 80 degrees. The tilt-table test is often used to assess the efficacy of prophylactic pacing in some patients with vasopressor syncope. It is also used to evaluate the impact of posture with some forms of tachyarrhythmias. Normally, a minimal drop in systolic blood pressure, rise in diastolic blood pressure, and increase in heart rate occur in the tilted position. Patients with vasopressor syncope demonstrate these changes in an exaggerated fashion and become lightheaded and dizzy on assuming the tilted position.

Contraindications

- Patients who are uncooperative
- Patients with acute myocardial infarction

Potential complications
- Cardiac arrhythmias leading to ventricular tachycardia or fibrillation
- Perforation of the myocardium
- Catheter-induced embolic cerebrovascular accident (stroke) or myocardial infarction
- Peripheral vascular problems
- Hemorrhage
- Phlebitis at the venipuncture site

Interfering factors
- Patients with dehydration or hypovolemia demonstrate similar changes in blood pressure and heart rate with tilt-table testing. This is especially true in elderly patients.
- Patients on antihypertensive medications or diuretics also may demonstrate similar changes when placed in the tilt position.
- Drugs that may interfere with test results include analgesics, sedatives, and tranquilizers.

Procedure and patient care
Before
- **PT** Instruct the patient to fast for 6 to 8 hours before the procedure. Usually fluids are permitted until 3 hours before.
- Obtain an informed consent from the patient.
- **PT** Encourage the patient to verbalize any fears.
- Prepare the catheter insertion site as directed.
- Collect a blood sample for potassium or drug levels if indicated.
- Obtain peripheral IV access for the administration of drugs.
- Inquire as to whether the patient has had excessive fluid loss (diarrhea or vomiting) in the previous 24 hours.
- Record the use of antihypertensive or diuretic medicines.

During
- Note the following procedural steps:

Electrophysiologic study
   1. In the cardiac catheterization laboratory, the patient has electrocardiographic (ECG) leads attached.
   2. The catheter insertion site, usually the femoral vein, is prepared and draped in a sterile manner.
   3. Under fluoroscopic guidance, the catheter is passed to the atrium and ventricle.

4. Baseline surface intracardiac ECGs are recorded.
5. Various parts of the cardiac electroconduction system are stimulated by atrial or ventricular pacing.
6. Mapping of the electroconduction system is performed.
7. Arrhythmias are identified.
8. Drugs may be administered to assess their efficacy in preventing EPS-induced arrhythmias.
9. Because dangerous arrhythmias can be prolonged, cardioversion must be immediately available.
10. Not only are vital signs and the heart monitored, but the patient is also constantly engaged in light conversation to assess mental status and consciousness.

Tilt-table test

1. The patient lies supine on a horizontal tilt table.
2. Obtain the patient's blood pressure and pulse as baseline values before tilting is carried out.
3. Monitor these vital signs during the procedure.
4. Question the patient as to the presence of symptoms of dizziness and lightheadedness.
5. The table is progressively tilted 60 to 80 degrees while the patient is being monitored. Alternatively, the patient is asked to sit or stand.

PT Tell the patient that he or she may experience palpitations, lightheadedness, or dizziness when arrhythmias are induced. Report these sensations to the physician. For most patients, this is an anxiety-producing experience.

PT Inform the patient that discomfort from catheter insertion is minimal.

After

• Keep the patient on bed rest for approximately 6 to 8 hours.
• Evaluate the venous/arterial access site for swelling and bleeding.
• Monitor the patient's vital signs for at least 2 to 4 hours for hypotension and arrhythmias. Additional monitoring is especially important for certain medications that the patient received during the test.
• Continue cardiac monitoring to identify arrhythmias. Transfer arrangements to a monitored unit may be necessary.
• Cover the area with sterile dressings if the electrical catheter is left in place for subsequent studies.

Abnormal findings

Electroconduction defects
Cardiac arrhythmias
Sinoatrial node defects (e.g., sick sinus syndrome)
Atrioventricular node defects and heart blocks
Vasomotor syncope syndrome
Inducible arrhythmias (e.g., ventricular tachycardia and Wolff-
  Parkinson-White syndrome)

notes

endometrial biopsy

Type of test Microscopic examination of tissue

Normal findings

No pathologic conditions
Presence of a secretory-type endometrium 3 to 5 days before
  normal menses

Test explanation and related physiology

An endometrial biopsy can determine whether ovulation has
occurred. A biopsy specimen taken 3 to 5 days before normal
menses should demonstrate a *secretory-type* endometrium on
histologic examination if ovulation and corpus luteum formation have occurred. If not, only a preovulatory *proliferative-type*
endometrium will be seen.

This test can determine if a woman has adequate ovarian
estrogen and progesterone levels. Another major use of endometrial biopsy is to diagnose endometrial cancer, tuberculosis,
polyps, or inflammatory conditions and to evaluate dysfunctional
uterine bleeding.

Contraindications

- Patients with infections (e.g., trichomonal, candidal, or suspected gonococcal) of the cervix or vagina
- Patients in whom the cervix cannot be visualized (e.g.,
  because of abnormal position or previous surgery)
- Patients who are or may be pregnant because the procedure
  may induce labor or abortion.

Potential complications

- Perforation of the uterus
- Uterine bleeding
- Interference with early pregnancy
- Infection

Procedure and patient care

Before

PT Explain the procedure to the patient.
- Ensure that written and informed consent is obtained.
PT Tell the patient that neither fasting nor sedation is usually
  required.

During

- Note the following procedural steps:
  1. The patient is placed in the lithotomy position, and a pelvic examination is performed to determine the position of the uterus.
  2. The cervix is exposed and cleansed.
  3. A biopsy instrument is inserted into the uterus, and specimens are obtained from the anterior, posterior, and lateral walls. This can be performed as part of a dilation and curettage or hysteroscopy (p. 548).
  4. The specimens are placed in a solution containing 10% formalin solution and sent to pathology.
- Note that this procedure is performed by an obstetrician/gynecologist in approximately 10 to 30 minutes.
- **PT** Tell the patient that this procedure may cause momentary discomfort (menstrual-type cramping).

After

- Assess the patient's vital signs at regular intervals. Any temperature elevation should be reported to the physician because this procedure may activate pelvic inflammatory disease.
- **PT** Advise the patient to wear a pad because some vaginal bleeding is to be expected. Tell the patient to call her physician if there is excessive bleeding (>1 pad per hour).
- **PT** Inform the patient that douching and intercourse are not permitted for 72 hours after the biopsy.
- **PT** Instruct the patient to rest during the next 24 hours and to avoid heavy lifting to prevent uterine hemorrhage.

Abnormal findings

Anovulation
Tumor
Tuberculosis
Polyps
Inflammatory condition

notes

endoscopic retrograde cholangiopancreatography (ERCP)

Type of test   Endoscopy

Normal findings

Normal size of biliary and pancreatic ducts
No obstruction or filling defects in the biliary or pancreatic ducts

Test explanation and related physiology

With the use of a fiberoptic endoscope, ERCP provides radiographic visualization of the biliary and pancreatic ducts. This is especially useful in patients with jaundice. If a partial or total obstruction of those ducts exists, characteristics of the obstructing lesion can be demonstrated. Stones, benign strictures, cysts, ampullary stenosis, anatomic variations, and malignant tumors can be identified.

Incision of the papillary muscle in the ampulla of Vater can be performed through the scope at the time of ERCP. This incision widens the distal common duct so that common bile duct gallstones can be removed. Stents can be placed through narrowed bile ducts with the use of ERCP, and the bile of jaundiced patients can be internally drained. Pieces of tissue and brushings of the common bile duct can be obtained by ERCP for pathologic review. Manometric studies of the sphincter of Oddi and pancreaticobiliary ducts can be performed at the time of ERCP. These are used to investigate unusual functional abnormalities of these structures.

Another less commonly used method of visualizing the biliary tree is *percutaneous transhepatic cholangiography (PTHC)*. PTHC is performed by passing a needle through the skin into the liver and into an intrahepatic bile duct. Iodinated x-ray contrast dye is directly injected into the biliary system. The intrahepatic and extrahepatic biliary ducts and occasionally the gallbladder can be visualized. If the jaundice is found to result from extrahepatic obstruction, a catheter can be left in the bile duct and used for external drainage of bile. Furthermore, with the assistance of ERCP, a stent can be placed across a stricture to decompress the biliary system internally.

Contraindications

• Patients who are uncooperative
Cannulation of the ampulla of Vater requires that the patient lie very still.

- Patients whose ampulla of Vater is not accessible endoscopically because of previous upper gastrointestinal surgery
- Patients with esophageal diverticula
  The scope can fall into a diverticulum and perforate its wall.
- Patients with known acute pancreatitis

Potential complications

- Perforation of the esophagus, stomach, or duodenum
- Gram-negative sepsis
  This results from introducing bacteria through the biliary system and into the blood.
- Pancreatitis
  This results from pressure of the dye injection.
- Aspiration of gastric contents into the lungs
- Respiratory arrest as a result of oversedation

Interfering factors

- Barium in the abdomen as a result of a previous upper GI series or barium enema x-ray study precludes adequate visualization of the biliary and pancreatic ducts.

Procedure and patient care

Before

PT Explain the procedure to the patient.
- Obtain informed consent from the patient.

PT Inform the patient that breathing will not be compromised by the insertion of the endoscope.
- Keep the patient NPO as of midnight the day of the test.
- Administer appropriate premedication (e.g., midazolam, atropine) if ordered.

During

- Note the following procedural steps:
  1. A flat plate of the abdomen is taken to ensure that any barium from previous studies will not obscure visualization of the bile duct.
  2. The patient is placed in the supine position or on the left side.
  3. The patient is usually sedated with a narcotic and a sedative/hypnotic.
  4. The pharynx is sprayed with a local anesthetic to inactivate the gag reflex and to lessen the discomfort.
  5. A fiberoptic duodenoscope is inserted through the oral pharynx and passed through the esophagus and stomach and then into the duodenum (Figure 19).

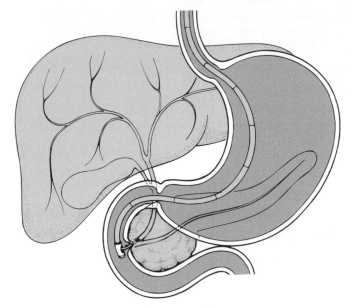

FIGURE 19 Endoscopic retrograde cholangiopancreatography. The fiberoptic scope is passed into the duodenum. Note the small catheter being advanced into the biliary duct.

6. Glucagon is often administered intravenously to minimize the spasm of the duodenum and to improve visualization of the ampulla of Vater.

7. Through the accessory lumen within the scope, a small catheter is passed through the ampulla of Vater and into the common bile or pancreatic ducts.

8. Radiographic dye is injected, and x-ray images are taken.

- Note that the test usually takes approximately 1 hour and is performed by a physician trained in endoscopy. The x-ray images are interpreted by a radiologist.

PT Tell the patient that no discomfort is associated with the dye injection but that minimal gagging may occur during the initial introduction of the scope into the oral pharynx.

After

- Do *not* allow the patient to eat or drink until the gag reflex returns. Encourage light eating for the next 12 to 24 hours.

- Observe the patient closely for development of abdominal pain, nausea, and vomiting. This may herald the onset of ERCP-induced pancreatitis or gastroduodenal perforation.
- Observe safety precautions until the effects of the sedatives have worn off.
- Monitor the patient for signs of respiratory depression. Medication (e.g., naloxone) should be available to counteract serious respiratory depression.
- Assess the patient for signs and symptoms of septicemia, which may indicate the onset of ERCP-induced cholangitis.

PT Inform the patient that he or she may be hoarse and have a sore throat for several days. Drinking cool fluids and gargling will help relieve some of this soreness.

PT Instruct the patient to notify the physician immediately of fever or shaking chills. This may indicate possible cholangitis.

Abnormal findings

Tumor, strictures, or gallstones of the common bile duct
Sclerosing cholangitis
Biliary sclerosis
Cysts of the common bile duct
Tumor, strictures, or inflammation of the pancreatic duct
Pseudocyst of the pancreatic duct
Chronic pancreatitis
Anatomic biliary or pancreatic duct variations
Cancer of the duodenum or ampulla of Vater

notes

Epstein-Barr virus testing (EBV antibody titer)

Type of test Blood

Normal findings

Titers ≤1:10 are nondiagnostic.
Titers of 1:10 to 1:60 indicate infection at some undetermined time.
Titers of ≥1:320 suggest active infection.
Fourfold increase in titer in paired sera drawn 10 to 14 days apart is usually indicative of an acute infection.

Test explanation and related physiology

EBV infects 80% of the U.S. population. After infection occurs, the virus becomes latent but can be reactivated later. EBV infection can produce infectious mononucleosis. Mononucleosis is seen most often in children, adolescents, and young adults. Clinical features include acute fatigue, fever, sore throat, lymphadenopathy, and splenomegaly. Laboratory findings of lymphocytosis, atypical lymphocytes, and transient serum heterophil antibodies are seen in patients with acute EBV infection. Most patients with infectious mononucleosis recover uneventfully and return to normal activity within 4 to 6 weeks. In Africa, EBV has been associated with Burkitt lymphoma. In China, EBV infection has been associated with nasopharyngeal carcinoma.

After recovery from primary EBV infection, patients are lifelong, latent EBV carriers. Specific immunologic tests to identify EBV activity indicate that latent EBV can reactivate and become associated with a constellation of chronic signs and symptoms resembling infectious mononucleosis. Clinical manifestations of chronic EBV are variable and include nonspecific symptoms, such as profound fatigue (chronic fatigue syndrome), pharyngitis, myalgia, arthralgia, low-grade fever, headache, paresthesia, and loss of abstract thinking.

The majority of EBV infections can be recognized, however, by testing the patient's serum for heterophile antibodies (rapid latex slide agglutination test or mononucleosis [mono] spot test; see page 645). Other more specific immunologic tests are recommended only when a mononucleosis screening procedure is negative and infectious mononucleosis or a complication of EBV infection is suspected. Also, more specific tests can more precisely define the acuity of the infection (Table 16). When EBV is suspected but the heterophile antibody is not detected, an evaluation of the EBV-specific antibody profile (e.g., EBV viral capsid antigen [VCA] IgM, EBV VCA IgG, and EBV nuclear antigen [EBNA]) may be useful (Table 17). The viral capsid antigen-antibodies (VCAs) can be

TABLE 16 Serologic studies and the timing of infections

Serologic study	Appears/disappears	Clinical significance
Monospot heterophil	5 days/2 weeks	Acute or convalescent infection
VCA-IgM	7 days/3 months	Acute or convalescent infection
VCA-IgG	7 days/exists for life	Acute, convalescent, or old infection
EBNA-IgG	3 weeks/exists for life	Old infection
EA-D	7 days/2 weeks	Acute or convalescent infection

TABLE 17 EBV antibodies and the timing of infections

Possible results

VCA IgG	VCA IgM	EBNA IgG	EA	Interpretation
−	−	−	−	No previous exposure
+	+	−	±	Acute infection
+	−	+	−	Past infection
+	±	±	±	Recent infection
+	±	+	+	Reactivation

immunoglobulin (Ig) G or IgM. The EBV nuclear antigen (EBNA) is located in the nuclei of the infected lymphocyte. Another EBV antigen is called the early antigen (EA). There are two EA antigens. One is EA-D and is commonly associated with nasopharyngeal cancer. EA-R is commonly associated with Burkitt lymphoma.

The interpretation of EBV antibody tests is based on the following assumptions:

1. After the person becomes infected with EBV, the anti-VCA IgG antibodies appear first.
2. Anti-EA (EA-D or EA-R) antibodies appear next or are present with anti-VCA antibodies early in the course of illness. An anti-EA antibody titer greater than 80 in a patient 2 years after acute infectious mononucleosis indicates chronic EBV syndrome.
3. As the patient recovers, anti-VCA IgG and anti-EA antibodies decrease, and anti-EBNA antibodies appear. Anti-EBNA antibodies persist for life and reflect a past infection.

4. After the patient is well, anti-VCA IgG and anti-EBNA antibodies are always present but at lower ranges. Occasionally, anti-EA antibodies also may be present after the patient recovers.

In an acute infection, heterophile antibodies usually appear on Monospot within the first 3 weeks of illness, but then decline rapidly within a few weeks. The heterophile antibody, however, fails to develop in about 10% of adults, more frequently in children, and almost uniformly in infants with primary EBV infections. If EBV infection is suspected to have occurred more than a few weeks before testing, the Monospot test result may be negative. Detecting anti-VCA IgG or EBNA will not be helpful because they indicate that an EBV infection has occurred sometime in the patient's life but not necessarily recently. But detecting anti-VCA IgM would indicate that the syndrome of complaints the patient experienced a few weeks prior was because of EBV.

In immunosuppressed patients (i.e., AIDS, transplantation, or long-term chemotherapy), EBV infection can be much more serious, instigating extranodal lymphoma and posttransplant lymphoproliferative disorders. These patients may have serologic negative tests because of their immunosuppression.

Procedure and patient care

- See inside front cover for Routine Blood Testing.
- Fasting: no.
- Blood tube commonly used: verify with lab.
- Obtain serum samples as soon as possible after the onset of the illness.
- Obtain a second blood specimen 14 to 21 days later.

Abnormal findings

Infectious mononucleosis
Chronic fatigue syndrome
Chronic EBV carrier state
Burkitt lymphoma
Nasopharyngeal cancer
Posttransplant lymphoproliferative disease

notes

erythrocyte fragility (Osmotic fragility [OF], Red blood cell fragility)

Type of test Blood

Normal findings

Hemolysis begins at 0.5% NaCl.
Hemolysis complete at 0.3% NaCl.

E

Test explanation and related physiology

Red blood cells (RBCs) are bound by a membrane that allows water to pass through while generally restricting the solutes. This process, called *osmosis*, causes RBCs to absorb water when in a hypotonic medium. This results in swelling and, ultimately, hemolysis when the cell bursts. The osmotic fragility (OF) test uses this fact to determine the concentration of solute inside the cell by subjecting it to salt solutions of different concentrations. The ability of the normal RBC to withstand hypotonicity results from its biconcave shape, which allows the cell to increase its volume by 70% before the surface membrane is stretched. When this limit is reached, lysis occurs. When intravascular hemolysis is identified, OF is used to determine if the RBCs have increased fragility (tend to burst open when exposed to a higher-concentrated NaCl solution) or decreased fragility (tend to burst open in lower-concentrated, and thus more hypotonic, NaCl solution).

This test is performed to detect hereditary spherocytosis and thalassemia when intravascular hemolysis is identified. Round cells (spherocytes) have increased OF compared to normal indented RBCs. In hereditary spherocytosis, there is abnormal morphology due to a lack of spectrin, a key RBC cytoskeletal membrane protein. This produces membrane instability, which forces the cell to the smallest volume—that of a sphere. This common disorder is associated with intravascular hemolysis. This is shown by increased osmotic fragility. Thalassemia, on the other hand, is associated with thinner leptocytes whose OF is decreased. A single-tube osmotic fragility test has been proposed for thalassemia screening with a range of different saline concentrations.

Interfering factors

- Acute hemolysis

  The osmotically labile cells are already hemolyzed and, therefore, not found in the blood specimen. Testing is recommended during a state of prolonged homeostasis with stable hematocrit.

- Dapsone can increase OF.

Procedure and patient care

- See inside front cover for Routine Blood Testing.
- Fasting: no.
- Blood tube commonly used: green.

Abnormal findings

▲ **Increased erythrocyte**
Acquired hemolytic anemia
Hereditary spherocytosis
Hemolytic disease of the newborn
Pyruvate kinase deficiency
Malaria

▼ **Decreased erythrocyte fragility**
Thalassemia
Hemoglobinopathies (C and S disease)
Iron deficiency anemia
Reticulocytosis

notes

erythrocyte sedimentation rate (ESR, Sed rate test)

Type of test Blood

Normal findings

Westergren method
Male: up to 15 mm/hr
Female: up to 20 mm/hr
Child: up to 10 mm/hr
Newborn: 0-2 mm/hr

Test explanation and related physiology

ESR is a measurement of the rate with which the red blood cells (RBCs) settle in saline or plasma over a specified time period. It is nonspecific and therefore not diagnostic for any particular organ disease or injury. Because acute and chronic infection, inflammation (collagen-vascular diseases), advanced neoplasm, and tissue necrosis or infarction increase the protein (mainly fibrinogen) content of plasma, RBCs have a tendency to stack up on one another, increasing their weight and causing them to descend faster. Therefore, in these diseases the ESR is increased. ESR is considered an *acute-phase* or a *reactant* protein (i.e., it occurs as a reaction to acute illnesses as described previously).

The test can be used to detect occult disease. Many physicians use the ESR test in this way for routine patient evaluation for vague symptoms. Other physicians regard this test as so nonspecific that it is useless as a routine study. The ESR test occasionally can be helpful in differentiating disease entities or complaints. For example, in the patient with chest pain, the ESR may be increased with myocardial infarction but may be normal in patients with musculoskeletal chest pain.

The ESR is a fairly reliable indicator of the course of disease and can be used to monitor disease therapy, especially for inflammatory autoimmune diseases (e.g., temporal arteritis or polymyalgia rheumatica). In general, as the disease worsens, the ESR increases; as the disease improves, the ESR decreases. If the results of the ESR are equivocal or inconsistent with clinical impressions, the C-reactive protein test (p. 306) is often performed.

Interfering factors

- Artificially low results can occur when the collected specimen is allowed to stand longer than 3 hours before the testing.

- Pregnancy (second and third trimesters) can cause elevated levels.
- Menstruation can cause elevated levels.
- Polycythemia is associated with decreased ESR.
✔ Drugs that may cause *increased* ESR levels include dextran, methyldopa, oral contraceptives, penicillamine, procainamide, theophylline, and vitamin A.
✔ Drugs that may cause *decreased* levels include aspirin, cortisone, and quinine.

Procedure and patient care

- See inside front cover for Routine Blood Testing.
- Fasting: no.
- Blood tube commonly used: lavender (verify with lab).

Abnormal findings

▲ **Increased levels**
  Chronic renal failure
  Malignant diseases
  Bacterial infection
  Inflammatory diseases
  Necrotic tissue diseases
  Hyperfibrinogenemia
  Macroglobulinemia
  Severe anemias (e.g., iron
    deficiency or B_{12} deficiency)

▼ **Decreased levels**
  Sickle cell anemia
  Spherocytosis
  Hypofibrinogenemia
  Polycythemia vera

notes

erythropoietin (EPO)

Type of test Blood

Normal findings 5-35 IU/L

Test explanation and related physiology

Erythropoietin (EPO) is a hormone produced by the kidney. In response to decreased oxygen, the production of EPO is increased. EPO stimulates the bone marrow to increase RBC production. This improves oxygenation in the kidney, and the stimulus for EPO is reduced. This feedback mechanism is very sensitive to minimal persistent changes in oxygen levels. In patients with normal renal function, EPO levels are inversely proportional to the hemoglobin concentration.

As a hormone, EPO is often administered to patients who experience anemia as a result of chemotherapy. Occasionally athletes, in order to improve oxygen-carrying capacity and thereby improve performance, abuse this hormone.

EPO testing is performed to assist in the differential diagnosis of patients with anemia or polycythemia. EPO is elevated in patients who have low hemoglobin due to failure of marrow production or with increased RBC destruction (iron-deficiency or hemolytic anemia, respectively). However, patients with anemia due to renal diseases (or bilateral nephrectomy) do not have elevated EPO levels. The renal cells are damaged by disease. EPO levels fall and these patients develop anemia.

Patients who have polycythemia as an appropriate response to chronic hypoxemia have elevated EPO levels. Yet patients who have malignant marrow causes of polycythemia vera may have reduced EPO levels. Some renal cell or adrenal carcinomas can produce elevated EPO levels.

Interfering factors

- Pregnancy is associated with elevated EPO levels.
- The use of transfused blood decreases EPO levels.
- ✗ Drugs that may *increase* EPO levels include ACTH, oral contraceptives, and steroids.

Procedure and patient care

- See inside front cover for Routine Blood Testing.
- Fasting: no.
- Blood tube commonly used: red or gel separator.

Abnormal findings

▲ **Increased levels**
  Iron deficiency anemia
  Megaloblastic anemia
  Hemolytic anemia
  Myelodysplasia
  Chemotherapy
  AIDS
  Pheochromocytoma
  Renal cell carcinoma
  Adrenal carcinoma

▼ **Decreased levels**
  Polycythemia vera
  Renal diseases
  Renal failure

notes

E

Type of test Manometric

Normal findings

Lower esophageal sphincter pressure: 10-20 mm Hg
Swallowing pattern: normal peristaltic waves
Acid reflux: negative
Acid clearing: <10 swallows
Bernstein test: negative

Test explanation and related physiology

Esophageal function studies include the following:

- Determination of the *lower esophageal sphincter (LES)* pressure (manometry)
- Graphic recording of esophageal swallowing waves, or *swallowing pattern* (manometry)
- Detection of reflux of gastric acid back into the esophagus (acid reflux)
- Detection of the ability of the esophagus to clear acid (acid clearing)
- An attempt to reproduce symptoms of heartburn (Bernstein test)

Manometry studies

Two manometry studies are used in assessing esophageal function: measurement of LES pressure and graphic recording of swallowing waves (motility). The LES is a sphincter muscle that acts as a valve to prevent reflux of gastric acid into the esophagus. Free reflux of gastric acid occurs when sphincter pressures are low. An example of such a disorder in adults is gastroesophageal reflux; in children it is called chalasia (incompetent or relaxed LES).

With increased sphincter pressure, as found in patients with achalasia (failure of the LES to relax normally with swallowing) and diffuse esophageal spasms, food cannot pass from the esophagus into the stomach. Increased LES pressures are noted on manometry. In achalasia, few if any swallowing waves are detected. In contrast, diffuse esophageal spasm is characterized by strong, frequent, asynchronous, and nonpropulsive waves.

Acid reflux with pH probe

Acid reflux is the primary component of gastroesophageal reflux. Patients with an incompetent LES will regurgitate gastric acid into the esophagus. This will then cause a drop in the esophageal pH during *esophageal pH monitoring*. With the newer and smaller catheters, 24-hour pH monitoring can be performed. Episodes of acid reflux are evident. If they coincide with patient symptoms of chest pain, esophagitis can be incriminated. Trans-nasal pH catheters can cause discomfort in patients, sometimes resulting in the avoidance of pH testing. This limits the ability to definitively diagnose and ultimately treat gastroesophageal reflux (GERD).

With the *wireless pH probes*, patients can eat and drink normally as well as engage in their usual activities while having their pH levels tested. A wireless pH probe capsule is now being used with increasing frequency. It collects pH data in the esophagus and transmits them via radio frequency telemetry to an external, pager-sized receiver worn by the patient. This allows patients to maintain regular diet and activities during the monitoring period (24 to 48 hours). This small pH capsule is attached to the wall of the esophagus by esophagoscopy (p. 401). Within days, the capsule spontaneously sloughs off the wall of the esophagus and passes through the patient's gastrointestinal tract. After the study is completed, the patient returns the receiver, and the data are downloaded to a computer for analysis.

Acid clearing

Patients with normal esophageal function can completely clear hydrochloric acid from the esophagus in less than 10 swallows. Patients with decreased esophageal motility (frequently caused by severe esophagitis) require a greater number of swallows to clear the acid.

Bernstein test (acid perfusion)

The Bernstein test is simply an attempt to reproduce the symptoms of gastroesophageal reflux. If the patient suffers pain with the instillation of hydrochloric acid into the esophagus, the test is positive and proves that the patient's symptoms are caused by reflux esophagitis. If the patient has no discomfort, a cause other than esophageal reflux must be sought to explain the patient's symptoms.

Contraindications

- Patients who cannot cooperate
- Patients who are medically unstable

Potential complications

- Aspiration of gastric contents

Interfering factors

- Eating shortly before the test may affect results.
- ☤ Drugs such as sedatives can alter test results.

Procedure and patient care

Before

PT Explain the procedure to the patient.

PT Instruct the patient not to eat or drink anything for at least 8 hours before the test.

PT Allay any fears and allow the patient to verbalize concerns. Be sensitive to the patient's fears about choking.

During

- Note the following procedural steps:
  1. Esophageal studies are usually performed in the endoscopy laboratory.
  2. The fasting, unsedated patient is asked to swallow two or three very tiny tubes. The tubes are equipped so that pressure measurements can be taken at 5-cm intervals (Figure 20).
  3. The outer ends of the tubes are attached to a pressure transducer.
  4. All tubes are passed into the stomach; then three tubes are slowly pulled back into the esophagus. A rapid and extreme increase in the pressure readings indicates the high-pressure zone of the LES.
  5. The LES pressure is recorded.
  6. With all tubes in the esophagus, the patient is asked to swallow. Motility wave patterns are recorded.
  7. The pH indicator probe is placed in the esophagus.
  8. The patient's stomach is filled with approximately 100 mL of 0.1-N hydrochloric acid. A decrease in the pH of the esophageal pH probe indicates gastroesophageal reflux.
  9. Hydrochloric acid is instilled into the esophagus, and the patient is asked to swallow. The number of swallows is counted to determine acid clearing. More than 10 swallows to clear the acid (as determined by the pH probe) indicates decreased esophageal motility.
  10. Finally, 0.1-N hydrochloric acid and saline solution are alternately instilled into the esophagus for the Bernstein test. The patient is not told which solution is being infused. If the patient volunteers symptoms of discomfort while the acid is running, the test is considered positive. If no discomfort is recognized, the test is negative.

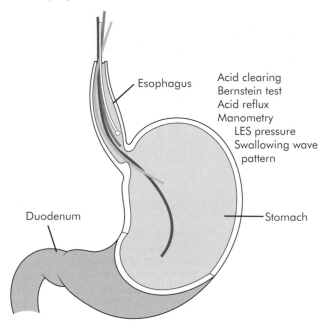

Esophagus

Acid clearing
Bernstein test
Acid reflux
Manometry
    LES pressure
    Swallowing wave
        pattern

Duodenum

Stomach

FIGURE 20 Esophageal function studies demonstrating placement of manometry tubes and a pH probe in the esophagus. *LES*, Lower esophageal sphincter.

- Note that these tests are performed by an esophageal technician in approximately 30 minutes.
PT Inform the patient that the test results are interpreted by a physician and will be available in a few hours.
PT Tell the patient that, except for some initial gagging when swallowing the tubes, these tests are not uncomfortable.

After
PT Inform the patient that it is not unusual to have a mild sore throat after placement of the tubes.

Abnormal findings

Presbyesophagus   Achalasia
Diffuse esophageal spasm   Gastroesophageal reflux
Chalasia   Reflux esophagitis

notes

esophagogastroduodenoscopy (EGD, Upper gastrointestinal [UGI] endoscopy, Gastroscopy)

Type of test   Endoscopy

Normal findings   Normal esophagus, stomach, and duodenum

Test explanation and related physiology

Endoscopy enables direct visualization of the upper gastrointestinal (GI) tract by means of a long, flexible, fiberoptic-lighted scope. The esophagus, stomach, and duodenum are examined for tumors, varices, mucosal inflammations, hiatal hernias, polyps, ulcers, and obstructions. The endoscope has one to three channels. The first channel is used for viewing; the second for insufflation of air and aspiration of fluid; and the third for passing cable-activated instruments to perform a biopsy of suspected pathologic tissue. Probes also can be passed through the third channel to allow for coagulation or injection of sclerosing agents to areas of active GI bleeding. A laser beam can pass through the endoscope to perform endoscopic surgery (e.g., obliteration of tumors or polyps, control of bleeding). Video images and still pictures can be taken.

This test is used to visualize the lumen of the esophagus, stomach, and duodenum. It is used to evaluate patients with dysphagia, weight loss, early satiety, upper abdominal pain, ulcer symptoms, or dyspepsia. It is also used to detect esophageal varices in cirrhotic patients. Suspicious barium swallow or upper GI x-ray findings can be corroborated by EGD.

With upper GI endoscopy, one can also visualize and perform a biopsy of tissue in most of the small intestinal tract. This procedure is referred to as *enteroscopy*. Abnormalities of the small intestine, such as arteriovenous (AV) malformations, tumors, enteropathies (e.g., celiac disease), and ulcerations, can be diagnosed with enteroscopy.

Capsule endoscopy (or *wireless capsule endoscopy*) uses a capsule containing a miniature camera that records images of the entire digestive tract, particularly the small intestine. This capsule is about the size of a large vitamin and contains a color video camera, a radiofrequency transmitter, four LED lights, and enough battery power to take 50,000 color images during an 8-hour journey through the digestive tract. It moves through the digestive tract naturally with the aid of peristaltic activity. During the 6- to 10-hour exam, the images are continuously transmitted to special antenna pads placed on the body and are captured on a recording device about the size of a portable radio that is worn around the patient's waist. After the exam, the patient returns to the doctor's office and the recording device is removed. Patients are not required to retrieve and return the video capsule to the physician. It is disposable and is expelled normally and effortlessly with the next bowel movement. The most common reason for doing capsule endoscopy is to search for a cause of bleeding from the small intestine. It may also be useful for detecting polyps, inflammatory bowel disease (Crohn disease), ulcers, and tumors of the small intestine.

An experienced endoscopist often can control active GI bleeding by electrocoagulation, laser coagulation, or the injection of sclerosing agents (such as alcohol for esophageal varices). Also, with the endoscope, benign and malignant strictures can be dilated to reestablish patency of the upper GI tract. Biliary, esophageal, and duodenal stents and percutaneous gastrostomy can be placed with the use of EGD.

Contraindications

- Patients with severe upper GI bleeding
  The viewing lens will become covered with blood clots.
- Patients with esophageal diverticula
  The scope can easily fall into the diverticulum and perforate the wall of the esophagus.
- Patients with suspected perforation
  The perforation can be worsened by the insufflation of pressurized air into the GI tract.
- Patients who have had recent GI surgery
  The anastomosis may not be able to withstand the pressure of the required air insufflation.

Potential complications

- Perforation of the esophagus, stomach, or duodenum
- Bleeding from a biopsy site or scope trauma
- Pulmonary aspiration of gastric contents
- Oversedation from the medication administered during the test
- Hypotension induced by the sedative medication

Interfering factors

- Food in the stomach
- Excessive GI bleeding

Procedure and patient care

Before

PT Explain the procedure to the patient.

• Obtain informed consent if required by the institution.

PT Instruct the patient to abstain from eating for 8 to 10 hours prior to the test.

• If capsule endoscopy is to be performed, apply the recording mechanism to the patient's abdomen and waist.

PT Reassure the patient that this test is not painful but may be mildly uncomfortable. Tell the patient that the throat will be anesthetized with a spray to depress the gag reflex.

• Encourage the patient to verbalize fears. Provide support.

• Remove the patient's dentures and eyewear before testing.

PT Remind the patient that he or she will not be able to speak during the test but that respiration will not be affected.

PT Instruct the patient not to bite down on the endoscope.

PT Instruct the patient as to appropriate oral hygiene, because the tube will be passed through the mouth.

During

• Note the following procedural steps:

1. The patient is placed on the endoscopy table in the left lateral decubitus position.

2. The throat is topically anesthetized with viscous lidocaine or another anesthetic spray.

3. The patient is usually sedated. This minimizes anxiety and allows the patient to experience a light sleep.

4. The endoscope is gently passed through the mouth and finally into the esophagus.

5. Air is insufflated to distend the upper GI tract for adequate visualization.

6. The esophagus, stomach, and duodenum are evaluated.

7. During enteroscopy, the upper small bowel is visualized and a biopsy is performed if needed.

8. Biopsy or any endoscopic intervention is performed with direct visualization.

9. On completion of direct inspection and surgery, the excess air and GI secretions are aspirated through the scope.

• Note that the test is performed in the endoscopy laboratory by a physician trained in GI endoscopy and takes approximately 20 to 30 minutes.

PT Instruct the patient that eating is allowed about 2 to 4 hours after swallowing the capsule for capsule endoscopy.

PT For capsule endoscopy, instruct the patient to return to the physician's office in 6 to 10 hours to return the recording device and have all recording wires removed.

PT For capsule endoscopy, instruct the patient that he or she can continue regular activities throughout the examination and will not feel any sensations resulting from the capsule's passage.

After

PT Inform the patient that he or she may have hoarseness or a sore throat after the test. A soothing mouthwash may help.

- Withhold any fluids until the patient is alert and the swallowing reflex returns to normal, usually 2 to 4 hours.
- Observe the patient's vital signs. Evaluate the patient for bleeding, fever, abdominal pain, dyspnea, or dysphagia.
- Observe safety precautions until the effects of the sedatives have worn off.

PT For capsule endoscopy, instruct the patient that there is no need to retrieve the capsule/camera from the stool.

PT Inform the patient that it is normal to have some bloating, belching, and flatulence after the procedure.

PT Inform the patient that the sedation may cause some retrograde and antegrade amnesia for a few hours.

Abnormal findings

Tumor (benign or malignant) of the esophagus, stomach, or duodenum

Esophageal diverticula

Hiatal hernia

Esophagitis, gastritis, duodenitis

Gastroesophageal varices

Peptic ulcer

Peptic stricture and subsequent scarring

Extrinsic compression by a cyst or tumor outside the upper GI tract

Source of upper GI bleeding

Helicobacter pylori infection

notes

estrogen fractions (Estriol excretion, Estradiol, Estrone)

Type of test Urine (24-hour); blood

Normal findings

	Serum	Urine mcg/24 hours
Estradiol		
Child <10 years old	<15 pg/mL	0-6
Adult male	10-50 pg/mL	0-6
Adult female		
Follicular phase	20-350 pg/mL	0-13
Midcycle peak	150-750 pg/mL	4-14
Luteal phase	30-450 pg/mL	4-10
Postmenopause	≤20 pg/mL	0-4
Estriol		
Male or child <10 years old	N/A	1-11
Female, adult		
Follicular phase	N/A	0-14
Ovulatory phase	N/A	13-54
Luteal phase	N/A	8-60
Postmenopausal	N/A	0-11
Female, pregnant		
1st trimester	<38 ng/mL	0-800
2nd trimester	38-140 ng/mL	800-12,000
3rd trimester	31-460 ng/mL	5000-12,000
Total estrogen		
Male or child <10 years old	N/A	4-25
Female, nonpregnant	N/A	4-60
Female, pregnant		
1st trimester	N/A	0-800
2nd trimester	N/A	800-5000
3rd trimester	N/A	5000-50,000

Possible critical values Values 40% below the average of two previous values demand immediate evaluation of fetal well-being during pregnancy.

Test explanation and related physiology

There are three major estrogens. Estradiol (E_2), the most potent estrogen, is produced predominantly in the ovary. In females, there is a feedback mechanism for the secretion of E_2.

Low levels of E_2 stimulate the hypothalamus to produce gonadotropin-releasing factors. These hormone factors stimulate the pituitary to produce follicle-stimulating hormone (FSH) and luteinizing hormone (LH). LH and FSH stimulate the ovary to produce E_2, which peaks during the ovulatory phase of the menstrual cycle. This hormone is measured most often to evaluate menstrual and fertility problems, menopausal status, sexual maturity, gynecomastia, feminization syndromes, or as a tumor marker for patients with certain ovarian tumors.

Estrone (E_1) is also secreted by the ovary, but most is converted from androstenedione in peripheral tissues. E_1 is the major circulating estrogen after menopause.

Estriol (E_3) is the major estrogen in the pregnant female. Serial urine and blood studies for E_3 excretion provide objective means of assessing placental function and fetal normality in high-risk pregnancies. Unfortunately, only severe placental distress will decrease urinary E_3 sufficiently to reliably predict fetoplacental stress. Furthermore, plasma and urinary E_3 levels are normally associated with significant daily variation, which may confuse serial results. Most clinicians now use nonstress fetal monitoring (see p. 432) to indicate fetoplacental health.

E_3 excretion studies can be done using urine tests or blood studies. A serially increasing estriol/creatinine ratio is a favorable sign in pregnancy. The advantage of the plasma E_3 determination is that it is more easily obtained than a urine specimen and less affected by medications. E_3 is one of the components of the "quad screen" that is obtained in the 2nd trimester of pregnancy to screen for Down syndrome.

Interfering factors

- Recent administration of radioisotopes may alter test results.
- Glycosuria and urinary tract infections can increase urine E_3 levels.
- ✔ Drugs that may *increase* levels include adrenocorticosteroids, ampicillin, estrogen-containing drugs, phenothiazines, and tetracyclines.
- ✔ Drugs that may *decrease* levels include clomiphene.

Procedure and patient care

- See inside front cover for Routine Blood Testing.
- Fasting: no.
- Blood tube commonly used: red.
- See inside front cover for Routine Urine Testing for spot urine.

Abnormal findings

▲ **Increased levels**
Feminization syndromes
Precocious puberty
Ovarian tumor
Testicular tumor
Adrenal tumor
Normal pregnancy
Hepatic cirrhosis
Hepatic necrosis
Hyperthyroidism

▼ **Decreased levels**
Failing pregnancy
Turner syndrome
Hypopituitarism
Primary and secondary
  hypogonadism
Stein-Leventhal syndrome
Menopause
Anorexia nervosa

E

notes

estrogen receptor assay (ER assay, ERA, Estradiol receptor)

Type of test Microscopic examination

Normal findings

Immunohistochemistry
Negative: <5% of the cells stain for receptors
Positive: >5% of the cells stain for receptors

Reverse-transcriptase polymerase chain reaction (RT-PCR)
Negative: <6.5 units
Positive: >6.5 units

Test explanation and related physiology

The ER assay is useful in determining the prognosis and treatment of breast cancer. The assay is used to determine whether a tumor is likely to respond to endocrine therapy. Tumors with a positive ER assay are more than twice as likely to respond to endocrine therapy than ER-negative tumors. Hormone receptor assay should be performed on all breast cancers. Breast tumors in postmenopausal women tend to be positive more often than in premenopausal women. In general, ER-positive tumors have a better prognosis than ER-negative tumors.

Slightly more than 50% of patients with breast carcinoma who are ER positive respond to endocrine therapy (e.g., tamoxifen, estrogens, aromatase inhibitors, oophorectomy). The response is greater when the progesterone receptors (p. 748) are also positive. Patients whose breast cancers lack these hormone receptors (i.e., are ER negative) have a much lower chance of tumor response to hormone therapy and may not be candidates for this form of treatment.

Specimens are obtained from surgical specimens by a pathologist. Results are usually available in about 1 week.

Interfering factors

- Delay in tissue fixation or too long in fixative solution may cause deterioration of receptor proteins and produce lower values.

Procedure and patient care

Before

PT Explain the procedure to the patient.

PT Instruct the patient to discontinue hormones before breast biopsy is performed.

- Before biopsy, a gynecologic history is obtained, including menopausal status and exogenous hormone use.

During

- The surgeon obtains tumor tissue.
- This tissue should be placed on ice or in formalin.
- Part of the tissue is used for routine histology. A portion of the paraffin block or a slide containing cancer is used for IHC staining.

After

- Results are usually available in 1 week.

Abnormal findings

Nonapplicable

notes

ethanol (Ethyl alcohol, Blood alcohol, Blood EtOH)

Type of test Blood; urine; gastric; breath

Normal findings Blood: 0-50 mg/dL, or 0%-0.05%

Possible critical values Blood: >300 mg/dL

Test explanation and related physiology

Ethanol depresses the central nervous system and may lead to coma and death. This test is usually performed to evaluate alcohol-impaired driving or alcohol overdose. Proper collection, handling, and storage of blood alcohol are important for medicolegal cases involving sobriety. Legal testing must be done by specially trained people and must have a strict chain of custody (a paper trail that records sample movement and handling).

Samples tested for legal purposes may include blood, breath, urine, or saliva. Blood is the specimen of choice. Blood is taken from a peripheral vein in living patients and from the aorta in cadavers. Results are given as mg/dL, grams/100 mL, or a percentage. Each represents the same amount of alcohol. Blood alcohol concentrations (BACs) greater than 80 mg/dL (0.08%) may cause flushing, slowing of reflexes, and impaired visual activity. Depression of the CNS occurs with BACs over 0.1%, and fatalities are reported with levels greater than 0.4%. Persons with BACs less than 0.05% are not considered under the influence of alcohol. Levels greater than 0.05% to 0.10% are considered in most states to be illegal for the operation of motor vehicles, and as definite evidence of intoxication.

For legal purposes, when outside of a laboratory/hospital, taking a blood sample for later analysis in the laboratory is not practical or efficient. Breath testing is the most common test performed on automobile drivers. It uses the tail end sample of breath from deep in the lungs and uses a conversion factor to estimate the amount of alcohol in the blood. Blood alcohol testing may be ordered to confirm or refute findings. Alcohol that a person drinks shows up in the breath because it gets absorbed from the intestinal tract into the bloodstream. The alcohol is not metabolized on first pass through the liver. As the blood goes through the lungs, some of the volatile alcohol moves across the alveolar membranes and is exhaled.

Urine testing may also be performed as an alternative to blood. Usually, a patient collects and discards a urine sample and then collects a second sample 20 to 30 minutes later. Saliva alcohol testing is not as widely used, but may be used as an alternate screening test. Alcohol stays in the saliva for 6 to 12 hours. Finally, hair testing is used but represents a more chronic use of alcohol.

Interfering factors

- Elevated blood ketones (as with diabetic ketoacidosis) can cause false elevations of blood and breath test results.
- Bacteria in the urine of diabetic patients with glucosuria can metabolize the glucose to alcohol.
- Alcohols other than ethanol (e.g., isopropyl [rubbing alcohol] or methanol [grain alcohol]) will cause positive results.
- **PT** The use of alcohol-based mouthwash or cough syrup may cause false positives on a breath test.

Procedure and patient care

- See inside front cover for Routine Blood Testing.
- Fasting: no.
- Blood tube commonly used: gray or red.
- Follow the institution's chain-of-custody protocol.
- Follow the agency's protocol regarding specimen collection.
- Use a povidone-iodine wipe instead of an alcohol wipe for cleansing the venipuncture site.
- If a gastric or urine specimen is indicated, approximately 20 to 50 mL of fluid is necessary.
- Breath analyzers are taken at the end of expiration after a deep inspiration.
- The exact time of specimen collection should be indicated.

Abnormal findings

Alcohol intoxication or overdose

notes

evoked potential studies (EP studies, Evoked brain potentials, Evoked responses)

Type of test Electrodiagnostic

Normal findings No neural conduction delay

Test explanation and related physiology

EP studies are indicated for patients who are suspected of having a sensory deficit but are unable to or cannot reliably indicate recognition of a stimulus. These may include infants, comatose patients, or patients with an inability to communicate. These tests are also used to evaluate specific areas of the cortex that receive incoming stimuli from the eyes, ears, and lower/upper extremity sensory nerves. They are used to monitor natural progression or treatment of deteriorating neurologic diseases. Finally, they are used to identify histrionic or malingering patients who have sensory deficit complaints.

EP studies focus on changes and responses in brain waves that are evoked from stimulation of a sensory pathway. The study of EPs grew out of early work with the electroencephalogram (EEG, p. 365). The EEG measures spontaneous brain electrical activity, whereas the sensory EP study measures minute voltage changes produced in response to a specific stimulus such as a light pattern, a click, or a shock. In contrast to the EEG, which records signals that reach amplitudes of up to 50 to 100 millivolts (mV), EP signals are usually less than 5 mV. Because of this, they can be detected only with an averaging computer. The computer averages out (or cancels) unwanted random waves to sum the evoked response that occurs at a specific time after a given stimulus.

Evoked potential studies measure and assess the entire sensory pathway from the peripheral sensory organ all the way to the brain cortex (recognition of the stimulus). These tests also monitor progressive neurologic diseases.

Clinical abnormalities are usually detected by an increase in *latency*, which refers to the delay between the stimulus and the wave response. Normal latency times are calculated depending on body size, position of the body where the stimulus is applied, conduction velocity of axons in the neural pathways, number of synapses in the system, location of nerve generators of EP components (brainstem or cortex), and presence of central nervous system pathology. Conduction delays indicate damage or disease anywhere along the neural pathway from the sensory organ to the cortex. Sensory stimuli used for the EP study can be visual, auditory, or somatosensory. The sensory stimulus chosen depends on which sensory system is suspected of being pathologic (e.g., questionable blindness, deafness, or numbness). Also, the sensory stimulus chosen may depend on the area of the brain where pathology is suspected (auditory stimuli check the brainstem and temporal lobes of the brain; visual stimuli test the optic nerve, central neural visual pathway, and occipital parts of the brain; and somatosensory stimuli check the peripheral nerves, spinal cord, and parietal lobe of the brain). Increased latency indicates pathology of the sensory organ or the specific neural pathway as described earlier.

Visual-evoked responses (VERs) are usually stimulated by a strobe light flash, reversible checkerboard pattern, or retinal stimuli. Ninety percent of patients with multiple sclerosis show abnormal latencies of VERs, a phenomenon attributed to demyelination of nerve fibers. In addition, patients with other neurologic disorders (e.g., Parkinson disease) show an abnormal latency of VERs. The degree of latency seems to correlate with the severity of the disease. Abnormal results also may be seen in patients with lesions of the optic nerve, optic tract, visual center, and the eye itself. Absence of binocularity, which is a neurologic developmental disorder in infants, can be detected and evaluated by VERs. Eyesight problems or blindness can be detected in infants through VERs or *electroretinography*. This test can also be used during eye surgery to provide a warning of possible damage to the optic nerve. The gross visual acuity of infants can even be checked via VERs.

Auditory brainstem-evoked potentials (ABEPs) are usually stimulated by clicking sounds to evaluate the central auditory pathways of the brainstem. Either ear can be evoked to detect lesions in the brainstem that involve the auditory pathway without affecting hearing. One of the most successful applications of ABEPs has been screening low–birth-weight newborns and other infants for hearing disorders. Recognition of deafness enables infants to be fitted with corrective devices as soon as possible before learning to speak (to prevent speech pathology). ABEPs also have great therapeutic implications in the early detection of posterior fossa brain tumors.

Somatosensory-evoked responses (SERs) are usually stimulated by sensory stimulus to an area of the body. The time is then measured for the current of the stimulus to travel along the nerve to the cortex of the brain. SERs are used to evaluate patients with spinal cord injuries and to monitor spinal cord functioning during spinal surgery. They are also used to monitor treatment of diseases (e.g., multiple sclerosis); to evaluate the location and extent of areas of brain dysfunction after head injury; and to pinpoint tumors at an early stage. These tests can also be used to identify malingering or hysterical numbness (e.g., that latency is normal in these patients despite the fact that patients indicate numbness).

One of the main benefits of EPs is their objectivity, because voluntary patient response is not needed. This objectivity makes EPs useful with nonverbal and uncooperative patients. It permits the distinction of organic from psychogenic problems. This is invaluable in settling lawsuits concerning workers' compensation insurance.

Procedure and patient care
Before
PT Explain the procedure to the patient.
PT Instruct the patient to shampoo his or her hair before the test.
PT Tell the patient that no fasting or sedation is required.

During
- Note that the position of the electrode depends on the type of EP study to be done:
  - *VERs* are measured using electrodes placed on the scalp along the vertex and cortex lobes. Stimulation occurs by using a strobe light, checkerboard pattern, or retinal stimuli.
  - *ABEPs* are stimulated with clicking noises or tone bursts delivered via earphones. The responses are detected by scalp electrodes placed along the vertex and on each earlobe.
  - *SERs* are stimulated using electrical stimuli applied to nerves at the wrist (medial nerve) or knee (peroneal nerve). The response is detected by electrodes placed over the sensory cortex of the opposite hemisphere on the scalp.
- Note that this study is performed by a physician or technician in less than 30 minutes.

PT Tell the patient that little or no discomfort is associated with this study.

After
- If gel was used for the adherence of the electrodes, remove it.

Abnormal findings
Prolonged latency for ABEP
Demyelinating diseases (e.g., multiple sclerosis)
Tumor (e.g., acoustic neuroma)
Cerebrovascular accident
Auditory nerve damage
Deafness

Abnormal latency for SER
Spinal cord injury
Cervical disc disease
Spinal cord demyelinating diseases
Peripheral nerve injury, transection, or disease
Parietal cortical tumor or CVA

Prolonged latency for VER
Parkinson disease
Demyelinating diseases (e.g., multiple sclerosis)
Optic nerve damage
Ocular disease or injury
Blindness
Optic tract disease
Occipital lobe tumor or CVA
Absence of binocularity
Visual field defects
Occipital lobe tumor or CVA
Absence of binocularity
Visual field defects

notes

E

factor V Leiden (FVL, Mutation analysis)

Type of test Blood

Normal findings

Negative for factor V Leiden

Test explanation and related physiology

Factor V is an important factor in reaction 4 (common pathway) of normal hemostasis (p. 261). The term *factor V Leiden* (FVL) refers to an inherited abnormal form of the gene for factor V. That genetic mutation causes a single amino acid replacement at one of three cleavage sites in the factor V molecule. The endogenous anticoagulant protein C (p. 765) is normally able to break down factor V at one of these cleavage sites. However, protein C cannot inactivate this same cleavage site on FVL. Therefore, FVL is inactivated at a rate approximately ten times slower than that of normal factor V and persists longer in the circulation. This results in increased thrombin generation and a mild, hypercoagulable state reflected by elevated levels of prothrombin fragment F1+2 and other activated coagulation markers. This test is used to diagnose FVL-associated thrombophilia.

Individuals *heterozygous* for the FVL mutation have a slightly increased risk for venous thrombosis. *Homozygous* individuals have a much greater thrombotic risk (e.g., deep vein thrombosis [DVT], arterial thrombosis, or pulmonary embolism).

Individuals who are candidates for FVL testing include patients who:

- Experienced a thrombotic event without any predisposing factors
- Have a strong family history of thrombotic events
- Experienced a thrombotic event while 30 years of age
- Experienced DVT during pregnancy or while taking birth control pills
- Had venous thrombosis at unusual sites (e.g., cerebral, mesenteric, portal, and hepatic veins)
- Experienced an arterial clot

FVL is the most common hereditary blood coagulation disorder in the United States. It is present in 5% of the Caucasian population and 1.2% of the African American population. Only about 10% of patients who have FVL will experience a thrombotic event.

Testing for FVL is sometimes preceded by a coagulation screening test called the *activated protein C (APC) resistance test*. This test identifies resistance of factor V to activated protein C (APC). If APC resistance is identified, the patient then may choose to undergo mutation testing by DNA analysis of the F5 gene, which encodes the factor V protein. This testing should be accompanied by professional genetic counseling for the patient and family members.

Procedure and patient care

- See inside front cover for Routine Blood Testing.
- Fasting: no.
- Blood tube commonly used: purple.
- If the patient is having FVL mutation analysis, anticoagulants will not interfere with testing.
- As an alternative, genetic testing can be done on the patient's cells obtained by a smear of the oral surface of the cheek.
- Remember, if the patient is receiving anticoagulants, the bleeding time will be increased.

Abnormal findings

Activated protein C resistance
Factor V Leiden genetic mutation (homozygous or heterozygous)

notes

febrile antibodies (Febrile agglutinins)

Type of test Blood

Normal findings titers ≤1:80

Test explanation and related physiology

Febrile antibodies are used to support the diagnosis and monitoring of infectious diseases (e.g., salmonellosis, rickettsial diseases, brucellosis, and tularemia). Neoplastic diseases, such as leukemias and lymphomas, are also associated with febrile agglutinins. Appropriate antibiotic treatment of the infectious agent is associated with a drop in the titer activity of febrile antibodies. Rickettsial species produce antibodies that agglutinate proteus vulgaris antigens. This test is nonspecific and insensitive. More specific testing for these infective agents provides more sensitive and specific laboratory testing. Temperature regulation is important for the performance of these tests. Under no circumstances should the febrile agglutinin be heated before delivery to the laboratory.

Procedure and patient care

- See inside front cover for Routine Blood Testing.
- Fasting: no.
- Blood tube commonly used: red.

Abnormal findings

▲ **Increased febrile antibodies**
Salmonellosis infection
Rickettsial disease
Brucellosis
Tularemia leukemia
Lymphoma
Systemic lupus erythematosus

notes

fecal fat (Fat absorption, Quantitative stool fat determination)

Type of test   Stool

Normal findings

Fat: 2-6 g/24 hr or 7-21 mmol/day (SI units)
Retention coefficient: ≥95%

Test explanation and related physiology

This qualitative or quantitative test is performed to confirm the diagnosis of steatorrhea. Steatorrhea occurs when fat content in the stool is high. It is suspected when the patient has large, greasy, and foul-smelling stools. Determining an abnormally high fecal fat content confirms the diagnosis. Short-gut syndrome and any condition that may cause malabsorption (e.g., sprue, Crohn disease, Whipple disease) or maldigestion (e.g., bile duct obstruction, pancreatic duct obstruction secondary to tumor or gallstones) are also associated with increased fecal fat. Neutral fats include the monoglycerides, diglycerides, and triglycerides whereas split fats are the free fatty acids that are liberated from them. Impaired synthesis or secretion of pancreatic enzymes or bile may cause an increase in neutral fats. An increase in split fats suggests impaired absorption of nutrients.

The total output of fecal fat can be tested on a random stool specimen but is more accurate when total 24-, 48-, or 72-hour collection is carried out. Abnormal results from a random specimen should be confirmed by submission of a timed collection. Test values for random fecal fat collections are reported in terms of percent fat.

Interfering factors

☛ Drugs that may alter test results include enemas and laxatives, especially mineral oil.

☛ Drugs that may *decrease* levels of fecal fat include barium and psyllium fiber (e.g., Metamucil).

Procedure and patient care

Before

PT Explain the procedure to the patient.

PT Instruct the patient to abstain from alcohol ingestion for 3 days prior to testing.

PT Give the patient instructions regarding the appropriate diet (a diet diary may be requested by the laboratory):
  o For adults, usually 100 g of fat per day is suggested for 3 days before and during the collection period.
  o Children, and especially infants, cannot ingest 100 g of fat. Therefore, a *fat retention coefficient* is determined by measuring the difference between ingested fat and fecal fat and then expressing that difference (the amount of fat retained) as a percentage of the ingested fat:

$$\frac{\text{Ingested fat} - \text{Fecal fat}}{\text{Ingested fat}} \times 100\% = \text{Fat retention coefficient}$$

- Note that the normal fat retention coefficient is 95% or greater. A low value indicates steatorrhea.
PT Instruct the patient to defecate in a dry, clean container.
- Occasionally, a tongue blade is required to transfer the stool to the specimen container.
PT Tell the patient not to urinate in the stool container.
PT Inform the patient that even diarrheal stools should be collected.
PT Instruct the patient that toilet paper should not be placed in the stool container.
PT Tell the patient not to take any laxatives or enemas during this test because they will interfere with intestinal motility and alter test results.

During
- Collect each stool specimen and send immediately to the laboratory during the 24- to 72-hour testing period. Label each specimen and include the time and date of collection.
- If the specimen is collected at home, give the patient a large stool container to keep in the freezer.

After
PT Inform the patient that a normal diet can be resumed.

Abnormal findings

▲ **Increased levels**
  Cystic fibrosis
  Malabsorption secondary to sprue, celiac disease, Whipple disease, Crohn disease, or radiation enteritis
  Maldigestion secondary to obstruction of the pancreatico-biliary tree (e.g., cancer, stricture, gallstones)
  Short-gut syndrome secondary to surgical resection, surgical bypass, or congenital anomaly

notes

ferritin

Type of test   Blood

Normal findings

Male: 12-300 ng/mL or 12-300 mcg/L (SI units)
Female: 10-150 ng/mL or 10-150 mcg/L (SI units)
Children
    Newborn: 25-200 ng/mL
    ≤1 month: 200-600 ng/mL
    2-5 months: 50-200 ng/mL
    6 months-15 years: 7-142 ng/mL

Test explanation and related physiology

The serum ferritin study is a good indicator of available iron stores in the body. Ferritin, the major iron storage protein, is normally present in the serum in concentrations directly related to iron storage. In normal patients, 1 ng/mL of serum ferritin corresponds to approximately 8 mg of stored iron. Ferritin levels rise with age in males and postmenopausal females. In premenopausal females, levels stay about the same.

Decreases in ferritin levels indicate a decrease in iron storage associated with iron deficiency anemia. A ferritin level less than 10 ng/100 mL is diagnostic of iron deficiency anemia. The decrease in serum ferritin level often precedes other signs of iron deficiency, such as decreased iron levels or changes in red blood cell size, color, and number. Only when protein depletion is severe can ferritin be decreased by malnutrition. Increased levels are a sign of iron excess, as seen in hemochromatosis, hemosiderosis, iron poisoning, or recent blood transfusions. Increased ferritin is also noted in patients with megaloblastic anemia, hemolytic anemia, and chronic hepatitis. Furthermore, ferritin is factitiously elevated in patients with chronic disease states, such as neoplasm, alcoholism, uremia, collagen diseases, or chronic liver diseases. Ferritin is also used in patients with chronic renal failure to monitor iron stores.

A limitation of this study is that ferritin levels also can act as an acute phase reactant protein and may be elevated in conditions not reflecting iron stores (e.g., acute inflammatory diseases, infections, metastatic cancer, lymphomas). Elevations in ferritin occur 1 to 2 days after onset of the acute illness and peak at 3 to 5 days. If iron deficiency were to coexist in patients with these diseases, it may not be recognized because the levels of ferritin would be factitiously elevated by the concurring disease.

Interfering factors

- Recent transfusions and recent ingestion of a meal with high iron content may cause elevated ferritin levels.
- Recent administration of a radionuclide can cause abnormal levels if testing is performed by radioimmunoassay.
- Hemolytic diseases may be associated with an artificially high iron content.
- Disorders of excessive iron storage (e.g., hemochromatosis, hemosiderosis) are associated with high ferritin levels.
- Iron-deficient menstruating women may have decreased ferritin levels.
- Acute and chronic inflammatory conditions and Gaucher disease can falsely increase ferritin levels.
- ✄ Iron preparations may *increase* ferritin levels.

Procedure and patient care

- See inside front cover for Routine Blood Testing.
- Fasting: no.
- Blood tube commonly used: red.

Abnormal findings

▲ **Increased levels**
Hemochromatosis
Hemosiderosis
Megaloblastic anemia
Hemolytic anemia
Alcoholic/inflammatory
    hepatocellular disease
Inflammatory disease
Advanced cancers
Chronic illnesses
    (e.g., leukemias, cirrhosis,
    chronic hepatitis)
Collagen vascular diseases
Hemophagocytic syndromes
Congenital and acquired
    sideroblastic anemias

▼ **Decreased levels**
Severe protein deficiency
Iron deficiency anemia
Hemodialysis

notes

fetal biophysical profile (Biophysical profile [BPP])

Type of test Ultrasound; fetal activity study

Normal findings Score of 8-10 points (if amniotic fluid volume is adequate)

Possible critical values Score of less than 4 points may necessitate immediate delivery.

Test explanation and related physiology

The BPP is a method of evaluating fetal status during the antepartal period based on five variables originating within the fetus: fetal heart rate, fetal breathing movement, gross fetal movements, fetal muscle tone, and amniotic fluid volume. Fetal heart rate reactivity is measured by the nonstress test (NST) (p. 432); the other four parameters are measured by ultrasound scanning. BPP is often done to assess fetal well-being in the face of a nonreactive NST.

The major premise behind the BPP is that variable assessments of fetal biophysical activity are more reliable than an examination of a single parameter (e.g., fetal heart rate). Indications for this test include such factors as postdate pregnancy, maternal hypertension, diabetes mellitus, vaginal bleeding, maternal Rh sensitization, maternal history of stillbirth, and premature rupture of membranes. The BPP is probably more useful in identifying a fetus in distress than in predicting future fetal well-being.

The five parameters are briefly described here. Each parameter is scored and contributes either a 2 or a 0 to the score. Therefore, 10 is the perfect score, and 0 is the lowest score. Gestational age influences these results. For example, fetal breathing movements are the latest parameter to develop.

- *Fetal heart rate reactivity.* This is measured and interpreted in the same way as the nonstress test (p. 432). The fetal heart rate is considered reactive when there are movement-associated fetal heart rate accelerations of at least 15 beats/min above baseline and 15 seconds in duration over a 20-minute period. A score of 2 is given for reactivity; a score of 0 indicates that the fetal heart rate is nonreactive.
- *Fetal breathing movements.* This parameter is assessed based on the assumption that fetal breathing movements indicate fetal well-being and their absence may indicate hypoxemia. To earn a score of 2, the fetus must have at least one episode of fetal breathing lasting at least 60 seconds within a 30-minute observation. Absence of this breathing pattern is scored a 0 on the BPP. It is important to note that several factors can

alter fetal breathing movements. For example, fetal breathing movements increase during the second and third hours after maternal meals and at night. Fetal breathing movements may decrease in such conditions as hypoxemia, hypoglycemia, nicotine use, and alcohol ingestion.

- *Fetal body movements.* Fetal activity is a reflection of neurologic integrity and function. The presence of at least three discrete episodes of fetal movements within a 30-minute observation period is given a score of 2. A score of 0 is given with two or fewer fetal movements in this time period. It is important to note that fetal activity is greatest 1 to 3 hours after the mother has consumed a meal.
- *Fetal tone.* In the uterus, the fetus is normally in a position of flexion. However, the fetus also stretches, rolls, and moves in the uterus. The arms, legs, trunk, and head may be flexed and extended. A score of 2 is earned when there is at least one episode of active extension with return to flexion. An example of this would be the opening and closing of a hand. A score of 0 is given for slow extension with a return to only partial flexion, fetal movement not followed by return to flexion, limbs or spine in extension, and an open fetal hand.
- *Amniotic fluid volume.* Amniotic fluid volume has been demonstrated to be an effective method of predicting fetal distress and in particular is an indicator of chronic hypoxemia. Oligohydramnios (too little amniotic fluid) has been associated with fetal anomalies, intrauterine growth retardation, and postterm pregnancy. A score of 2 is given for this parameter when there is at least one pocket of amniotic fluid that measures 1 cm in two perpendicular planes. A score of 0 indicates either that fluid is absent in most areas of the uterine cavity or that the largest pocket measures 1 cm or less in the vertical axis.

A score of 8 or 10 with a normal amount of amniotic fluid indicates a healthy fetus. A score of 8 with oligohydramnios or a score of 4 to 6 is equivocal. An equivocal test result is interpreted as possibly abnormal. A score of 0 or 2 is abnormal and indicates the need for assessment of immediate delivery.

Modifications can be made to the BPP. Some physicians omit the nonstress test if the ultrasound parameters are normal. Some physicians have added placental grading as a sixth parameter.

Another measure of fetal well-being is the *amniotic fluid index (AFI)*. Ultrasound is used to measure the largest collection of amniotic fluid in each of the four quadrants within the uterus. The numbers are added together, and the sum is the AFI. The normal range for the AFI is 8 to 18 cm. The sum is plotted on a graph where the age of gestation also is taken into account. If the AFI is less than the 2.4 percentile, oligohydramnios is present. If AFI exceeds the 97th percentile, polyhydramnios exists. An abnormally low AFI observed in antepartum testing is associated with an increased risk of intrauterine growth restriction and overall adverse perinatal outcome. The percentile value seems to be a better indicator than an absolute fluid volume. Oligohydramnios is associated with placental failure or fetal renal problems. Polyhydramnios is associated with maternal diabetes or fetal upper gastrointestinal malformation/obstruction.

Doppler ultrasound evaluations of the placenta and the *umbilical artery velocity* can recognize alterations in umbilical artery flow and direction that may indicate fetal stress or illness.

Interfering factors

- Occasionally no movement is noted. If no eye movement or respiratory movement is noted, the fetus may be sleeping. Testing is then extended.
- Central nervous system stimulants (e.g., catecholamine) can *increase* BPP activities.
- Antenatal steroids can *increase* BPP activities.
- Sedatives and narcotic analgesics can *decrease* BPP activities.

Procedure and patient care

Before

PT Explain the procedure to the patient.
PT Inform the patient that no fasting is required.

During

- Fetal heart rate reactivity is measured and interpreted from a nonstress test (p. 432).
- Fetal breathing movements, fetal body movements, fetal tone, and amniotic fluid volume are determined by ultrasound imaging (see obstetric ultrasonography, p. 697).

After

- If the test results are abnormal or equivocal, support the patient in the next phase of the fetal evaluation process.

Abnormal findings

Fetal asphyxia
Congenital anomalies
Oligohydramnios
Intrauterine growth retardation

Postterm pregnancyv
Fetal stress
Fetal death

notes

fetal contraction stress test (Contraction stress test [CST], Oxytocin challenge test [OCT])

Type of test Electrodiagnostic

Normal findings Negative

Test explanation and related physiology

CST is used to evaluate the viability of a fetus. It documents the function of the placenta in its ability to supply adequate blood to the fetus.

The CST, frequently called the *oxytocin challenge test (OCT)*, is a relatively noninvasive test of fetoplacental adequacy used in the assessment of high-risk pregnancy. For this study, a temporary stress in the form of uterine contractions is applied to the fetus after the IV administration of oxytocin. The reaction of the fetus to the contractions is assessed by an external fetal heart monitor. Uterine contractions cause a transient impediment of placental blood flow. If the placental reserve is adequate, the maternal-fetal oxygen transfer is not significantly compromised during the contractions and the fetal heart rate (FHR) remains normal (a *negative* test). The fetoplacental unit can then be considered adequate for the next 7 days.

If the placental reserve is inadequate, the fetus does not receive enough oxygen during the contraction. This results in intrauterine hypoxia and late deceleration of the FHR. The test is considered to be *positive* if consistent, persistent, late decelerations of the FHR occur with two or more uterine contractions. False-positive results caused by uterine hyperstimulation can occur in 10% to 30% of patients. Thus, positive test results warrant a complete review of other studies (e.g., amniocentesis) before the pregnancy is terminated by delivery.

The test is considered to be *unsatisfactory* if the results cannot be interpreted (e.g., because of hyperstimulation of the uterus, excessive movement of the mother, or deceleration of unknown meaning). In the case of unsatisfactory results, other means of management should be considered.

Although this test can be performed reliably at 32 weeks of gestation, it usually is done after 34 weeks. CST can induce labor, and a fetus at 34 weeks is more likely to survive an unexpectedly induced delivery than a fetus at 32 weeks. Nonstress testing (p. 432) of the fetus is the preferred test in almost every instance and can be performed more safely at 32 weeks; it can then be followed 2 weeks later by CST if necessary. The CST may be performed weekly until delivery terminates pregnancy.

Contraindications

- Patient pregnant with multiple fetuses, because the myometrium is under greater tension and is more likely to be stimulated to premature labor
- Patient with a prematurely ruptured membrane, because labor may be stimulated by the CST
- Patient with placenta previa, because vaginal delivery may be induced
- Patient with abruptio placentae, because the placenta may separate from the uterus as a result of the oxytocin-induced uterine contractions
- Patient with a previous hysterotomy, because the strong uterine contractions may cause uterine rupture
- Patient with a previous vertical or classic cesarean section, because the strong uterine contractions may cause uterine rupture (the test can be performed, however, if it is carefully monitored and controlled)
- Patient with pregnancy of less than 32 weeks, because early delivery may be induced by the procedure

Potential complications

- Premature labor

Interfering factors

- Hypotension may cause false-positive results.

Procedure and patient care

Before
- **PT** Explain the procedure to the patient.
- Obtain informed consent for the procedure.
- **PT** Teach the patient breathing and relaxation techniques.
- Record the patient's blood pressure and FHR before the test as baseline values.
- If the CST is performed on an elective basis, the patient may be kept NPO in case labor occurs.

During
- Note the following procedural steps:
  1. After the patient empties her bladder, place her in a semi-Fowler position and tilted slightly to one side to avoid vena caval compression by the enlarged uterus.
  2. Check her blood pressure every 10 minutes to avoid hypotension, which may cause diminished placental blood flow and a false-positive test result.

3. Place an external fetal monitor over the patient's abdomen to record the fetal heart tones. Attach an external tokodynamometer to the abdomen at the fundal region to monitor uterine contractions.
4. Record the output of the fetal heart tones and uterine contractions on a two-channel strip recorder.
5. Monitor baseline FHR and uterine activity for 20 minutes.
6. If uterine contractions are detected during this pretest period, withhold oxytocin and monitor the response of the fetal heart tone to spontaneous uterine contractions.
7. If no spontaneous uterine contractions occur, administer oxytocin (Pitocin) by IV infusion pump.
8. Increase the rate of oxytocin infusion until the patient is having moderate contractions; then record the FHR pattern.
9. After the oxytocin infusion is discontinued, continue FHR monitoring for another 30 minutes until the uterine activity has returned to its preoxytocin state. The body metabolizes oxytocin in approximately 20 to 25 minutes.

- Note that the CST is performed safely on an outpatient basis in the labor and delivery unit, where qualified nurses and necessary equipment are available. The test is performed by a nurse with a physician available.
- Note that the duration of this study is approximately 2 hours.
- **PT** Tell the patient that the discomfort associated with the CST may consist of mild labor contractions. Usually, breathing exercises are sufficient to control any discomfort. Administer analgesics if needed.

After
- Monitor the patient's blood pressure and FHR.
- Discontinue the IV line and assess the site for bleeding.

Abnormal findings
Fetoplacental inadequacy

notes

fetal fibronectin (fFN)

Type of test Fluid analysis

Normal findings Negative: ≤0.05 mcg/mL

Test explanation and related physiology

Fibronectin may help with implantation of the fertilized egg into the uterine lining. Normally, fibronectin cannot be identified in vaginal secretions after 22 weeks of pregnancy. However, concentrations are very high in the amniotic fluid. If fibronectin is identified in vaginal secretions after 24 weeks, the patient is at high risk for preterm delivery. The use of fFN is limited to symptomatic women with contractions whose membranes are intact and who have cervical dilatation of less than 3 cm.

Procedure and patient care

Before

PT Explain the procedure to the patient.

PT Tell the patient that no fasting is required.

- Determine whether the patient has had a cervical exam or intercourse within the past 24 hours. Results may be inaccurate.

During

- Note the following procedural steps:
  1. The patient is placed in the lithotomy position.
  2. A vaginal speculum is inserted to expose the cervix.
  3. Vaginal secretions are collected from the posterior vagina and paracervical area using a swab from a kit.
  4. The container with appropriate medium is labeled with the patient's name, age, and estimated date of confinement.

PT Tell the patient that no discomfort, except for insertion of the speculum, is associated with this procedure.

- Note that this procedure is performed by a physician or other licensed health care provider in several minutes.

After

PT Tell the patient results will be available the same or next day.

PT Educate the patient about the signs of preterm labor.

Abnormal findings

High risk for preterm premature delivery

notes

fetal hemoglobin (Kleihauer-Betke)

Type of test Blood

Normal findings <1% of RBCs

Test explanation and related physiology

Fetal hemoglobin may be present in the mother's blood because of fetal–maternal hemorrhage (FMH), which causes leakage of fetal cells into the maternal circulation. When large volumes of fetal blood are lost in this way, neonatal outcomes can be serious and potentially fatal. Massive FMH may be the cause of about 1 in every 50 stillbirths.

Leakage of fetal RBCs can begin any time after the middle of the first trimester. It presumably results from a breach in the integrity of the placental circulation. As pregnancy continues, more women will show evidence of fetal RBCs in their circulation; by term, about 50% will have detectable fetal cells. Most of these, however, are the result of very small leaks. In 96% to 98% of pregnancies, the total fetal blood volume lost in this way is 2 mL or less. Small leaks are not implicated in intrauterine death.

Risk factors correlated with the increasing risk of massive FMH include maternal trauma, placental abruption, placental tumors, third trimester amniocentesis, fetal hydrops, pale fetal organs, antecedent sinusoidal fetal heart tracing, and twinning. Having one or more of these features should be an indication for fetal hemoglobin testing.

The standard method of detecting FMH is the *Kleihauer-Betke test*. This takes advantage of the differential resistance of fetal hemoglobin to acid. The *flow cytometric method* for fetal hemoglobin determination offers several advantages over the traditional Kleihauer-Betke method. This more objective method has been shown to improve sensitivity, precision, and linearity over traditional methods.

FMH becomes of even greater significance when the mother is Rh negative, because this is the mechanism through which Rh sensitization could develop if the fetus has paternal Rh-positive blood cells. If this is known to exist, RhoGAM (RhIG) antibodies directed to Rh-positive fetal cells are given to the pregnant mother at the time of any invasive procedure in which the mother may be exposed to fetal blood or upon delivery. The RhoGAM antibodies kill the fetal RBCs in the maternal bloodstream before the mother can develop antibodies to fetal Rh-positive RBCs. This precludes more aggressive antifetal RBC occurrences in the future. By determination of the amount and volume of fetal blood loss, a dose of RhoGAM can be calculated using the following formula:

$$\text{Vials of RhIG} = \frac{\text{mL of fetal blood}}{30}$$

This test is often performed on women who have delivered a stillborn baby to see if FMH was a potential cause of fetal death.

Interfering factors

- Any maternal condition (e.g., sickle cell disease) that involves persistence of fetal hemoglobin in the mother will cause a false positive.
- If the blood is drawn after C-section, a false positive could occur. Vaginal delivery results in higher frequency of detection of FMH.

Procedure and patient care

- See inside front cover for Routine Blood Testing.
- Fasting: no.
- Blood tube commonly used: red.
- Provide emotional support in the event this test is performed after a stillborn delivery.

Abnormal findings

Fetal–maternal hemorrhage
Hereditary persistence of fetal hemoglobin
Intrachorionic thrombi

notes

fetal nonstress test (Nonstress test, NST, Fetal activity determination)

Type of test Electrodiagnostic

Normal findings Reactive fetus (heart rate acceleration associated with fetal movement)

Test explanation and related physiology

The NST is a method of evaluating the viability of a fetus. It documents the function of the placenta in its ability to supply adequate blood to the fetus. The NST can be used to evaluate any high-risk pregnancy in which fetal well-being may be threatened.

The NST is a noninvasive study that monitors acceleration of the fetal heart rate (FHR) in response to fetal movement. This FHR acceleration reflects the integrity of the central nervous system and fetal well-being. Fetal activity may be spontaneous, induced by uterine contraction, or induced by external manipulation. Oxytocin stimulation is not used. Fetal response is characterized as *reactive* or *nonreactive*. The NST indicates a reactive fetus when, with fetal movement, two or more FHR accelerations are detected, each of which must be at least 15 beats/min for 15 seconds or more within any 10-minute period. The test is 99% reliable in indicating fetal viability and negates the need for the contraction stress test (CST, p. 426). If the test detects a nonreactive fetus (i.e., no FHR acceleration with fetal movement) within 40 minutes, the patient is a candidate for the CST. A 40-minute test period is used because this is the average duration of the sleep-wake cycle of the fetus. The cycle may vary considerably, however.

The NST is useful in screening high-risk pregnancies and in selecting patients who may require the CST. An NST is routinely performed before the CST to avoid the complications associated with oxytocin administration. No complications are associated with the NST.

Procedure and patient care

Before

PT Explain the procedure to the patient.

- Encourage verbalization of the patient's fears. The necessity for the study usually raises realistic fears in the expectant mother.

PT If the patient is hungry, instruct her to eat before the NST is begun. Fetal activity is enhanced with a high maternal serum glucose level.

During

- After the patient empties her bladder, place her in Sims position.
- Place an external fetal monitor on the patient's abdomen to record the FHR. The mother can indicate fetal movement by pressing a button on the fetal monitor whenever she feels the fetus move. FHR and fetal movement are concomitantly recorded on a two-channel strip graph.
- Observe the fetal monitor for FHR accelerations associated with fetal movement.
- If the fetus is quiet for 20 minutes, stimulate fetal activity by external methods, such as rubbing or compressing the mother's abdomen, ringing a bell near the abdomen, or placing a pan on the abdomen and hitting the pan.
- Note that a nurse performs the NST in approximately 20 to 40 minutes in the physician's office or a hospital unit.

PT Tell the patient that no discomfort is associated with the NST.

After

PT If the results detect a nonreactive fetus, inform the patient that she is a candidate for the CST. Provide appropriate education.

Abnormal findings

Fetal stress
Fetal death

notes

fetal scalp blood pH

Type of test Blood

Normal findings

pH: 7.25-7.35
O_2 saturation: 30%-50%
PO_2: 18-22 mm Hg
PCO_2: 40-50 mm Hg
Base excess: 0 to –10 mEq/L

Test explanation and related physiology

Measurement of fetal scalp blood pH provides valuable information on fetal acid-base status. This test is useful clinically for diagnosing fetal distress.

Although the oxygen partial pressure (PO_2), carbon dioxide partial pressure (PCO_2), and bicarbonate ion concentration can be measured with a fetal scalp blood sample, the pH is the most useful clinically. The pH normally ranges from 7.25 to 7.35 during labor; a mild decline within the normal range is noted with contractions and as labor progresses.

Fetal hypoxia causes anaerobic glycolysis, resulting in excess production of lactic acid. This causes an increase in hydrogen ion concentration (acidosis) and a decrease in pH. Acidosis reflects the effect of hypoxia on cellular metabolism. A high correlation exists between low pH levels and low Apgar scores.

Fetal oxygen saturation monitoring (FSpo2) also is available to assist the monitoring of fetal well-being during delivery. When the FHR becomes significantly abnormal, C-section is often performed because of concern for fetal well-being. However, with $FSpo_2$, an accurate measure of fetal oxygen saturation can be determined. After membranes are ruptured, and if the baby is in vertex position with good cervical dilatation, a specialized probe can be placed on the temple or cheek of the fetus for $FSpo_2$ monitoring. The oxygen saturation is displayed on a monitor screen as a percentage. The normal oxygen saturation for a baby in the womb receiving oxygenated blood from the placenta is usually between 30% and 70%.

Contraindications

- Patients with premature membrane rupture
- Patients with active cervical infection

Potential complications

- Continued bleeding from the puncture site
- Hematoma

- Ecchymosis
- Infection

Procedure and patient care
Before
PT Explain the procedure to the patient.
- Obtain informed consent for this procedure.
PT Tell the patient that no fasting or sedation is required.

During
- Note the following procedural steps for fetal scalp pH:
  1. Amnioscopy is performed with the mother in the lithotomy position.
  2. The cervix is dilated, and the endoscope (amnioscope) is introduced into the cervical canal.
  3. The fetal scalp is cleansed with an antiseptic and dried with a sterile cotton ball.
  4. A small amount of petroleum jelly is applied to the fetal scalp to cause droplets of fetal blood to bead.
  5. After the skin on the scalp is pierced with a small metal blade, beaded droplets of blood are collected in long, heparinized capillary tubes.
  6. The tube is sealed with wax and placed on ice to retard cellular respiration, which can alter the pH.
  7. The physician performing the procedure applies firm pressure to the puncture site to retard bleeding.
  8. Scalp blood sampling can be repeated as necessary.
- Note that this study is performed by a physician in approximately 10 to 15 minutes.
PT Tell the patient that she may be uncomfortable during the cervical dilation.

After
PT Inform the patient that she may have vaginal discomfort and menstrual-type cramping.

After delivery
- Assess the newborn and document the puncture site(s).
- Cleanse the fetal scalp puncture site with an antiseptic solution and apply an antibiotic ointment.

Abnormal findings
Fetal distress

notes

fetoscopy

Type of test Endoscopy

Normal findings No fetal distress

Test explanation and related physiology

Fetoscopy is an endoscopic procedure that allows direct visualization of the fetus via the insertion of a tiny, telescope-like instrument through the abdominal wall and into the uterine cavity (Figure 21). Direct visualization may lead to diagnosis of a severe malformation (e.g., a neural tube defect). During the procedure, fetal blood samples to detect congenital blood disorders (e.g., hemophilia, sickle cell anemia) can be drawn from a blood vessel in the umbilical cord for biochemical analysis. Fetal skin biopsies also can be done to detect primary skin disorders.

Fetoscopy is performed at approximately 18 weeks of gestation. At this time, the vessels of the placental surface are of adequate size, and the fetal parts are readily identifiable. A therapeutic abortion would not be as hazardous at this time as it would be if it were done later in the pregnancy. An ultrasound is usually performed the day after the procedure to confirm the adequacy of the amniotic fluid and fetal viability.

Potential complications

- Spontaneous abortion
- Premature delivery
- Amniotic fluid leak
- Intrauterine fetal death
- Amnionitis

Procedure and patient care

Before

PT Explain the procedure to the patient.
- Obtain informed consent.
- Assess the fetal heart rate (FHR) before the test to serve as a baseline value.
- Administer fentanyl, if ordered, before the test because it crosses the placenta and quiets the fetus. This prevents excessive fetal movement, which would make the procedure more difficult.

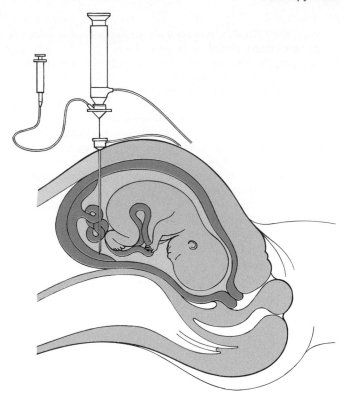

FIGURE 21 Fetoscopy for fetal blood sampling.

During
- Note the following procedural steps:
  1. The woman is placed in the supine position on an examining table.
  2. The abdominal wall is anesthetized locally.
  3. Ultrasonography is performed to locate the fetus and the placenta.
  4. The endoscope is inserted.
  5. Biopsies and blood samples may be obtained.
- Note that this procedure is performed by a physician in 1 to 2 hours.
- **PT** Tell the patient that the only discomfort associated with this study is the injection of the local anesthetic.

After

- Assess the FHR and compare with the baseline value to detect any side effects related to the procedure.
- Monitor the mother and fetus carefully for alterations in blood pressure, pulse, uterine activity, and fetal activity; vaginal bleeding; and loss of amniotic fluid.
- Administer RhoGAM to mothers who are Rh negative unless the fetal blood is found to be Rh negative.
- Note that a repeat ultrasound is usually performed the day after the procedure to confirm the adequacy of the amniotic fluid and fetal viability.
- If ordered, administer antibiotics prophylactically after the test to prevent amnionitis.

PT Instruct the mother to avoid strenuous activity for 1 to 2 weeks after the procedure.

PT Advise the mother to report any pain, bleeding, amniotic fluid loss, or fever.

Abnormal findings

Developmental defects (e.g., neural tube defects)
Congenital blood disorders (e.g., hemophilia, sickle cell anemia)
Primary skin disorders

notes

fibrinogen (Factor I, Quantitative fibrinogen)

Type of test Blood

Normal findings

Adult: 200-400 mg/dL or 2-4 g/L (SI units)
Newborn: 125-300 mg/dL

Possible critical values <100 mg/dL

Test explanation and related physiology

Fibrinogen is essential to the blood-clotting mechanism. It is part of the common pathway in the coagulation system. Fibrinogen is converted to fibrin by action of thrombin during the coagulation process. (See discussion of coagulating factors, p. 261.) Fibrinogen, which is produced by the liver, is also an acute-phase protein reactant. It rises sharply during instances of tissue inflammation or necrosis. High levels of fibrinogen have been associated with an increased risk of coronary heart disease, stroke, myocardial infarction, and peripheral arterial disease. This makes fibrinogen an important risk factor for cardiovascular disease.

Fibrinogen is used primarily to aid in the diagnosis of suspected bleeding disorders. This testing is used to detect increased or decreased fibrinogen (factor I) concentration of acquired or congenital origin. It is also used for monitoring the severity and treatment of disseminated intravascular coagulation and fibrinolysis.

Reduced levels of fibrinogen can be seen in patients with liver disease, malnourished states, and consumptive coagulopathies (e.g., disseminated intravascular coagulation). Large-volume blood transfusions are also associated with low levels of fibrinogen because banked blood does not contain fibrinogen. Reduced levels of fibrinogen will cause a prolonged pro-time and partial thromboplastin time.

Interfering factors

- Blood transfusions within the past month may affect test results.
- Diets rich in omega-3 and omega-6 fatty acids reduce fibrinogen levels.
- Drugs that may cause *increased* levels include estrogens and oral contraceptives.
- Drugs that may cause *decreased* levels include anabolic steroids, androgens, L-asparaginase, phenobarbital, streptokinase, tissue plasminogen activators (e.g., urokinase), and valproic acid.

Procedure and patient care

- See inside front cover for Routine Blood Testing.
- Fasting: no.
- Blood tube commonly used: blue.

Abnormal findings

▲ **Increased levels**

Acute inflammatory reactions (e.g., rheumatoid arthritis, glomerulonephritis)
Trauma
Acute infection (e.g., pneumonia)
Coronary heart disease
Cigarette smoking
Pregnancy
Cerebrovascular accident
Myocardial infarction
Peripheral arterial disease

▼ **Decreased levels**

Liver disease (e.g., hepatitis, cirrhosis)
Consumptive coagulopathy
Fibrinolysins
Congenital afibrinogenemia
Advanced carcinoma
Malnutrition
Large-volume blood transfusion
Hemophagocytic lymphohistiocytosis

notes

fluorescein angiography (FA, Ocular photography)

Type of test Other

Normal findings Normal retinal/choroidal vasculature

Test explanation and related physiology

With the use of fluorescein angiography, the patency and integrity of the retinal circulation can be determined. This test involves injection of sodium fluorescein into the systemic circulation followed by timed-interval photographs performed with a fundus camera. The timed images are then reviewed for specific patterns indicative of disease states. This test is performed to diagnose disease affecting the posterior eye, including the retina, choroid, and optic nerve. The test is often repeated at intervals to monitor treatment or disease progression.

Fluorescein is a member of the triphenylmethane dyes. When the fluorescein molecules absorb light toward the end of the blue spectrum (465 to 490 nm), the molecules transfer from a basal state to an excited state. In doing so, light of a different wavelength (450 to 465 nm, the yellow-green end of the light spectrum) is emitted. This light emission is then recorded by a specialized camera. With digital technology, color photographs can be obtained at specified times after dye injections. Baseline photographs are taken prior to fluorescein injection.

Fluorescein enters the ocular circulation from the internal carotid artery via the ophthalmic artery. Pathologic changes are recognized by the detection of either hyperfluorescence or hypofluorescence. Among the common groups of ophthalmologic disease, fluorescein angiography can detect diabetic retinopathy, vein occlusions, retinal artery occlusions, edema of the optic disc, and tumors.

Fluorescein angiography is often done to follow the course of a disease, such as diabetes or age-related macular degeneration, that can cause the blood vessels of the retina to leak blood or fluid. These abnormalities can be treated with a laser to help prevent loss of vision, and treatment results can be monitored using fluorescein angiography.

Potential complications

- Allergic reactions
  Allergies to fluorescein dye are rare. If they occur, they may cause a skin rash and itching. Severe allergic reactions (anaphylaxis) occur rarely but can be life threatening.

Procedure and patient care

Before

PT Explain the procedure to the patient.

• Obtain an informed consent.

PT Reinforce the need for the patient to remain still during the few seconds following fluorescein injection.

• Obtain an ocular history of cataracts, prior retinal surgery, or other disease that may inhibit photography.

PT Instruct the patient to remove any ocular lenses.

PT Inform the patient that there are no dietary restrictions.

• Note that pupil dilatation can improve access to the posterior eye. If ordered, administer appropriate mydriatic medications. Note, however, that these medications are contraindicated for patients with glaucoma because they may dangerously increase ocular pressures.

During

• Note the following procedural steps:
  1. The patient is positioned in the fundus camera with the chin on the bar.
  2. The patient is told to pick a spot in the far distance and to concentrate on that spot during the examination.
  3. Intravenous access is obtained.
  4. Fluorescein dye is injected with the assistance of an autoinjector.
  5. Photographs are taken by the ophthalmologist at timed intervals.

• The test is performed and interpreted by an ophthalmologist, usually in the office setting. Results are available in less than 30 minutes.

After

• Remove the intravenous access device and apply pressure to the venipuncture site.

PT Inform the patient that fluorescein dye is excreted by the kidneys and to expect very yellow urine for the next 24 hours.

Abnormal findings

▲ **Increased levels**
 Tumor
 Detached retina
 Trauma
 Inflammation
 Retinitis pigmentosa
 Papilledema
 Diabetic retinopathy

▼ **Decreased levels**
 Diabetes
 Vascular disease
 Radiation to the eye
 Hemorrhage
 Edema
 Prior photocoagulation
  therapy

folic acid (Folate)

Type of test Blood

Normal findings

Serum: 5-25 ng/mL or 11-57 nmol/L (SI units)
RBC folate: 360-1400 nmol/L

Test explanation and related physiology

Folic acid (folate), one of the B vitamins, is necessary for normal function of red and white blood cells (RBCs, WBCs). It is needed for the adequate synthesis of certain purines and pyrimidines, which are precursors for deoxyribonucleic acid (DNA). Blood folate levels require normal absorption by the intestinal tract. The finding of a low serum folate level means that the patient's recent diet has been subnormal in folate content and/or that recent absorption of folate has been subnormal.

Tissue folate is best tested by determining the content of folate in RBCs. A low RBC folate can mean either that there is tissue folate depletion due to folate deficiency, which requires folate therapy, or that the patient has primary vitamin B_{12} (p. 994) deficiency, which blocks the ability of cells to take up folate. In the latter case, the proper therapy would be with vitamin B_{12} rather than with folic acid.

Folic acid blood levels are performed to assess folate availability in pregnancy, to evaluate hemolytic disorders, and to detect anemia caused by folic acid deficiency (in which the RBCs are abnormally large, causing a megaloblastic anemia). These RBCs have a shortened life span and impaired oxygen-carrying capacity. If folic acid blood levels are low, RBC folate is measured.

Folate deficiency is present in about 33% of pregnant women; many alcoholics; and patients with a variety of malabsorption syndromes, including celiac disease, sprue, Crohn disease, and jejunal/ileal bypass procedure. Folate binds to aluminum hydroxide. Patients with a chronic use of antacids or H_2-receptor antagonists and with diets marginal in folate may experience low folate levels.

Elevated serum levels of folic acid may be seen in patients with pernicious anemia because vitamin B_{12} is needed to allow incorporation of folate into tissue cells. The folic acid tests are often done in conjunction with tests for vitamin B_{12} levels.

Interfering factors

- A falsely normal result may occur in a folate-deficient patient who has received a blood transfusion.
- ✘ Drugs that may cause *decreased* folic acid levels include alcohol, aminopterin, aminosalicylic acid, antimalarials, chloramphenicol, erythromycin, estrogens, methotrexate, oral contraceptives, penicillin derivatives, phenobarbital, phenytoins, and tetracyclines.

Procedure and patient care

- See inside front cover for Routine Blood Testing.
- Fasting: verify with lab.
- Blood tube commonly used: red.
- Some laboratories prefer an 8-hour fast.
- PT Instruct the patient not to consume alcoholic beverages before the test.
- Draw the specimen before starting folate therapy.

Abnormal findings

▲ Increased levels
Pernicious anemia
Vegetarianism
Recent blood transfusions

▼ Decreased levels
Folic acid deficiency
  anemia
Hemolytic anemia
Malnutrition
Malabsorption syndrome
  (e.g., sprue, celiac
  disease)
Malignancy
Pregnancy
Alcoholism
Anorexia nervosa

notes

fungal testing (Antifungal antibodies; Beta-D-glucan
(1,3)-ß-D-glucan, Fungitell, Fungal culture, Fungal antigen assay,
Fungal PCR testing)

Type of test Blood, microscopic examination

Normal findings No antibodies detected

β-D-glucan:

Negative	Less than 60 pg/mL
Indeterminate	60-79 pg/mL
Positive	≥80 pg/mL

Culture: no growth in 24 days

Gram stain: no fungus seen

Test explanation and related physiology

Few fungal diseases can be diagnosed clinically; many are diagnosed by isolating and identifying the infecting fungus in the clinical laboratory. Fungal infections can be superficial, subcutaneous, or systemic (deep). The systemic fungal infections (mycoses) are the most important, for which serologic antibody testing is performed. Generally, mycoses are caused by the inhalation of airborne fungal spores. In the United States, the most serious fungal infections are coccidioidomycosis, blastomycosis, histoplasmosis, and paracoccidioidomycosis. These infections start out as primary pulmonary infections. *Aspergillus, Candida,* and *Cryptococcus* systemic infections usually affect only those with compromised immunity.

Fungal antibody testing is not highly reliable. In general, this testing is used for screening for antibodies to dimorphic fungi (*Blastomyces, Coccidioides, Histoplasma*) and the antigen of *Cryptococcus neoformans* during acute infection. Antibodies are present in only about 70% to 80% of infected patients. When positive, they merely indicate that the person has an active or has had a recent fungal infection. These antibodies can be identified in the blood or cerebrospinal fluid (CSF). In general, more specific antibodies are tested only after screening antibody testing (e.g., complement fixation studies) are performed. Antibodies can be tested singularly or as a fungal panel. Cross-reactions can occur (e.g., antibodies to blastomycosis can cross-react with histoplasmosis antigens).

(1,3)-ß-D-glucan is an enzyme immunoassay used to support the diagnosis of invasive fungal disease (IFD) in at-risk patients. Normally, serum contains low levels of (1,3)-ß-D-glucan, presumably from yeasts present in the alimentary and gastrointestinal tract. (1,3)-ß-D-glucan is produced by most invasive fungal organisms. D-glucan becomes elevated well in advance of

conventional clinical signs and symptoms of IFD. As opportunistic infections, IFDs are common among patients with hematologic malignancies or AIDS. They account for a growing number of nosocomial infections, particularly among organ transplant recipients and other patients receiving immunosuppressive treatments. $(1,3)$-β-D-glucan is produced by most invasive fungal organisms. *Blastomyces* and *Cryptococcus* produce very low levels of $(1,3)$-β-D-glucan. Mucormycetes do not produce $(1,3)$-β-D-glucan. It is important to note that negative results do not exclude fungal etiology, especially in the early stages of infection.

Fungal antigen assays are available to detect a portion of the infecting fungus such as *Aspergillus* galactomannan. Fungal organisms can be identified by culture growth and macro- or microscopy. Fungi components can occasionally be seen on Gram stain. Fungi can be pathogens, colonizers, or contaminants. Correlation of the patient clinical condition with culture results is necessary. Fungus can be cultured from blood, body fluids, CSF, fresh tissue, bronchopulmonary secretions, or swabs of the ear, nose, and throat or from urine. Accurate fungal culture is labor intensive and requires a highly experienced laboratory. Results are not available quickly.

Interfering factors

- False-positive results can occur if a patient's intestinal tract is colonized with *Candida*.
- False-positive results occur in patients on hemodialysis using cellulose membranes.
- False-negative results occur in serum that is hemolyzed, icteric, lipemic, or turbid.

Procedure and patient care

- See inside front cover for Routine Blood Testing.
- Fasting: no.
- Blood tube commonly used: red or serum separator.
- Indicate on the laboratory slip the particular antibody or panel of antibodies that are to be tested.
- Because some patients with fungal infection may be immunocompromised, instruct them to check for signs of infection at the venipuncture site.

Abnormal findings

▲ **Increased levels**
  Acute fungal infection
  Previous systemic exposure to fungal disease

notes

galectin-3 (GAL-3)

Type of test Blood

Normal findings ≤22.1 ng/mL

Test explanation and related physiology

Heart failure progresses primarily by dilatation of the ventricular cardiac chamber through remodeling in fibrosis as a response to cardiac injury and/or overload. Galectin-3 (GAL-3) is a biomarker that appears to be actively involved in both the inflammatory and fibrotic pathways involved in remodeling. GAL-3 is a carbohydrate-binding lectin whose expression is associated with inflammatory cells, including macrophages, neutrophils, and mast cells. GAL-3 has been linked to cardiac remodeling in the setting of heart failure and a variety of other cardiac insults. Elevated levels are associated with increased risk of mortality.

Interfering factors

- Hemolysis increases GAL-3 levels.
- Heterophile antibodies (page 645) increase GAL-3 levels.

Procedure and patient care

- See inside front cover for Routine Blood Testing.
- Fasting: no.
- Blood tube commonly used: lavender.

Abnormal findings

▲ Increased levels

Congestive heart failure

notes

gallbladder nuclear scanning (Hepatobiliary scintigraphy, Cholescintigraphy, DISIDA scanning, HIDA scanning)

Type of test Nuclear scan

Normal findings Gallbladder, common bile duct, and duodenum visualized within 60 minutes after radionuclide injection. (This confirms patency of the cystic and common bile ducts.)

Test explanation and related physiology

Through the use of iminodiacetic acid analogues (IDAs) labeled with technetium-99 m (^{99m}Tc), the biliary tract can be evaluated in a safe, accurate, and noninvasive manner. These radionuclide compounds are extracted by the liver and excreted into the bile. Gamma rays emitted from the bile are detected by a scintillator, and a realistic image of the biliary tree is apparent.

Failure to visualize the gallbladder 60 to 120 minutes after injection of the radionuclide dye is virtually diagnostic of an obstruction of the cystic duct (acute cholecystitis). Delayed filling of the gallbladder is associated with chronic or acalculous cholecystitis. The identification of the radionuclide in the biliary tree, but not in the bowel, is diagnostic of common bile duct obstruction.

With cholescintigraphy, gallbladder function can be numerically determined by calculating the capability of the gallbladder to eject its contents after the injection of a cholecystokinetic drug (e.g., sincalide). It is believed that an ejection fraction below 35% indicates chronic cholecystitis or functional obstruction of the cystic duct. Ultrasound has largely replaced this test for the diagnosis of acute cholecystitis.

Occasionally, morphine sulfate is given intravenously during nuclear scanning. The morphine causes increased ampullary contraction. This reproduces the patient's symptoms of biliary colic and forces the bile containing the radionuclide into the gallbladder, shortening the expected time of visualization of the gallbladder. If no radionuclide is seen in the gallbladder with the use of morphine within 15 to 30 minutes, the diagnosis of acute cholecystitis is nearly certain.

Contraindications

- Patients who are pregnant, because of the risk of fetal damage

Interfering factors

- If the patient has not eaten for more than 24 hours, the radionuclide may not fill the gallbladder. This would produce a false-positive result.

✗ The administration of opiates can prolong the time for gall-bladder identification.

Procedure and patient care
Before
PT Explain the procedure to the patient.
PT Assure the patient that he or she will not be exposed to large amounts of radioactivity.
PT Instruct the patient to fast for at least 2 to 4 hours before the test. This fasting is preferable but not mandatory.

During
- Note the following procedural steps:
  1. After IV administration of a ^{99m}Tc-labeled IDA analogue (e.g., mebrofenin, disofenin), the right upper quadrant of the abdomen is scanned.
  2. Serial images are obtained over 1 hour.
  3. Subsequent images can be obtained at 15- to 30-minute intervals.
  4. If the gallbladder, common bile duct, or duodenum is not visualized within 60 minutes after injection, delayed images are obtained up to 4 hours later.
  5. When an *ejection fraction* is to be determined, the patient is given a fatty meal or cholecystokinin to evaluate emptying of the gallbladder. The gallbladder is continually scanned to measure the percentage of isotope ejected.
- Note that a radiologist performs this study in 1 to 4 hours in the nuclear medicine department.
PT Tell the patient that the only discomfort associated with this procedure is the IV injection of radionuclide.

After
- Obtain a meal for the patient if indicated.

Abnormal findings
Acute cholecystitis
Chronic cholecystitis
Acalculous cholecystitis
Common bile duct obstruction secondary to gallstones, tumor, or stricture
Cystic duct syndrome

notes

gallium scan

Type of test Nuclear scan

Normal findings

Diffuse, low level of gallium uptake, especially in the liver and spleen
No increased gallium uptake within the body

Test explanation and related physiology

A gallium scan of the total body may be performed 24, 48, and 72 hours after an IV injection of radioactive gallium. Most commonly, a single scan is performed 2 to 4 days after the gallium injection. Gallium is a radionuclide that is concentrated by areas of inflammation and infection, abscesses, and benign and malignant tumors. However, not all types of tumors will concentrate gallium. Lymphomas are particularly gallium avid. Other tumors that can be detected by a gallium scan include sarcomas; hepatomas; and carcinomas of the gastrointestinal tract, kidney, uterus, stomach, and testicle.

This test is useful in detecting metastatic tumor. However, to a large degree, PET scans (p. 731) have replaced gallium scans for the identification of malignancy. The gallium scan is useful in demonstrating a source of infection in patients with a fever of unknown origin. Gallium can be used to identify noninfectious inflammation within the body in patients who have an elevated sedimentation rate. Unfortunately, this test is not specific enough to differentiate among tumor, infection, inflammation, or abscess. PET scans are more commonly used to identify areas of acute infection.

Another method of scanning is called *single-photon emission computed tomography (SPECT) imaging.* With SPECT scanning, the patient lies supine on a table surrounded by a doughnut-like gantry. The photon detection camera rotates around the patient to obtain proton counts from 360 degrees. This provides a more detailed image.

Contraindications

- Patients who are pregnant, unless the benefits outweigh the risks of fetal damage

Interfering factors

- Recent barium studies will interfere with visualization of gallium within the abdomen.

Procedure and patient care

Before
PT Explain the procedure to the patient.
- If ordered, administer a cathartic or enema to the patient to minimize increased gallium uptake in the bowel.

During
- Note the following procedural steps:
  1. The unsedated patient is injected with gallium.
  2. A total-body scan may be performed 4 to 6 hours later by slowly passing a radionuclide detector over the body.
  3. Additional scans are usually taken 24, 48, and 72 hours later.
  4. During the scanning process, the patient is placed in the supine position and occasionally in the lateral position.
- Note that a nuclear medicine technologist performs each scan in approximately 30 to 60 minutes. Repeated scanning is required. Repeated injections are not necessary.

PT Inform the patient that test results are interpreted by a physician trained in nuclear medicine and are usually available 72 hours after the injection.

After
PT Assure the patient that only tracer doses of radioisotopes have been used and that no precautions against radioactive exposure to others are necessary.

Abnormal findings
Tumor
Noninfectious inflammation
Infection
Abscess

notes

gamma-glutamyl transpeptidase (GGTP, γ-GTP, Gamma-glutamyl transferase [GGT])

Type of test Blood

Normal findings

Male and female age 45 and older: 8-38 units/L or 8-38 international units/L (SI units)

Female younger than age 45: 5-27 units/L or 5-27 international units/L (SI units)

Elderly: slightly higher than adult level

Child: similar to adult level

Newborn: 5 times higher than adult level

Test explanation and related physiology

The enzyme GGTP participates in the transfer of amino acids and peptides across the cellular membrane and possibly participates in glutathione metabolism. The highest concentrations of this enzyme are found in the liver and biliary tract. Lesser concentrations are found in the kidney, spleen, heart, intestine, brain, and prostate gland. This test is used to detect liver cell dysfunction, and it very accurately indicates even the slightest degree of cholestasis. This is the most sensitive liver enzyme in detecting biliary obstruction, cholangitis, or cholecystitis. As with leucine aminopeptidase and 5-nucleotidase, the elevation of GGTP generally parallels that of alkaline phosphatase; however, GGTP is more sensitive. Also, as with 5-nucleotidase and leucine aminopeptidase, GGTP is not increased in bone diseases as is alkaline phosphatase. A normal GGTP level with an elevated alkaline phosphatase level implies skeletal disease. Elevated GGTP and alkaline phosphatase levels imply hepatobiliary disease. GGTP is also not elevated in childhood or pregnancy.

Another important clinical aspect of GGTP is that it can detect chronic alcohol ingestion. Therefore, it is very useful in the screening and evaluation of alcoholic patients. GGTP is elevated in approximately 75% of patients who chronically drink alcohol.

Why this enzyme is elevated after an acute myocardial infarction is not clear. It may represent the associated hepatic insult (if elevation occurs in the first 7 days) or the proliferation of capillary endothelial cells in the granulation tissue that replaces the infarcted myocardium. The elevation usually occurs 1 to 2 weeks after infarction.

Interfering factors

- Values may be decreased in late pregnancy.
- ⚑ Drugs that may cause *increased* GGTP levels include alcohol, phenobarbital, and phenytoin.
- ⚑ Drugs that may cause *decreased* levels include clofibrate and oral contraceptives.

Procedure and patient care

- See inside front cover for Routine Blood Testing.
- Fasting: yes.
- Blood tube commonly used: red.
- Patients with liver dysfunction often have prolonged clotting times.

Abnormal findings

▲ **Increased levels**

Hepatitis
Cirrhosis
Hepatic necrosis
Hepatic tumor or metastasis
Hepatotoxic drugs
Cholestasis
Jaundice
Myocardial infarction
Alcohol ingestion
Pancreatitis
Cancer of the pancreas
Epstein-Barr virus (infectious mononucleosis)
Cytomegalovirus infections
Reye syndrome

notes

gastric emptying scan

Type of test Nuclear scan

Normal findings

Normal values are determined by type and quantity of radio-labeled ingested food.

Time	Lower normal limits	Upper normal nimits
0 minutes		
30 minutes	70%	
1 hour	30%	90%
2 hours		60%
3 hours		30%
4 hours		10%

Values lower than normal represent abnormally fast gastric emptying. Values higher than upper limits represent delayed gastric emptying.

Test explanation and related physiology

In this study, the patient ingests a solid or liquid "test meal" containing a radionuclide such as technetium (Tc). The stomach is then scanned until gastric emptying is complete. This study is used to assess the stomach's ability to empty solids or liquids and to evaluate disorders that may cause a delay in gastric emptying, such as obstruction (caused by peptic ulcers or gastric malignancies) and gastroparesis. This scan is also useful in determining the rate of gastric emptying. This is helpful in the diagnosis of gastric obstruction secondary to gastroparesis or gastric obstruction. It is helpful in evaluating patients who have postcibal nausea, vomiting, bloating, early satiety, belching, or abdominal pain.

Contraindications

- Patients who are pregnant or lactating, unless the benefits outweigh the risk of fetal or newborn injury

Interfering factors

☒ Drugs that *decrease* gastric emptying time include anticholinergics, opiates, and sedative-hypnotics. These medications should be withheld for 2 days before testing.

Procedure and patient care

Before

PT Explain the procedure to the patient.

PT Inform the patient that only a small dose of nuclear material is ingested. Reassure the patient that this is a safe dose.

PT Instruct the patient to keep on nothing by mouth (NPO) status after midnight on the day of the test.

PT Tell the patient that smoking is prohibited on the day of examination because exposure to tobacco can inhibit gastric emptying.

During

- Note the following procedural steps:
    1. In the nuclear medicine department, the patient is asked to ingest a test meal. In the *solid-emptying* study, the patient eats scrambled egg whites containing Tc. In the *liquid-emptying* study, the patient drinks orange juice or water containing technetium-99 m diethylenetriamine pentaacetic acid (DTPA) or indium-111 DTPA.
    2. After ingestion of the test meal, the patient is imaged by a gamma camera that records gastric images. Images are obtained for 2 minutes every 30 to 60 minutes until gastric emptying is complete. This may take several hours, although each particular timed scan takes only a few minutes.
- With the use of computer calculations of timed images, the rate of gastric emptying can be determined.

After

PT Assure the patient that no radiation precautions need to be taken.

Abnormal findings

Gastric obstruction caused by gastric ulcer or cancer
Nonfunctioning GI anastomosis
Gastroparesis

notes

gastrin

Type of test Blood

Normal findings

Adult: 0-180 pg/mL or 0-180 ng/L (SI units)

 Levels are higher in elderly patients.

Child: 0-125 pg/mL

Test explanation and related physiology

 Gastrin is a hormone produced by the G cells located in the distal part of the stomach (antrum). Gastrin is a potent stimulator of gastric acid. In normal gastric physiology, an alkaline environment (created by food or antacids) stimulates the release of gastrin. Gastrin then stimulates the parietal cells of the stomach to secrete gastric acid. The pH environment in the stomach is thereby reduced. By negative feedback, this low-pH environment suppresses further gastrin secretion.

 Zollinger-Ellison (ZE) syndrome (gastrin-producing pancreatic tumor) and G-cell hyperplasia (overfunctioning of G cells in the distal stomach) are associated with high serum gastrin levels. Patients with these tumors have aggressive peptic ulcer disease. Unlike a patient with routine peptic ulcers, a patient with ZE syndrome or G-cell hyperplasia has a high incidence of complicated and recurrent peptic ulcers. It is important to identify this latter group of patients to institute more appropriate, aggressive medical and surgical therapy. The serum gastrin level is normal in patients with routine peptic ulcer and greatly elevated in patients with ZE syndrome or G-cell hyperplasia.

 It is important to note that patients who are taking antacid peptic ulcer medicines, have had peptic ulcer surgery, or have atrophic gastritis will have a high serum gastrin level. However, levels usually are not as high as in patients with ZE syndrome or G-cell hyperplasia.

 Not all patients with ZE syndrome exhibit increased levels of serum gastrin. Some may have *top normal* gastrin levels, which makes these patients difficult to differentiate from patients with routine peptic ulcer disease. ZE syndrome or G-cell hyperplasia can be diagnosed in these top normal patients by *gastrin stimulation tests* with the use of calcium or secretin. Patients with these diseases have greatly increased serum gastrin levels associated with the infusion of these drugs.

Interfering factors

- Peptic ulcer surgery creates a persistent alkaline environment, which is the strongest stimulant to gastrin.
- Ingestion of high-protein food can result in an increase in serum gastrin two to five times the normal level.
- ✗ Patients with diabetes who take insulin may have falsely *increased* levels.
- ✗ Drugs that may *increase* serum gastrin levels include antacids and H_2-blocking agents (e.g., esomeprazole, lansoprazole, omeprazole, pantoprazole, rabeprazole).
- ✗ Drugs that may *decrease* levels include anticholinergics and tricyclic antidepressants.

Procedure and patient care

- See inside front cover for Routine Blood Testing.
- Fasting: yes.
- Blood tube commonly used: red.
- **PT** Tell the patient to avoid alcohol for at least 24 hours.
- For the *calcium infusion test*, administer calcium gluconate intravenously. A preinfusion serum gastrin level is then compared with specimens taken every 30 minutes for 4 hours.
- For the *secretin test*, administer secretin intravenously. Preinjection and postinjection serum gastrin levels are taken at 15-minute intervals for 1 hour after injection.

Abnormal findings

▲ **Increased levels**

Zollinger-Ellison syndrome
G-cell hyperplasia
Pernicious anemia
Atrophic gastritis
Gastric carcinoma

Chronic renal failure
Pyloric obstruction or gastric outlet obstruction
Retained antrum after gastric surgery

notes

gastroesophageal reflux scan (GE reflux scan, Aspiration scan)

Type of test   Nuclear scan

Normal findings   No evidence of gastroesophageal reflux

Test explanation and related physiology

GE reflux scans are used to evaluate patients with symptoms of heartburn, regurgitation, vomiting, and dysphagia. They are also used to evaluate the medical or surgical treatment of patients with GE reflux. Finally, *aspiration scans* may be used to detect aspiration of gastric contents into the lungs.

Contraindications

- Patients who cannot tolerate abdominal compression
- Patients who are pregnant or lactating, unless the benefits outweigh the risks

Procedure and patient care

Before

PT   Explain the procedure to the patient.

PT   Assure the patient that no pain is associated with this test.

PT   Instruct the patient not to eat anything after midnight.

During

- Note the following procedural steps:

GE reflux scan

1. The patient is placed in the supine position and asked to swallow a tracer cocktail (e.g., orange juice, diluted hydrochloric acid, and technetium-99 m–labeled colloid).
2. Images are taken of the patient's esophageal area.
3. The patient is asked to assume other positions to determine whether GE reflux occurs and, if so, in what position.
4. A large abdominal binder that contains an air-inflatable cuff is placed on the patient's abdomen. This is insufflated to increase abdominal pressure.
5. Images are again taken over the esophageal area to determine whether any GE reflux occurs.

Aspiration scans

- Delayed images are made over the lung fields 24 hours after injection of technetium to detect esophagotracheal aspiration of the tracer.
- Note that this procedure is performed in the nuclear medicine department in approximately 30 minutes.

PT Remind the patient that no discomfort is associated with this test.

- For infants being evaluated for chalasia, note that the tracer is added to the feeding or formula. Nuclear tracer films are then taken over the next hour, with 24-hour delayed films as needed.

After

PT Assure the patient that he or she has ingested only a small dose of nuclear material. No radiation precautions need to be taken against the patient or his or her bodily secretions.

Abnormal findings

Gastroesophageal reflux
Pulmonary aspiration

notes

gastrointestinal bleeding scan
(Abdominal scintigraphy, GI scintigraphy)

Type of test   Nuclear scan

Normal findings   No collection of radionuclide in GI tract

Test explanation and related physiology

The GI bleeding scan is a test used to localize the site of bleeding in patients who are having active GI hemorrhage. The scan also can be used in patients who have suspected intraabdominal hemorrhage from an unknown source.

Arteriography has limitations in its evaluation of GI bleeding. Arteriography can determine the site of bleeding only if the rate of bleeding exceeds 0.5 mL/min for detection. The GI bleeding scan has several advantages over arteriography. It can detect bleeding if the rate is greater than 0.05 mL/min. Also, with the use of ^{99m}Tc-labeled red blood cells (RBCs), delayed films (as long as 24 hours) can be obtained indicating the site of an intermittent or extremely slow intestinal bleed.

A GI scintigram is sensitive in locating the area of GI bleeding; however, it is not very specific in pinpointing the site or cause of bleeding. It is important to realize that this test can take 1 to 4 hours to obtain useful information. An unstable patient may need to go to surgery in minutes.

Contraindications

- Patients who are pregnant or lactating, unless the benefits outweigh the risks
- Medically unstable patients

Interfering factors

- Barium in the GI tract may mask a small source of bleeding.

Procedure and patient care

Before

PT Explain the procedure to the patient.

PT Inform the patient that no pretest preparation is required.

PT Assure the patient that only a small amount of nuclear material will be administered.

PT Instruct the patient to notify the nuclear medicine technologist if he or she has a bowel movement during the test. Blood in the GI tract can act as a cathartic.

During

- Note the following procedural steps:
  1. Ten millicuries of freshly prepared ^{99m}Tc-labeled sulfur colloid is administered intravenously to the patient. If ^{99m}Tc-labeled RBCs are to be used, 3 to 5 mL of the patient's own blood is combined with the ^{99m}Tc and reinjected into the patient.
  2. Immediately after administration of the radionuclide, the patient is placed under a scintillation camera.
  3. Multiple images of the abdomen are obtained at short intervals (5 to 15 minutes).
  4. Detection of radionuclide in the abdomen indicates the site of bleeding. If no bleeding sites are noted in the first hour, the scan may be repeated at hourly intervals for as long as 24 hours.
- Note that areas of the bowel hidden by the liver or spleen may not be adequately evaluated by this procedure. Also, the rectum cannot be easily evaluated because other pelvic structures (e.g., the bladder) obstruct the view.
- Note that this test is usually performed in approximately 60 minutes by a technologist in nuclear medicine.
- **PT** Tell the patient that the only discomfort associated with this study is the injection of the radioisotope.

After

PT Assure the patient that only tracer doses of radioisotopes have been used and that radiation precautions are not necessary.

Abnormal findings

Ulcer
Tumor
Angiodysplasia
Polyps
Diverticulosis
Inflammatory bowel disease
Aortoduodenal fistula

notes

genetic testing (Breast cancer [BRCA] and ovarian cancer, Colon cancer, Cardiovascular disease, Tay-Sachs disease, Cystic fibrosis, Melanoma, Hemochromatosis, Thyroid cancer, Paternity [parentage analysis], Forensic genetic testing)

Type of test Blood; miscellaneous

Normal findings No genetic mutation

Test explanation and related physiology

Genetic testing is used to identify a predisposition to disease, to establish the presence of a disease, to establish or refute paternity, or to provide forensic evidence used in criminal investigations. As research progresses and the Human Genome Project provides more information, precise and accurate methods of identification of normal and mutated genes are becoming more common.

Tests for defective genes known to be associated with certain diseases are now commonly used in screening people who have certain phenotypes and family histories compatible with a genetic mutation. Genetic testing is done in addition to a family history (pedigree). Whereas a family history is not always reliable, accurate, or available, genetic testing is very accurate in its determination of risks. Preventive medicine or surgery can be provided to eliminate disease development. Reproductive counseling and pregnancy prevention can preclude the conception of children who are likely to suffer the consequence of disease.

The ethics and disadvantages to this genetic testing are presently being discussed. Patients may face financial discrimination for health or life insurance or employment if the results are positive. The Health Insurance Portability and Accountability Act (HIPAA) protects patients from discrimination based on genetic information. This testing may be expensive and not covered by insurance. The information obtained by testing may cause great emotional turmoil in affected individuals or their family. The information obtained by medical genetic testing should be shared with the patient only. If the patient chooses to allow others to know the information, the patient must direct that release of information. Voluntary genetic testing should always be associated with aggressive counseling and support. Because of the potential changes in life for other family members, each person receiving the genetic information must be counseled separately.

Breast cancer and ovarian cancer genetic testing

Inherited mutations in BRCA (BReast CAncer) genes indicate an increased susceptibility for development of breast cancer. The two genes in which mutations are most commonly seen are BRCA1 and BRCA2. The BRCA1 gene exists on chromosome 17, and BRCA2 is on chromosome 13. These genes encode tumor suppressor proteins. More than half of women who inherit mutations will develop breast cancer by the age of 50 compared with less than 2% of women without the genetic defect. (See Table 18.)

The BRCA genes also confer an increased susceptibility for ovarian cancer. In the normal population, less than 2% of women develop ovarian cancer by age 70. Of women with mutations of the BRCA1 gene, 44% develop ovarian cancer by that age. Ovarian cancer is less commonly associated with the BRCA2 gene (20%). Furthermore, a woman with a BRCA mutation who has already had breast cancer has a 65% chance of developing a

TABLE 18 Who should be tested for BRCA mutations?

Patient with breast cancer	Family history (with at least one characteristic)
Diagnosed at <40 years of age	• No other family history
Diagnosed around 50 years of age with 2 primary breast cancers	• 1 relative around 50 years of age with breast cancer • 1 relative with ovarian cancer
Diagnosed at any age	• 2 relatives with ovarian cancer • 2 relatives with breast cancer • Male with breast cancer • Personal history of ovarian cancer • Ashkenazi Jewish heritage • 1st/2nd degree relative with BRCA mutation
Male breast cancer at any age	• 1 relative with breast cancer or ovarian cancer • Ashkenazi Jewish heritage • 1st/2nd degree relative with BRCA mutation

contralateral breast cancer in her lifetime (compared with less than 15% of women without the genetic defect). A woman with breast cancer and a BRCA genetic defect has a 10 times greater risk of developing ovarian cancer as a second primary cancer when compared with similar women without the mutated form of the gene.

These mutations have an autosomal dominant inheritance pattern, indicating that women who inherit just one genetic defect can develop the phenotypic cancers. Men with BRCA genetic mutations (most commonly BRCA2) are at an increased risk for the development of breast, prostate, and colon cancer. In addition, they can pass the mutation to their daughters. Because BRCA is an autosomal dominant gene, 50% of the children are at risk.

Colon cancer genetic testing

There are multiple forms of colon cancer strongly associated with family history. These genetic defects are inherited in an autosomal dominant fashion and are important for genome mismatch repair.

The most common form is familial adenomatous polyposis (FAP). The patient presents with over one hundred polyps in his or her colon—one or more of which may degenerate into cancer. FAP is caused by a genetic mutation in the 5q 21-22 (APC) gene on chromosome 5. These genes encode tumor suppression proteins. Less common forms of polyposis syndromes include attenuated FAP (AFAP) and MYH associated polyposis (MAP). MAP is associated with mutations in the MYH gene.

Hereditary nonpolyposis colorectal cancer (HNPCC) syndrome is also known as Lynch syndrome. These patients are more difficult to recognize because they may have few polyps. HNPCC is associated most often with mutations (defective DNA mismatch repair) of MLH1, MLH2, and MSH6. HNPCC is associated with several other cancers (endometrial, gastric, and ovarian).

Tay-Sachs disease genetic testing

Tay-Sachs disease is a GM2 gangliosidosis characterized by the onset of severe mental and developmental retardation in the first few months of life. Affected children become totally debilitated by 2 to 5 years of age and die by ages 5 to 8. Another form of the same disease is *late-onset Tay-Sachs* or chronic GM2, also known as gangliosidosis. The basic defect in affected patients is a mutation in the hexosaminidase A gene, which is on chromosome 15. This gene is responsible for the synthesis of hexosaminidase (HEX), an enzyme that normally breaks down a fatty substance called GM2 gangliosides. Ashkenazi (Eastern European) Jews and non-Jewish French Canadians, particularly those in the Cajun population in Louisiana, are affected most. This gene is inherited as an autosomal recessive gene. Carriers have one affected gene. Affected individuals have both defective genes. A *carrier couple* has a 25% chance of having a child affected with the disease.

At present there is no treatment for the disease; it is important to identify carriers so that reproductive counseling can be provided. HEX A protein testing (p. 513) has been extremely effective for identification of carriers and affected individuals. Both the test for the protein and that for the gene mutation are performed on a blood sample or on chorionic villus samples obtained during amniocentesis (p. 49).

Cystic fibrosis genetic testing

Cystic fibrosis (CF) is caused by a mutation in the cystic fibrosis transmembrane conductance regulator (CFTR) gene located on chromosome 7. This gene encodes the synthesis of a protein that serves as a channel through which chloride enters and leaves some types of epithelial cells. A mutation in this gene alters the cell's ability to regulate the chloride transport (p. 246).

Currently more than 1000 mutations can cause CF; several dozens of these account for 90% of the mutations in European Americans. However, the most common mutation, which accounts for 70% of the CF cases, is known as Delta F508.

CF is an autosomal recessive disease. A carrier has one mutated CFTR gene. The person affected by CF has mutations on both copies of CFTR. Genetic testing is now used to identify both carriers of CF and neonates with the disease, as well as to detect fetal disease during pregnancy. The sweat chloride test (p. 875) is more easily performed and is a cheaper way to diagnose the disease in affected children. The use of genetic testing for CF is often limited to those with a family history of CF, partners of CF patients, and pregnant couples with a family history of CF. The main purpose of CF genetic testing is to identify carriers who could conceive a child with CF.

It is important to recognize that not all patients who have a CFTR genetic mutation will develop the disease. Furthermore, because not all mutations that may cause CF can be detected, a negative test does not necessarily eliminate the possibility of being affected by the disease. Genetic testing can be performed on blood samples or on samples taken during chorionic villus sampling (CVS, p. 254) or during amniocentesis (p. 49).

Melanoma genetic testing

Recent progress in the genetics of cutaneous melanoma has led to the identification of two melanoma susceptibility genes:

- The tumor suppressor gene CDKN2A encoding the p16 protein on chromosome 9 p21
- The CDK4 gene on chromosome 12 q13

The p16 genetic mutation is by far the most common form of hereditary melanoma. Characteristics of familial melanoma include frequent multiple primary melanomas, early age of onset of first melanoma, and frequently the presence of atypical or dysplastic nevi (moles). Family members with the following characteristics may consider testing for p16 genetic mutations:

- Multiple diagnoses of primary melanoma
- Two or more family members with melanoma
- Melanoma and pancreatic cancer
- Melanoma and a personal or family history of multiple atypical nevi
- Relatives of a patient with a confirmed p16 genetic mutation

Approximately 20% to 40% of families with three or more affected first-degree relatives show inheritance of mutations in the p16 gene. Fifteen percent of patients with multiple melanoma will have a p16 mutation. The average age at diagnosis is 35 years for those with a mutation in p16 versus 57 years in the general population. P16 carriers also have an increased risk for pancreatic cancer.

Hemochromatosis genetic testing

The diagnosis of hemochromatosis is traditionally made by using serum iron studies. When hereditary hemochromatosis (HH) is suspected, mutation analysis of the *hemochromatosis-associated HFE genes* (*C282Y* and *H63D*) is done. HH is an iron overload disorder that is considered to be the most common inherited disease in Caucasians; it affects 1 in 500 individuals. Increased intestinal iron absorption and intracellular iron accumulation lead to progressive damage of the liver, heart, pancreas, joints, reproductive organs, and endocrine glands. Without therapy, males may develop symptoms between 40 and 60 years of age and women after menopause.

A large, but as yet undefined, fraction of homozygotes for this disease do not develop clinical symptoms (i.e., penetrance is low). Patients with symptoms and early biochemical signs of iron overload consistent with HH should be tested. Relatives of individuals with HH should also be studied. HFE genotyping could improve disease outcomes of the disease. Serum iron markers are monitored at more frequent intervals if an HFE mutation is detected and phlebotomy therapy is initiated earlier. Early initiation of phlebotomy therapy reduces the frequency or severity of hemochromatosis-related symptoms and organ damage.

Thyroid cancer genetic testing

The RET proto-oncogene, located on chromosome subband 10 q11.2, encodes a receptor tyrosine kinase expressed in tissues and tumors derived from the neural crest. Genetic testing for RET germline mutations has shown 100% sensitivity and specificity for identifying those at risk for developing inherited medullary thyroid cancer (multiple endocrine neoplasia [MEN] 2 A, MEN 2 B, or familial medullary thyroid carcinoma [FMTC]).

Use of the genetic assay allows earlier and more definitive identification and clinical management of those with a risk for FMTC. FMTC is surgically curable if detected before it has spread to regional lymph nodes. However, lymph node involvement at diagnosis may be found in up to 75% of patients for whom a thyroid nodule is the first sign of disease. Thus, there is an emphasis on early detection and intervention in families that are affected by MEN types 2 A and 2 B and FMTC, which account for one fourth of medullary thyroid cancer cases.

Cardiac genetic testing

Mutations in sarcomeric genes cause early onset cardiac channelopathies and cardiomyopathies. These are rare but potentially lethal heart conditions that include long QT syndrome (LQTS), catecholaminergic polymorphic ventricular tachycardia (CPVT), hypertrophic cardiomyopathy (HCM), arrhythmogenic right ventricular cardiomyopathy, and dilated cardiomyopathy (DCM). Patients with a sarcomeric gene mutation are nearly three times more likely to suffer an adverse cardiac outcome (cardiovascular death, nonfatal ischemic stroke, or progression to severe heart failure). Identifying patients with these genetic mutations can help diagnose a patient's disease, guide treatment options, and determine whether family members are at risk.

Paternity genetic testing (parentage analysis)

DNA testing is the most accurate form of testing to prove or exclude paternity when the identity of the biological father of a child is in doubt. By comparing DNA variants in the mother and child, it is possible to determine variants that the child inherited from the biological mother. Thus, any remaining DNA variation must have come from the biological father. If the DNA from the tested man is found to contain these paternal characteristics, then the probability of paternity can be determined. Testing is more than 99% accurate.

Testing is so reliable that it is admissible in court. Testing can be done on a mouth swab or blood. Results are usually available in 1 to 3 weeks.

Many parents are given misinformation at the time of twin births as to whether the twins are identical or fraternal. DNA samples from siblings can be analyzed to indicate whether twins are identical or fraternal with an accuracy of greater than 99%.

Unfortunately, prenatal testing of the fetal components for paternity testing requires invasive testing such as chorionic villus sampling or amniocentesis. There are times, particularly in circumstances of rape, when early pregnancy paternity identification is desired. *Noninvasive prenatal paternity testing* can now be performed accurately by extracting and amplifying fetal chromosome alleles from maternal blood.

Forensic genetic testing

Forensic DNA testing is used with increasing frequency in today's courtrooms because of its accuracy. In a courtroom, the reliability of the evidence can protect the individual and society as a whole. Furthermore, DNA testing can be so conclusive that it often motivates plea-bargaining and thereby reduces court time. It can quickly establish guilt or innocence beyond a reasonable doubt. Because DNA does not change and deteriorates very slowly even after death, testing can be performed on any body part, cadaver, or live person. Specimens considered adequate for DNA testing include blood, teeth, semen, saliva, bone, nails, skin scrapings, and hair. Forensic testing is also used for body identification.

Contraindications

- Patients who are not emotionally able to deal with the results

Procedure and patient care

Before

PT Explain the procedure to the patient.

PT Tell the patient that no fasting is required.

- It is recommended that all patients who undergo testing receive genetic counseling.

PT Tell the patient the time it will take to have the results back.

PT Inform the patient of the high costs of genetic testing and that it may not be covered by all medical insurance plans.

During

- Obtain the specimen in a manner provided by the specialized testing laboratory.
- **Blood:** A venous blood sample is collected in a lavender-top tube. Cord blood can be used for infants.
- **Buccal swab:** A cotton swab is placed between the lower cheek and gums. It is twisted and then placed on a special paper or in a special container. Usually two to four swabs are requested.
- **Amniotic fluid:** At least 20 mL of fluid is preferred.
- **Chorionic villus sampling:** 10 mg of cleaned villi are sent as prescribed by the testing laboratory.
- **Product of conception:** 10 mg of placental tissue are preserved in a sterile medium.
- **Other body parts:** As much tissue as is available is sent for testing.

After

- Apply pressure or a pressure dressing to the venipuncture site.
- Make sure that the patient has an appointment scheduled for obtaining the results. It is very upsetting for a patient and family to wait for the results.
- Arrangements should be made to ensure genetic and emotional counseling after results are obtained.

Abnormal findings

Genetic carrier state
Affected state

notes

gliadin, endomysial, and tissue transglutaminase antibodies

Type of test Blood

Normal findings

	Age	Normal
Gliadin IgA/IgG	0-2 years	<20 EU
	3 years and older	<25 EU
Endomysial IgA	All	Negative
Tissue transglutaminase IgA	All	<20 EU

Test explanation and related physiology

Gliadin and gluten are proteins found in wheat and wheat products. Patients with celiac disease cannot tolerate ingestion of these proteins or any products containing wheat. These proteins are toxic to the mucosa of the small intestine and cause characteristic pathologic lesions. These patients experience severe intestinal malabsorption symptoms. The only treatment is for the patient to abstain from wheat and wheat-containing products.

When an affected patient ingests wheat-containing foods, gluten and gliadin build up in the intestinal mucosa. These gliadin and gluten proteins (and their metabolites) cause direct mucosal damage. Furthermore, IgA immunoglobulins (antigliadin, antiendomysial, and antitissue transglutaminase [tTG-ab]) are made, appearing in the gut mucosa and in the serum of severely affected patients. The identification of these antibodies in the blood of patients with malabsorption is helpful in supporting the diagnosis of celiac sprue or dermatitis herpetiformis. However, a definitive diagnosis of celiac disease can be made only when a patient with malabsorption is found to have the pathologic intestinal lesions characteristic of celiac disease. Also, the patient's symptoms must be improved with a gluten-free diet. Both are needed for the diagnosis. Because of the high specificity of IgA endomysial antibodies (EMA) for celiac disease, the test may obviate the need for multiple small bowel biopsies to verify the diagnosis. This may be particularly advantageous in the pediatric population, including the evaluation of children with failure to thrive.

In patients with known celiac disease, these antibodies can be used to monitor disease status and dietary compliance. Furthermore, these antibodies identify successful treatment because they will become negative in patients on a gluten-free diet.

Interfering factors

- Other GI diseases (e.g., Crohn disease, colitis, and severe lactose intolerance) can cause elevated gliadin antibodies.

Procedure and patient care

- See inside front cover for Routine Blood Testing.
- Fasting: no.
- Blood tube commonly used: red.
- Obtain a list of foods that have been ingested in the last 48 hours.
- Assess how many malabsorption symptoms the patient has been experiencing in the last few weeks.

Abnormal findings

Celiac disease
Celiac sprue
Dermatitis herpetiformis

notes

glucagon

Type of test Blood

Normal findings 50-100 pg/mL or 50-100 ng/L (SI units)

Test explanation and related physiology

Glucagon is a hormone secreted by the alpha cells of the pancreatic islets of Langerhans. It is secreted in response to hypoglycemia and increases the blood glucose. As serum glucose levels rise in the blood, glucagon is inhibited by a negative feedback mechanism.

Elevated glucagon levels may indicate the diagnosis of a *glucagonoma* (i.e., an alpha islet cell neoplasm). Glucagon deficiency occurs with extensive pancreatic resection or with burned-out pancreatitis. Arginine is a potent stimulator of glucagon. If glucagon levels fail to rise even with arginine infusion, a diagnosis of glucagon deficiency as a result of pancreatic insufficiency is confirmed.

In an insulin-dependent patient with diabetes, glucagon stimulation caused by hypoglycemia does not occur. To differentiate the causes of glucagon insufficiency between pancreatic insufficiency and diabetes, *arginine stimulation* is performed. Patients with diabetes will have an exaggerated elevation of glucagon with arginine. In pancreatic insufficiency, glucagon is not stimulated with arginine. Furthermore, in patients with diabetes, hypoglycemia fails to stimulate glucagon release as would occur in a nondiabetic person.

Because glucagon is thought to be metabolized by the kidneys, renal failure is associated with high glucagon and, as a result, high glucose levels. When rejection of a transplanted kidney occurs, one of the first signs of rejection may be increased serum glucagon levels.

Interfering factors

- Test results may be invalidated if a patient has undergone a radioactive scan within the previous 48 hours.
- Levels may be elevated after prolonged fasting or moderate to severe exercise.
- ✘ Drugs that may cause *increased* levels include some amino acids (e.g., arginine), danazol, gastrin, glucocorticoids, insulin, and nifedipine.
- ✘ Drugs that may cause *decreased* levels include atenolol, propranolol, and secretin.

Procedure and patient care
- See inside front cover for Routine Blood Testing.
- Fasting: yes.
- Blood tube commonly used: lavender.

Abnormal findings

▲ **Increased levels**
  Familial hyperglucagonemia
  Glucagonoma
  Diabetes mellitus
  Chronic renal failure
  Severe stress including
    infection, burns, surgery,
    and acute hypoglycemia
  Acromegaly
  Hyperlipidemia
  Acute pancreatitis
  Pheochromocytoma

▼ **Decreased levels**
  Idiopathic glucagon
    deficiency
  Cystic fibrosis
  Chronic pancreatitis
  Postpancreatectomy
  Cancer of the pancreas
  Diabetes mellitus

G

notes

glucose, blood (Blood sugar, Fasting blood sugar [FBS])

Type of test Blood

Normal findings

Cord: 45-96 mg/dL or 2.5-5.3 mmol/L (SI units)
Premature infant: 20-60 mg/dL or 1.1-3.3 mmol/L
Neonate: 30-60 mg/dL or 1.7-3.3 mmol/L
Infant: 40-90 mg/dL or 2.2-5.0 mmol/L
Child <2 years: 60-100 mg/dL or 3.3-5.5 mmol/L
Child >2 years to adult:
    Fasting: 70-110 mg/dL or <6.1 mmol/L (Fasting is defined as no caloric intake for at least 8 hours.)
    Casual: ≤200 mg/dL (<11.1 mmol/L) (Casual is defined as any time of day regardless of food intake.)
Adult: 74-106 mg/dL or 4.1-5.9 mmol/L
Elderly:
    60-90 years: 82-115 mg/dL or 4.6-6.4 mmol/L
    >90 years: 75-121 mg/dL or 4.2-6.7 mmol/L

Possible critical values

Adult male: <50 and >400 mg/dL
Adult female: <40 and >400 mg/dL
Infant: <40 mg/dL
Newborn: <30 and >300 mg/dL

Test explanation and related physiology

Through an elaborate feedback mechanism, glucose levels are controlled by insulin and glucagon. In the fasting state, glucose levels are low. In response, glucagon is secreted. Glucagon causes glucose levels to rise.

After eating, glucose levels are elevated. Insulin is secreted. Insulin drives glucose into the cells to be metabolized to glycogen, amino acids, and fatty acids. Blood glucose levels diminish. Other hormones, such as adrenocorticosteroids, adrenocorticotropic hormone, epinephrine, growth hormone, and thyroxine, can also affect glucose metabolism.

Serum glucose levels must be evaluated according to the time of day they are performed. For example, a glucose level of 135 mg/dL may be abnormal if the patient is in the fasting state, but this level would be within normal limits if the patient had eaten a meal within the previous hour.

In general, true glucose elevations indicate diabetes mellitus; however, one must be aware of many other possible causes of hyperglycemia. Similarly, hypoglycemia has many causes. The most common cause is inadvertent insulin overdose in patients with brittle diabetes. If diabetes is suspected by elevated fasting blood levels, glycosylated hemoglobin (p. 483) or glucose tolerance tests (p. 479) can be performed.

Glycosylated hemoglobin (page 483) is now being performed more frequently to identify diabetes because this blood test represents blood sugar levels over the previous 120 days. That being said, the diagnosis of diabetes should be confirmed with a repeat of the same tests initially performed but on a different day to guard against laboratory error.

Glucose determinations must be performed frequently in new patients with diabetes to monitor closely and adjust the insulin dosage to be administered. Fingerstick blood glucose determinations are often performed before meals and at bedtime. Patients with diabetes can then adjust their insulin doses of rapid-acting subcutaneous insulin.

For patients with diabetes who experience recurrent episodes of severe hypoglycemia or who require more than three doses of insulin per day, minimally invasive glucose monitoring is available. A small, sterile, disposable glucose-sensing device is inserted into the subcutaneous tissue (usually the arm). This sensor measures the change in glucose in the interstitial fluid. This information is recorded in a small beeper-sized monitor for 3 to 4 days. The monitor is taken to the doctor's office, where it is connected to a standard personal computer. Specialized software then downloads the stored information, and a more effective insulin regimen can be developed.

Interfering factors

- Many forms of stress (e.g., general anesthesia, cerebrovascular accident, myocardial infarction, shock, strenuous exercise, burns) can cause increased serum glucose levels.
- Many pregnant women experience some degree of glucose intolerance. If significant, it is called gestational diabetes.
- Most IV fluids contain dextrose, which is quickly converted to glucose. Therefore, most patients receiving IV fluids will have *increased* glucose levels.
- Drugs that may cause *increased* levels include antidepressants (tricyclics), antipsychotics, beta-adrenergic blocking agents, corticosteroids, cyclosporine, dextrose IV infusion, dextrothyroxine, diazoxide, diuretics, epinephrine, estrogens, glucagon, isoniazid, lithium, niacin, phenothiazines, phenytoin, salicylates (acute toxicity), triamterene, and statins.

✄ Drugs that may cause *decreased* levels include acetaminophen, alcohol, alpha-glucosidase inhibitors, anabolic steroids, biguanides, clofibrate, disopyramide, gemfibrozil, incretin mimetics, insulin, meglitinides, monoamine oxidase inhibitors, pentamidine, propranolol, sulfonylureas, and thiazolidinediones.

Procedure and patient care

- See inside front cover for Routine Blood Testing.
- Fasting: yes.
- Blood tube commonly used: red or gray.
- **PT** For FBS, instruct the patient to fast for 8 hours. Water is permitted.
- **PT** To prevent starvation, which may artificially raise the glucose levels, tell the patient not to fast much longer than 8 hours.
- Withhold insulin or oral hypoglycemics until after blood is obtained.
- Glucose levels also can be evaluated by performing a finger stick and using either a *visually read test* or a *reflectance meter*. The advantage of the visually read test is that it does not require an expensive machine. However, the patient must be able to visually interpret the color of the reagent strip. Using reflectance meters (e.g., glucometer, Accu-Chek bG, Stat-Tek) improves the accuracy of the blood glucose determination.

Abnormal findings

▲ **Increased levels (hyperglycemia)**
Diabetes mellitus
Acute stress response
Cushing syndrome
Pheochromocytoma
Chronic renal failure
Glucagonoma
Acute pancreatitis
Diuretic therapy
Corticosteroid therapy
Acromegaly

▼ **Decreased levels (hypoglycemia)**
Insulinoma
Hypothyroidism
Hypopituitarism
Addison disease
Extensive liver disease
Insulin overdose
Starvation

notes

glucose, postprandial (2-Hour postprandial glucose [2-Hour PPG], 1-Hour glucose screen)

Type of test Blood

Normal findings

2-Hour PPG
  0-50 years: <140 mg/dL or <7.8 mmol/L (SI units)
  50-60 years: <150 mg/dL
  60 years and older: <160 mg/dL
1-Hour glucose screen for gestational diabetes
  <140 mg/dL

Test explanation and related physiology

For this study, a meal acts as a glucose challenge to the body's metabolism. Normally, insulin is secreted immediately after a meal in response to the elevated blood glucose level, causing the level to return to the premeal range within 2 hours. In patients with diabetes, the glucose level usually is still elevated 2 hours after the meal. The PPG is an easily performed screening test for diabetes mellitus. If the results are greater than 140 mg/dL and less than 200 mg/dL, a glucose tolerance test (GTT, p. 479) may be performed to confirm the diagnosis. If the 2-hour PPG is greater than 200 mg/dL, a diagnosis of diabetes mellitus is confirmed.

The *1-hour glucose screen* is used to detect gestational diabetes mellitus (GDM). The detection and treatment of GDM may reduce the risk for several adverse perinatal outcomes (e.g., excessive fetal growth and birth trauma, fetal death, and neonatal morbidity).

Screening for GDM is performed with a 50- to 100-g oral glucose load, followed by a glucose level determination 1 hour later. This is called the *O'Sullivan test*. Screening is done between weeks 24 and 28 of gestation. However, patients with risk factors, such as a previous history of GDM, may benefit from earlier screening. Patients whose serum glucose levels equal or exceed 140 mg/dL may be evaluated by a 3-hour glucose tolerance test (p. 479). A 100-g oral glucose load is indicated for the diagnosis of gestational diabetes when results of the 50-g oral glucose load 1-hour screening test are abnormal.

Interfering factors

- Stress can increase glucose levels.
- If the patient is not able to eat the entire test meal or vomits some or all of the meal, levels will be falsely decreased.

Procedure and patient care

- See inside front cover for Routine Blood Testing.
- Fasting: yes.
- Blood tube commonly used: red or gray.
- **PT** For the *2-hour PPG*, instruct the patient to eat the entire meal (with at least 75 g of carbohydrates) and then not to eat anything else until the blood is drawn.
- For the *1-hour glucose screen for GDM*, give the fasting or non-fasting patient a 50-g oral glucose load.
- **PT** Instruct the patient not to smoke during the testing. Smoking may increase glucose levels.
- **PT** Inform the patient that he or she should rest during the 1- or 2-hour interval.

Abnormal findings

▲ **Increased levels**
  Diabetes mellitus
  Gestational diabetes mellitus
  Malnutrition
  Hyperthyroidism
  Acute stress response
  Cushing syndrome
  Pheochromocytoma
  Chronic renal failure
  Glucagonoma
  Diuretic therapy
  Corticosteroid therapy
  Acromegaly
  Extensive liver disease

▼ **Decreased levels**
  Insulinoma
  Hypothyroidism
  Hypopituitarism
  Addison disease
  Insulin overdose
  Malabsorption or
    maldigestion

notes

glucose tolerance test (GTT, Oral glucose tolerance test [OGTT])

Type of test Blood; urine

Normal findings

Plasma test

Fasting: <110 mg/dL or <6.1 mmol/L (SI units)
1 hour: <180 mg/dL or <10.0 mmol/L
2 hours: <140 mg/dL or <7.8 mmol/L

Urine test

Negative

Test explanation and related physiology

A diagnosis of diabetes mellitus can be made on the basis of the results from two tests—fasting blood glucose (p. 474) and GTT—performed on separate days that are close in time. The American Diabetes Association (ADA), the International Diabetes Federation, and the European Association for the Study of Diabetes all suggest that two abnormal glycosylated hemoglobin assays should be used whenever possible instead of the fasting glucose and GTT. Nevertheless, the GTT is used when diabetes is suspected (retinopathy, neuropathy, diabetic-type renal diseases). It is also suggested for the following:

- Patients with a family history of diabetes
- Patients who are markedly obese
- Patients with a history of recurrent infections
- Patients with delayed healing of wounds (especially on the lower legs or feet)
- Women who have a history of delivering large babies, stillbirths, or neonatal births
- Patients who have transient glycosuria or hyperglycemia during pregnancy or following myocardial infarction, surgery, or stress

In the GTT, the patient's ability to tolerate a standard oral glucose load (usually 75 g of glucose) is evaluated by obtaining plasma and urine specimens for glucose level determinations before glucose administration and then at 1 hour and 2 hours afterward. Normally, there is a rapid insulin response to the ingestion of a large oral glucose load. This response peaks in 30 to 60 minutes and returns to normal in about 3 hours. Patients with an appropriate insulin response are able to tolerate the glucose load quite easily, with only a minimal and transient rise in plasma glucose levels within 1 to 2 hours after ingestion. In normal patients, glucose does not spill over into the urine.

Patients with diabetes will not be able to tolerate this load. As a result, their serum glucose levels will be greatly elevated from 1 to 5 hours (Figure 22). Also, glucose can be detected in their urine. It is important to note that intestinal absorption may vary among individuals. For this reason, some centers prefer the glucose load to be administered intravenously.

The ADA recommends that pregnant women who have not previously had an abnormal GTT be tested at weeks 24 and 28 of gestation with a 75-g dose of glucose. A glucose level of more than 180 mg/100 mL one hour later is consistent with gestational diabetes.

Glucose intolerance also may exist in patients with oversecretion of hormones that have an ancillary effect on glucose, as in patients with Cushing syndrome, pheochromocytoma, acromegaly, aldosteronism, or hyperthyroidism. Patients with chronic renal failure, acute pancreatitis, myxedema, type IV lipoproteinemia, infection, or cirrhosis can also have an abnormal GTT. Certain drugs can also cause abnormal GTT results, as discussed in the interfering factors section.

The GTT also is used to evaluate patients with reactive hypoglycemia. This may occur as late as 5 hours after the initial glucose load.

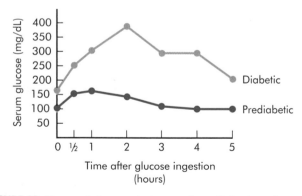

FIGURE 22 Glucose tolerance test curve for a diabetic and a prediabetic patient.

Contraindications
- Patients with serious concurrent infections or endocrine disorders, because glucose intolerance will be observed even though these patients may not have diabetes

Potential complications
- Dizziness, tremors, anxiety, sweating, euphoria, or fainting during testing.
  If these symptoms occur, a blood specimen is obtained. If the glucose level is too high, the test may need to be stopped and insulin administered.

Interfering factors
- Smoking during the testing period stimulates glucose production because of the nicotine.
- Stress (e.g., from surgery, infection) can increase glucose levels.
- Exercise during the testing can affect glucose levels.
- Fasting or reduced caloric intake before GTT can cause glucose intolerance.
- ✗ Drugs that may cause glucose intolerance include antihypertensives, antiinflammatory drugs, aspirin, beta-blockers, furosemide, nicotine, oral contraceptives, psychiatric drugs, steroids, and thiazide diuretics.

Procedure and patient care
Before
- PT Explain the procedure to the patient.
- PT Educate the patient about the importance of having adequate food intake with adequate carbohydrates (150 g) for at least 3 days before the test.
- PT Instruct the patient to fast for 12 hours before the test.
- PT Instruct the patient to discontinue drugs (including tobacco) that could interfere with the test results. This should be done in consultation with the physician.
- PT Give the patient written instructions explaining the pretest dietary requirement.
- Obtain the patient's weight to determine the appropriate glucose loading dose (especially in children).

During
- Obtain fasting blood and urine specimens.
- Administer the prescribed oral glucose solution, usually a 75- to 100-g carbohydrate load.

- Give pediatric patients a carbohydrate load based on their body weight.
- ^{PT} Instruct the patient to ingest the entire glucose load.

PT Tell the patient that he or she cannot eat anything until the test is completed. However, encourage the patient to drink water. No other liquids should be taken.

PT Inform the patient that tobacco, coffee, and tea are not allowed because they cause physiologic stimulation.

- Collect a venous blood sample in a gray-top tube at 30 minutes and at hourly periods. Apply pressure or a pressure dressing to the sites.
- Collect urine specimens at hourly periods.
- Mark on the tubes the time that the specimens are collected.
- Assess the patient for such reactions as dizziness, sweating, weakness, and giddiness. (These are usually transient.)
- For the IV-GTT, administer the glucose load intravenously over 3 to 4 minutes.

After

- Send all specimens promptly to the laboratory.
- Allow the patient to eat and drink normally.
- Administer insulin or oral hypoglycemics if ordered.
- Apply pressure to the venipuncture site.

Abnormal findings

Diabetes mellitus
Acute stress response
Cushing syndrome
Pheochromocytoma
Chronic renal failure
Glucagonoma
Acute pancreatitis
Diuretic therapy
Corticosteroid therapy
Acromegaly
Myxedema
Somogyi response to hypoglycemia
Postgastrectomy

notes

glycosylated hemoglobin (GHb, GHB, Glycohemoglobin, Glycolated hemoglobin, Hemoglobin [HbA$_{1c}$], Diabetic control index)

Type of test Blood

Normal findings

Nondiabetic adult/child: 4%-5.9%
Good diabetic control: <7%
Fair diabetic control: 8%-9%
Poor diabetic control: >9%
(Values vary with laboratory method used.)

Test explanation and related physiology

This test is used to diagnose and monitor diabetes treatment. It measures the amount of hemoglobin A$_{1c}$ (HbA$_{1c}$) in the blood and provides an accurate long-term index of the patient's average blood glucose level. In adults, about 98% of the hemoglobin in the red blood cells (RBCs) is hemoglobin A. About 7% of hemoglobin A consists of a type of hemoglobin (HbA$_1$) that can combine strongly with glucose in a process called *glycosylation*. When glycosylation occurs, it is not easily reversible.

HbA$_1$ is actually made up of three components: A$_{1a}$, A$_{1b}$, and A$_{1c}$. HbA$_{1c}$ is the component that combines most strongly with glucose. Therefore, HgA$_{1c}$ is the most accurate measurement because it contains the majority of glycosylated hemoglobin. If the total HbA$_1$ is measured, its value is 2% to 4% higher than the HbA$_{1c}$ component.

The amount of glycosylated hemoglobin (glycohemoglobin [GHb]) depends on the amount of glucose available in the bloodstream over an RBC's 120-day life span. Therefore, determination of the GHb value reflects the average blood sugar level for the 100- to 120-day period before the test. The more glucose the RBC was exposed to, the greater the GHb percentage. One important advantage of this test is that the sample can be drawn at any time because it is not affected by short-term variations (e.g., food intake, exercise, stress, hypoglycemic agents).

As mentioned, the average life span of an RBC is 120 days, so the GHb may not reflect more recent changes in glucose levels. Because the turnover rate of proteins is much faster than hemoglobin, the measurement of serum *glycated proteins* (e.g., *glycated albumin* or *fructosamine*) provides more recent information about glucose levels. Glycated proteins reflect an average blood glucose level of the past 15 to 20 days. Although an initial single

G

glycated protein result may not separate good glucose control from poor control, serial testing provides a much better indication of glucose control.

The GHb or glycated protein tests are particularly beneficial for the following:

- Evaluating patient compliance and success of treatment
- Comparing and contrasting the success of past and new forms of diabetic therapy
- Determining the duration of hyperglycemia in patients with newly diagnosed diabetes
- Providing a sensitive estimate of glucose imbalance in patients with mild diabetes
- Individualizing diabetic control regimens
- Providing a feeling of reward for many patients when the test shows achievement of good diabetic control
- Evaluating the diabetic patient whose glucose levels change significantly day to day (brittle diabetic)
- Differentiating short-term hyperglycemia in patients who do not have diabetes (e.g., recent stress or myocardial infarction) from those who have diabetes (where the glucose has been persistently elevated)

A diagnosis of diabetes mellitus can be made on the basis of the results from two tests—fasting blood glucose (p. 474) and GTT—performed on separate days that are close in time. The American Diabetes Association (ADA), the International Diabetes Federation, and the European Association for the Study of Diabetes all indicate that two abnormal GHb assays should be used whenever possible instead of the fasting glucose and GTT.

By a relatively simple calculation, GHb can be accurately correlated with the daily *mean plasma glucose (MPG)* level, which is the average glucose level throughout the day. This has been very helpful for diabetics and health care professionals in determining and evaluating daily glucose goals. Each 1% change in GHb represents a change of approximately 35 mg/dL MPG. See Table 19.

Interfering factors

- Hemoglobinopathies can affect results because the quantity of hemoglobin A (and, as a result, HbA_1) varies considerably.
- Falsely elevated values occur when the RBC life span is lengthened.
- Abnormally low levels of proteins may falsely indicate normal glycated protein levels despite high glucose levels.
- Ascorbic acid may falsely indicate low levels of fructosamine.

TABLE 19   Correlation between GHb and MPG

A_{1c}(%)	Approximate MPG (mg/dL)	Interpretation
4	65	Nondiabetic range
5	100	Nondiabetic range
6	135	Nondiabetic range
7	170	ADA target
8	205	Action suggested

Procedure and patient care

- See inside front cover for Routine Blood Testing.
- Fasting: no.
- Blood tube commonly used: gray or lavender.

Abnormal findings

▲ **Increased levels**
   Newly diagnosed diabetic patient
   Poorly controlled diabetic patient
   Nondiabetic hyperglycemia (e.g., acute stress response, Cushing syndrome, pheochromocytoma, glucagonoma, corticosteroid therapy, or acromegaly)
   Splenectomized patients
   Pregnancy

▼ **Decreased levels**
   Hemolytic anemia
   Chronic blood loss
   Chronic renal failure

notes

growth hormone (GH, Human growth hormone [HGH], Somatotropin hormone [SH])

Type of test   Blood

Normal findings

Men: <5 ng/mL (mcg/L [SI units])
Women: <10 ng/mL (mcg/L [SI units])
Children:
   Newborn: 5-23 ng/mL (mcg/L [SI units])
   1 week: 2-27 ng/mL (mcg/L [SI units])
   1-12 mos: 2-10 ng/mL (mcg/L [SI units])
   >1 year female: 0-10 ng/mL (mcg/L [SI units])
   >1 year male: 0-6 ng/mL (mcg/L [SI units])

Test explanation and related physiology

This test is used to identify growth hormone (GH) deficiency in adolescents who have short stature, delayed sexual maturity, or other growth deficiencies. It is also used to document the diagnosis of GH excess in gigantic or acromegalic patients. GH is used to identify and follow patients with ectopic growth hormone production by neoplasm. Finally, it is often used as a screening test for pituitary hypofunction or hyperfunction.

Because GH release is episodic, a random measurement of GH is unreliable to predict GH deficiency in adolescents. Measurement of free IGF 1 and IGF BP 3 (see Insulin-Like Growth Factor, p. 556) is preferred in cases of short stature.

GH, or somatotropin, is secreted by the acidophilic cells in the anterior pituitary gland. It plays a central role in modulating growth from birth until the end of puberty. GH exerts its effects on many tissues through a group of peptides called *somatomedins*. The most commonly tested somatomedin is somatomedin C (also known as IGF-1), which is produced by the liver and has its major effect on cartilage.

If GH secretion is insufficient during childhood, limited growth and dwarfism may result. Also, a delay in sexual maturity may be a result in adolescents with reduced GH levels. Conversely, overproduction of GH during childhood results in gigantism, with the person sometimes reaching nearly 7 to 8 feet in height. An excess of GH during adulthood (after closure of long bone end plates) results in acromegaly, which is characterized by an increase in bone thickness and width but no increase in height.

Normal GH levels overlap significantly with deficient levels. Low GH levels may indicate deficiency or may be normal for certain individuals at certain times of the day. To negate time variables in GH testing, GH can be drawn 1 to 1 1/2 hours after deep sleep has occurred. Levels increase during sleep. Also, strenuous exercise can be performed for 30 minutes in an effort to stimulate GH production.

To negate the common variations in GH secretion, screening for *insulin-like growth factor (IGF-1)* or *somatomedin C* (p. 556) provides a more accurate reflection of the mean plasma concentration of growth hormone. These proteins are not affected by the time of day or food intake like GH is. A *GH stimulation test* (p. 489) can be performed to evaluate the body's ability to produce GH. *Growth hormone suppression testing* is used to identify gigantism in children or acromegaly in the adult. If GH can be suppressed to <2 ng/mL, neither of these conditions exists. The most commonly used suppression test is the oral glucose tolerance test (p. 479). GH is normally suppressed when the glucose level increases. In acromegalic patients, only a slight decrease in GH occurs.

Interfering factors

- Random measurements of GH are not adequate determinants of GH deficiency, because hormone secretion is episodic.
- GH secretion is increased by stress, exercise, and low blood glucose levels.
- Drugs that may cause *increased* levels include amphetamines, arginine, dopamine, estrogens, glucagon, histamine, insulin, levodopa, methyldopa, and nicotinic acid.
- Drugs that may cause *decreased* levels include corticosteroids and phenothiazines.

Procedure and patient care

Before

PT Explain the procedure to the patient.
- The patient should not be emotionally or physically stressed because this can increase GH levels.
- It is preferred that the patient be fasting and well rested. Water is permitted.
- For *GH suppression testing*, the patient is kept NPO after midnight.

During
Growth hormone test
- Collect a venous blood sample in a red-top tube.
- Because approximately two-thirds of the total release of GH occurs during sleep, GH secretion also can be measured during hospitalization by obtaining blood samples while the patient is sleeping.

Growth hormone suppression test
- Obtain peripheral venous access with Normal saline solution.
- Obtain baseline GH and glucose levels as described previously.
- Administer the prescribed dose of glucose over 5 minutes.
- Obtain GH and glucose levels at 10, 60, and 120 minutes after glucose ingestion.

After
- Indicate the patient's fasting status and the time the blood is collected on the laboratory slip. Include the patient's recent activity (e.g., sleeping, walking, eating).
- Send the blood to the laboratory immediately after collection.

Abnormal findings

▲ **Increased levels**
Gigantism
Acromegaly
Diabetes mellitus
Anorexia nervosa
Stress
Major surgery
Hypoglycemia
Starvation
Deep-sleep state
Exercise

▼ **Decreased levels**
Pituitary insufficiency
Dwarfism
Hyperglycemia
Failure to thrive
Growth hormone
  deficiency

notes

growth hormone stimulation test (GH provocation test, Insulin tolerance test [ITT], Arginine test)

Type of test Blood

Normal findings Growth hormone levels >10 ng/mL or >10 mcg/L (SI units)

Insulin-like growth factor 1 (IGF1) >80 ng/mL

Test explanation and related physiology

Because growth hormone (GH, p. 486) secretion is episodic, a random measurement of plasma GH is not adequate to make a diagnosis of GH deficiency. IGF-1 screening (page 556) followed by GH stimulation is indicated for children and adults suspected of GH deficiency. To diagnose GH deficiency, GH stimulation tests are sometimes needed. One of the most reliable GH stimulators is insulin-induced hypoglycemia, in which the blood glucose declines to less than 40 mg/dL. Other GH stimulants include vigorous exercise and drugs (e.g., arginine, clonidine, glucagon, levodopa). Glucagon is more widely used for GH stimulation because of safety concerns with insulin-induced hypoglycemia).

Usually a *double-stimulated test* is performed using an arginine infusion followed by insulin-induced hypoglycemia. A GH concentration of more than 10 mcg/L after stimulation effectively excludes the diagnosis of GH deficiency. Hypothyroidism should be excluded prior to GH stimulation testing.

Contraindications

- Patients with epilepsy
- Patients with cerebrovascular disease
- Patients with myocardial infarction
- Patients with low basal plasma cortisol levels

Potential complications

- Hypoglycemia so significant and severe as to cause ketosis, acidosis, and shock
  With close observation, this is unlikely.

Procedure and patient care

Before
- **PT** Explain the procedure very carefully to the patient and, if appropriate, to the parents.
- **PT** Instruct the patient to remain NPO after midnight on the morning of the test. Water is permitted.

During
- Note the following procedural steps:
  1. A saline lock IV line is inserted for the administration of medications and for the withdrawal of frequent blood samples.
  2. Baseline blood levels are obtained for GH, glucose, and cortisol.
  3. Venous samples for GH are obtained at 60 and 90 minutes after injection of arginine, insulin, or glucagon.
  4. Blood glucose levels are monitored at 30-minute intervals with a glucometer. The blood sugar should drop to less than 40 mg/dL for effective measurement of GH reserve.
- Monitor the patient for signs of hypoglycemia, postural hypotension, somnolence, diaphoresis, and nervousness. Ice chips are often given during the test for patient comfort.
- This procedure is usually performed by a nurse with a physician in proximity.
- This test takes approximately 2 hours to perform.
- **PT** Tell the patient that the minor discomfort associated with this test results from the insertion of the IV line and the hypoglycemic response induced by the insulin injection.
- GH also can be stimulated by vigorous exercise. This entails running or stair-climbing for 20 minutes. Blood samples of GH are obtained at 0, 20, and 40 minutes.

After
- Observe the venipuncture site for bleeding.
- Send the blood to the laboratory immediately after collection.
- Give the patient cookies and punch or an IV glucose infusion.
- **PT** Inform the patient and family that results may not be available for approximately 7 days. Some laboratories run GH tests only once per week.

Abnormal findings
Growth hormone deficiency
Pituitary deficiency

notes

haptoglobin

Type of test Blood

Normal findings

Adult: 50-220 mg/dL or 0.5-2.2 g/L (SI units)
Newborn: 0-10 mg/dL or 0-0.1 g/L (SI units)

Possible critical values <40 mg/dL

Test explanation and related physiology

The serum haptoglobin test is used to detect intravascular destruction (lysis) of red blood cells (RBCs), also called *hemolysis*. Haptoglobins, which are glycoproteins produced by the liver, are powerful, free hemoglobin–binding proteins. In hemolytic anemias associated with the hemolysis of RBCs, the released hemoglobin is quickly bound to haptoglobin, and the new complex is quickly catabolized. This results in a diminished amount of free haptoglobin in the serum; this decrease cannot be quickly compensated for by normal liver production. As a result, the patient demonstrates a transient, reduced level of haptoglobin in the serum. Megaloblastic anemias can reduce the haptoglobin level because of increased destruction of megaloblastic RBC precursors in the bone marrow.

Haptoglobins are also decreased in patients with primary liver disease not associated with hemolytic anemias. This occurs because the diseased liver is unable to produce these glycoproteins. Hematoma can reduce haptoglobin levels by the absorption of hemoglobin into the blood and binding with haptoglobin.

Elevated haptoglobin concentrations are found in many inflammatory diseases and can be used as a nonspecific acute-phase protein in much the same way as a sedimentation rate test is used (p. 393). That is, levels of haptoglobin increase with severe infection, inflammation, tissue destruction, acute myocardial infarction, burns, and some cancers.

Interfering factors

- A slight decrease in haptoglobin levels is noted in normal pregnancy.
- Ongoing infection can cause falsely elevated test results.
- ✗ Drugs that may cause *increased* haptoglobin levels include androgens and steroids.

- Drugs that may cause *decreased* levels include chlorpromazine, diphenhydramine, indomethacin, isoniazid, nitrofurantoin, oral contraceptives, quinidine, and streptomycin.

Procedure and patient care

- See inside front cover for Routine Blood Testing.
- Fasting: no.
- Blood tube commonly used: red.

Abnormal findings

▲ **Increased levels**
Collagen vascular disease
Infection
Tissue destruction
Biliary obstruction
Nephritis
Pyelonephritis
Ulcerative colitis
Peptic ulcer
Myocardial infarction
Acute rheumatic disease
Neoplasia

▼ **Decreased levels**
Hemolytic anemia
Transfusion reactions
Prosthetic heart valves
Systemic lupus erythematosus
Primary liver disease not associated with hemolytic anemia
Hemolytic disease of the newborn
Hematoma
Tissue hemorrhage
Megaloblastic anemia
Severe malnutrition

notes

Heinz body preparation

Type of test Blood

Normal findings No Heinz bodies detected

Test explanation and related physiology

Heinz bodies are water-insoluble precipitates of oxidated-denatured hemoglobin that form within red blood cells (RBCs). They occur as a result of exposure to oxidative chemicals and drugs. Mutations of hemoglobin, thalassemias, and defects in the hemoglobin reductive defense system against oxidation lead to an enhanced tendency toward oxidative hemolysis. The diagnosis of these problems can be established by the detection of Heinz bodies in RBCs.

Heinz bodies are often associated with hemolytic anemias and the presence of spherocytosis. The pathophysiology of these anemias starts with oxidative injury to hemoglobin. As a result, RBC inclusions (Heinz bodies) of variable size and usually eccentric location adhere to the RBC membrane. Smooth movement of the membrane over the cytosol is reduced. These RBCs are selectively blocked from leaving the splenic cords and entering the sinuses. Splenic macrophages attack these RBCs and cause hemolysis.

Procedure and patient care

- See inside front cover for Routine Blood Testing.
- Fasting: no.
- Blood tube commonly used: lavender, pink, or green.

Abnormal findings

▲ **Increased levels**

Unstable hemoglobinopathies (e.g., Hb Gun Hill)
Red blood cell enzymopathies (e.g., G6PD)
Thalassemia
Heinz body hemolytic anemia

notes

Helicobacter pylori testing (Anti-*Helicobacter pylori* antibody, *Campylobacter*-like organism [CLO] test, *H. pylori* stool antigen)

Type of test Blood; microscopic examination of antral or duodenal biopsy specimen; breath test; stool

Normal findings

Blood test

IgM	IgG
≤30 U/mL (negative)	<0.75 (negative)
30.01-39.99 U/mL (equivocal)	0.75-0.99 (equivocal)
≥40 U/mL (positive)	≥1 (positive)

Breath test No evidence of *H. pylori*

Stool test No evidence of *H. pylori*

Test explanation and related physiology

H. pylori, a bacterium found in the mucus overlying the gastric mucosa and in the mucosa (cells that line the stomach), is a risk factor for gastric and duodenal ulcers, chronic gastritis, or even ulcerative esophagitis. This gram-negative bacillus is also a class I gastric carcinogen. Gastric colonization by this organism has been reported in about 90% to 95% of patients with a duodenal ulcer, in 60% to 70% of patients with a gastric ulcer, and in about 20% to 25% of patients with gastric cancer.

Approximately 10% of healthy persons younger than age 30 have gastric colonization with *H. pylori*. Gastric colonization increases with age, with people older than age 60 having rates at a percentage similar to their age. Most patients with gastric colonization by *H. pylori* remain asymptomatic and never develop ulceration. Testing should only be performed on symptomatic patients because a large percentage of *H. pylori*–colonized individuals could have positive results. It is estimated that as many as 40% to 60% of asymptomatic Caucasians older than 60 years are colonized with this bacteria and are without disease.

There are several methods of detecting the presence of this organism. The organism can be cultured from a specimen of mucus obtained through a gastroscope (p. 401). The organism can also be detected on a gastric mucosal biopsy (from the antrum and greater curvature of the corpus). This is very accurate.

The gold standard for diagnosis of *H. pylori* disease is identifying the infected tissue by Gram, silver, Giemsa, or acridine orange stains.

It often takes several weeks before the results from cultures are available. It is preferable to start treatment before that time on a patient with symptomatic or active ulcer disease. For that reason, *rapid urease testing* for *H. pylori* was developed. *H. pylori* can break down large quantities of urea because of its ability to produce great amounts of an enzyme called urease. In the *CLO test*, a small piece of gastric mucosa (obtained through gastroscopy) is placed onto a specialized testing gel. If *H. pylori* organisms are present in the gastric mucosa, the urease (made by the *H. pylori*) will change the colors of the test material.

A *breath test* is also available for the detection of *H. pylori*. In the breath test, radioactive carbon (^{13}C) is administered orally. The urea is absorbed through the gastric mucosa, where, if *H. pylori* is present, the urea will be converted to $^{13}CO_2$ (where the carbon is radiolabeled). The $^{13}CO_2$ is then taken up by the capillaries in the stomach wall and delivered to the lungs. There the $^{13}CO_2$ is exhaled.

Although *H. pylori* does not survive in the stool, an enzyme-linked immunosorbent assay (ELISA) using a polyclonal anti-*H. pylori*–capture antibody can detect the presence of *H. pylori* antigen in a fresh stool specimen. Negative results indicate the absence of detectable antigen but do not eliminate the possibility of infection due to *H. pylori*.

Serologic testing is an inexpensive and noninvasive way of screening and diagnosing *H. pylori* infection. It is also used as a supportive diagnostic where no preparation or abstinence from antacids is required. The IgG anti-*H. pylori* antibody is most commonly used. It becomes elevated 2 months after infection and stays elevated for more than 1 year after treatment. The IgA anti-*H. pylori* antibody, like IgG, becomes elevated 2 months after infection but decreases 3 to 4 weeks after treatment. The IgM anti-*H. pylori* antibody is the first to become elevated (about 3 to 4 weeks after infection) and is not detected 2 to 3 months after treatment. These antibody titers are fast becoming the gold standard for *H. pylori* detection. These antibodies can be detected with the use of a small amount of blood obtained by finger stick. Serologic testing is often used several months after treatment in order to document cure of *H. pylori* infection. Serologic testing is also used to corroborate the findings of other *H. pylori* testing methods.

H

Contraindications

- Patients who are pregnant or are children
  The breath tests use radioactive carbon to which children should not be exposed.

Interfering factors

- *H. pylori* can be transmitted by contaminated endoscopic equipment during endoscopic procedures.
- ✔ Rapid urease tests can be falsely negative if the patient uses antacid therapy within the week prior to testing.

Procedure and patient care

Before

- **PT** Explain the procedure to the patient.
- **PT** Tell the patient that no fasting is required for the blood test.
- If a biopsy or culture will be obtained by endoscopy, see discussion of esophagogastroduodenoscopy (EGD, p. 401).
- If culture is to be performed, be sure the patient has not had any antibiotic, antacid, or bismuth treatment for 5 to 14 days prior to the endoscopy.

During

- Collect a venous blood sample according to the protocol of the laboratory performing the test.
- A gastric or duodenal biopsy can be obtained by endoscopy. Keep the specimen moist by the addition of approximately 5 mL of sterile saline.
- For the breath test, a dose of radioactive ^{14}C or nonradioactive ^{13}C urea is given by mouth.

After

- Apply pressure to the venipuncture site.
- If endoscopy was used to obtain a culture, see procedure for EGD (p. 401). The specimen should be transported to the laboratory within 30 minutes after collection.

Abnormal findings

▲ **Increased levels**
  Acute and chronic gastritis
  Duodenal ulcer
  Gastric ulcer
  Gastric carcinoma

notes

hematocrit (Hct, Packed red blood cell volume, Packed cell volume [PCV])

Type of test Blood

Normal findings

Male: 42%-52% or 0.42-0.52 volume fraction (SI units)
Female: 37%-47% or 0.37-0.47 volume fraction (SI units)
Pregnant female: >33%
Elderly: values may be slightly decreased
Children (%)
    Newborn: 44-64
    2-8 weeks: 39-59
    2-6 months: 35-50
    6 months-1 year: 29-43
    1-6 years: 30-40
    6-18 years: 32-44

Possible critical values <15% or >60%

Test explanation and related physiology

The Hct is a measure of the percentage of the total blood volume that is made up by the red blood cells (RBCs). The height of the RBC column is measured after centrifugation. It is compared with the height of the column of the total whole blood (Figure 23). The ratio of the height of the RBC column compared with the original total blood column is multiplied by 100%. This is the Hct value. It is routinely performed as part of a complete blood count. The Hct closely reflects the hemoglobin (Hgb) and RBC values. The Hct in percentage points usually is approximately three times the Hgb concentration in grams per deciliter when RBCs are of normal size and contain normal amounts of Hgb.

Abnormal values indicate the same pathologic states as abnormal RBC counts and Hgb concentrations (p. 500). Decreased levels indicate anemia (reduced number of RBCs). Increased levels can indicate erythrocytosis. Like other RBC values, the Hct can be altered by many factors, such as hydration status and RBC morphology.

Interfering factors

- Abnormalities in RBC size may alter Hct values.
- Extremely elevated white blood cell (WBC) counts may affect values.
- Hemodilution and dehydration may affect the Hct level.

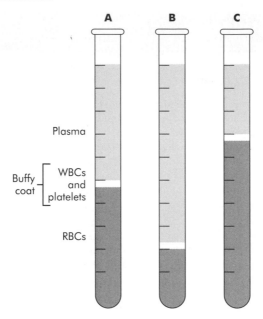

FIGURE 23 Tubes showing hematocrit levels of normal blood, blood with evidence of anemia, and blood with evidence of polycythemia. Note the buffy coat located between the packed red blood cells (RBCs) and the plasma. **A,** A normal percentage of RBCs. **B,** Anemia (low percentage of RBCs). **C,** Polycythemia (high percentage of RBCs).

- Pregnancy usually causes slightly decreased values because of hemodilution.
- Living in high altitudes causes increased values.
- Values may not be reliable immediately after hemorrhage.
- ✗ Drugs that may cause *decreased* levels include chloramphenicol and penicillin.

Procedure and patient care

- See inside front cover for Routine Blood Testing.
- Fasting: no.
- Blood tube commonly used: lavender.

Abnormal findings

▲ **Increased levels**
Congenital heart disease
Polycythemia vera
Severe dehydration
Erythrocytosis
Eclampsia
Burns
Chronic obstructive
pulmonary disease

▼ **Decreased levels**
Anemia
Hyperthyroidism
Cirrhosis
Hemolytic reaction
Hemorrhage
Dietary deficiency
Bone marrow failure
Normal pregnancy
Rheumatoid arthritis
Multiple myeloma
Leukemia
Hemoglobinopathy
Prosthetic valves
Renal disease
Lymphoma
Hodgkin disease

H

notes

hemoglobin (Hb, Hgb)

Type of test Blood

Normal findings

Male: 14-18 g/dL or 8.7-11.2 mmol/L (SI units)
Female: 12-16 g/dL or 7.4-9.9 mmol/L (SI units)
Pregnant female: >11 g/dL
Elderly: values are slightly decreased
Children
    Newborn: 14-24 g/dL
    0-2 weeks: 12-20 g/dL
    2-6 months: 10-17 g/dL
    6 months–1 year: 9.5-14 g/dL
    1-6 years: 9.5-14 g/dL
    6-18 years: 10-15.5 g/dL

Possible critical values <5.0 g/dL or >20 g/dL

Test explanation and related physiology

The Hgb concentration is a measure of the total amount of Hgb in the peripheral blood, which reflects the number of red blood cells (RBCs) in the blood. The test is normally performed as part of a complete blood count. Hgb serves as a vehicle for oxygen and carbon dioxide transport.

The hematocrit (Hct) in percentage points usually is approximately three times the Hgb concentration in grams per deciliter when RBCs are of normal size and contain normal amounts of Hgb. Abnormal values indicate the same pathologic states as abnormal RBC counts and Hct concentrations (pp. 497). Decreased levels indicate anemia (reduced number of RBCs). Increased levels can indicate erythrocytosis. In addition, however, changes in plasma volume are more accurately reflected by the Hgb concentration. Slight decreases in the values of Hgb and the Hct during pregnancy reflect both the expanded blood volume due to a chronic state of overhydration and an increased number of RBCs. Hemoglobinopathies, such as sickle cell disease and Hgb C disease, are also associated with reduced Hgb levels.

Interfering factors

- Slight Hgb decreases normally occur during pregnancy because of the expanded blood volume.
- Living in high-altitude areas causes high Hgb values.
- Heavy smokers have higher levels than nonsmokers.

- Drugs that may cause *increased* levels include gentamicin and methyldopa.
- Drugs that may cause *decreased* levels include antibiotics, antineoplastic drugs, aspirin, indomethacin, rifampin, and sulfonamides.

Procedure and patient care

- See inside front cover for Routine Blood Testing.
- Fasting: no.
- Blood tube commonly used: lavender.

Abnormal findings

▲ **Increased levels**
Congenital heart disease
Polycythemia vera
Hemoconcentration of the blood
Chronic obstructive pulmonary disease
Congestive heart failure
High altitudes
Severe burns
Dehydration

▼ **Decreased levels**
Anemia
Hemorrhage
Hemolysis
Hemoglobinopathies
Nutritional deficiency
Lymphoma
Systemic lupus erythematosus
Sarcoidosis
Kidney disease
Chronic hemorrhage
Splenomegaly
Neoplasia

notes

hemoglobin electrophoresis (Hgb electrophoresis)

Type of test Blood

Normal findings

Adult/elderly: percentage of total hemoglobin

Hgb A_1: 95%-98%

Hgb A_2: 2%-3%

Hgb F: 0.8%-2%

Hgb S: 0%

Hgb C: 0%

Hgb E: 0%

Children: Hgb F

Newborn: 50%-80%

<6 months: <8%

>6 months: 1%-2%

Test explanation and related physiology

Hgb electrophoresis is a test that identifies and quantifies normal and abnormal forms of Hgb (hemoglobinopathies). Although many different forms of Hgb have been described, the more common types are A_1, A_2, F, S, E, and C. Each major Hgb type is electrically charged to varying degrees. When Hgb from lysed RBCs is placed on electrophoresis paper and placed in an electromagnetic field, the Hgb variants migrate at different rates and spread apart from each other. The migrations of the various forms of Hgb make up a series of bands on the paper. The bands correspond to the various forms of Hgb present. The pattern of bands is compared with normal and other well-known abnormal patterns. Furthermore, each band can be quantitated as a percentage of the total Hgb, indicating the severity of any recognized abnormality.

The form *Hgb A_1* constitutes the major component of Hgb in the normal RBC. *Hgb A_2* is only a minor component (2% to 3%) of the normal Hgb total. *Hgb F* is the major hemoglobin component in a fetus but normally exists in only minimal quantities in a normal adult. Levels of Hgb F greater than 2% in patients older than age 3 are considered abnormal. Hgb F is able to transport oxygen when only small amounts of oxygen are available (as in fetal life). In patients requiring compensation for prolonged chronic hypoxia (as in congenital cardiac abnormalities), Hgb F may be found in increased levels to assist in the transport of the available oxygen.

Hgb S and *Hgb C* are abnormal forms of Hgb that occur predominantly in African Americans. Hgb E occurs predominantly in Southeast Asians. The Hgb contents of some common disorders affecting Hgb, as determined by electrophoresis, are indicated in Table 20 (p. 504). Hgb E is produced less efficiently by RBC precursors; if there is an increased Hgb E content in the RBCs, those cells will have a low mean corpuscular volume (MCV, p. 788).

Quantifying abnormal hemoglobins is helpful in determining the zygosity of a familial hemoglobinopathy. Furthermore, quantification of abnormal hemoglobin proteins provides a method of monitoring treatments designed to increase more effective hemoglobin variants and decrease abnormal variants.

Interfering factors

- Blood transfusions within the previous 12 weeks may alter test results.
- Glycosylated hemoglobin can blur the peak of Hgb F and cause falsely low levels of Hgb F.

Procedure and patient care

- See inside front cover for Routine Blood Testing.
- Fasting: no.
- Blood tube commonly used: lavender.

Abnormal findings

Sickle cell disease
Sickle cell trait
Hemoglobin C disease
Hemoglobin H disease
Thalassemia major
Thalassemia minor
Hemoglobin E disease

notes

TABLE 20 Hemoglobin contents of some common hemoglobinopathies

| | Percentage range | | | | | | |
	Hgb A$_1$	Hgb A$_2$	Hgb F	Hgb S	Hgb H	Hgb C	Hgb E
Sickle cell disease	0	2-3	2	95-98	0	0	0
Sickle cell trait	50-65	2-3	2	35-45	0	0	0
Hemoglobin C disease	0	2-3	2	0	0	90-100	0
Three gene deletion α-Thalassemia (Hgb H disease)	65-90	0.3-1.5	0.6-4.5	0	0-30	0	0
β-Thalassemia major	0	0-15	85-100	0	0	0	0
β-Thalassemia trait	50-85	4-8	1-5	0	0	0	0
Hemoglobin E disease	0	0	0	0	0	0	100

hepatitis virus studies

Type of test Blood

Normal findings Negative

Test explanation and related physiology

Hepatitis is an inflammation of the liver caused by viruses, alcohol ingestion, drugs, toxins, or overwhelming bacterial sepsis. The three common viruses now recognized to cause disease are hepatitis A, hepatitis B, and hepatitis C (also called non-A/non-B) viruses. Hepatitis D and E viruses are much less common in the United States. Hepatitis D can infect the liver only by entering into a hepatitis B virus, which it uses as a carrying vehicle. Therefore, hepatitis D cannot cause disease unless patients have hepatitis B virus in their bloodstream in the active, chronic, or carrier forms. The clinical presentations are similar in that they all include low-grade fever, malaise, anorexia, and fatigue. Most often they are all associated with elevations of hepatocellular enzymes, such as aspartate aminotransferase (AST) and alanine aminotransferase (ALT).

Hepatitis A virus (HAV) was originally called *infectious hepatitis.* It has a short incubation period of 2 to 6 weeks and is highly contagious. During active infection, HAV is excreted in the stool and transmitted via oral-fecal contamination of food and drink. Most infections are not associated with symptoms severe enough to warrant medical evaluation. IgG and IgM antibodies to HAV are routinely used when HAV infection is suspected.

The first HAV antibody to appear is the IgM antibody *(HAV-Ab/IgM)* in approximately 3 to 4 weeks after exposure or just before hepatocellular enzyme elevations occur. These IgM levels usually return to normal in approximately 8 weeks. The next HAV antibody to rise is IgG *(HAV-Ab/IgG),* which appears approximately 2 weeks after the IgM begins to increase and slowly returns to normal levels. The IgG antibody can remain detectable for more than 10 years after the infection. If the IgM antibody is elevated in the absence of the IgG antibody, acute hepatitis is suspected. If, however, IgG is elevated in the absence of IgM elevation, a convalescent or chronic stage of HAV viral infection is indicated.

These antibodies may not be positive soon after infection occurs, which delays the investigation of infectious outbreaks. The HAV virus can be detected directly by measuring *HAV RNA* in the sera of patients suspected of acute infection.

Hepatitis B virus (HBV) is commonly known as *serum hepatitis*. It has a long incubation period of 5 weeks to 6 months. HBV is most frequently transmitted by blood transfusion; however, it also can be contracted via exposure to other body fluids. HBV may cause a severe and unrelenting form of hepatitis culminating in liver failure and death. The incidence is increased among blood transfusion recipients, male homosexuals, dialysis patients, transplant patients, IV drug abusers, and patients with leukemia or lymphoma. Hospital personnel are also at increased risk of infection mostly due to needlestick contamination.

HBV, also called the *Dane particle*, is made up of an inner core surrounded by an outer capsule. The outer capsule contains the *hepatitis B surface antigen (HBsAg)*, formerly called *Australian antigen*. The inner core contains *HBV core antigen (HBcAg)*. The *hepatitis B e-antigen (HBeAg)* is also found in the core. Antibodies to these antigens are called HBsAb, HBcAb, and HBeAb. The tests used to detect these antigens and antibodies include (Table 21):

- *Hepatitis B surface antigen (HBsAg)*. This is the most frequently and easily performed test for hepatitis B, and it is the first test to become abnormal. HBsAg rises before the onset of clinical symptoms, peaks during the first week of symptoms, and returns to normal by the time jaundice subsides. HBsAg generally indicates active infection by HBV. If the level of this antigen persists in the blood, the patient is considered to be a carrier or have chronic active hepatitis.
- *Hepatitis B surface antibody (HBsAb)*. This antibody appears approximately 4 weeks after the disappearance of the surface antigen and signifies the end of the acute infection phase. HBsAb also signifies immunity to subsequent infection. Concentrated forms of this agent constitute the hyperimmunoglobulin given to patients who have come in contact with HBV-infected patients. HBsAb is the antibody that denotes immunity after administration of hepatitis B vaccine.
- *Hepatitis B core antigen (HBcAg)*. No tests are currently available to detect this antigen.
- *Hepatitis B core antibody (HBcAb)*. This antibody appears approximately 1 month after infection with HBsAg and declines (although it remains elevated) over several years. HBcAb is also present in patients with chronic hepatitis. The HBcAb level is elevated during the time lag between the disappearance of HBsAg and the appearance of HBsAb. This interval is called the *core window*. During the core window, HBcAb is the only detectable marker of a recent hepatitis infection.

TABLE 21 Hepatitis testing

Serologic findings	Appearance/disappearance	Application
HAV-Ab/IgM	4-6 weeks/3-4 months	Acute HAV infection
HAV-Ab/IgG	8-12 weeks/10 years	Previous HAV exposure/immunity
HAV RNA	First week of infection	Acute infection/carrier state
HBeAg	1-3 weeks/6-8 weeks	Acute HBV infection/chronic active hepatitis
HBeAb	4-6 weeks/4-6 years	Acute HBV infection ended/precore/core promoter mutant chronic infection
HBsAg	4-12 weeks/1-3 months	Acute/chronic HBV infection
HBsAb total	3-10 months/6-10 years	Previous HBV infection/immunity indicated
HBVc-Ab/IgM	2-12 weeks/3-6 months	Acute HBV infection
HBVc-Ab total	3-12 weeks/life	Previous HBV infection/convalescent stage
HBV DNA	First week of infection	Acute/chronic infection
HCV-Ab/IgG	3-4 months/2 years	Previous HCV infection
HCV RNA	First week of infection	Acute/chronic infection
HDV-Ag	1-3 days/3-5 days	Acute HDV infection/chronic infection
HDV-Ab/IgM	10 days/1-3 months	Acute HDV infection
HDV-Ab total	2-3 months/7-14 months	Chronic HDV infection

H

- *Hepatitis B e-antigen (HBeAg).* This antigen generally is not used for diagnostic purposes but rather as an index of infectivity. The presence of HBeAg correlates with early and active disease, as well as with high infectivity in acute HBV infection. The persistent presence of HBeAg in the blood predicts the development of chronic HBV infection.
- *Hepatitis B e-antibody (HBeAb).* This antibody indicates that an acute phase of HBV infection is over, or almost over, and that infectivity is greatly reduced.

Hepatitis B DNA can be quantified and is a direct measurement of the HBV viral load. A one- or two-log decrease in viral load in a hepatitis B–infected patient means that antiviral therapy is working. A one- or two-log increase in a similar patient means an antiviral has stopped working and that viral resistance may have developed. High levels of HBV DNA, ranging from 100,000 to more than 1 billion viral copies per milliliter, indicate a high rate of HBV replication. Low or undetectable levels, about 300 copies per milliliter or less, indicate an inactive infection. The World Health Organization established the international unit (IU) or copies per milliliter (mL), written as IU/mL or copies/mL, to measure HBV DNA.

Hepatitis C (HCV) (non-A/non-B [NANB] hepatitis) is transmitted in a manner similar to HBV. Most cases of hepatitis C are caused by blood transfusion. The incubation period is 2 to 12 weeks after exposure, and the clinical manifestations of the illness parallel those of HBV. However, unlike with HBV, HCV infection is chronic in more than 60% of infected persons. Although the disease course is variable, it is slowly progressive. Twenty percent of HCV patients develop cirrhosis and hepatocellular cancers associated with this chronic infection.

The screening test for detecting HCV infection is the detection of *anti-HCV antibodies* to HCV recombinant core antigen, NS3 gene, NS4 antigen, and NS5 antigen. The antibodies can be detected within 4 weeks of infection. With *HCV RNA testing*, the HCV virus can be directly detected and quantified. Like HBV DNA testing, HCV RNA viral load is usually expressed as units per milliliter or copies per milliliter. Although a higher viral load may not necessarily be a sign of more severe or more advanced disease, it does correlate with likelihood to respond to treatment. HCV RNA tests can also be used to monitor response to hepatitis C treatment.

Hepatitis D virus (HDV) is known to cause *delta hepatitis.* As stated earlier, HDV must enter the HBV to gain access to the liver and be infective. The patient must have HBV in the blood from a past or synchronously occurring infection. In the United States, this is most commonly transmitted through tainted blood. The *HDV antigen* can be detected by immunoassay within a few days after infection. The IgM and total antibodies to HDV are also detected early in the disease. A persistent elevation of these antibodies indicates a chronic or carrier state.

Hepatitis E virus (HEV) was initially included in the non-A/non-B virus group but was isolated several years ago as an etiologic virus of short incubation. No antigen or antibody tests are currently available.

Procedure and patient care

- See inside front cover for Routine Blood Testing.
- Fasting: no.
- Blood tube commonly used: red.
- Usually a hepatitis profile that includes several HBV antigens and antibodies is performed.

Abnormal findings

▲ **Increased levels**

Hepatitis A

Hepatitis B

Hepatitis C

Chronic carrier state, hepatitis B

Chronic hepatitis B

Hepatitis D

notes

herpes simplex (Herpesvirus types 1 and 2, Herpes simplex virus types 1 and 2 [HSV 1, HSV 2], Herpes genitalis)

Type of test Blood; microscopic

Normal findings

No virus present
No HSV antibodies present

Test explanation and related physiology

HSV can be classified as either type 1 or type 2. *Type 1* is primarily responsible for oral lesions (blisters on the lips, or "cold sores") or even corneal lesions. About half of the patients with HSV 1 develop recurrent infections. HSV 2 is a sexually transmitted viral infection of the urogenital tract. Vesicular lesions may occur on the penis, scrotum, vulva, perineum, perianal region, vagina, or cervix. Initial infections are often associated with generalized symptoms of fever and malaise.

Because most infants become infected if they pass through a birth canal containing HSV, determining its presence at delivery is necessary. Congenital infections may result in problems such as microcephaly, chorioretinitis, and mental retardation in the newborn. Disseminated neonatal herpes virus infections carry a high incidence of infant mortality. A vaginal delivery is possible if no virus is present, but birth by cesarean section is necessary if HSV is present. Viral testing can be performed on males or females to determine the risk for sexual transmission.

Culture is still the standard criterion for HSV. Culture can be performed only during an outbreak. Serologic tests are more easily and conveniently available for detection of HSV 1 and HSV 2 antibodies. *Serologic tests for herpes simplex* are useful to supplement cultures or molecular detection for acute infection. Only about 85% of patients who are culture positive have positive serologies. The advantage of serology tests is that results can be available in a day. Serologic tests for IgG antibodies are available to help differentiate type 1 from type 2 infection. IgG antibodies indicate a previous exposure. IgM antibodies indicate an acute infection but do not differentiate well between types 1 and 2. Perhaps more than 50% of people in the United States have positive herpes antibodies. Serologic tests for antibodies require repeated blood tests during the acute and convalescent phases of an acute viral outbreak (about 2 weeks apart). A fourfold rise in titer is expected to diagnose acute initial herpes infection. Recurrent infections are far less likely to demonstrate titer elevations.

Fresh tissue is the definitive specimen for detection of HSV by molecular detection, particularly in infections involving oral, genital, CNS, ocular, and other sites.

Procedure and patient care

Before

PT Explain the procedure to the patient.

PT Tell the female patient to refrain from douching and tub bathing before the cervical culture is performed.

- Obtain the urethral specimen from the male patient before voiding.

During

- Obtain cultures as follows:

Urethral culture

1. A culture is taken by inserting a sterile swab gently into the anterior urethra (see Figure 40, p. 832) or genital skin lesion of the male patient.
2. Place the male patient in the supine position to prevent falling if vasovagal syncope occurs during introduction of the cotton swab or wire loop into the urethra.
3. The patient is observed for hypotension, bradycardia, pallor, sweating, nausea, and weakness.

Cervical culture

1. The female patient is placed in the lithotomy position, and a vaginal speculum is inserted.
2. Cervical mucus is removed with a cotton ball.
3. A sterile cotton-tipped swab is inserted into the endocervical canal and moved from side to side to obtain the culture. If a genital lesion is present, swabs from that area will be more sensitive in indicating infection.

   o For pregnant women with herpes genitalis, note that the cervix is cultured weekly for the herpes virus beginning 4 to 6 weeks before the due date. Vaginal delivery is possible if the following criteria are met:
   - The two most recent cultures are negative.
   - The woman is not experiencing any symptoms.
   - No lesions are visible on inspection of the vagina and vulva.
   - Throughout pregnancy, the woman has not had more than one positive culture, during which she was symptom free.

Blood for serology

- Obtain a venous blood sample in a red-top tube.

Molecular PCR tissue and other fluids
- Obtain CSF (p. 596) or other fluids by sterile technique as described elsewhere in this book.
- Obtain tissue by appropriate biopsy techniques.
- Place specimen in an appropriate container designated by the reference laboratory.

After

PT Inform the patient how to obtain the test results.

Abnormal findings

Herpesvirus infection

notes

hexosaminidase (Hexosaminidase A, Hex A, Total hexosaminidase, Hexosaminidase A and B)

Type of test Blood

Normal findings

Hexosaminidase A: 7.5-9.8 units/L (SI units)
Total hexosaminidase: 9.9-15.9 units/L (SI units)
(Check with the lab due to the variety of testing methods.)

Test explanation and related physiology

Tay-Sachs disease (TSD) is a lysosomal storage disease (GM2 gangliosidosis), which, in infancy and early childhood, is characterized by loss of motor skills. Death usually occurs by age 4. TSD is a result of a mutation in an autosomal recessive gene. Thus, the affected person must have inherited a mutated gene from each parent in order to have TSD. One of 25 Ashkenazi (Eastern European) Jews is a carrier for a mutation. Eighty different mutations inhibit the function of this important gene. This gene encodes the synthesis of an enzyme called hexosaminidase. Without this enzyme, lysosomes of GM2 accumulate, particularly in the central nervous system.

Two clinically important isoenzymes of hexosaminidase have been detected in the serum: hexosaminidase A (hex A, made up of 1 alpha subunit and 1 beta subunit) and hexosaminidase B (hex B, made up of 2 beta subunits). Any genetic mutation that affects the alpha unit will cause a deficiency of hexosaminidase A, resulting in TSD. A mutation that affects the beta unit will cause a deficiency in hex A and B. Sandhoff disease, an uncommon variant of TSD, occurs with deficiency of both of these enzymes.

Because TSD is uniformly untreatable and fatal, significant effort has gone into the development of biochemical testing to identify carriers of the genetic mutation (persons who carry one of the recessive genetic defective genes). Hex A has been found to be abnormally low in carriers, whereas hex B is high. Therefore, testing for total hexosaminidase is not useful. A carrier has a 25% chance of having a child with TSD if the other biological parent is also a carrier. Pregnancy should occur only with thorough genetic counseling. In communities where the Ashkenazi Jewish population is high, hex A screening has been very effective for identifying carriers. Furthermore, hex A is used to diagnose TSD in infants, young children, and adults. Genetic testing (p. 462) is useful to corroborate the identification of an affected person or a carrier.

H

Interfering factors

- Hemolysis of the blood sample can cause inaccurate test results.
- Pregnancy can cause markedly increased values. For this reason, blood tests are not done during pregnancy.
- ☑ Oral contraceptives can falsely *increase* levels.

Procedure and patient care

- See inside front cover for Routine Blood Testing.
- Fasting: no.
- Blood tube commonly used: red.
- **PT** Emphasize the importance of this test to Jewish couples of Eastern European ancestry who plan to have children. Explain that both must carry the defective gene to transmit TSD to their offspring.
- Professional genetic counseling should be provided to every person considering undergoing this test.
- Check with the lab regarding withholding contraceptives.
- Note that pregnant women can be evaluated by amniocentesis (p. 49) or chorionic villus biopsy (p. 254).
- Note that infants may have blood obtained by heel sticks. Neonates often have blood drawn through the umbilical cord.

Abnormal findings

▼ **Decreased hexosaminidase A**
Tay-Sachs disease

▼ **Decreased hexosaminidase A and B**
Sandhoff disease

notes

HIV drug resistance testing (HIV genotype)

Type of test Blood

Normal findings No resistant HIV

Test explanation and related physiology

There are several factors that affect the success of HIV antiviral medications, including patient compliance, access to adequate care, optimal dosing, and drug pharmacology issues (e.g., absorption, elimination, and drug interactions). Another significant factor that determines a patient's response to antiviral HIV drugs is the percentage of an HIV viral population that is resistant to the drugs that are administered. HIV resistance to therapy develops in 78% of patients. HIV genotyping is able to detect changes in the viral genome that are associated with drug resistance and is particularly able to predict HIV-1 resistance to protease and reverse-transcriptase inhibitor antiretroviral drugs.

HIV genotyping is particularly useful when failure of the most active antiviral therapy is suspected from decreasing CD4 counts (p. 234). HIV genotyping can also be performed in conjunction with *HIV drug sensitivity testing*. HIV sensitivity testing estimates the ability of a cloned copy of the patient's virus to replicate in a cell culture in the presence of a particular antiviral drug. This same testing can help determine the amount of drug needed to inhibit viral replication. It is generally reported as the concentration of drug required to inhibit (inhibiting concentration, IC) viral replication by 50%, or the IC_{50}. This is particularly helpful when considering the use of expensive drugs or where frequent hypersensitivity to a particular drug is possible.

Interfering factors

- If the plasma HIV-1 RNA viral load is less than 1000 HIV-1 RNA copies per mL of plasma, genotyping may be inaccurate.
- Minor HIV-1 populations that are less than approximately 20% of the total population may not be identified by this test.

Procedure and patient care

- See inside front cover for Routine Blood Testing.
- Fasting: no.
- Blood tube commonly used: lavender or pink.

PT Instruct the patient to observe the venipuncture site for infection. Patients with AIDS are immunocompromised and susceptible to infection.

Abnormal findings

Drug resistance

notes

HIV RNA quantification (HIV viral load)

Type of test   Blood

Normal findings   Undetected

Test explanation and related physiology

Quantification of HIV RNA in the blood of patients infected with HIV can be used as an FDA approved or supplementary test after serologic tests (p. 521) are positive. Quantification is also helpful when confirmatory tests are indeterminate or cannot be accurately interpreted. Direct viral testing is helpful in differentiating newborn HIV infection from passive transmission of HIV antibodies from an HIV-infective mother. Finally HIV RNA quantification testing determines HIV viral load. Determining viral load is used:

- Before initiating anti–HIV-1 drug therapy (baseline viral load)
- To identify HIV-1 drug resistance while on anti-HIV therapy
- To identify noncompliance with anti–HIV-1 drug therapy
- To monitor HIV-1 disease progression while on or off anti–HIV-1 drug therapy
- To recommend the initiation of antiretroviral treatment (Table 22)
- To indicate the course of the disease because it is more accurate than any other test, including CD4 T-cell counts (p. 234)
- As a determinant of patient survival (see Table 23).

HIV viral load is most accurately determined by quantifying the amount of genetic material of the virus in the blood. There are several different laboratory methods for measuring HIV viral load. It is important that the same method be used in monitoring the course of the disease. A common method uses a *reverse-transcriptase polymerase chain reaction (RT-PCR)* using gene amplification. This method can quantify HIV-1 or HIV-2 RNA to ranges less than 50 copies/mL.

In general, it is recommended to determine the baseline viral load by obtaining two measurements 2 to 4 weeks apart after HIV infection. Monitoring may continue with testing every 3 to 4 months in conjunction with CD4 counts. Both tests provide data used to determine when to start antiviral treatment. The viral load test can be repeated every 4 to 6 weeks after starting or changing antiviral therapy. Usually, antiviral treatment is continued until the HIV viral load is less than 500 copies/mL. It is

TABLE 22   Recommendations for antiretroviral therapy based on viral load and CD4 count

CD 4 count, ×10⁵/L	HIV RNA viral load, copies/mL		
	<5000	5000–30,000	>30,000
<350	Recommend therapy	Recommend therapy	Recommend therapy
350–500	Consider therapy	Recommend therapy	Recommend therapy
>500	Defer therapy	Consider therapy	Recommend therapy
Symptomatic		Recommend therapy	

TABLE 23   Using the viral load to predict disease course

	HIV RNA viral load, copies/mL					
	<500	501–3000	3001–10,000	10,001–30,000	>30,000
% Developing AIDS	5.4	16.6	31.7	55.2	80
% Dying of AIDS	0.9	6.3	18.1	34.9	69.5

H

important to recognize that a *nondetectible* result does not mean no virus is left in the blood after treatment; it means that the viral load has fallen below the limit of detection by the test. However, the clinical implications of a viral load below 50 copies/mL remain unclear. Possible causes of such a result include very low plasma HIV-1 viral load present (e.g., in the range of 1 to 19 copies/mL), very early HIV-1 infection (i.e., <3 weeks from the time of infection), or absence of HIV-1 infection (i.e., false-positive test result). A significant (greater than threefold) rise of viral load should warrant reevaluation of therapy.

Interfering factors

- Incorrect handling and processing of the specimen can cause inconsistent results.
- Recent vaccinations may affect viral levels.
- Concurrent infections can cause inconsistent results.
- Variable compliance to therapy may alter test results.

Procedure and patient care

- See inside front cover for Routine Blood Testing.
- Fasting: no.
- Blood tube commonly used: lavender.
- Specimens are often sent to a central laboratory.
- **PT** Instruct the patient to observe the venipuncture site for infection. Patients with AIDS are immunocompromised and susceptible to infection.
- **PT** Encourage the patient to discuss his or her concerns regarding the prognostic information that may be obtained by these results.
- Do not give test results over the phone. Increasing viral load results can have devastating consequences.
- Because test results vary according to the laboratory test method, it is important to use the same laboratory method for monitoring the course of the disease.
- Viral loads are usually repeated after starting or changing antiviral therapy. A significant rise in viral load should warrant immediate reevaluation of therapy.

Abnormal findings

HIV infection

notes

HIV serologic and virologic testing (AIDS serology, Acquired immunodeficiency serology, AIDS screen, Human immunodeficiency virus [HIV] antibody test, Western blot test, p24 direct antigen, HIV-RNA viral test)

Type of test Blood or fluid analysis (saliva)

Normal findings No evidence of HIV antigen or antibodies

Test explanation and related physiology

There are two active types of human immunodeficiency viruses, types 1 and 2. HIV-1 is the most prevalent type within the United States and Western Europe while HIV-2 is mostly limited to Western African nations. Serologic testing identifies antibodies developed as a result of HIV-1 or HIV-2 infections. Virologic tests identify RNA (or DNA) specific to HIV. Virologic tests can identify HIV infection in the first 11 days after infection. Serologic tests can identify HIV infection only after about 3 weeks. This 3-week time period is called the *seroconversion window*.

Serologic testing for HIV is divided into "screening tests" and "confirmatory" tests. See Table 24 below.

In the past, serologic screening of patients suspected of having HIV-1 or HIV-2 infection usually began with an HIV antibody "screening test." If positive, a confirmatory test was required to make the diagnosis of HIV infection. HIV serologic qualitative screening tests (for HIV-1 and HIV-2) were used to screen high- and low-risk individuals Box 5, p. 523 or for donor blood products. Because these rapid screening qualitative antibody immunoassays do

TABLE 24   Serologic testing for HIV

Screening tests	Confirmatory/Discriminatory tests
HIV-1 p24 antigen	WB HIV-1 antibody
HIV-1 antibody	WB HIV-2 antibody
HIV-2 antibody	Immunoblot–HIV-2 antibody
HIV-1/HIV-2 antibody	Immunofluoresence HIV-1 antibody (IFA)
Combined HIV-1/ HIV-2+HIV-1 p24 antigen	HIV RNA NAAT qualitative testing
Rapid HIV-1 antibody	
Rapid HIV-2 antibody	
Rapid HIV-1/HIV-2 antibody	

WB, Western blot.

TABLE 25 Centers for Disease Control and Prevention HIV screening recommendations

Who	How often
All adults ages 18-64 years	Once in a lifetime
All adults with known risk factors	Yearly
All pregnant women	Once
Pregnant women at risk for HIV	2nd test in 3rd trimester
Newborns if mother is HIV positive or HIV status is unknown	Frequent repeated testing through 1st 6 months of life

not detect viral antigens, they could not detect infection in its earliest stage (before antibodies are formed). Because some persons who undergo HIV testing do not return to learn their test results, "point of service" rapid HIV antibody serologic screening testing in which results can be available in less than 1 hour are available. This is particularly helpful in urgent or emergent care points of service where HIV transmission could occur from blood or body fluid contamination. Furthermore, rapid antibody testing is helpful during labor in women whose HIV status is unknown. Point-of-care home kits are also available. Confirmatory tests for HIV-1 and HIV-2 antibodies include the Western blot assay and the indirect immunofluorescence assay (IFA). See screening recommendations (Table 25).

The *p24 direct serologic antigen assay* detects the viral protein p24 in the peripheral blood of HIV-infected individuals in which it exists either as a free (core) antigen or complexed to anti-p24 antibodies. The p24 antigen may be detectable as early as 16 days after infection. The p24 antigen test can be used to assess the antiviral activity of anti-HIV therapies. The p24 antigen test can also be used to differentiate active neonatal HIV infection from passive HIV antibody present from the mother's blood. It is also used to detect HIV infection before antibody seroconversion, to detect HIV in donor blood, and to monitor therapy.

The use of oral fluids for serologic HIV testing is as an alternative to serum testing. These HIV-1 antibody tests use *oral mucosal transudate (OMT)*, a serum-derived fluid that enters saliva from the gingival crevice and across oral mucosal surfaces. Another alternative to blood testing is *urine testing for HIV*. Only a spot urine collection is required. Testing urine for HIV antibodies is valuable, especially when venipuncture is inconvenient, difficult, or unacceptable. Insurance companies also commonly

> **BOX 5   Risk factors for HIV infection**
>
> Sexually active male homosexuals
> Bisexual males
> Women with at-risk male partner
> Women with multiple male partners
> IV drug abusers
> Persons receiving blood products containing HIV
> Infants of HIV-positive mothers or mothers of unknown HIV status

use it. It is important to note that all urine HIV tests are detecting antibodies and not the HIV particles. Urine does not contain the virus and is not a body fluid capable of infecting others. *HIV antigen/antibody (Ag/Ab) combination assays* are now available that can detect HIV infection on average 5 to 7 days earlier than assays that only detect antibodies.

The serologic tests described above detect HIV infection based on demonstration of antibodies to HIV or to HIV viral protein (page 23). HIV viral RNA particles can be detected. A person with positive HIV test results does not have AIDS until the patient develops the clinical features of diminished immune ability. Positive confirmatory HIV antibody test results are required under laws in many states to be reported to the departments of health of the respective states in which the patients reside.

Interfering factors

- False-positive results can occur in patients who have autoimmune disease, lymphoproliferative disease, leukemia, lymphoma, syphilis, or alcoholism.
- False-positive results can occur in non-infected pregnant woman.
- HIV-2 infection can cause positive HIV-1/HIV-2 screening antibody test and an indeterminate WB HIV-1 confirmatory test.
- False-negative results can occur in the early incubation stage or end stage of AIDS.

Procedure and patient care

- See inside front cover for Routine Blood Testing.
- Fasting: no.
- Blood tube commonly used: red.
- Obtain an informed consent if required by the institution for all "opt in" testing.

- The blood is often sent to an outside laboratory for testing, although rapid antibody testing kits are becoming increasingly available in hospital laboratories and even in homes.
- If the patient wishes to remain anonymous, use a number with the patient's name; be sure to record it accurately.
- Note that if the serologic test is reactive (i.e., test is positive twice consecutively), the Western blot test is performed on the same blood sample.

PT Instruct the patient to observe the venipuncture site for infection. Patients with AIDS are immunocompromised and susceptible to infection.

- Follow the institution's policy regarding test result reporting. Do not give results over the telephone. Remember that positive results may have devastating consequences, including loss of job, insurance, relationships, and housing.

PT Explain to the patient that a positive Western blot test merely implies HIV infection. It does not mean that the patient has clinical AIDS. Not all patients with positive antibodies will acquire the disease.

PT Encourage patients who test positive to inform their sexual contacts so that they can be tested. Most new cases of HIV infection are transmitted from patients who are unaware of their HIV status.

PT Inform the patient that subsequent sexual contact will put new partners at high risk for contracting AIDS.

Abnormal findings

▲ **Increased levels**
AIDS
HIV infection

notes

Holter monitoring

Type of test Electrodiagnostic

Normal findings Normal sinus rhythm

Test explanation and related physiology

Holter monitoring is a continuous recording of the electrical activity of the heart. This can be performed for periods of up to 72 hours. With this technique, an electrocardiogram (ECG) is recorded continuously on magnetic tape during unrestricted activity, rest, and sleep (Figure 24). The Holter monitor is equipped with a clock that permits accurate time monitoring on the ECG tape. The patient is asked to carry a diary and to record daily activities as well as any cardiac symptoms that may develop during the period of monitoring.

Most units are equipped with an *event marker*. This is a button the patient can push when such symptoms as chest pain, syncope, or palpitations are experienced. This type of monitor is referred to as an *event recorder*.

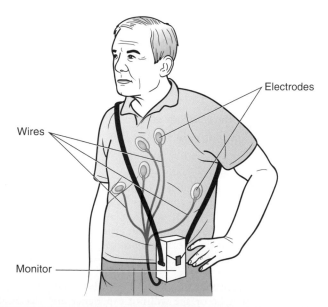

Electrodes

Wires

Monitor

FIGURE 24 Electrical activity of the heart is recorded on a Holter monitor.

The Holter monitor is used primarily to identify suspected cardiac rhythm disturbances and to correlate these disturbances with symptoms (e.g., dizziness, syncope, palpitations, or chest pain). The monitor is also used to assess pacemaker function and the effectiveness of antiarrhythmic medications.

After completion of the determined time period, usually 24 to 72 hours, the Holter monitor is removed from the patient, and the record tape is played back at high speeds. The ECG tracing is usually interpreted by computer, which can detect any significant, abnormal waveform patterns that occurred during the testing.

Implantable loop recorders (ILRs) are used when long-term monitoring is required. These recorders are implanted subcutaneously via a small incision. ILRs can record electrocardiographic tracings continuously or only when purposefully activated by the patient. The ILR can be automatically activated by a predefined arrhythmia that will trigger device recording. If nothing irregular happens, then the information is subsequently erased. But if an arrhythmia does occur, the device locks it in and saves it to memory. ILRs can provide a diagnosis in many patients with unexplained syncope or presyncope.

Contraindications

- Patients who are unable to cooperate with maintaining the lead placement from the monitor to the body
- Patients who are unable to maintain an accurate diary of significant activities or events

Interfering factors

- Interruption in the electrode contact with the skin

Procedure and patient care

Before

PT Explain the procedure to the patient.

PT Instruct the patient about care of the Holter monitor.

PT Inform the patient about the necessity of ensuring good contact between the electrodes and the skin.

PT Teach the patient how to maintain an accurate diary. Stress the need to record significant symptoms.

PT Instruct the patient to note in the diary if any interruption in Holter monitoring occurs.

PT Assure the patient that the electrical flow is coming from the patient and that he or she will not experience any electrical stimulation from the machine.

PT Instruct the patient not to bathe during the period of cardiac monitoring.

PT Tell the patient to minimize the use of electrical devices (e.g., electric toothbrushes, shavers) that may cause artificial changes in the ECG tracing.

During

- Prepare the sites for electrode placement with alcohol. (This is usually done in the cardiology department by a technologist.)
- Place the gel and electrodes at the appropriate sites. Usually the chest and abdomen are the most appropriate locations for limb-lead electrode placement. The precordial leads also may be placed.
- Usually do not use the extremities for electrode placement to minimize alterations in tracing that occur with normal physical activity.

PT Encourage the patient to call if he or she has any difficulties.

After

- Gently remove the tape and other paraphernalia securing the electrodes.
- Wipe the patient clean of electrode gel.

PT Inform the patient when the Holter monitoring interpretation will be available.

Abnormal findings

Cardiac arrhythmia
Ischemic changes

notes

homocysteine (Hcy)

Type of test Blood

Normal findings 4-14 µmol/L

(Levels may increase with age.)

Test explanation and related physiology

Homocysteine is an intermediate amino acid formed during the metabolism of methionine. Increasing evidence suggests that elevated blood levels of homocysteine may act as an independent risk factor for ischemic heart disease, cerebrovascular disease, peripheral arterial disease, and venous thrombosis. Homocysteine appears to promote the progression of atherosclerosis by causing endothelial damage, promoting low-density lipoprotein (LDL) deposition, and promoting vascular smooth muscle growth.

Dietary deficiency of vitamins B_6, B_{12}, or folate is the most common cause of elevated homocysteine. These vitamins are essential for the enzymatic metabolism of homocysteine to methionine (a protein). Because of the relationship of homocysteine to these vitamins, homocysteine blood levels are helpful in the diagnosis of deficiency syndromes associated with these vitamins. Homocysteine levels are elevated in patients with megaloblastic anemia. Some practitioners recommend homocysteine testing in patients with known poor nutritional status (alcoholics, drug abusers) and the elderly. Homocysteine is elevated in children with inborn errors of methionine metabolism. Some researchers believe that elevated levels of homocysteine can be treated by administration of vitamins B_6, B_{12}, and folate.

Both fasting and postmethionine loading levels of homocysteine can be measured. In general, homocysteine levels less than 12 are considered optimal, levels from 12 to 15 are borderline, and levels greater than 15 are associated with high risk of vascular disease. When blood levels are elevated, urine homocysteine levels are also increased.

Contraindications

- Patients whose creatinine levels exceed 1.5 mg/dL are not candidates for methionine loading. Elevated creatinine levels indicate malfunctioning kidneys that cannot effectively filter methionine.

Interfering factors

- Patients with renal impairment have elevated levels of homocysteine due to poor excretion of the protein.

- Men usually have higher levels of homocysteine than women. Most likely, this is due to higher creatinine values and greater muscle mass. Values also increase with age.
- Patients with a low intake of B vitamins have higher levels of homocysteine.
- Smoking is associated with increased homocysteine levels.
- ✠ Drugs that may cause *increased* levels include azaribine, carbamazepine, methotrexate, nitrous oxide, and phenytoin.
- ✠ Oral contraceptives containing estrogen may alter the metabolism of homocysteine.

Procedure and patient care

- See inside front cover for Routine Blood Testing.
- Fasting: yes (10 to 12 hours).
- Blood tube commonly used: purple, green, or blue.
- For *methionine loading*, the patient ingests approximately 100 mg/kg of methionine after fasting for 10 to 12 hours. A blood sample is obtained. Repeat blood samples are collected at 2, 4, 8, 12, and 24 hours to compare levels of B vitamins and amino acids in the plasma.
- In the laboratory, the blood should be spun down within 30 minutes in order to avoid false elevation caused by release of homocysteine from red blood cells (RBCs).

Abnormal findings

▲ **Increased levels**
Cardiovascular disease
Cerebrovascular disease
Peripheral vascular disease
Cystinuria
Vitamin B_6 or B_{12} deficiency
Folate deficiency

notes

human chorionic gonadotropin (hCG, Pregnancy tests, hCG beta subunit)

Type of test   Blood; urine

Normal findings

Negative: <5 IU/L
Indeterminate: 5-25 IU/L
Positive: >25 IU/L
Males and nonpregnant females: <2 IU/L

Test explanation and related physiology

All pregnancy tests are based on the detection of human chorionic gonadotropin (hCG), which is secreted by the placental trophoblast after the ovum is fertilized. hCG appears in the blood and urine of pregnant women within days after conception. In the first few weeks of pregnancy, hCG rises markedly, and serum levels are higher than urine levels. After about 1 month, hCG is about the same in either specimen.

hCG is made up of alpha and beta subunits. The alpha subunit is the same for many other glycoprotein hormones, including TSH, FSH, and LH. The beta subunit is specific for hCG. Immunologic tests are performed by using commercially prepared antibodies against the hCG and its subunits (particularly the beta subunit).

With the development of hCG sandwich-type immunoassay, very small levels of hCG can be detected, and pregnancy can be determined 3 to 7 days after conception. Furthermore, this method eliminates any crossover reactivity with other non-hCG glycoprotein hormones and thereby increases accuracy and specificity. The diagnostic cutoff for pregnancy is >25 IU/L. Values between 5 and 25 IU/L are indeterminate for pregnancy. Results can be confirmed with a repeat test in 72 hours. Values in pregnancy should double every 3 days for the first 6 weeks. When an embryo is first large enough to be visible on transvaginal ultrasonography (page 697), the patient generally will have hCG concentrations between 1000 and 2000 IU/L. If the hCG value is high and gestational contents are not visible in the uterus, an ectopic pregnancy is suggested.

There are qualitative serum and urine hCG assays and quantitative serum hCG assays (Table 26). All assays use the same sandwich immunoassays. There are different point-of-care testing devices for hospital/laboratory use and for use by the general public. In the home setting, the urine is applied to a testing

TABLE 26 Recommended uses for hCG testing

Test name	Recommended use
Qualitative beta hCG	Rapid pregnancy test
Quantitative hCG	More accurate pregnancy test
	Used to monitor high-risk pregnancy
Quantitative hCG (tumor marker)	Monitor patients with hCG-secreting tumors

apparatus, and the color change is compared with a standard. If the color matches that standard, pregnancy is present. Other test kits use the development of a line or plus symbol that may appear indicating pregnancy. These tests take only a few minutes to perform and to obtain results. They are best if performed a few days after a missed menses. However, they can be positive on the day of an expected menses.

hCG is synthesized in the placenta and maintains the corpus luteum, and hence progesterone production, during the first trimester. Thereafter the placenta produces steroid hormones, diminishing the role of hCG. Concentrations of hCG fall, leveling off around week 20, significantly above prepregnancy levels. After delivery, miscarriage, or pregnancy termination, hCG falls until prepregnancy levels are reached.

Normally, hCG is not present in nonpregnant women. In a very small number of women (<5%), hCG exists in minute levels. The presence of hCG does not necessarily indicate a normal pregnancy. Ectopic pregnancy, hydatidiform mole of the uterus, recent abortion, and choriocarcinoma can all produce hCG. However, hCG levels in ectopic pregnancy typically fail to double appropriately, and decreased levels eventually result relative to the values expected in normal intrauterine pregnancies of similar gestational age. hCG may be secreted by seminomatous and nonseminomatous testicular tumors, ovarian germ cell tumors, and benign or malignant nontesticular teratomas. Serial measurement of hCG after treatment is used to monitor therapeutic response in these tumors and will detect persistent or recurrent neoplastic disease.

Interfering factors

- Tests performed too early in the pregnancy, before a significant hCG level exists, may cause false-negative results.

- Hematuria and proteinuria in the urine may cause false-positive results.
- Hemolysis of blood may interfere with test results.
- Urine pregnancy tests can vary according to the dilution of the urine. hCG levels may not be detectable in dilute urine but may be detectable in concentrated urine.
- Drugs that may cause false-negative urine results include diuretics (by causing diluted urine) and promethazine.
- Drugs that may cause false-positive results include anticonvulsants, antiparkinsonian drugs, hypnotics, and tranquilizers (especially promazine and its derivatives).

Procedure and patient care

Before
- PT Explain the procedure to the patient.
- If a urine specimen will be collected, give the patient a urine container the evening before so that she can provide a first-voided morning specimen. This specimen generally contains the greatest concentration of hCG.

During
- Collect the first-voided urine specimen for urine testing.
- Collect a venous blood sample in a red-top tube for serum testing. Avoid hemolysis.

After
- Apply pressure to the venipuncture site.
- PT Emphasize to the patient the importance of antepartal health care.

Abnormal findings

▲ **Increased levels**
Pregnancy
Ectopic pregnancy
Hydatidiform mole of the uterus
Choriocarcinoma of the uterus, testes, or ovaries
Tumor

▼ **Decreased levels (inappropriate rise in hCG levels)**
Spontaneous abortion
Fetal death
Ectopic pregnancy

notes

human lymphocyte antigen B27 (HLA-B27 antigen, Human leukocyte A antigen, White blood cell antigens, Histocompatibility leukocyte A antigen)

Type of test Blood

Normal findings Negative

Test explanation and related physiology

The HLA antigens exist on the surface of white blood cells and on the surface of all nucleated cells in other tissues. These antigens can be detected most easily on the cell surface of lymphocytes. The presence or absence of these antigens is determined genetically. Each gene controls the presence or absence of HLA A, B, C, or D.

The HLA system is used to assist in the diagnosis of certain other diseases. For example, HLA-B27 is present in 80% of patients with Reiter syndrome. When a patient has recurrent and multiple arthritic complaints, the presence of HLA-B27 supports the diagnosis of Reiter syndrome. HLA-B27 is found in 5% to 7% of normal patients. Other HLA-disease associations are mentioned in the abnormal findings section.

The HLA system of antigens has been used to indicate tissue compatibility in transplantation. Because HLA antigens are genetically determined, they can also be used to resolve *paternity investigations*.

Procedure and patient care

- See inside front cover for Routine Blood Testing.
- Fasting: no.
- Blood tube commonly used: verify with lab.

Abnormal findings

▲ **Increased levels (HLA-B27 antigens present)**
Ankylosing spondylitis
Reiter syndrome
Yersinia enterocolitica arthritis
Anterior uveitis
Graves disease
Celiac disease/gluten enteropathy

Chronic active hepatitis
Multiple sclerosis
Myasthenia gravis
Dermatitis herpetiformis
Psoriasis
Juvenile diabetes
Hemochromatosis
Rheumatoid arthritis

notes

human papillomavirus (HPV test, HPV DNA testing)

Type of test Fluid analysis

Normal findings No HPV present

Test explanation and related physiology

An HPV test is performed to identify genital HPV infection in a woman with an abnormal PAP smear (p. 680). HPV is a small, nonenveloped, double-stranded, circular deoxyribonucleic acid (DNA) tumor virus, classified in the genus *Papillomavirus* of the Papovaviridae family of viruses. HPV DNA incorporates itself into the cervical cell genome, promoting its effects through activation of oncogenes and suppression of host-cell immune response. HPV protein products prevent DNA repair and programmed cell death, which can lead to instability and unchecked cell growth.

HPV infects the genital epithelium and is spread via skin-to-skin contact. Some strains of HPV cause genital warts, but HPV infections often produce no signs or symptoms. As a result, infected persons are frequently unaware that they are carriers, and transmission occurs unknowingly.

Genital HPV strains are divided into two groups (low, or nononcogenic risk, and high, or oncogenic risk), based on their oncogenic potential and ability to induce viral-associated tumors. Low-risk strains (HPV 6, 11, 42, 43, and 44) are associated with condylomata (genital warts) and low-grade cervical changes, such as mild dysplasia. Lesions caused by low-risk HPV infection have a high likelihood of regression and little potential for progression and are considered of no or low oncogenic risk. High-risk strains (HPV 16, 18, 31, 33, 35, 39, 45, 51, 52, 56, 58, 59, and 68) are associated with intraepithelial neoplasia and are more likely to progress to severe lesions and cervical cancer.

A clear causal relationship has been established between HPV infection and cervical cancer. HPV is found in almost all cases of cervical malignancies worldwide. Of the high-risk HPV strains, HPV 16 and 18 are the most carcinogenic and most prevalent (>90% of cervical cancers are related particularly to HPV 16 and 18). HPV 16 is the predominant strain in the world. High-grade cervical intraepithelial lesions are most commonly associated with HPV 16 and 18, yet these strains are also frequently found to be the etiologic factor in minor lesions and mild dysplasia.

The latency period between initial HPV exposure and development of cervical cancer may be months or years. Women who have normal PAP tests results and no HPV infection are at a very low risk (0.2%) for developing cervical cancer.

Gardasil is a vaccine that will guard against HPV 6, 11, 16, and 18. The Centers for Disease Control and Prevention (CDC) recommends Gardasil for all girls and boys ages 11 or 12 years old. The vaccine is also recommended in men and women ages 13 through 26 years old who have not already received the vaccine or have not completed all booster shots.

The HPV test is performed on women who have an abnormal PAP smear. PAP smear results such as "atypical squamous cells of undetermined significance" or "low-grade squamous intraepithelial lesion" should prompt a routine HPV test.

Numerous sources indicate that more than 60% of women with an abnormal PAP smear will test positive for high-risk HPV. If the HPV test is positive, the woman should undergo colposcopy to look for a more serious cervical lesion, such as cancer. It is well known that HPV infection in younger women is more prevalent and will often spontaneously regress, particularly in those younger than the age of 30 years. In contrast, persistent high-risk infection peaks in women older than 30 years. As a result, recent screening guidelines recommend that HPV testing be reserved for clinical use in the evaluation of women older than the age of 30 years or for younger women with high-grade squamous intraepithelial lesions. Most recent studies have suggested that HPV testing is more sensitive than PAP testing in the detection of serious cervical disease.

Several clinical professional societies have made recommendations as to the appropriate use of high-risk HPV testing. Testing for high-risk (oncogenic) HPV is summarized in Table 27.

Interfering factors

- Cervical specimens with low cellularity may diminish sensitivity of the test.
- High concentrations of antifungal cream or contraceptive jelly may diminish sensitivity of the test.

Procedure and patient care

Before

PT Explain the procedure for PAP smear.

PT Instruct the patient not to douche or bathe in a tub during the 24 hours before the test.

TABLE 27 **American Cancer Society recommendations for cervical screening**

Population by age	Recommended screening
<21 years	No screening
21-29 years	PAP or thin prep alone every 3 years
30-65 years	HPV and PAP/thin prep co-testing every 5 years
>65 years	No screening after adequate negative prior screening
After hysterectomy	No screening
HPV vaccinated	Follow above recommendations (? delay screening for 3-5 years)

PT Instruct the patient to empty her bladder.

PT Instruct the patient to reschedule testing if she is menstruating.

PT Tell the patient that no fasting or sedation is required.

During
- Note the following procedural steps:
  1. The patient is placed in the lithotomy position.
  2. With the use of either a cytology brush or a wooden spatula, a cervical mucous specimen is obtained by placing the instrument into the cervical os and rotating 3 to 5 times in clockwise and counterclockwise directions.
  3. After specimen collection, rotate the broomlike device or spatula and Cytobrush several times in the collection vial to remove the specimen. Firmly cap the vial and discard the collection devices.
  4. Affix a patient identification label to the vial.
  5. Seal the vial and place in a plastic specimen bag along with a properly filled-out cytology requisition form, and send to the laboratory.
- Note that a smear is obtained by a nurse or a physician in approximately 10 minutes.

PT Tell the patient that no discomfort, except for insertion of the speculum, is associated with this procedure.

After

PT Inform the patient that usually she will not be notified unless further evaluation is necessary.

PT Instruct the patient that HPV is a sexually transmitted disease. Proper precautions should be taken to prevent infecting sexual partners.

Abnormal findings

HPV infection

notes

human placental lactogen (hPL, Human chorionic somatomammotropin [HCS])

Type of test Blood

Normal findings

Weeks of pregnancy	hPL concentration (mg/L = mcg/mL)
up to 20	0.05-1
up to 22	1.5-3
up to 26	2.5-5
up to 30	4-6.5
up to 34	5-8
up to 38	5.5-9.5
up to 42	5-7

Test explanation and related physiology

The human placenta produces several hormones that are homologous to hormones of the anterior pituitary. Human placental lactogen (hPL), which maintains the pregnancy, is structurally similar to both human prolactin and growth hormone. Not surprisingly, hPL demonstrates both lactogenic and growth-stimulating activity. Serum levels of hPL rise very early in normal pregnancy and continue to increase until a plateau is reached at about the 35th week after conception. Assays for maternal serum levels of hPL are useful in monitoring placental function. Measurements of hPL also are used in pregnancies complicated by hypertension, proteinuria, edema, postmaturity, placental insufficiency, or possible miscarriage.

A decreased serum concentration of hPL is pathognomonic for a malfunction of the placenta, which may cause intrauterine growth retardation, intrauterine death of the fetus, or imminent miscarriage. Pregnant women with hypertonia also show low serum concentrations of hPL. Because of the short biological half-life of hPL in serum, the determination of hPL always gives a very accurate picture of the present situation.

Increased serum concentrations of hPL are found in women with diabetes mellitus and, because of the higher placental mass, in multiple pregnancies. In contrast to estriol, the hPL concentration depends only on the placental mass and not on fetal function. The simultaneous determination of hPL and estriol can be helpful in the differential evaluation of placental function.

Interfering factors
- Prior nuclear medicine scans, because they can interfere with interpretation of test results

Procedure and patient care
- See inside front cover for Routine Blood Testing.
- Fasting: no.
- Blood tube commonly used: red.
- Indicate the date of the patient's last menstrual period on the laboratory slip.
- **PT** Explain the possibility that serial testing is often required.

Abnormal findings
▲ **Increased levels**
Multiple pregnancies
Placental site trophoblastic tumor
Intact molar pregnancy
Diabetes
Rh incompatibility

▼ **Decreased levels**
Placental insufficiency
Toxemia
Preeclampsia
Hydatidiform mole
Choriocarcinoma

notes

human T-cell lymphotrophic virus (HTLV) I/II antibody

Type of test Blood

Normal findings Negative

Test explanation and related physiology

Several forms of HTLV, a human retrovirus, affect humans. HTLV-I is associated with adult T-cell leukemia/lymphoma. HTLV-II is associated with adult hairy-cell leukemia and neurologic disorders (e.g., tropical spastic paraparesis).

The human immunodeficiency viruses (HIVs), which are known to be the cause of acquired immunodeficiency syndrome (AIDS), are also retroviruses; however, HTLV infection is not associated with AIDS. HTLV transmission is similar, though, to HIV transmission (e.g., body fluid contamination, intravenous drug use, sexual contact, breastfeeding).

Blood and organ donors are routinely tested for the presence of anti-HTLV-I/II antibodies by enzyme immunoassays (EIAs), which are highly sensitive but lack specificity. For accurate diagnosis of HTLV-I/II infection, all initially EIA-positive results should be verified by a confirmatory test, such as Western blot or line immunoassay. HTLV-I/II can also be directly detected by real-time amplification of the specific HTLV genomic DNA sequences from the blood of infected patients.

Procedure and patient care

- See inside front cover for Routine Blood Testing.
- Fasting: no.
- Blood tube commonly used: red.

Abnormal findings

Acute HTLV infection
Adult T-cell leukemia
Hairy-cell leukemia
Tropical spastic paraparesis

notes

17-hydroxycorticosteroids (17-OCHS)

Type of test Urine (24-hour)

Normal findings

Adult
  Male: 3-10 mg/24 hr or 8.3-27.6 μmol/day (SI units)
  Female: 2-8 mg/24 hr or 5.2-22.1 μmol/day (SI units)
Elderly: values slightly lower than adult
Children
  <8 years: <1.5 mg/24 hr
  8-12 years: <4.5 mg/24 hr

Test explanation and related physiology

H

Elevated levels of 17-OCHS are seen in patients with hyperfunctioning of the adrenal gland (Cushing syndrome), whether this condition is caused by a pituitary or adrenal tumor, bilateral adrenal hyperplasia, or ectopic tumors producing adrenocorticotropic hormone (ACTH). Low levels of 17-OCHS are seen in patients who have a hypofunctioning adrenal gland (Addison disease) as a result of destruction of the adrenals (by hemorrhage, infarction, metastatic tumor, or autoimmunity), surgical removal of an adrenal gland, congenital enzyme deficiency, hypopituitarism, or adrenal suppression after prolonged exogenous steroid ingestion.

Testing the urine for this hormone metabolite is only an indirect measure of adrenal function. Urine and plasma levels of cortisol (p. 301) provide a much more accurate measurement of adrenal function. Because the excretion of cortisol metabolites follows a diurnal variation, a 24-hour collection is necessary.

Interfering factors

- Emotional and physical stress (e.g., infection) and licorice ingestion may cause increased adrenal activity.
- Drugs that may cause *increased* 17-OCHS levels include acetazolamide, chloral hydrate, chlorpromazine, colchicine, erythromycin, meprobamate, paraldehyde, quinidine, quinine, and spironolactone.
- Drugs that may cause *decreased* levels include estrogens, oral contraceptives, phenothiazines, and reserpine.

Procedure and patient care

- See inside front cover for Routine Urine Testing.
- Note that drugs are usually withheld several days before the urine collection. Check with the physician and laboratory for specific guidelines.
- Assess the patient for signs of stress and report these to the physician.
- Do not administer to the patient any drugs that may interfere with test results.

Abnormal findings

▲ **Increased levels**
  Cushing syndrome
  Ectopic ACTH-producing tumors
  Stress
  Adrenal adenoma or carcinoma
  Hyperthyroidism
  Obesity

▼ **Decreased levels**
  Adrenal hyperplasia (adrenogenital syndrome)
  Addison disease
  Adrenal suppression from steroid therapy
  Hypopituitarism
  Hypothyroidism

notes

5-hydroxyindoleacetic acid (5-HIAA)

Type of test Urine (24-hour)

Normal findings

2-8 mg/24 hr or 10-40 μmol/day (SI units)
Female levels lower than male levels

Test explanation and related physiology

Quantitative analysis of urine levels of 5-HIAA is used to detect and follow the clinical course of patients with carcinoid tumors. Carcinoid tumors are serotonin-secreting tumors that may grow in the appendix, intestine, lung, or any tissue derived from the neuroectoderm. These tumors contain *argentaffin-staining (enteroendocrine)* cells, which produce serotonin and other powerful neurohormones that are metabolized by the liver to 5-HIAA and excreted in the urine. These powerful neurohormones are responsible for the clinical presentation of carcinoid syndrome (bronchospasm, flushing, diarrhea).

This test is used not only to identify patients with carcinoid tumor but also to reevaluate those with known tumor by using serial levels of urinary 5-HIAA. Rising levels of 5-HIAA indicate progression of tumor; falling levels of 5-HIAA indicate a therapeutic response of the tumor to antineoplastic therapy.

Interfering factors

- Bananas, plantains, pineapples, kiwifruit, walnuts, plums, pecans, eggplant, tomatoes, and avocados can factitiously elevate 5-HIAA levels.
- Drugs that may cause *increased* 5-HIAA levels include acetaminophen, acetanilid, acetophenetidin, glyceryl guaiacolate, methocarbamol, and reserpine.
- Drugs that may cause *decreased* levels include aspirin, chlorpromazine, ethyl alcohol, heparin, imipramine, isoniazid, levodopa, MAO inhibitors, methenamine, methyldopa, phenothiazines, promethazine, and tricyclic antidepressants.

Procedure and patient care

- See inside front cover for Routine Urine Testing for 24-hour collection.
- **PT** Instruct the patient to refrain from eating foods containing serotonin (e.g., plums, pineapples, bananas, eggplant, tomatoes, avocados, walnuts, plantains, kiwifruit, and pecans) for several days (usually 3) before and during testing.

- Keep the specimen on ice or in a refrigerator during the 24-hour collection. A preservative is needed to keep the specimen at an appropriate pH.

Abnormal findings

▲ **Increased levels**
Carcinoid tumors
Noncarcinoid illness
Cystic fibrosis
Intestinal malabsorption

▼ **Decreased levels**
Mental depression
Migraine headaches

notes

21-hydroxylase antibodies

Type of test Blood

Normal findings <1 U/mL

Test explanation and related physiology

Chronic primary adrenal insufficiency (Addison disease) is most commonly caused by the insidious autoimmune destruction of the adrenal cortex and is characterized by the presence of adrenal cortex autoantibodies in the serum. It can occur sporadically or in combination with other autoimmune endocrine diseases. This antibody may precipitate this disease. Measurement of this antibody is used in the investigation of causes of adrenal insufficiency.

Procedure and patient care

- See inside front cover for Routine Blood Testing.
- Fasting: no.
- Blood tube commonly used: red.

Abnormal findings

▲ **Increased levels**

Autoimmune adrenal insufficiency

Autoimmune polyglandular syndrome

notes

hysterosalpingography (Uterotubography, Uterosalpingography, Hysterogram)

Type of test   X-ray with contrast dye

Normal findings

Patent fallopian tubes
No defects in uterine cavity

Test explanation and related physiology

In hysterosalpingography, the uterine cavity and fallopian tubes are visualized radiographically after the injection of contrast material through the cervix. Uterine tumors, intrauterine adhesions, and developmental anomalies can be seen. Tubal obstruction caused by internal scarring, tumor, or kinking also can be detected. A possible therapeutic effect of this test is that passage of dye through the tubes may clear mucous plugs, straighten kinked tubes, or break up adhesions. This test also may be used to document adequacy of surgical tubal ligation.

Contraindications

- Patients with infections of the vagina, cervix, or fallopian tubes, because there is risk of extending the infection
- Patients with suspected pregnancy, because contrast material might induce abortion

Potential complications

- Infection of the endometrium (endometritis)
- Infection of the fallopian tubes (salpingitis)
- Uterine perforation
- Allergic reaction to iodinated dye
  This rarely occurs because the dye is not administered intravenously.

Procedure and patient care

Before
PT Explain the procedure to the patient.
- Determine pregnancy status of the patient.
- Administer sedatives (e.g., midazolam) or antispasmodics, if ordered, before the test.
PT Tell the patient that no food or fluid restrictions are needed.

During
- Note the following procedural steps:
  1. After voiding, the patient is placed on the fluoroscopy table in the lithotomy position.

2. With a speculum in the vagina, contrast material is injected through the cervix. The dye fills the entire upper genital tract (uterus and tubes).

3. Fluoroscopy is performed, and x-ray images are taken.

- Note that this procedure is performed by a physician in approximately 15 to 30 minutes.

PT Tell the patient that she may feel occasional transient menstrual-type cramping and that she may have shoulder pain caused by subphrenic irritation from the dye as it leaks into the peritoneal cavity.

After

PT Inform the patient that a vaginal discharge (sometimes bloody) may be present for 1 to 2 days after the test.

PT Instruct the patient on the signs and symptoms of infection (e.g., fever, increased pulse rate, pain).

Abnormal findings

Uterine tumor (e.g., leiomyoma, cancer) or polyps
Developmental anomaly (e.g., uterus bicornis) of the uterus
Intrauterine adhesions or polyps
Uterine fistula
Obstruction, kinking, or twisting of the fallopian tubes
Extrauterine pregnancy
Tumor of the fallopian tubes

notes

hysteroscopy

Type of test Endoscopy

Normal findings Normal structure and function of the uterus

Test explanation and related physiology

Hysteroscopy is an endoscopic procedure that provides direct visualization of the uterine cavity by inserting a hysteroscope (a thin, telescope-like instrument) through the vagina and cervix and into the uterus (Figure 25). Hysteroscopy can be used to identify the cause of abnormal uterine bleeding, infertility, and repeated miscarriages. It is also used to identify, evaluate, and perform biopsies of uterine adhesions (Asherman syndrome), polyps, cancer, fibroids, and to detect displaced intrauterine devices (IUDs).

In addition to diagnosing and evaluating uterine problems, hysteroscopy can also correct uterine problems. For example, uterine adhesions and small fibroids can be removed through the hysteroscope, thus avoiding open abdominal surgery. Hysteroscopy can also be used to perform endometrial ablation, which destroys the uterine lining to treat some cases of heavy dysfunctional uterine bleeding.

Contraindications

- Patients with pelvic inflammatory disease
- Patients with vaginal discharge

Potential complications

- Uterine perforation
- Infection

Procedure and patient care

Before

PT Explain the procedure to the patient.
- Obtain informed consent for this procedure.
- Assess the pregnancy status of the patient.
PT Instruct the patient to be NPO for at least 8 hours before the test.

During

- Note the following procedural steps:
  1. Hysteroscopy may be performed in the operating room or the doctor's office. Local, regional, general, or no anesthesia may be used. (The type of anesthesia depends on other procedures that may be done at the same time.)

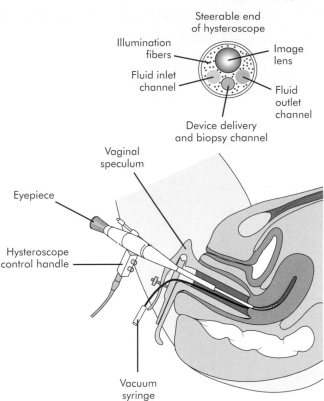

FIGURE 25 Hysteroscopy.

2. The patient is placed in the lithotomy position. The vaginal area is cleansed with an antiseptic solution.
3. The cervix may be dilated before this procedure.
4. The hysteroscope is inserted through the vagina and cervix and into the uterus.
5. A liquid or gas is released through the hysteroscope to expand the uterus for better visualization.
6. If minor surgery is to be performed, small instruments will be inserted through the hysteroscope.
7. For more detailed or complicated procedures, a laparoscope (p. 578) may be used to concurrently view the outside of the uterus.

- Note that hysteroscopy is performed by a physician in approximately 30 minutes.

After

PT Tell the patient that it is normal to have slight vaginal bleeding and cramps for a day or two after the procedure.

PT Inform the patient that signs of fever, severe abdominal pain, or heavy vaginal discharge or bleeding should be reported to her physician.

Abnormal findings

Endometrial cancer, polyps, or hyperplasia
Uterine fibroids
Asherman syndrome
Septate uterus
Displaced IUD

notes

immunoglobulin quantification

Type of test Blood

Normal findings Results vary by age and methods.

IgG (mg/dL)
  Adults: 565-1765
  Children: 250-1600

IgA (mg/dL)
  Adults: 85-385
  Children: 1-350

IgM (mg/dL)
  Adults: 55-375
  Children: 20-200

IgD and IgE: minimal

Test explanation and related physiology

Proteins in the blood are made up of albumin and globulin. Several types of globulin exist, one of which is gamma globulin. Antibodies are made up of gamma globulin protein and are called *immunoglobulins.* There are many classes of immunoglobulins. *Immunoglobulin G (IgG)* constitutes approximately 75% of the serum immunoglobulins; therefore, it constitutes the majority of circulating blood antibodies. *IgA* constitutes approximately 15% of the immunoglobulins in the body and is present primarily in secretions of the respiratory and gastrointestinal tracts, in saliva, in colostrum, and in tears. IgA is also present to a smaller degree in the blood. *IgM* is an immunoglobulin primarily responsible for ABO blood grouping and rheumatoid factor; it is also involved in the immunologic reaction to many infections. IgM does not cross the placenta, so an elevation of IgM in a newborn indicates in utero infection (e.g., rubella, cytomegalovirus [CMV], or sexually transmitted disease [STD]). *IgE* often mediates an allergic response and is measured to detect allergic diseases. *IgD*, which constitutes the smallest part of the immunoglobulins, is rarely evaluated or detected.

Serum protein quantification is used to detect and monitor the course of hypersensitivity diseases, immune deficiencies, autoimmune diseases, chronic infections, and intrauterine fetal infections. Although *electrophoresis* is usually required to interpret an elevated immunoglobulin class as polyclonal versus monoclonal, *immunofixation* is usually required to characterize a monoclonal protein.

Increased serum immunoglobulin concentrations occur due to polyclonal or oligoclonal immunoglobulin proliferation in hepatic disease, connective tissue diseases, and acute and chronic infections. Elevation of immunoglobulins may occur in monoclonal gammopathies (e.g., multiple myeloma, primary systemic amyloidosis, and monoclonal gammopathies of undetermined significance). Decreased immunoglobulin levels are found in patients with acquired or congenital immune deficiencies. It can be used to monitor therapy and recurrence. Testing can determine the type of connective tissue disease, its severity, its clinical course, and its response to therapy.

Interfering factors

☒ Drugs that may cause *increased* immunoglobulin levels include hydralazine, isoniazid (INH), phenytoin, procainamide, tetanus toxoid/antitoxin, and gamma globulin.

Procedure and patient care

- See inside front cover for Routine Blood Testing.
- Fasting: no.
- Blood tube commonly used: red.
- Indicate on the laboratory slip if the patient has received any vaccinations or immunizations in the past 6 months.

Abnormal findings

▲ **Increased IgA levels**
Chronic liver diseases
(e.g., primary biliary
cirrhosis)
Chronic infections
Inflammatory bowel
disease

▼ **Decreased IgA levels**
Ataxia/telangiectasia
Congenital isolated
deficiency
Hypoproteinemia (e.g.,
nephrotic syndrome
or protein-losing
enteropathies)
Immunosuppressive
drugs (e.g., steroids,
dextran)

▲ **Increased IgG levels**
Chronic granulomatous
infections (e.g., tuberculosis,
Wegener granulomatosis,
sarcoidosis)
Hyperimmunization reactions
Chronic liver disease
Multiple myeloma (mono-
clonal IgG type)
Autoimmune diseases (e.g.,
rheumatoid arthritis, Sjögren
disease, systemic lupus
erythematosus)
IUD devices

▲ **Increased IgM levels**
Waldenström
macroglobulinemia
Chronic infections (e.g.,
hepatitis, mononucleosis,
sarcoidosis)
Autoimmune diseases
(e.g., systemic lupus
erythematosus, rheumatoid
arthritis)
Acute infections
Chronic liver disorders (e.g.,
biliary cirrhosis)

▲ **Increased IgE levels**
Allergy reactions (e.g., hay
fever, asthma, eczema,
anaphylaxis)
Allergic infections (e.g.,
aspergillosis or parasites)

▼ **Decreased IgG levels**
Wiskott-Aldrich
syndrome
Agammaglobulinemia
AIDS
Hypoproteinemia
(e.g., nephrotic
syndrome, protein-
losing enteropathies)
Drug immunosuppression
(e.g., steroids, dextran)
Non-IgG multiple
myeloma
Leukemia

▼ **Decreased IgM levels**
Agammaglobulinemia
AIDS
Hypoproteinemia (e.g.,
nephrotic syndrome,
protein-losing
enteropathies)
Drug immunosuppression
(e.g., steroids, dextran)
IgG or IgA multiple
myeloma
Leukemia

▼ **Decreased IgE levels**
Agammaglobulinemia

notes

insulin assay

Type of test Blood

Normal findings

6-26 µU/mL or 43-186 pmol/L (SI units)

Newborn: 3-20 µU/mL

Possible critical values >30 µU/mL

Test explanation and related physiology

Insulin assay is used to diagnose insulinoma (tumor of the islets of Langerhans). It is also used in the evaluation of patients with fasting hypoglycemia.

Some investigators believe that measuring the ratio of the blood sugar and insulin on the same specimen obtained during the oral glucose tolerance test (GTT, p. 479) is more reliable than measuring insulin levels alone. Combined with the oral GTT, the insulin assay can show characteristic curves. For example, patients with juvenile diabetes have low fasting insulin levels and display flat GTT insulin curves because of little or no increase in insulin levels. Patients who have mild cases of diabetes have normal fasting insulin levels and display GTT curves with a delayed rise.

Type 2 diabetes (adult onset) is characterized by an excess of insulin production in response to GTT. This hyperresponse of insulin may precede hyperglycemia by many years, allowing the patient time and opportunity to take action to reduce the incidence of outright diabetes through diet management and lifestyle changes.

When combined with fasting blood sugar, insulin assay is very accurate in detecting insulinoma. After the patient fasts 12 to 14 hours, the insulin/glucose ratio should be less than 0.3. Patients with insulinoma have ratios greater than this. To increase the sensitivity and specificity of these combined tests for insulinoma, Turner and others have proposed the *amended* insulin/glucose ratios using variable mathematical *fudge factors*:

$$\frac{\text{Serum insulin level} \times 100}{\text{Serum glucose} - 30\,\text{mg}/100\,\text{mL}}$$

A Turner amended ratio of more than 50 suggests insulinoma.

Interfering factors

- Antiinsulin antibodies can interfere with radioimmunoassay.
- Food intake and obesity may cause increased insulin levels.
- Recent administration of radioisotopes may affect test results.
- ✄ Drugs that may cause *increased* insulin levels include corticosteroids, levodopa, and oral contraceptives.

Procedure and patient care

- See inside front cover for Routine Blood Testing.
- Fasting: yes.
- Blood tube commonly used: red.
- If the serum insulin level will be measured during the GTT, collect the blood sample before oral ingestion of the glucose load and often at designated intervals after glucose ingestion.

Abnormal findings

▲ **Increased levels**
Insulinoma
Cushing syndrome
Acromegaly
Obesity
Fructose or galactose
   intolerance

▼ **Decreased levels**
Diabetes mellitus
Hypopituitarism

notes

insulin-like growth factor (IGF-1, Somatomedin C, Insulin-like growth factor binding proteins [IGF BP])

Type of test   Blood

Normal findings

Adults: 42-110 ng/mL
Children:

Age (yr)	Girls (ng/mL)	Boys (ng/mL)
0-8	5-128	2-118
9-10	24-158	15-148
11-13	65-226	55-216
14-15	124-242	114-232
16-17	94-231	84-211
18-19	66-186	56-177

Test explanation and related physiology

Growth hormone (GH) exerts its effects on many tissues through a group of peptides called *somatomedins*. The most commonly tested somatomedins are insulin-like growth factor 1 (IGF-1) and IGF-3. Measurement of free IGF-1 and IGF binding proteins (BP) 3 is preferred to growth hormone measurements in cases of short stature in early adolescence. IGF is the test of choice in identifying and monitoring treatment of acromegaly.

Great variation in GH secretion occurs during the day. A random GH assay result may significantly overlap between normal and abnormal values. To diminish the common variations in GH secretion, screening for IFG-1 provides a more accurate reflection of the mean plasma concentration of GH. Somatomedins are not affected (as GH is) by the time of day, food intake, or exercise because they circulate bound to proteins that are durable or long-lasting. As a result, there is no overlap of results of IGF-1 between normal and abnormal values. Normally there is a large increase during the pubertal growth spurt.

Levels of IGF-1 depend on levels of GH. As a result, IGF-1 levels are low when GH levels are deficient. (See GH [p. 486] for a discussion of causes of and diseases associated with GH deficiency.) Nonpituitary causes of reduced IGF-1 levels include malnutrition, severe chronic illnesses, severe liver disease, hypothyroidism, renal failure, inflammatory bowel disease, and Laron dwarfism. Abnormally low test results require an abnormally reduced or absent GH during a GH-stimulation test (p. 487) to make the diagnosis of GH deficiency.

Pediatricians commonly use *insulin-like growth factor binding proteins (IGF BPs)* to even further diminish the impact of the variables affecting GH and somatomedin levels. Specifically, IGF BP 2 and IGF BP 3 are the most commonly measured. However, if GH deficiency is strongly suspected yet documentation using GH or somatomedins is questionable, IGF BP determinations are helpful. IGF BP 3 is less age-dependent and is the most accurate (97% sensitivity and specificity). These proteins help to evaluate GH deficiencies and GH-resistant syndromes (e.g., Laron dwarfism). Finally, these binding proteins are very useful in predicting responses to therapeutic exogenous GH administration.

Interfering factors

- A radioactive scan performed within the week before the test may affect test results.
- ✘ Drugs that may cause *decreased* levels include high doses of estrogens.

Procedure and patient care

- See inside front cover for Routine Blood Testing.
- Fasting: yes.
- Blood tube commonly used: lavender or red.

Abnormal findings

▲ Increased levels
Acromegaly
Gigantism
Hyperpituitarism
Obesity
Pregnancy
Precocious puberty

▼ Decreased levels
Growth hormone deficiency/resistance
Laron dwarfism (growth hormone resistance)
Inactive growth hormone
Resistance to somatomedins
Nutritional deficiency
Delayed puberty
Pituitary tumor
Hypopituitarism
Cirrhosis of the liver

notes

intravascular ultrasound (IVUS)

Type of test Ultrasound

Normal findings Normal coronary arteries

Test explanation and related physiology

Percutaneous intravascular ultrasound (IVUS) imaging requires very small, specially made transducers that are mounted on the tip of an intravascular catheter. The ultrasound catheter tip is slid in over the guidewire and positioned using angiographic techniques, so that the tip is in the blood vessel to be studied. Sound waves are emitted from the catheter tip. The catheter receives and conducts the echo information from the blood vessel out to the external digital ultrasound equipment. The machine then constructs and displays a real-time ultrasound image of a thin section of the blood vessel currently surrounding the catheter tip.

Unlike arteriography, which shows a shadow of the arterial lumen, IVUS shows a tomographic, cross-sectional view of the vessel. This orientation enables direct measurements of lumen dimensions, which are considered to be more accurate than angiographic dimensions. The guidewire is kept stationary and the ultrasound catheter tip is slid backward, usually under motorized control at a pullback speed of 0.5 mm/s. The data obtained can be restructured into a longitudinal image by the ultrasound machine software to create a three-dimensional image of the particular segment of artery.

IVUS is an important technology for studying the progression, stabilization, and potential regression of coronary atherosclerosis. IVUS permits imaging of the lumen size, vessel wall structure, and any atheroma that may be present. It allows characterization of atheroma size, plaque distribution, and lesion composition and enables accurate visualization of not only the lumen of the coronary arteries, but also the atheroma that may be hidden within the vessel wall. In this way, IVUS has enabled advances in clinical research, providing a more thorough perspective and better understanding of vascular disease. It provides a reproducible, safe, and sensitive method for assessing the development and extent of atherosclerosis, particularly in its earlier, presymptomatic stages. This procedure is predominantly used in the coronary arteries.

IVUS is used in the following clinical situations:

o Assessment of coronary stent placement and determination of minimum luminal diameter within the stent o Determination of the mechanism of stent restenosis and selection of appropriate therapy (plaque ablation versus repeat balloon expansion)

o Evaluation of coronary obstruction at a location difficult to image by angiography

o Assessment of a suboptimal angiographic result following stent placement in cases in which the degree of stenosis of a coronary artery is unclear

o Guidance and assessment for vascular atherectomy

o Determination of plaque location and circumferential distribution for guidance of directional coronary atherectomy

o Determination of the extent of atherosclerosis in patients with characteristic anginal symptoms and a positive functional study with no focal stenoses or mild coronary artery disease on angiography. IVUS can directly quantify the percentage of stenosis and give insight into the anatomy of the plaque.

o Preinterventional assessment of lesion characteristics and vessel dimensions as a means to select an optimal revascularization device

o Assessment of the changes in plaque volume after lipid-lowering therapy

Interfering factors

• The accuracy of ultrasonography is dependent on the skills of the sonographer.

Procedure and patient care

Before

PT Explain the procedure to the patient.

PT Tell the patient that fasting is required.

During

• The IVUS probe is placed by coronary angiographic procedures (p. 214).

• The test is completed in approximately 1 hour, usually by a cardiologist.

After

• See cardiac catheterization (p. 214) for postprocedure care.

Abnormal findings

Coronary occlusive disease

notes

intrinsic factor antibody (IF ab)

Type of test   Blood

Normal findings   Negative

Test explanation and related physiology

The intrinsic factor antibody (IF ab) is used to diagnose pernicious anemia (PA). PA is one of the major causes of vitamin B_{12} deficiency and megaloblastic anemia. It is a disease of the stomach in which secretion of IF is severely reduced or absent, resulting in malabsorption of B_{12}. PA appears to be an autoimmune process.

Approximately 50% to 75% of adult patients have IF abs. There are two types of this antibody. Type I, blocking antibody, is more common and prevents the binding of vitamin B_{12} and IF. Type II antibody, binding antibody, is less specific for PA and affects the binding of IF in the ileum. The blocking antibody is extremely specific for PA and is more sensitive than the binding antibody. In the context of a low or borderline B_{12} result, where other clinical and hematologic findings are compatible with a diagnosis of B_{12} deficiency, the presence of IF blocking antibody can be taken as confirmation of this diagnosis and, at the same time, as an indication of its cause. A negative result, on the other hand, cannot rule out the possibility of PA because blocking antibody is not demonstrable in nearly 50% of all patients with this disorder.

Interfering factors

- IF ab levels are *decreased* if an injection of vitamin B_{12} is administered within 48 hours of testing.

Procedure and patient care

- See inside front cover for Routine Blood Testing.
- Fasting: no.
- Blood tube commonly used: red.

Abnormal findings

▲ Increased levels

   Pernicious anemia

notes

iron level and total iron-binding capacity (Fe and TIBC, Transferrin saturation, Transferrin)

Type of test Blood

Normal findings

Iron

Male: 80-180 mcg/dL or 14-32 μmol/L (SI units)
Female: 60-160 mcg/dL or 11-29 μmol/L (SI units)
Newborn: 100-250 mcg/dL
Child: 50-120 mcg/dL

TIBC

250-460 mcg/dL or 45-82 μmol/L (SI units)

Transferrin

Adult male: 215-365 mg/dL or 2.15-3.65 g/L (SI units)
Adult female: 250-380 mg/dL or 2.50-3.80 g/L (SI units)
Newborn: 130-275 mg/dL
Child: 203-360 mg/dL

Transferrin saturation

Male: 20%-50%
Female: 15%-50%

Test explanation and related physiology

Serum iron

Abnormal levels of iron are characteristic of many diseases, including iron deficiency anemia and hemochromatosis. Seventy percent of iron in the body is found in the hemoglobin of red blood cells (RBCs). The other 30% is stored iron in the form of *ferritin* (p. 421) and hemosiderin. Iron is supplied by the diet. Iron is bound to a globulin protein called *transferrin*. Transferrin exists in relationship to the need for iron. When iron stores are low, transferrin levels increase. Transferrin is low when there is too much iron. Usually about one third of the transferrin is being used to transport iron. Because of this, the blood serum has considerable extra iron-binding capacity, which is the *unsaturated iron-binding capacity (UIBC)*. The TIBC equals UIBC plus the serum iron measurement. Some laboratories measure UIBC, some measure TIBC, and some measure transferrin. The serum iron determination is a measurement of the quantity of iron bound to transferrin.

Iron deficiency anemia is a result of reduced serum iron. Iron deficiency anemia has many causes, including the following:

- Insufficient iron intake
- Inadequate gut absorption
- Increased requirements (e.g., in growing children)
- Loss of blood (e.g., menstruation, bleeding peptic ulcer)

Iron deficiency results in decreased production of hemoglobin, which in turn results in small, pale (microcytic, hypochromic) RBCs. A decreased serum iron level, elevated TIBC, and low transferrin saturation (TS) value are characteristic of iron deficiency anemia.

Acute iron poisoning due to accidental or intentional overdose is characterized by a serum iron level that exceeds the TIBC. Chronic iron overload or poisoning is called *hemochromatosis* or *hemosiderosis*. Excess iron is usually deposited in the brain, liver, and heart and causes severe dysfunction of these organs. Massive blood transfusions also may cause elevated serum iron levels, although only transiently. Transfusions should be avoided before serum iron level blood specimens are obtained in the evaluation of anemia.

Total iron-binding capacity and transferrin

TIBC is a measurement of all proteins available for binding mobile iron. Transferrin represents the largest quantity of iron-binding proteins. Therefore, TIBC is an indirect yet accurate measurement of transferrin. Ferritin is not included in TIBC because it binds only stored iron. TIBC is increased in 70% of patients with iron deficiency.

Transferrin is a *negative* acute-phase reactant protein. That is, in various acute inflammatory reactions, transferrin levels diminish. Transferrin also is diminished in the face of chronic illnesses, such as malignancy, collagen vascular diseases, or liver diseases. Hypoproteinemia is also associated with reduced transferrin levels.

TIBC varies minimally according to iron intake and is more of a reflection of liver function (transferrin is produced by the liver) and nutrition than of iron metabolism.

Total iron-binding capacity and transferrin saturation

The percentage of transferrin and other mobile iron-binding proteins saturated with iron is calculated by dividing the serum iron level by the TIBC:

$$TS\ (\%) = \frac{\text{Serum iron level}}{\text{TIBC}} \times 100\%$$

The normal value for TS is 20% to 50%. TS is decreased to less than 15% in patients with iron deficiency anemia. It is increased in patients with hemolytic, sideroblastic, or megaloblastic anemias. TS is also increased in patients with iron overload or poisoning. Increased intake or absorption of iron (as in hemochromatosis) leads to elevated iron levels. In such cases, TIBC is unchanged; as a result, the percentage of TS is very high. UIBC has been proposed as an inexpensive alternative to transferrin saturation.

Chronic illness is characterized by a low serum iron level, decreased TIBC, and normal TS. Pregnancy is marked by high levels of protein, including transferrin. Because iron requirements are high, it is not unusual to find low serum iron levels, high TIBC, and a low percentage of TS in late pregnancy.

Contraindications

- Patients with hemolytic diseases, because they may have an artificially high iron content

Interfering factors

- Recent blood transfusions may affect test results.
- Recent ingestion of a meal containing high iron content may affect test results.
- Hemolytic diseases may be associated with an artificially high iron content.
- Drugs that may cause *increased* iron levels include chloramphenicol, dextran, estrogens, ethanol, iron preparations, methyldopa, and oral contraceptives.
- Drugs that may cause *decreased* iron levels include adrenocorticotropic hormone (ACTH), chloramphenicol, cholestyramine, colchicine, deferoxamine, methicillin, and testosterone.
- Drugs that may cause *increased* TIBC levels include fluorides and oral contraceptives.
- Drugs that may cause *decreased* TIBC levels include ACTH and chloramphenicol.

Procedure and patient care

- See inside front cover for Routine Blood Testing.
- Fasting: yes (12 hours).
- Blood tube commonly used: red.
- Avoid hemolysis, because the iron contained in the RBCs will pour out into the serum and cause artificially high iron levels.

Abnormal findings

▲ **Increased serum iron levels**
Hemosiderosis
Hemochromatosis
Hemolytic anemia
Hepatitis
Hepatic necrosis
Lead toxicity
Iron poisoning
Massive transfusion

▼ **Decreased serum iron levels**
Insufficient dietary iron
Chronic blood loss
Inadequate absorption of iron
Pregnancy (late)
Iron deficiency anemia
Neoplasia
Chronic gastrointestinal blood loss
Chronic hematuria
Chronic heavy physiologic or pathologic menstruation

▲ **Increased TIBC/transferrin levels**
Oral contraceptives
Pregnancy (late)
Polycythemia vera
Iron deficiency anemia

▼ **Decreased TIBC/transferrin levels**
Hypoproteinemia
Inflammatory diseases
Cirrhosis
Hemolytic anemia
Pernicious anemia
Sickle cell anemia

▲ **Increased TS or TIBC saturation**
Hemochromatosis
Hemosiderosis
Acute iron overdose
Hemolytic anemia

▼ **Decreased TS or TIBC saturation**
Iron deficiency anemia
Chronic illnesses (e.g., malignancy)

notes

ischemia-modified albumin (IMA)

Type of test Blood

Normal findings <85 international units/mL

Test explanation and related physiology

When albumin is exposed to an ischemic environment, its *N* terminal is altered; this causes an alteration of the albumin called *ischemia-modified albumin (IMA)*. This has become particularly helpful in identifying cardiac ischemia in patients with chest pain. When combined with troponins (p. 931), myoglobin (p. 650), and ECG, the diagnosis of an ischemic cardiac event can be corroborated or ruled out. IMA is produced continually during the period of ischemia. Blood levels rise within 10 minutes of the initiation of the ischemic event and stay elevated for 6 hours after ischemia has resolved.

IMA may also be elevated in patients with pulmonary embolus or acute stroke. False positives can occur in other clinical circumstances, such as advanced cancers, acute infections, and end-stage renal or liver disease.

Procedure and patient care

- See inside front cover for Routine Blood Testing.
- Fasting: no.
- Blood tube commonly used: yellow.
- This test is usually done after the initial onset of chest pain, then 12 hours later, and then daily testing for 3 to 5 days.
- Record the exact time and date of venipuncture on each laboratory slip. This aids in the interpretation of the temporal pattern of blood level elevations.

Abnormal findings

▲ **Increased levels**
  Myocardial ischemia
  Brain ischemia
  Pulmonary ischemia

notes

laboratory genetics

Type of test Blood, fluid analysis, microscopic examination

Normal findings No genetic/chromosomal abnormalities

Test explanation and related physiology

Genetic laboratory testing has become a vital part of identifying diseases of inborn errors in metabolism such as phenylketonuria (PKU). These genetic laboratory tests have also proven to be helpful in the identification, classification, and prognostication of many oncologic diseases such as leukemias. The heredity of diseases can be more accurately traced with the use of laboratory genetics.

There are many different laboratory methods used in genetic testing, and each is particularly helpful for study of a particular disease. It is not the intent of this reference book to explain the details of commonly used genetic laboratory methods. However, it is important to be aware of the availability and ability of genetic laboratory testing in clinical medicine.

Molecular genetics is utilized to detect mutation carriers, diagnose genetic disorders, test at-risk fetuses, and identify patients at high risk of developing adult-onset conditions such as Huntington disease or familial cancers. In addition, full-gene analysis is available for tests such as cystic fibrosis, beta globin, and hereditary hemorrhagic telangiectasia. When a mutation is identified in a family, family-specific mutation microarray testing can be performed.

Biochemical genetics is frequently used to diagnose one of many metabolic disorders that affect the body's ability to produce or break down amino acids, organic acids, and fatty acids. Early identification of such a metabolic disorder may prevent serious health problems as well as death. Biochemical genetic testing can be used as a supplemental newborn screening for inborn errors of metabolism (e.g., PKU and creatine or tyrosine disorders). Biochemical genetics is also helpful in the evaluation of malabsorption syndromes. For some of these disorders, such as MCAD, more precise DNA testing for causative mutations is also available. Biochemical testing can differentiate heterozygous carriers from non-carriers of genes by metabolite and enzymatic analysis of physiological fluids and tissues.

Cytogenetics is used to identify chromosomal disorders that cause spontaneous abortuses, congenital malformations, mental retardation, or infertility. It is used to evaluate women with gonadal dysgenesis and couples with repeated spontaneous miscarriages. Additionally, the field of cytogenetics is very important in the diagnosis and classification of leukemias, lymphomas, myeloma, and myeloproliferative diseases. This laboratory method also helps with decisions about treatment and for monitoring disease status and recovery.

Fluorescence in situ hybridization (FISH) testing utilizes genomic microarray probes to identify well-characterized hereditary genetic microdeletion, microduplication, or rearrangement inherited disorders, such as DiGeorge syndrome. It is also helpful in the evaluation of oncology specimens (see breast cancer tumor analysis, p. 184). Many disease-specific FISH panels target subtelomeric and pericentromeric sites and locations of known microdeletion syndromes. FISH testing can assist in the diagnosis and monitoring of patients with cancer (e.g., breast, leukemia, lymphomas). It can help determine the specific type of cancer present, predict disease course, or determine a course of treatment.

Microarray genetic testing can identify diseases associated with oligonucleotide and SNP-based genetic diseases. Single nucleotide polymorphisms (SNPs, snips, or snippets) are variations in the genetic code at a specific point in the DNA. Like cytogenetic techniques, microarray analysis identifies unbalanced chromosomal abnormalities (loss and/or gain of DNA) in patients with unexplained abnormal phenotypes such as mental retardation, developmental delay, dysmorphic features, congenital anomalies, and autism. But the SNP-based array will also identify long contiguous stretches of homozygosity that may suggest an increased likelihood for a recessive condition or uniparental disomy.

Microarray FISH testing is also utilized to determine the presence of a genetic deletion or duplication in a family with a known inheritable disease. FISH testing is used to determine ploidy status of newborns or of cancers. FISH techniques are often used in the evaluation of amniotic fluid, products of conception, and chorionic villi.

Contraindications

- Individuals or families not prepared to deal with the social and medical issues of inherited disease

Procedure and patient care

Before

PT Explain the procedure to the patient.

- When testing for inheritable diseases, obtain the services of a licensed genetic counselor to inform the patient and family of the testing methods and potential results. The counselor will also provide the patient and family with potential actions that may need to be taken if the results are positive.

During

- Provide the appropriate specimen to the laboratory.
- Collect a venous sample of blood in a green-top (sodium heparin) tube.
- Testing is performed in a central reference laboratory, but special specimen preparation may be required.

After

- When testing for inheritable diseases, ensure that arrangements have been made with the genetics counselor to provide the results to the patient and family members.

Abnormal findings

Genetic errors in metabolism
Inheritable chromosomal abnormalities
Cancer
Autism
Mental retardation
Spontaneous abortion

notes

lactic acid (Lactate)

Type of test Blood

Normal findings

Venous blood: 5-20 mg/dL or 0.6-2.2 mmol/L (SI units)
Arterial blood: 3-7 mg/dL or 0.3-0.8 mmol/L (SI units)

Test explanation and related physiology

Under conditions of normal oxygen availability to tissues, glucose is metabolized to CO_2 and H_2O for energy. When oxygen to the tissues is diminished, anaerobic metabolism of glucose occurs, and lactate (lactic acid) is formed instead of CO_2 and H_2O. To compound the problem of lactic acid buildup, when the liver is hypoxic, it fails to clear the lactic acid. Lactic acid levels accumulate, causing lactic acidosis (LA). Therefore, blood lactate is a fairly sensitive and reliable indicator of tissue hypoxia. The hypoxia may be caused by local tissue hypoxia (e.g., mesenteric ischemia, extremity ischemia) or generalized tissue hypoxia (e.g., that which exists in shock). Lactic acid blood levels are used to document the presence of tissue hypoxia, determine the degree of hypoxia, and monitor the effect of therapy.

Type I LA is caused by diseases or factors that increase lactate but are not hypoxic related (e.g., glycogen storage diseases, liver diseases, or drugs). LA caused by hypoxia is classified as type II. Shock, convulsions, and extremity ischemia are the most common causes of type II LA. Type III LA is idiopathic and is most commonly seen in nonketotic patients with diabetes. The pathophysiology of lactic acid accumulation in type III is not known.

Interfering factors

- The prolonged use of a tourniquet or clenching of hands increases lactate levels.
- ☛ Drugs that *increase* levels include aspirin, cyanide, ethanol (chronic use), nalidixic acid, and phenformin.

Procedure and patient care

- See inside front cover for Routine Blood Testing.
- Fasting: no.
- Blood tube commonly used: red.
- **PT** Instruct the patient to avoid making a fist before and while blood is being withdrawn.
- Avoid the use of a tourniquet if possible.
- Collect a venous blood sample or arterial blood sample in a red-top tube.

Abnormal findings

▲ **Increased levels**
Shock
Tissue ischemia
Carbon monoxide poisoning
Severe liver disease
Genetic errors of metabolism
Diabetes mellitus (nonketotic)

notes

lactic dehydrogenase (LDH, Lactate dehydrogenase)

Type of test   Blood

Normal findings

Total

Adult/elderly: 100-190 units/L at 37 °C (lactate → pyruvate) or 100-190 units/L (SI units)

Child: 60-170 units/L (30 °C)

Infant: 100-250 units/L

Newborn: 160-450 units/L

Isoenzymes

Adult/elderly:

LDH-1: 17%-27%

LDH-2: 27%-37%

LDH-3: 18%-25%

LDH-4: 3%-8%

LDH-5: 0%-5%

Test explanation and related physiology

LDH is found in the cells of many body tissues, especially the heart, liver, red blood cells, kidneys, skeletal muscles, brain, and lungs. When disease or injury affects the cells that contain LDH, the cells lyse and LDH is spilled into the bloodstream, where it is identified in higher than normal levels. The LDH test is a measure of total LDH. There are actually five separate fractions (isoenzymes) that make up the total LDH.

In general, isoenzyme LDH-1 comes mainly from the heart; LDH-2 comes primarily from the reticuloendothelial system; LDH-3 comes from the lungs and other tissues; LDH-4 comes from the kidney, placenta, and pancreas; and LDH-5 comes mainly from the liver and striated muscle. In normal persons, LDH-2 makes up the greatest percentage of total LDH.

With myocardial injury, the serum LDH level rises within 24 to 48 hours after a myocardial infarction (MI), peaks in 2 to 3 days, and returns to normal in approximately 5 to 10 days. Other cardiac markers (e.g., CK-MB, p. 308; and troponin, p. 931) have replaced the indications for LDH in the MI patient. LDH-1 is generally not as useful as troponin or creatine kinase-MB for detection of MI, unless the MI occurred 24 hours or more prior to the assay. LDH-5 is usually not as reliable as the transaminases as a liver function test.

LDH is also measured in other body fluids. Elevated urine levels of total LDH indicate neoplasm or injury to the urologic system. When the LDH in an effusion (pleural, cardiac, or peritoneal) is >60% of the serum total LDH (i.e., effusion LDH/serum LDH ratio is greater than 0.6), the effusion is said to be an *exudate* and not a transudate.

Interfering factors

- Strenuous exercise may cause an elevation of total LDH, specifically LDH-1, -2, and -5.
- Hemolysis of blood will cause false-positive LDH levels.
- ☛ Drugs that may cause *increased* LDH levels include alcohol, anesthetics, aspirin, clofibrate, fluorides, mithramycin, narcotics, and procainamide.
- ☛ Drugs that may cause *decreased* levels include ascorbic acid.

Procedure and patient care

- See inside front cover for Routine Blood Testing.
- Fasting: no.
- Blood tube commonly used: red.

Abnormal findings

▲ **Increased values**

Myocardial infarction

Pulmonary disease (e.g., embolism, infarction, pneumonia)

Hepatic disease (e.g., hepatitis, active cirrhosis, neoplasm)

Red blood cell disease (e.g., hemolytic or megaloblastic anemia or red blood cell destruction from prosthetic heart valves)

Skeletal muscle disease and injury (e.g., muscular trauma)

Renal parenchymal disease (e.g., infarction, glomerulonephritis, acute tubular necrosis)

Intestinal ischemia and infarction

Testicular tumors (seminoma or dysgerminomas)

Lymphoma and other reticuloendothelial system tumors

Advanced solid tumor malignancies

Pancreatitis

Diffuse disease or injury (e.g., heatstroke)

notes

lactoferrin

Type of test Stool

Normal findings None detected

Test explanation and related physiology

Lactoferrin is a glycoprotein expressed by activated neutrophils. The detection of lactoferrin in a fecal sample therefore serves as a surrogate marker for inflammatory white blood cells (WBCs) in the intestinal tract. WBCs in the stool are not stable and may be easily destroyed by temperature changes, delays in testing, and toxins within the stool. As a result, WBCs may not be detected by common microscopic methods. Lactoferrin assay has allowed the identification of inflammatory cells in the stool without the use of microscopy.

Detection of fecal lactoferrin allows for the differentiation of inflammatory and noninflammatory intestinal disorders in patients with diarrhea. Usually the test is used as a diagnostic aid to help identify patients with active inflammatory bowel disease (e.g., Crohn disease or ulcerative colitis) and to rule out those with active irritable bowel syndrome, which is noninflammatory. Lactoferrin is also present in patients with bacterial enteritis (e.g., *Shigella, Salmonella, Campylobacter jejuni,* and *Clostridium difficile*). Diarrhea caused by viruses and most parasites is not associated with elevated lactoferrin levels.

The lactoferrin analyte may be qualitatively detected by two distinct methods: (1) a latex agglutination procedure (the most commonly used) and (2) a microwell enzyme immunoassay procedure. The former method has been used primarily in the evaluation of patients with diagnoses of bacterial infectious gastroenteritis, whereas the latter method has been developed primarily as a diagnostic aid to distinguish between active inflammatory bowel disease and active noninflammatory irritable bowel syndrome.

Interfering factors

- The stool specimen should be examined immediately. In some instances a specific stool preservative–enteric transport media can be used.
- Breastfeeding can affect test results in breastfed infants.

Procedure and patient care

Before

PT Explain the procedure to the patient.

PT Instruct the patient not to mix urine or toilet paper with the specimen.

During

- Stool is collected in a clean bedpan.
- Place at least 5 g of stool in a clean specimen container.

After

- Observe appropriate contamination precautions.
- Transfer the specimen to the laboratory immediately.

PT Inform the patient that results are usually available in less than 1/2 hour.

Abnormal findings

Bacterial enteritis
Crohn disease
Ulcerative colitis

notes

lactose tolerance test (Hydrogen breath test)

Type of test Blood

Normal findings

Blood: Adult/elderly: rise in plasma glucose levels >20 mg/dL
  No abdominal cramps or diarrhea
Breath: <50 ppm hydrogen increase over baseline

Test explanation and related physiology

This test is performed to detect lactose intolerance, intestinal malabsorption, maldigestion, or bacterial overgrowth in the small intestine. Because lactose-intolerant patients have an absence of lactase, any lactose (the common sugar in dairy products) ingested will not be digested in the small bowel. Thus, the colon is flooded with a high lactose load. Bacterial metabolism of the lactose occurs within the colon, creating a strong cathartic effect. Symptoms of lactose intolerance include abdominal cramping, flatus, abdominal bloating, and diarrhea.

Although all adults have some degree of lactase reduction, severe lactose intolerance can occur in patients with inflammatory bowel disease, short-gut syndrome, and other malabsorption syndromes. Lactase deficiency can be congenital and become apparent in the newborn. These infants present with vomiting, diarrhea, malabsorption, and failure to thrive.

In this test, the patient is given an oral lactose load. If lactase is not present in sufficient quantities, lactose is not metabolized to glucose and galactose. Plasma levels of glucose do not rise as expected. Therefore, lower than expected serum glucose levels suggest intestinal lactase deficiency. Patients who have malabsorption without lactase deficiency will also fail to elevate the blood glucose levels.

There is a breath test portion of this diagnostic test in which exhaled air is analyzed for hydrogen content. This is called the *lactose breath test* (or *hydrogen breath test*). The bacteria in the colon produce hydrogen when exposed to unabsorbed food, particularly the lactose load that was not absorbed in the small intestine. Large amounts of hydrogen may also be produced when the colonic bacteria move back into the small intestine, a condition called bacterial overgrowth of the small bowel. In this instance, the bacteria overgrowth are exposed to the lactose load that has not had a chance to completely traverse the small intestine to be fully digested and absorbed. Large amounts of the hydrogen produced by the bacteria are absorbed into the blood flowing through the

L

wall of the small intestine and colon. This hydrogen-containing blood travels to the lungs, where the hydrogen is released and exhaled in the breath in measurable quantities.

Prior to lactose hydrogen breath testing, individuals must fast for at least 12 hours. At the start of the test, the individual blows into a hydrogen analyzer. The individual then ingests a small amount of the test sugar (e.g., lactose, sucrose, sorbitol, fructose, lactulose, depending on the purpose of the test). Additional samples of breath are collected and analyzed for hydrogen every 15 minutes for 1 to 5 hours. When rapid intestinal transit is present, the test dose of nondigestible lactulose reaches the colon more quickly than normal; therefore, hydrogen is produced by the colonic bacteria soon after the sugar is ingested. When bacterial overgrowth of the small bowel is present, ingestion of lactulose results in two separate periods during the test in which hydrogen is produced: an earlier period caused by the bacteria in the small intestine and a later one caused by the bacteria in the colon.

Interfering factors

- Enterogenous steatorrhea
- Strenuous exercise
- Smoking may increase blood glucose levels.
- Ethnicity has a major impact on primary lactose deficiency.
- Patients with diabetes may have glucose levels that exceed 20 mg/dL despite lactase insufficiency.
- ☛ Antibiotics can *decrease* the bacteria in the intestine and may cause false-negative breath tests and thus should not be taken for 1 month prior to testing.

Procedure and patient care

Before

- **PT** Explain the procedure to the patient. Inform the patient that four blood samples will be needed.
- **PT** Instruct the patient to fast for 12 hours before testing.
- **PT** Instruct the patient to avoid strenuous exercise for 8 hours before testing because exercise may factitiously affect the blood glucose level.
- **PT** Inform the patient that smoking is prohibited for approximately 8 hours before testing because smoking can increase the blood glucose level.

During

- Collect a venous blood sample in a gray-top tube from the fasting patient.

- Provide a specified dose of lactose for the patient. Usually dilute 50-100 g of lactose with 200 mL of water for ingestion in adults.
- Note that pediatric doses of lactose are based on weight.
- Collect three more blood samples at 30, 60, and 120 minutes after the ingestion of lactose.
PT Tell the patient that the only discomfort is the venipuncture; however, patients with lactase deficiency may have symptoms of lactose intolerance (e.g., cramps and diarrhea).
- If the breath test is being done, the exhaled air is evaluated for hydrogen content before ingestion of lactose and every 15 minutes thereafter. Hydrogen levels are recorded.

After
- Apply pressure to the venipuncture site.
- Note that patients with abnormal test results may receive a monosaccharide tolerance test (e.g., glucose or galactose tolerance test).

Abnormal findings

▼ **Decreased levels**
   Lactase insufficiency
   Intestinal malabsorption/maldigestion
   Small bowel overgrowth of bacteria

notes

laparoscopy

Type of test Endoscopy

Normal findings Normal-appearing abdominal and pelvic organs

Test explanation and related physiology

Laparoscopy is used to visualize directly the abdominal and pelvic organs when pathology is suspected. It is used to evaluate patients with:

- Acute abdominal/pelvic pain
- Chronic abdominal/pelvic pain
- Suspected advanced cancer
- Abdominal mass of uncertain etiology
- Unexplained infertility

During laparoscopy, the abdominal organs can be visualized by inserting a scope through the abdominal wall and into the peritoneum (Figure 26). A camera is attached to the scope, and the view of the scope is seen on color monitors. This is particularly helpful in diagnosing abdominal and pelvic adhesions, tumors, and cysts affecting any abdominal organ and tubal and uterine causes of infertility. Endometriosis, ectopic pregnancy, a ruptured ovarian cyst, and salpingitis can be detected during an evaluation for pelvic pain. This procedure is also used to

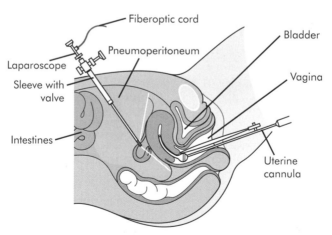

FIGURE 26 Laparoscopy directed toward the pelvis.

stage cancers and determine their resectability. Surgical procedures (e.g., cholecystectomy, appendectomy, hernia repair, tubal ligation, oophorectomy, colectomy, liver biopsy, nephrectomy, gastrectomy, and bowel resection) can be performed with the laparoscope.

Contraindications

- Patients who have had multiple abdominal surgical procedures, because adhesions may have formed
- Patients with suspected intraabdominal hemorrhage

Potential complications

- Perforation of the bowel or bladder
- Hemorrhage
- Umbilical hernia due to inadequate repair of the hole in the fascia made by the trocar used to insert the laparoscope

Interfering factors

- Adhesions or extreme obesity may obstruct the field of vision.

Procedure and patient care

Before

- **PT** Explain the procedure to the patient.
- **PT** Ensure that an informed consent for this procedure is obtained.
- If enemas are ordered to clear the bowel, assist the patient as needed and record the results.
- Because the procedure is usually performed with the patient under general anesthesia, follow general anesthesia precautions.
- Keep the patient NPO after midnight on the day of the test. IV fluids may be given.
- **PT** Instruct the patient to void before going to the operating room because a distended bladder can be easily penetrated.

During

- After general anesthesia is induced, a catheter and nasogastric tube are inserted to minimize the risk of penetrating a distended stomach or bladder with the initial needle placement.
- Note the following procedural steps:
  1. Laparoscopy is performed in the operating room. The patient is initially placed in the supine position. Other positions may be assumed to maximize visibility.
  2. After the abdominal skin is cleansed, a blunt-tipped (Verres) needle is inserted through a small incision in

the periumbilical area and into the peritoneal cavity. Alternatively, a slightly larger incision is placed in the skin, and the abdominal wall is separated under direct vision. The peritoneal cavity is entered directly. Adhesions can be lysed under direct vision.

3. The peritoneal cavity is filled with approximately 2 to 3 L of carbon dioxide to separate the abdominal wall from the intraabdominal viscera, enhancing visualization of pelvic and abdominal structures.

4. A laparoscope is inserted through a trocar to examine the abdomen (see Figure 26). Other trocars can be placed as conduits for other instrumentation.

5. After the desired procedure is completed, the laparoscope is removed, and the carbon dioxide is allowed to escape.

6. The incision(s) is closed with a few skin stitches and covered with an adhesive bandage.

• Note that laparoscopy is performed by a surgeon.

PT Most patients will have mild incisional pain later and also may complain of shoulder or subcostal discomfort from pneumoperitoneum. Inform the patient, if applicable.

After

• Note that fever and chills may indicate a bowel perforation.

• Assess the patient frequently for signs of bleeding (increased pulse rate, decreased blood pressure) and perforated viscus (abdominal tenderness, guarding, decreased bowel sounds). Report any significant findings to the physician.

PT Inform the patient that the carbon dioxide inserted into the peritoneal cavity during the procedure may cause discomfort in the shoulder area or under the ribs.

PT If patients have shoulder or subcostal discomfort from pneumoperitoneum, assure them that this usually lasts only 24 hours. Minor analgesics usually relieve this discomfort.

Abnormal findings

Abdominal adhesions	Abscess or infection
Ovarian tumor or cyst	Cancer
Endometriosis	Ascites
Ectopic pregnancy	Portal hypertension
Pelvic inflammatory disease	Other abdominal pathology
Uterine fibroids	

notes

lead

Type of test Blood

Normal findings <10 mcg/dL

Critical values
  Pediatrics (≤15 years): ≥20 mcg/dL
  Adults (≥16 years): ≥70 mcg/dL

Test explanation and related physiology

Lead poisoning is a preventable condition that results from environmental exposure to lead. This exposure, indicated by elevated blood lead levels, can result in permanent damage of almost all parts of the body. However, its effects are most pronounced on the central nervous system and kidneys, causing symptoms ranging from mild learning disabilities and behavioral problems to encephalopathy. Children less than 6 years of age are the most likely to be exposed and affected by lead. Blood lead levels are the best test for detecting and evaluating recent acute and chronic exposure. Blood lead samples are used to screen for exposure and to monitor the effectiveness of treatment. Lead can also be measured in human urine, bones, teeth, or hair.

Procedure and patient care

- See inside front cover for Routine Blood Testing.
- Fasting: no.
- Blood tube commonly used: verify with lab.
- A finger stick can be performed to obtain nearly 1 mL of blood.
- The blood sample is usually sent to a central diagnostic laboratory. The results are available in about 7 to 10 days.

Abnormal findings

▲ **Increased levels**
  Lead exposure

notes

legionnaires disease antibody test

Type of test Blood

Normal findings No *Legionella* antibody titer

Test explanation and related physiology

Legionnaires disease was originally described as a fulminating pneumonia caused by *Legionella pneumophila*, a tiny gram-negative, rod-shaped bacterium. This organism can also cause an influenza-type illness called *Pontiac fever*.

The diagnosis of legionnaires disease can be made by culturing this organism from suspected infected fluids (e.g., blood, sputum, lung tissue, and pleural fluid). Sputum for this test is best obtained by transtracheal aspiration or from bronchial washings. Another method of diagnosis is by directly identifying the organism in a microscopic smear of infected fluid with the use of direct fluorescent antibody methods. If positive, this allows for a rapid diagnosis of *Legionella*.

The most common and easiest method for diagnosis is detection of the antibody directed against the *Legionella* bacterium in the patient's blood. A presumptive diagnosis of legionnaires disease can be made in a symptomatic person when a single antibody titer is 1:256 or greater. A fourfold rise in titer to at least 1:128 between the acute-phase (1-week) and the convalescent-phase (3-week) titer is diagnostic.

Procedure and patient care

- See inside front cover for Routine Blood Testing.
- Fasting: no.
- Blood tube commonly used: red.
- For culture: Obtain sputum as indicated in sputum culture (p. 858).

Abnormal findings

▲ Increased levels

Legionnaires disease

leucine aminopeptidase (LAP)

Type of test Blood; urine (24-hour)

Normal findings

Blood

Male: 80-200 units/mL or 19.2-48.0 units/L (SI units)
Female: 75-185 units/mL or 18.0-44.4 units/L (SI units)

Urine: 2-18 units/24 hr

Test explanation and related physiology

LAP is an intracellular enzyme that exists in the hepatobiliary system and, to a much smaller degree, in the pancreas and small intestine. When disease or injury affects these organs, the cells lyse, and LAP is spilled out into the bloodstream. LAP is mainly used in diagnosing liver disorders and in the differential diagnosis of increased levels of alkaline phosphatase (ALP, p. 29). LAP levels tend to parallel ALP levels in hepatic disease. LAP is a sensitive indicator of cholestasis; however, unlike ALP, LAP remains normal in bone disease.

Interfering factors

- Pregnancy may cause increased values.
- ✘ Estrogens and progesterones may cause *increased* LAP levels.

Procedure and patient care

- See inside front cover for Routine Blood Testing.
- Fasting: no.
- Blood tube commonly used: red.
- If a urine sample is needed, See inside front cover for Routine Urine Testing.

Abnormal findings

▲ **Increased levels**

Hepatitis
Cirrhosis
Hepatic necrosis, ischemia, tumor
Hepatotoxic drugs
Cholestasis
Gallstones

notes

lipase

Type of test Blood

Normal findings 0-160 units/L or 0-160 units/L (SI units) (Values are method dependent.)

Test explanation and related physiology

The most common cause of an elevated serum lipase level is acute pancreatitis. Lipase is an enzyme secreted by the pancreas into the duodenum to break down triglycerides into fatty acids. As with amylase (p. 56), lipase appears in the bloodstream following damage to or disease affecting the pancreatic acinar cells.

Because lipase was thought to be produced only in the pancreas, elevated serum levels were considered to be specific to pathologic pancreatic conditions. It is now apparent that other conditions can be associated with elevated lipase levels. Lipase is excreted through the kidneys. Therefore, elevated lipase levels are often found in patients with renal failure. Intestinal infarction or obstruction also can be associated with lipase elevation. However, the lipase elevations in nonpancreatic diseases are less than three times the upper limit of normal compared with those in pancreatitis, where they are often five to ten times normal values.

In acute pancreatitis, elevated lipase levels usually parallel serum amylase levels. The lipase levels usually rise a little later than amylase (24 to 48 hours after the onset of pancreatitis) and remain elevated for 5 to 7 days. Because lipase peaks later and remains elevated longer than serum amylase, it is more useful in the diagnosis of acute pancreatitis later in the course of the disease. Lipase levels are less useful in more chronic pancreatic diseases (e.g., chronic pancreatitis, pancreatic carcinoma).

Interfering factors

- ✗ Drugs that may cause *increased* lipase levels include bethanechol, cholinergics, codeine, indomethacin, meperidine, methacholine, and morphine.
- ✗ Drugs that may cause *decreased* levels include calcium ions.

Procedure and patient care

- See inside front cover for Routine Blood Testing.
- Fasting: yes.
- Blood tube commonly used: red.

Abnormal findings

Acute pancreatitis
Chronic relapsing pancreatitis
Pancreatic cancer
Pancreatic pseudocyst
Acute cholecystitis
Cholangitis
Extrahepatic duct obstruction
Renal failure
Bowel obstruction or infarction
Salivary gland inflammation or tumor
Peptic ulcer disease

notes

L

lipoprotein-associated phospholipase A₂ (Lp-PLA₂ PLAC test)

Type of test Blood

Normal findings

Average value for females: 174 ng/mL (range: 120-342)
Average value for males: 251 ng/mL (range: 131-376)

Test explanation and related physiology

Lipoprotein-associated phospholipase A₂ (Lp-PLA₂) promotes vascular inflammation through the hydrolysis of oxidized LDL within the intima of the blood vessel, contributing directly to the atherogenic process. Lp-PLA₂ is an independent predictor of cardiovascular disease. When combined with CRP (p. 306), testing for Lp-PLA₂ markedly increases the predictive value in determining risks for a cardiac event, especially in patients whose ATP III cardiac risks are moderate. A Lp-PLA₂ level greater than 200 ng/mL would warrant reclassifying the patient to the next highest risk category, which would require more aggressive use of cholesterol-lowering agents. Lp-PLA₂ may play an important role in the progression of atherosclerosis and overall plaque stability.

Lp-PLA₂ is also an accurate aid in assessing the risk for ischemic stroke associated with atherosclerosis at all levels of blood pressure. The PLAC test is an enzyme-linked immunosorbent assay (ELISA) using two highly specific monoclonal antibodies to measure the level of Lp-PLA₂ in the blood.

Procedure and patient care

- See inside front cover for Routine Blood Testing.
- Fasting: no.
- Blood tube commonly used: red.

Abnormal findings

▲ **Increased levels**
 Atherosclerosis

notes

lipoproteins (High-density lipoproteins [HDLs, HDL-C], Low-density lipoproteins [LDLs, LDL-C], Very-low-density lipoproteins [VLDLs], Lipoprotein electrophoresis, Lipoprotein phenotyping, Lipid fractionation, Non-HDL cholesterol, Lipid profile)

Type of test Blood

Normal findings

HDL

Male: >45 mg/dL or >0.75 mmol/L (SI units)
Female: >55 mg/dL or >0.91 mmol/L (SI units)
LDL
Adult: <130 mg/dL
Children: <110 mg/dL
VLDL: 7-32 mg/dL

Test explanation and related physiology

Lipoproteins are considered to be an accurate predictor of heart disease. As part of the lipid profile, these tests are performed to identify persons at risk for developing heart disease and to monitor the response to therapy if abnormalities are found.

Lipoproteins are proteins in the blood whose main purpose is to transport cholesterol, triglycerides, and other insoluble fats. They are used as markers indicating the levels of lipids within the bloodstream. The lipid profile usually measures total cholesterol, triglycerides, HDL, LDL, and VLDL. With the use of *segmented gradient gel electrophoresis (SGGE)*, lipoproteins can be subclassified to more accurately indicate cardiovascular risks and familial risks of heart disease. Levels of lipoproteins are genetically influenced; however, these levels can be altered by diet, lifestyle, and medications.

HDLs (good cholesterol) are carriers of cholesterol. They are produced in the liver and, to a smaller degree, in the intestines. In general, the purpose of HDLs is believed to be removal of the cholesterol from the peripheral tissues and transportation to the liver for excretion. The function of removing lipids from the endothelium (reverse cholesterol transport) provides a protective effect against heart disease.

Clinical and epidemiologic studies have shown that total HDL cholesterol is an independent, inverse risk factor for coronary artery disease (CAD). Low levels (<35 mg/dL) are believed to increase a person's risk for CAD, while high levels (>60 mg/dL) are considered protective. When HDL and total cholesterol measurements are combined in a ratio fashion, the accuracy of

L

predicting CAD is increased. The total cholesterol/HDL ratio should be at least 5:1, with 3:1 being ideal.

With the use of SGGE, five subclasses of HDL (2a, 2b, 3a, 3b, and 3c) have been identified, but only 2b is cardioprotective. HDL 2b is the most efficient form of HDL in reverse cholesterol transport. Patients with low total HDL levels often have low levels of HDL 2b. When levels of total HDL are between 40 and 60, cardioprotective levels of HDL 2b are minimal. However, when levels of total HDL are greater than 60, levels of HDL 2b predominate, and efficient reverse cholesterol transport takes place. This protects the coronary arteries from disease. The other subclasses of HDL are not capable of reverse cholesterol transport and therefore are not cardioprotective. Levels of HDL 2b can be increased by niacin supplements but not by statin drugs (i.e., HMG CoA reductase inhibitors [simvastatin, lovastatin]).

LDLs (bad cholesterol) are also cholesterol rich. However, most cholesterol carried by LDLs can be deposited into the lining of the blood vessels and is associated with an increased risk of arteriosclerotic heart and peripheral vascular disease. Therefore, high levels of LDLs are atherogenic. The LDL level should be <70 mg/dL in patients at high risk for heart disease. For patients at moderately high risk, the LDL should be ≤100 mg/dL (depending on other cardiac risk factors). LDL can be difficult to measure. Therefore, the LDL level is usually calculated using the Friedwald formula. In this formula, subtracting the HDL plus one fifth of the triglycerides from the total cholesterol derives LDL level.

$$LDL = total\ cholesterol - (HDL + [triglycerides \div 5])$$

There are other formulas for deriving LDL, which may account for different sets of normal values. Furthermore, the formula is inaccurate if the triglycerides exceed 400 mg/dL.

With the use of SGGE, LDL has been divided into seven classes based on particle size. These subclasses include (from largest to smallest) LDL I, LDL IIa, LDL IIb, LDL IIIa, LDL IIIb, LDL IVa, and LDL IVb. The most commonly elevated forms of LDL (IIIa and IIIb) are small enough to get between the endothelial cells and cause atheromatous disease. The larger LDL particles (LDL I, LDL IIa, and LDL IIb) cannot get into the endothelial layer and therefore are not associated with increased risk of disease. LDL IVa and IVb, however, are very small and are associated with aggressive arterial plaques that are particularly vulnerable to ulceration and vascular occlusion. Nearly all patients with levels of LDL IVa and IVb greater than 10% of total LDL have vascular events within months.

LDL patterns can be identified, and they are associated with variable risks of coronary artery disease (CAD). LDL pattern A is seen in patients with mostly large LDL particles and does not carry increased risks for CAD. LDL pattern B is seen in patients with mostly small LDL particles and is associated with an increased risk of CAD. An intermediate pattern is noted in a large number of patients; they have small and large LDL particles and experience an intermediate risk of CAD. LDL levels can be lowered with diet, exercise, and statins.

VLDLs, though carrying a small amount of cholesterol, are the predominant carriers of blood triglycerides. To a lesser degree, VLDLs are also associated with an increased risk of CAD by virtue of their capability to be converted to LDL by lipoprotein lipase in skeletal muscle. The VLDL value is sometimes expressed as a percentage of total cholesterol. Levels in excess of 25% to 50% are associated with increased risk of coronary disease.

Interfering factors

- Smoking and alcohol ingestion decrease HDL levels.
- Binge eating can alter lipoprotein values.
- HDL values are age and sex dependent.
- HDL values, like cholesterol, tend to decrease significantly for as long as 3 months following myocardial infarction.
- HDL is elevated in hypothyroid patients and diminished in hyperthyroid patients.
- High triglyceride levels can make LDL calculations inaccurate.
- ✗ Drugs that may cause altered lipoprotein levels include alpha-blockers, aspirin, beta-blockers, phenytoin, estrogens, phenothiazines, steroids, and sulfonamides.

Procedure and patient care

- See inside front cover for Routine Blood Testing.
- Fasting: yes (12-14 hours).
- Blood tube commonly used: red.
- PT Inform the patient that dietary indiscretion within the previous few weeks may influence lipoprotein levels.
- PT Instruct patients with high lipoprotein levels regarding diet, exercise, and appropriate body weight.

Abnormal findings

▲ **Increased HDL levels**
Familial HDL
lipoproteinemia
Excessive exercise

▼ **Decreased HDL levels**
Metabolic syndrome
Familial low HDL
Hepatocellular disease
(e.g., hepatitis or
cirrhosis)
Hypoproteinemia
(e.g., nephrotic
syndrome or
malnutrition)

▲ **Increased LDL and
VLDL levels**
Familial LDL
lipoproteinemia
Nephrotic syndrome
Glycogen storage diseases
(e.g., von Gierke disease)
Hypothyroidism
Alcohol consumption
Chronic liver disease
(e.g., hepatitis or cirrhosis)
Hepatoma
Gammopathies
(e.g., multiple myeloma)
Familial hypercholesterolemia
type IIa
Cushing syndrome
Apoprotein CII deficiency

▼ **Decreased LDL and
VLDL levels**
Familial
hypolipoproteinemia
Hypoproteinemia
(e.g., malabsorption,
severe burns, or
malnutrition)
Hyperthyroidism

notes

liver biopsy

Type of test Microscopic examination of tissue

Normal findings Normal liver histology

Test explanation and related physiology

Liver biopsy is a safe, simple, and valuable method of diagnosing pathologic liver conditions. For this study, a specially designed needle is inserted through the abdominal wall and into the liver (Figure 27). A piece of liver tissue is removed for microscopic examination. Percutaneous liver biopsy is used in the diagnosis of various liver disorders (e.g., cirrhosis, hepatitis, drug reaction, granuloma, and tumor). Biopsy is indicated for the following:
- Patients with unexplained hepatomegaly
- Patients with persistently elevated liver enzymes

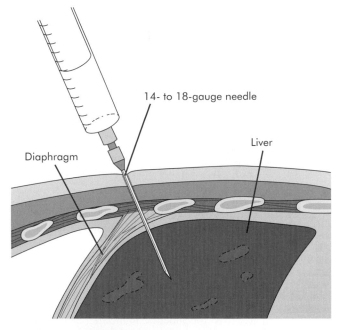

14- to 18-gauge needle

Liver

Diaphragm

FIGURE 27 Liver biopsy. Percutaneous liver biopsy requires the patient's cooperation. The patient must be able to lie quietly and hold his or her breath after exhaling.

○ Patients with suspected primary or metastatic tumor
○ Patients with unexplained jaundice
○ Patients with suspected hepatitis
○ Patients with suspected infiltrative diseases

The biopsy may be performed by a *blind stick* or directed with the use of computed tomography (CT), magnetic resonance imaging (MRI), or ultrasound.

Contraindications

- Uncooperative patients who cannot remain *still* and hold their breath during sustained exhalation
- Patients with impaired hemostasis
- Patients with anemia who could not tolerate blood loss associated with puncture of an intrahepatic blood vessel
- Patients with infections in the right pleural space or right upper quadrant
- Patients with obstructive jaundice
- Patients with a hemangioma
  Bleeding after a biopsy may be severe

Potential complications

- Hemorrhage caused by inadvertent puncture of a blood vessel
- Chemical peritonitis caused by inadvertent puncture of a bile duct, with subsequent leakage of bile
- Pneumothorax caused by improper placement of the biopsy needle into the adjacent chest cavity

Procedure and patient care

Before

PT Explain the procedure to the patient. Many patients are apprehensive about it.
- Obtain an informed consent.
- Ensure that all coagulation tests are normal.
PT Instruct the patient to keep NPO after midnight on the day of the test.
- Administer any sedative medications as ordered.

During

- Note the following procedural steps:
  1. The patient is placed in the supine or left lateral position.
  2. The skin area used for puncture is anesthetized locally.
  3. The patient is asked to exhale and hold the exhalation. This causes the liver to descend and reduces the possibility of a pneumothorax.

4. During the patient's sustained exhalation, the physician rapidly introduces the biopsy needle into the liver and obtains liver tissue.
   a. Several types of needles are available.
   b. Occasionally the biopsy needle is inserted under CT guidance. This is especially useful when tissue from a specific area of the liver is needed.
5. The needle is withdrawn from the liver.

- Note that this test is performed by a physician in approximately 15 minutes.

PT Inform the patient that he or she may have minor discomfort during injection of the local anesthetic and needle insertion.

After

- Place the tissue sample into a specimen bottle containing formalin and send it to the pathology department.
- Apply a small dressing over the needle insertion site.
- Place the patient on his or her right side for approximately 1 to 2 hours. In this position, the liver capsule is compressed against the chest wall, thereby decreasing the risk of hemorrhage or bile leak.
- Assess the patient's vital signs frequently for evidence of hemorrhage and peritonitis.
- Evaluate the rate, rhythm, and depth of respirations. Report chest pain and signs of dyspnea, cyanosis, and restlessness, which may be indicative of pneumothorax.

PT Tell the patient to avoid coughing or straining, which may cause increased intraabdominal pressure.

Abnormal findings

Benign tumor
Malignant tumor (primary or metastatic)
Abscess
Cyst
Hepatitis
Infiltrative diseases (e.g., amyloidosis, hemochromatosis, cirrhosis)

notes

liver/spleen scanning (Liver scanning)

Type of test Nuclear scan

Normal findings Normal size, shape, and position of the liver and spleen

Test explanation and related physiology

This radionuclide procedure is used to outline and detect structural changes of the liver and spleen. A radionuclide is administered intravenously. Later, a gamma ray scintillator is placed over the right and left upper quadrants of the patient's abdomen. This records the distribution of the radioactive particles emitted from the liver and spleen. Images are obtained and are recorded digitally or on an analogue film.

Single-photon emission computed tomography (SPECT) has significantly improved the quality and accuracy of liver scanning. With SPECT scanning, the radionuclide is injected, and the scintillator is placed to receive images from multiple angles (around the circumference of the patient). This greatly increases the accuracy of nuclear liver scanning. With the use of radioactive carbon, nitrogen, or oxygen, anatomic and biochemical changes can be visualized within the liver. This method of liver scanning is called PET scanning (p. 731).

This scan can also identify portal hypertension. Normally, most of the radionuclide administered during a liver scan is taken up by the liver. If the liver-to-spleen ratio is reversed (i.e., the spleen takes up more of the radionuclide), reversal of hepatic blood flow exists as a result of portal hypertension.

Contraindications

- Patients who are pregnant or lactating, unless the benefits of testing outweigh the risk of damage to the fetus or infant

Interfering factors

- Barium in the GI tract overlying the liver or spleen will produce defects on the scan that may be mistaken for masses.

Procedure and patient care

Before

PT Explain the procedure to the patient.

PT Tell the patient that no fasting or premedication is required.

PT Assure the patient that he or she will not be exposed to large amounts of radiation.

During

- Note the following procedural steps:
  1. The patient is taken to nuclear medicine, where the radionuclide is administered intravenously.
  2. Thirty minutes after injection, a gamma ray detector is placed over the right upper quadrant of the abdomen.
  3. The patient is placed in supine, lateral, and prone positions so that all surfaces of the liver can be visualized.
  4. The radionuclide image is recorded digitally or on an analogue film.
- Note that this procedure is performed by a trained technologist in approximately 1 hour. A physician trained in nuclear medicine interprets the results.
- **PT** Tell the patient that the only discomfort associated with this procedure is the IV injection of the radionuclide.

After

PT Because only tracer doses of radioisotopes are used, inform the patient that no radiation precautions are needed.

Abnormal findings

Primary or metastatic tumor of the liver or spleen
Abscess of the liver or spleen
Hematoma of the liver or spleen
Hepatic or splenic cyst
Hemangioma
Lacerations of the liver or spleen
Infiltrative processes (e.g., sarcoidosis, amyloidosis, tuberculosis, or granuloma of the liver or spleen)
Cirrhosis
Portal hypertension
Accessory spleen
Splenic infarction

notes

lumbar puncture and cerebrospinal fluid examination (LP and CSF examination, Spinal tap, Cerebrospinal fluid analysis)

Type of test Fluid analysis

Normal findings

Pressure: <20 cm H_2O

Color: clear and colorless

Blood: none

Cells:

  RBC: 0

  WBC

  Total

    Neonate: 0-30 cells/μL

    1-5 years: 0-20 cells/μL

    6-18 years: 0-10 cells/μL

    Adult: 0-5 cells/μL

  Differential

    Neutrophils: 0%-6%

    Lymphocytes: 40%-80%

    Monocytes: 15%-45%

Culture and sensitivity: no organisms present

Protein: 15-45 mg/dL CSF (up to 70 mg/dL in elderly adults and children)

Protein electrophoresis

  Prealbumin: 2%-7%

  Albumin: 56%-76%

  Alpha$_1$ globulin: 2%-7%

  Alpha$_2$ globulin: 4%-12%

  Beta globulin: 8%-18%

  Gamma globulin: 3%-12%

  Oligoclonal bands: none

  IgG: 0.0-4.5 mg/dL

Glucose: 50-75 mg/dL CSF or 60%-70% of blood glucose level

Chloride: 700-750 mg/dL

Lactic dehydrogenase (LDH): ≤40 units/L (adults), ≤70 units/L (neonates)

Lactic acid: 10-25 mg/dL

Cytology: no malignant cells

Serology for syphilis: negative

Glutamine: 6-15 mg/dL

Test explanation and related physiology

By placing a needle in the subarachnoid space of the spinal column, one can measure the pressure of that space and obtain CSF for examination and diagnosis. Lumbar puncture (LP) may also be used therapeutically to inject therapeutic or diagnostic agents and to administer spinal anesthetics. Furthermore, LP may be used to reduce intracranial pressure in patients with normal pressure hydrocephalus or in patients with pseudotumor cerebri.

Examination of the CSF includes evaluation for the presence of blood, bacteria, and malignant cells, along with quantification of the amount of glucose and protein present. Color is noted, and various other tests, such as a serologic test for syphilis (p. 877), are performed.

Pressure

By attaching a sterile manometer to the needle used for LP, the pressure within the subarachnoid space can be measured. A pressure greater than $20\,cm$ H_2O is considered abnormal and indicative of increased spinal pressure. Because the subarachnoid space surrounding the brain is freely connected to the subarachnoid space of the spinal cord, any increase in intracranial pressure will be directly reflected as an increase at the lumbar site. Tumors, infection, hydrocephalus, and intracranial bleeding can cause increased intracranial and spinal pressure. Intracranial pressure is related to the volume of CSF fluid. Also, because the cranial venous sinuses are connected to the jugular veins, obstruction of those veins or the superior vena cava increases intracranial pressure.

Pressures are routinely measured at the beginning and end of an LP. If there is a significant difference in these values, one must suspect a spinal cord obstruction (tumor). Large differences in opening and closing pressures are also seen in patients with hydrocephalus.

Color

Normal CSF is clear and colorless. Color differences can occur with hyperbilirubinemia, hypercarotenemia, melanoma, or elevated proteins. A cloudy appearance may indicate an increase in the white blood cell (WBC) count or protein. A red tinge to the CSF indicates the presence of blood.

Blood

Normally, CSF contains no blood. Blood may be present because of bleeding into the subarachnoid space or because the needle used in the LP has inadvertently penetrated a blood vessel on the way into the subarachnoid space. With a *traumatic puncture*, the blood within the CSF will clot. No clotting occurs in a patient with subarachnoid hemorrhage. Also, with a traumatic tap, the fluid clears toward the end of the procedure as successive CSF samples are obtained. This clearing does not occur with a subarachnoid hemorrhage.

Cells

The number of red blood cells (RBCs) is merely an indication of the amount of blood present within the CSF. Except for a few lymphocytes, the presence of WBCs in the CSF is abnormal. The presence of polymorphonuclear leukocytes (neutrophils) is indicative of bacterial meningitis or cerebral abscess. When mononuclear leukocytes are present, viral or tubercular meningitis or encephalitis is suspected. Leukemia or other primary or metastatic malignant tumors may cause elevated WBCs.

WBCs can be present in the CSF as a result of a traumatic tap, in which the spinal needle hits a blood vessel while performing the spinal tap. However, more than 1 WBC per 500 RBCs is considered pathologic and may indicate an infection, such as meningitis.

Culture and sensitivity

The organisms that cause meningitis or brain abscess can be cultured from the CSF. Organisms found also may include atypical bacteria, fungi, or *Mycobacterium tuberculosis*. A Gram stain (p. 858) of the CSF may give the clinician preliminary information about the causative infectious agent. This may allow appropriate antibiotic therapy to be initiated before the 24 to 72 hours necessary to complete the culture and sensitivity report.

Protein

Normally, very little protein is found in CSF because proteins are large molecules that do not cross the blood-brain barrier. Normally, the proportion of albumin to globulin is higher in CSF than in blood plasma (p. 761) because albumin is smaller than globulin and can pass more easily through the blood-brain barrier. Such diseases as meningitis, encephalitis, and myelitis can alter the permeability of the blood-brain barrier, allowing protein to leak into the CSF. Furthermore, central nervous system (CNS) tumors may produce and secrete protein into the CSF.

CSF protein electrophoresis is very important in the diagnosis of CNS diseases. Patients with multiple sclerosis, neurosyphilis, or other immunogenic degenerative central neurologic diseases have elevated immunoglobulins in their CSF. The detection of *oligoclonal gamma globulin bands* is highly suggestive of inflammatory and autoimmune diseases of the CNS, especially multiple sclerosis (MS). Myelin-basic protein, a component of myelin, may be elevated when demyelinating diseases (e.g., MS and amyotrophic lateral sclerosis) occur.

Glucose

The glucose level is decreased when bacteria, inflammatory cells, or tumor cells are present. A blood sample for glucose (p. 474) is usually drawn before the spinal tap is performed. A CSF glucose level of less than 60% of the blood glucose may indicate meningitis or neoplasm.

Chloride

The chloride concentration in CSF may be decreased in patients with meningeal infections, tubercular meningitis, and conditions of low blood chloride levels. CSF is not routinely evaluated for chloride; this test is done only if specifically requested.

Lactic dehydrogenase

Quantification of lactic dehydrogenase (LDH) (specifically fractions 4 and 5, p. 571) is helpful in diagnosing bacterial meningitis. The sources of LDH are the neutrophils that fight the invading bacteria. When the LDH level is elevated, infection or inflammation is suspected. The elevated WBC count associated with CNS leukemia is also associated with elevated LDH levels. The nerve tissue in the CNS is also high in LDH (isoenzymes 1 and 2). Therefore, disease directly affecting the brain or spinal cord (e.g., stroke) is associated with elevated LDH levels.

Lactic acid

Elevated levels indicate anaerobic metabolism associated with decreased oxygenation of the brain. CSF lactic acid is increased in both bacterial and fungal meningitis but not in viral meningitis.

Cytology

Examination of cells found in the CSF can determine whether they are malignant. Tumors in the CNS may shed cells from their surface. These cells can float freely in CSF.

Tumor markers

Increased levels of tumor markers (e.g., carcinoembryonic antigen, alpha-fetoprotein, and human chorionic gonadotropin) may indicate metastatic tumor.

Serology for syphilis

Latent syphilis is diagnosed by performing one of many presently available serologic tests on CSF. These include the Wasserman test, the Venereal Disease Research Laboratory test, and the fluorescent treponemal antibody (FTA) test (p. 877). When test results are positive, the diagnosis of neurosyphilis is made, and appropriate antibiotic therapy is initiated.

Glutamine

Elevated glutamine levels are helpful in the detection and evaluation of hepatic encephalopathy and hepatic coma. The glutamine is made by increased levels of ammonia, which are commonly associated with liver failure (see serum ammonia, p. 47). Levels of glutamine are also often increased in patients with Reye syndrome.

C-reactive protein

As noted on p. 306, C-reactive protein (CRP) is a nonspecific, acute-phase reactant used in the diagnosis of bacterial infections and inflammatory disorders. Elevated CSF levels of CRP have been useful in the diagnosis of bacterial meningitis. Failure to find elevated CSF levels of CRP appears to be strong evidence against bacterial meningitis. Some research studies have shown that CSF levels of CRP have been valuable in distinguishing bacterial meningitis from viral encephalitis, tuberculosis, meningitis, febrile convulsions, and other CNS disorders.

Contraindications

- Patients with increased intracranial pressure
  The LP may induce cerebral or cerebellar herniation through the foramen magnum.
- Patients who are anticoagulated
  Because of the risk of epidural hematoma, these patients need to have normal coagulation function prior to this procedure.
- Patients who have severe degenerative vertebral joint disease
  It is very difficult to pass the needle through the degenerated arthritic interspinal space.
- Patients with infection near the LP site
  Meningitis can result from contamination of CSF.

Potential complications

- Persistent CSF leak, causing severe headache
- Puncture of subcutaneous blood vessel during the procedure
- Introduction of bacteria causing meningitis

- Herniation of the brain through the tentorium cerebelli or herniation of the cerebellum through the foramen magnum
  In patients with increased intracranial pressure, the quick reduction of pressure in the spinal column by the LP may induce herniation of the brain, causing compression of the brainstem.
- Inadvertent puncture of the spinal cord caused by inappropriately high puncture of the spinal canal
- Puncture of the aorta or vena cava, causing serious retroperitoneal hemorrhage
- Transient back pain and pain or paresthesia in the legs
- Transient postural headache (worse when standing)

Procedure and patient care

Before

PT Explain the procedure to the patient. Many patients have misconceptions regarding LP.
- Obtain informed consent if required by the institution.
- Perform a baseline neurologic assessment of the legs by assessing the patient's strength, sensation, and movement.

PT Tell the patient that no fasting or sedation is required.

PT Instruct the patient to empty the bladder and bowels.

PT Explain to the patient that he or she must lie very still throughout this procedure. Movement may cause injury.

During

- Note the following procedural steps:
  1. This study can be easily performed at the bedside. The patient is usually placed in the lateral decubitus (fetal) position (Figure 28).
  2. The patient is instructed to clasp the hands on the knees to maintain this position. (A sitting position also may be used.)
  3. A local anesthetic is injected into the skin and subcutaneous tissues after the site has been aseptically cleaned.
  4. A spinal needle containing an inner obturator is placed through the skin and into the spinal canal.
  5. The subarachnoid space is entered.
  6. The insert (obturator) is removed, and CSF can be seen slowly dripping from the needle.
  7. The needle is attached to a sterile manometer, and the pressure (opening pressure) is recorded.
  8. Before the pressure reading is taken, the patient is asked to relax and straighten the legs to reduce the intraabdominal pressure.
  9. Three sterile test tubes are filled with 5 to 10 mL of CSF.
  10. The pressure (closing pressure) is measured.

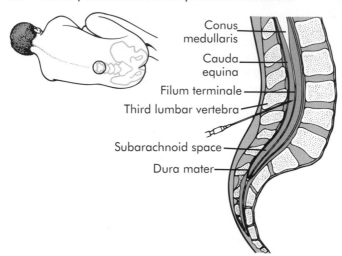

FIGURE 28 Patient position for lumbar puncture.

- Note that if blockage in CSF circulation in the spinal sub-arachnoid space is suspected, a *Queckenstedt-Stookey* test may be performed. For this test, the jugular vein is occluded either manually by digital pressure or by a medium-sized blood pressure cuff inflated to approximately 20 mm Hg. Within 10 seconds after jugular occlusion, CSF pressure should increase from 15 to 40 cm H_2O and then promptly return to normal within 10 seconds after release of the pressure. A sluggish rise or fall of CSF pressure suggests partial blockage of CSF circulation. No rise after 10 seconds suggests a complete obstruction within the spinal canal.
- Note that this procedure is performed by a physician in approximately 20 minutes.
- **PT** Inform the patient that this procedure is described as uncomfortable or painful by most patients.

After
- Apply digital pressure and an adhesive dressing to the puncture site.
- Place the patient in the prone position with a pillow under the abdomen to increase the intraabdominal pressure, which will indirectly increase the pressure in the tissues surrounding the spinal cord. This retards continued CSF flow from the spinal canal.

PT Encourage the patient to drink increased amounts of fluid with a straw to replace the CSF removed during the lumbar puncture.

PT Usually keep the patient in a reclining position for 1 hour or up to several hours to avoid the discomfort of potential post-puncture spinal headache. Instruct the patient to turn from side to side as long as the head is not raised.

• Label and number the specimen jars appropriately and deliver them immediately to the laboratory after the test. A delay between collection time and testing can invalidate results, especially cell counts.

PT Instruct the patient to report numbness, tingling, and movement of the extremities; pain at the injection site; drainage of blood or CSF at the injection site; and the inability to void. Notify the physician of any unusual findings.

Abnormal findings

Brain neoplasm
Spinal cord neoplasm
Cerebral hemorrhage
Encephalitis
Myelitis
Tumor
Neurosyphilis
Autoimmune disorder
Hepatic encephalopathy
Coma

Meningitis
Viral or tubercular meningitis
Cerebral abscess
Degenerative cord or brain disease
Multiple sclerosis
Acute demyelinating
    polyneuropathy
Subarachnoid bleeding
Reye syndrome
Metastatic tumor

notes

lung biopsy

Type of test Microscopic examination of tissue

Normal findings No evidence of pathology

Test explanation and related physiology

This invasive procedure is used to obtain a specimen of pulmonary tissue for a histologic examination by using either an open or a closed technique. The *open method* involves a limited thoracotomy. The *closed technique* includes methods such as transbronchial lung biopsy, transbronchial needle aspiration biopsy, transcatheter bronchial brushing, percutaneous needle biopsy, and video-assisted thoracotomy (VAT, p. 889).

Lung biopsy is indicated to determine the pathology of pulmonary parenchymal disease. Carcinomas, granulomas, infections, and sarcoidosis can be diagnosed with this procedure. The procedure is also useful in detecting environmental exposures, infections, or familial disease.

Contraindications

- Patients with bullae or cysts of the lung
- Patients with suspected vascular anomalies of the lung
- Patients with bleeding abnormalities
- Patients with pulmonary hypertension
- Patients with respiratory insufficiency

Potential complications

- Pneumothorax
- Pulmonary hemorrhage
- Empyema

Procedure and patient care

Before

PT Explain the procedure to the patient.
- Ensure that informed and signed consent is obtained.
PT Instruct the patient that fasting is usually ordered. The patient may be kept NPO after midnight on the day of the test.
PT Instruct the patient to remain still during the lung biopsy.

During

- Note that the patient's position depends on the method used and that the histologic lung specimen may be obtained by several different methods.

Transbronchial lung biopsy

o This technique is performed via flexible fiberoptic bronchoscopy by using cutting forceps.

o Fluoroscopy is used to ensure proper opening and positioning of the forceps on the lesions.

o Fluoroscopy also permits visualization of the tug of the lung as the specimen is removed.

Transbronchial needle aspiration

o The needle is inserted through the bronchoscope and into the tumor or desired area, where aspiration is performed with the attached syringe (Figure 29).

o The needle is retracted within its sheath, and the entire catheter is withdrawn from the fiberoptic scope.

Transbronchial brushing

o A small brush is moved back and forth over the suspicious area in the bronchus or its branches.

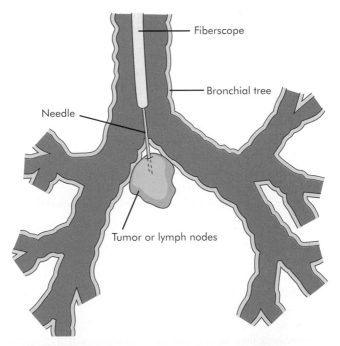

FIGURE 29 Transbronchial needle biopsy. The diagram shows a transbronchial needle penetrating the bronchial wall and entering a mass of subcarinal lymph nodes or tumor.

- o The cells adhere to the brush, which is then removed and used to make microscopic slides.

Percutaneous needle biopsy
- o In this method of obtaining a closed specimen, the biopsy is obtained after using fluoroscopic x-ray or CT scan.
- o The procedure is carried out by using a cutting needle or by aspiration with a spinal-type needle to obtain a specimen.

Open lung biopsy
- o The patient is taken to the operating room, and general anesthesia is provided.
- o An incision is made into the chest wall.
- o After a piece of lung tissue is removed, the lung is sutured.
- o Chest tube drainage is used for approximately 24 hours.

Thorascopic lung biopsy
- o The lung is collapsed with a double lumen endotracheal tube placed during induction of general anesthesia.
- o With the use of a thoracoscope, the lung is grasped, and a piece is cut off with the use of a cutting/stapling device.
- o The scope and trocars are removed, and a small chest tube is left in place.
- o The tiny incisions are closed.

- • Note that this procedure is performed by a surgeon, radiologist, or pulmonologist in 30 to 60 minutes.
- • During the lung biopsy procedure, assess the patient carefully for signs of respiratory distress.
- **PT** Tell the patient that most patients describe this procedure as painful.

After

- • Place biopsy specimens in appropriate containers for histologic and microbiologic examination.
- • Observe the patient's vital signs frequently for signs of bleeding and shortness of breath.
- • Assess the patient's breath sounds and report any decrease.
- • Obtain a chest x-ray image to check for complications.
- • Observe the patient for signs of pneumothorax (e.g., dyspnea, tachypnea, decrease in breath sounds, anxiety, restlessness).

Abnormal findings

Carcinoma
Granuloma
Exposure lung diseases (e.g., black lung, asbestosis)
Sarcoidosis
Infection

notes

lung scan (Ventilation/perfusion scanning [VPS], Pulmonary scintiphotography, V̇/Q̇ scan)

Type of test Nuclear scan

Normal findings Diffuse and homogeneous uptake of nuclear material by the lungs

Test explanation and related physiology

This nuclear medicine procedure is used to identify defects in blood *perfusion* of the lung in patients with suspected pulmonary embolism. Blood flow to the lungs is evaluated using a macroaggregated albumin (MAA) tagged with technetium (Tc^{99m}), which is injected into the patient's peripheral vein. Because the diameter of the radionuclide aggregates is larger than that of the pulmonary capillaries, the aggregates become temporarily lodged in the pulmonary vasculature. A scintillator (gamma camera) detects the gamma rays from within the lung microvasculature. With the use of light conversion, a realistic image of the lung is obtained on film.

A homogeneous uptake of particles that fills the entire pulmonary vasculature conclusively rules out pulmonary embolism. If a defect in an otherwise smooth and diffusely homogeneous pattern is seen, a perfusion abnormality exists. This can indicate pulmonary embolism. Unfortunately, many other serious pulmonary parenchymal lesions (e.g., pneumonia, pleural fluid, emphysematous bullae) also cause a defect in pulmonary blood perfusion. Therefore, although the scan may be sensitive, it is not specific, because many different pathologic conditions can cause the same abnormal results.

The chest x-ray image aids in assessing the perfusion scan, because a defect on the perfusion scan seen in the same area as an abnormality on the chest x-ray image does not indicate pulmonary embolism. Rather, the defect may represent pneumonia, atelectasis, effusion, and so on. However, when a perfusion defect occurs in an area of the lung that is normal on a chest x-ray study, pulmonary embolus is likely.

Specificity of a perfusion scan also can be enhanced by performance of a ventilation scan, which detects parenchymal abnormalities in ventilation (e.g., pneumonia, pleural fluid, emphysematous bullae). The *ventilation scan* reflects the patency of the pulmonary airways by using xenon gas or Tc-diethylenetriamine pentaacetic acid (DTPA) as an aerosol. When vascular obstruction (embolism) is present by perfusion scan, ventilation scans demonstrate a normal wash-in and wash-out of radioactivity from the embolized lung area. If parenchymal disease (e.g., pneumonia) is responsible for the perfusion abnormality, however, wash-in or wash-out will be abnormal. Therefore, the mismatch of perfusion and ventilation findings is characteristic of embolic disorders, whereas the match is indicative of parenchymal disease. When ventilation and perfusion scans are performed synchronously, this is called a *ventilation/perfusion (V̇/Q̇) scan*. Most nuclear physicians read the lung scan as one of several categories: negative for PE, low probability of PE, high probability of PE, or positive for PE.

Contraindications

- Patients who are pregnant, unless the benefits outweigh the risks

Interfering factors

- Pulmonary parenchymal problems (e.g., pneumonia, emphysema, pleural effusion, tumors) will give the picture of a perfusion defect and simulate pulmonary embolism.

Procedure and patient care

Before

PT Explain the procedure to the patient.
- Obtain informed consent if required by the institution.
PT Assure the patient that he or she will not be exposed to large amounts of radioactivity, because only tracer doses of isotopes are used.
PT Tell the patient that no fasting is required.
- Note that a recent chest x-ray image should be available.
PT Instruct the patient to remove jewelry around the chest.

During

- Note the following procedural steps for a ventilation/perfusion scan:
  1. The unsedated, nonfasting patient suspected of having a pulmonary embolism is taken to the nuclear medicine department.

Ventilation scan
  2. The patient breathes the tracer through a face mask with a mouthpiece.
  3. Ventilation scans require a cooperative patient.
  4. Tc-DTPA images are usually done before perfusion images and require patient cooperation with deep breathing and appropriate use of breathing equipment to prevent contamination.

Perfusion scan

5. The patient is given a peripheral IV injection of radionuclide-tagged MAA.

6. While the patient lies in the appropriate position, a gamma ray detector is passed over the patient and records radionuclide uptake on film.

7. The patient is placed in the supine, prone, and various lateral positions, which allow for anterior, posterior, lateral, and oblique views, respectively.

8. The results are interpreted by a physician trained in diagnostic nuclear medicine.

- Note that this test is usually performed by a technologist in approximately 30 minutes.
PT Tell the patient that no discomfort is associated with this test other than the peripheral venipuncture.

After

- Apply pressure to the venipuncture site.
PT Inform the patient that no radiation precautions are necessary.

Abnormal findings

Pulmonary embolism
Pneumonia
Tuberculosis
Emphysema
Tumor
Asthma
Atelectasis
Bronchitis
Chronic obstructive pulmonary disease

notes

luteinizing hormone (LH assay, Lutropin) and follicle-stimulating hormone (FSH) assay

Type of test Blood
Normal findings

	LH (IU/L)	FSH (IU/L)
Adult		
Male	1.24-7.8	1.42-15.4
Female		
Follicular phase	1.68-15	1.37-9.9
Ovulatory peak	21.9-56.6	6.17-17.2
Luteal phase	0.61-16.3	1.09-9.2
Postmenopause	14.2-52.3	19.3-100.6
Child (age 1-10 years)		
Male	0.04-3.6	0.3-4.6
Female	0.03-3.9	0.68-6.7

(Values may vary, depending on laboratory method.)

Test explanation and related physiology

LH and FSH are glycoproteins that are produced in the anterior pituitary gland. These two hormones then act on the ovary or testes. In the male, FSH stimulates Sertoli cell development and LH stimulates testosterone production from the Leydig cells. In the female, FSH stimulates the development of follicles in the ovary. LH stimulates follicular production of estrogen, ovulation, and formation of a corpus luteum. The midcycle peak of FSH is necessary for follicle/ovum formation. LH also must peak at about that same time to stimulate corpus luteal formation that could potentially support an embryo if fertilization were to occur.

Spot urine tests for LH have become very useful in the evaluation and treatment of infertility. Because LH is rapidly excreted into the urine, the plasma LH surge that precedes ovulation by 24 hours can be recognized quickly and easily. This is used to indicate the period when a woman is the most fertile. The best time to obtain a urine specimen is between 11 AM and 3 PM. Usually the woman begins to test her urine on the 10th day following the onset of her menses and continues to do so daily. Home kits in which a color change as an endpoint is used are used to make this process more convenient.

These hormones are used in the evaluation of infertility. Performing an LH assay is an easy way to determine whether ovulation has occurred. An LH surge in blood levels indicates that ovulation has taken place. Daily samples of serum LH around the woman's midcycle can detect the LH surge, which is believed to occur on the day of maximal fertility.

These assays (particularly FSH) also determine whether a gonadal insufficiency is primary (problem with the ovary/testicle) or secondary (caused by pituitary insufficiency resulting in reduced levels of FSH and LH). Elevated levels of FSH and LH in patients with gonadal insufficiency indicate primary gonadal failure, as may be seen in women with polycystic ovaries or menopause. In secondary gonadal failure, LH and FSH levels are low as a result of pituitary failure or some other pituitary-hypothalamic pathology.

Interfering factors

- Recent use of radioisotopes may affect test results if the testing method is performed by radioimmunoassay.
- Human chorionic gonadotropin (hCG) and thyroid-stimulating hormone may interfere with some immunoassay methods. Therefore, patients with hCG-producing tumors and hypothyroid patients should be expected to have falsely high LH levels.
- Drugs that may *increase* LH levels include anticonvulsants, clomiphene, naloxone, and spironolactone.
- Drugs that may *decrease* LH levels include digoxin, estrogens, oral contraceptives, phenothiazines, progesterones, and testosterone.

Procedure and patient care

- See inside front cover for Routine Blood Testing.
- Fasting: no.
- Blood tube commonly used: red.
- Note that the patient may also perform LH assays at home using a home urine test or a 24-hour urine test.
- Indicate the date of the last menstrual period on the laboratory slip. Note if the woman is postmenopausal.

Abnormal findings

▲ **Increased levels**
  Menopause
  Ovarian dysgenesis
    (Turner syndrome)
  Testicular dysgenesis
    (Klinefelter syndrome)
  Castration
  Anorchia
  Hypogonadism
  Polycystic ovaries
  Complete testicular
    feminization syndrome
  Precocious puberty
  Pituitary adenoma

▼ **Decreased levels**
  Pituitary failure
  Hypothalamic failure
  Stress
  Anorexia nervosa
  Malnutrition

notes

Lyme disease test

Type of test   Blood

Normal findings

Borrelia burgdorferi antibody EIA (Lyme index value [LIV])
   <0.90 = negative
   0.91-1.09 = equivocal
   >1.10 = positive

Western blot
   ≥5 different IgG antibodies reactive = positive
   ≥2 different IgM antibodies reactive = positive

PCR: negative

Cerebrospinal fluid: negative

Test explanation and related physiology

Lyme disease was first recognized in Lyme, Connecticut, in 1975. It is caused by a spirochete called *B. burgdorferi*. This is the most common tick-borne disease. The spirochete is spread by a bite from a black-legged tick *(Ixodes pacificus)* or deer tick *(Ixodes scapularis)*.

The clinical presentation of Lyme disease can either be localized or disseminated. Characteristic of early localized disease is the presence of erythema chronicum migrans (ECM), a round or oval erythematous skin lesion with a bull's-eye pattern that develops at the site of the tick bite; it is usually present 7 to 14 days after the tick bite and should be ≥5 cm in largest diameter for a firm Lyme disease diagnosis. Disseminated disease that may affect the musculoskeletal, cardiac, or nervous system can follow ECM within days or weeks and is considered early-stage disseminated disease. Meningoencephalitis, cranial or peripheral neuropathies, myocarditis, atrioventricular nodal block, and arthritis are some of the inflammatory changes that may occur.

Cultures of the ECM lesions can isolate the spirochete in half of the cases. However, it is difficult to culture and takes a long time to grow. Cultures of the blood or cerebrospinal fluid (CSF) are even less helpful. Currently, screening serologic studies are performed for the detection of Lyme disease. Enzyme-linked immunosorbent assay (ELISA) is the best diagnostic test for Lyme disease. This test determines titers of specific IgM and specific IgG antibodies to the *B. burgdorferi* spirochete. Levels of specific IgM antibody peak during the third to sixth week after disease onset and then gradually decline. Titers of specific IgG antibodies are generally low during the first several weeks of illness, reach maximal levels in 4 to 6 months, and often remain elevated for years.

Lyme disease can be confused with various viral infections. In these patients, a single titer of specific IgM antibody may suggest the correct diagnosis. Acute and convalescent sera can be tested to verify the diagnosis with a significant rise in positive antibody titers. The Food and Drug Administration recommends that all samples with positive or equivocal results in the *B. burgdorferi* antibody ELISA (screening) should be tested by Western blot. Positive or equivocal ELISA screening test results should not be interpreted as truly positive until verified with a confirmatory Western blot assay. The Western blot antibody assay can identify specifically the IgG or the IgM antibody. The Western blot assay is considered positive for IgG if 5 or more of the 10 significant electrophoretic bands are considered positive for *B. burgdorferi* specific IgG antibody. The Western blot IgM antibody assay is considered positive if two or more of three significant electrophoretic bands are considered positive for *B. burgdorferi* IgM antibody. However, the screening test or Western blot for *B. burgdorferi* antibodies may be falsely negative in early stages of Lyme disease, including the period when erythema migrans is apparent.

Patients with suspected Lyme disease should have the serologic test repeated if the initial test result is negative. Amplification of *Borrelia* genomic DNA by real-time polymerase chain reaction testing can be performed on CSF, synovial fluid, or urine to support the diagnosis. Ticks, after about 36 hours of attachment, may be tested by molecular methods to identify *B. burgdorferi*.

Interfering factors

- Previous infection with *B. burgdorferi* can cause positive serologic testing. These patients may no longer have Lyme disease.
- Other spirochete diseases (syphilis or leptospirosis) can cause false-positive results.

Procedure and patient care

- See inside front cover for Routine Blood Testing.
- Fasting: no.
- Blood tube commonly used: red.

Abnormal findings

Lyme disease

notes

magnesium

Type of test Blood

Normal findings

Adult: 1.3-2.1 mEq/L or 0.65-1.05 mmol/L (SI units)
Child: 1.4-1.7 mEq/L
Newborn: 1.4-2 mEq/L

Possible critical values <0.5 mEq/L or >3 mEq/L

Test explanation and related physiology

Most of the magnesium found in the body exists intracellularly; about half is in the bone. Most of the magnesium is bound to an adenosine triphosphate (ATP) molecule and is important in phosphorylation of ATP (important as the main source of energy for the body). Therefore, this electrolyte is critical in nearly all metabolic processes.

Most organ functions, including neuromuscular tissue, also depend on magnesium. It is especially important to monitor magnesium levels in cardiac patients. Low magnesium may increase cardiac irritability and aggravate cardiac arrhythmias. Hypermagnesemia retards neuromuscular conduction and is demonstrated as cardiac conduction slowing (widened PR and Q-T intervals, with wide QRS).

As intracellular elements, potassium, magnesium, and calcium (in order of quantity) are intimately tied together in maintaining a neutral intracellular electrical charge. That is why it is hard to maintain a normal potassium level when a patient has low magnesium blood levels.

Magnesium deficiency occurs in patients who are malnourished. Toxemia of pregnancy is also believed to be associated with reduced magnesium levels. Magnesium testing is used to monitor magnesium replacement therapy. Symptoms of magnesium depletion are mostly neuromuscular (i.e., weakness, irritability, tetany, electrocardiographic changes, delirium, and convulsions).

Increased magnesium levels most commonly are associated with ingestion of magnesium-containing antacids. Because most of the serum magnesium is excreted by the kidney, chronic renal diseases cause elevated magnesium levels. Symptoms of increased magnesium include lethargy, nausea and vomiting, and slurred speech.

M

Interfering factors

- Hemolysis should be avoided when collecting this specimen.
- Drugs that *increase* magnesium levels include aminoglycoside antibiotics, antacids, calcium-containing medications, laxatives, lithium, loop diuretics, and thyroid medication.
- Drugs that *decrease* magnesium levels include some antibiotics, diuretics, and insulin.

Procedure and patient care

- See inside front cover for Routine Blood Testing.
- Fasting: no.
- Blood tube commonly used: red.

Abnormal findings

▲ **Increased levels**
Renal insufficiency
Uncontrolled diabetes
Addison disease
Hypothyroidism
Ingestion of magnesium-containing antacids or salts

▼ **Decreased levels**
Malnutrition
Malabsorption
Hypoparathyroidism
Alcoholism
Chronic renal disease
Diabetic acidosis

notes

magnetic resonance imaging (MRI, Nuclear magnetic resonance imaging [NMRI])

Type of test Magnetic field study

Normal findings No evidence of pathology

Test explanation and related physiology

MRI is a noninvasive diagnostic scanning technique that provides valuable information about the body's anatomy by placing the patient in a magnetic field. MRI does not require exposure to ionizing radiation.

MRI is useful in the evaluation of the following areas:

- Head and surrounding structures
- Spinal cord and surrounding structures
- Face and surrounding structures
- Neck
- Mediastinum
- Heart and great vessels
- Liver and biliary tree
- Kidney
- Prostate
- Bones and joints
- Breast
- Extremities and soft tissues
- Pancreas

Cardiac monitoring or having metal implants, metal joint replacements, pins for open reduction of fractures, pacemakers, or cerebral aneurysm clips will result in image degradation and may endanger the patient.

MRI of the brain and meninges is particularly accurate in identifying benign and malignant neoplasms. It is able to identify and quantify brain edema, ventricular compression, hydrocephalus, and brain herniation. Intracranial hemorrhage can also be seen on MRI. *Magnetic resonance spectroscopy (MRS)* is a noninvasive procedure that generates high-resolution clinical images based on the distribution of chemicals in the body. This is particularly useful in the brain, where certain chemical metabolites will enhance the image of a high-grade malignancy. MRS has also been used to assess chemical abnormalities in the brain associated with HIV infection without having to perform a brain biopsy. This procedure has been used in a wide variety of disorders, including stroke, head injury, coma, Alzheimer disease, and multiple sclerosis.

M

MRI has revolutionized the practice of orthopedic surgery. It is particularly helpful in the determination of anatomic changes in muscle and joints (particularly knee and shoulder).

Magnetic resonance angiography (MRA) is a noninvasive procedure for viewing possible blockages in arteries. MRA has been useful in evaluation of the cervical carotid artery and large-caliber intracranial arterial and venous structures. Cardiac abnormalities, aortic aneurysm, and anatomic variants can be identified. This procedure also has proved useful in the noninvasive detection of intracranial aneurysms and vascular malformations, especially in renal artery stenosis. Coronary angiography with the resolution of most magnets is sufficient for the detection of stenosis in the large coronary arteries or venous bypass grafts but is inadequate for the detection of stenosis in smaller branches of the coronary tree.

MRI of the breast is more sensitive than mammography or ultrasonography of the breast. MRI of the breast is used for accurate localized staging of breast cancer by demonstrating an excellent three-dimensional image of a cancer and high sensitivity for other smaller synchronously occurring breast cancers that may be missed on mammography. MRI of the breast is helpful for preoperative surgical staging and for the identification of postoperative positive margins. This study is particularly helpful in differentiating postoperative scar tissue from breast cancer recurrence. MRI of the breast is the most accurate method of determining fracture of a breast implant. Most protocols use gadolinium contrast agents. With the addition of a needle-guiding system to the MRI, breast tumors can be nonoperatively and accurately localized and biopsied.

Significant improvement in *MRI of the heart* and great vessels has moved this noninvasive diagnostic procedure into the mainstream of clinical cardiology. Cardiac MRI already is considered the procedure of choice in the evaluation of pericardial disease and intracardiac and pericardiac masses; for imaging the right ventricle and pulmonary vessels; and for assessing many forms of congenital heart disease, especially after corrective surgery. The ventricle size, shape, and blood volumes can be evaluated. Cardiac valvular abnormalities, cardiac septal defects, and suspected intracardiac or pericardiac masses or thrombi can be identified. Pericardial disease (e.g., pericarditis or effusion) is easily identified. Ventricular muscle changes from ischemia or infarction can be determined. Finally, advanced MRI techniques are able to evaluate the coronary vessels directly.

Phase-contrast magnetic resonance imaging (PC-MRI) of the heart quantifies velocity and blood flow in the great arteries. Measurements of blood flow in the aorta and pulmonary trunk produce a wealth of information, including cardiac outputs of the left and right ventricles, regurgitant volumes and fraction of the aortic and pulmonary valves, and shunt ratio. Stress cardiac MRI can be performed using nitrates, dobutamine, and adenosine. When beta-blockers are added to electrocardiographic gating, cardiac volumes and images can be better portrayed.

Magnetic resonance cholangiopancreatography (MRCP) allows noninvasive imaging of the biliary tree, gallbladder, pancreas, and pancreatic duct. It is used to:

- Identify pancreatobiliary tumors, stones, inflammation, or infection
- Evaluate patients with pancreatitis to detect the underlying cause
- Help in the diagnosis of unexplained abdominal pain
- Provide a less invasive alternative to endoscopic retrograde cholangiopancreatography (ERCP)

Indications for the use of MRCP include unsuccessful or contraindicated ERCP, patient preference for noninvasive imaging, patients considered to be at low risk of having pancreatic or biliary disease, patients in which the need for therapeutic ERCP is considered unlikely, and those with a suspected neoplastic cause for pancreatic or biliary obstruction. Complication rates are much lower for MRCP than ERCP.

Magnetic resonance enterography (MRE) is used to identify inflammatory bowel disease. It is also helpful in determining extraluminal bowel pathology. MRI is an effective tool in liver imaging and in the staging of known prostate cancers.

One of the most common uses is *MRI of the cervical or lumbar spine*. The main purpose of this test is to determine the cause of neck or back pain, respectively. The MRI is the most accurate test to identify herniated disc disease. Using different MRI protocols, a *MRI myelogram* can be performed when the spinal fluid appears white and the solid tissue (discs or nerves) appears dark. Herniated discs are easily seen and graded as to their compression on the nerves. Furthermore, MRI of the spine is able to identify subtle changes associated with early infiltrating diseases such as metastatic cancer. An *upright MRI* can scan patients in any position. The upright MRI can scan patients in their positions of symptoms (e.g., pain or numbness) including weight-bearing positions, such as sitting, standing, or bending. The upright MRI can provide diagnostic images of the cervical spine, lumbar spine, and the joints over their full range of motion (such as cervical flexion/extension). The front-open and top-open design of the upright MRI nearly eliminates possible claustrophobia and accommodates larger patients.

MRI of the liver has improved significantly with the use of a gadolinium-like contrast agent called gadoxetate (Eovist). Imaging with this agent provides extremely sharp imaging that can identify liver and biliary tumors smaller than 1 cm.

Potential complications

- Gadolinium-based contrast agents (gadopentetate dimeglumine [Magnevist], gadobenate dimeglumine [MultiHance], gadodiamide [Omniscan], gadoversetamide [OptiMARK], and gadoteridol [ProHance]) have been linked to the development of nephrogenic systemic fibrosis (NSF) or nephrogenic fibrosing dermopathy (NFD). A creatinine, BUN, and/or estimated GFR (p. 312) may be obtained, especially on adults over the age of 60.

Contraindications

- Patients who are extremely obese, usually more than 300 lb
- Patients who are confused or agitated
- Patients who are claustrophobic, if an enclosed scanner is used. This can be overcome with the administration of anti-anxiety medication.
- Patients who are unstable and require continuous life-support equipment, because most monitoring equipment cannot be used inside the scanner room. Magnet-adaptive equipment is becoming available for use in the MRI scanner room.
- Patients with implantable metal objects (e.g., pacemakers, infusion pumps, aneurysm clips, inner ear implants, and metal fragments in one or both eyes), because the magnet may move the object in the body and injure the patient. Piercings, braces, and retainers need to be removed.

Interfering factors

- Movement during the scan may cause artifacts on MRI.
- Permanent retainers will cause an artifact on the scan.

Procedure and patient care

Before

PT Explain the procedure to the patient.

PT Inform the patient that there is no exposure to radiation.

- Obtain informed consent if required by the institution.

PT Tell the patient that he or she can drive without assistance after the procedure unless antianxiety medications are administered to treat claustrophobia.

PT Tell parents of young patients that they may read or talk to a child in the scanning room during the procedure. There is no risk of radiation from the procedure.

• Assess the patient for any contraindications for testing (e.g., aneurysm clips).

PT If available, show the patient a picture of the scanning machine and encourage verbalization of anxieties. Some patients may experience claustrophobia. Antianxiety medications may be helpful for those with mild claustrophobia. If possible, an open MRI system can be used for these patients.

PT Instruct the patient to remove all metal objects (e.g., dental bridges, jewelry, hair clips, belts), because they will create artifacts on the scan. The magnetic field can damage watches and credit cards. Also, movement of metal objects within the magnetic field can be detrimental to patients or staff within the field.

PT Tell the patient wearing a nicotine patch (or any other patch with a metallic foil backing) to remove it. These patches can become intensely hot during the MRI and cause burns.

PT Inform the patient that he or she will be required to remain motionless during this study. Any movement can cause artifacts on the scan.

PT Tell the patient that during the procedure he or she may hear a thumping sound. Earplugs are available if the patient wishes to use them.

PT Inform the patient that fluid or food restrictions may be required before abdominal MRI.

PT For comfort, instruct the patient to empty the bladder before the test.

• For some joint evaluations, patients have their joints injected in the x-ray department via fluoroscopy with a contrast dye prior to their *MRI arthrogram*.

During

• Note the following:
  1. The patient lies on a platform that slides into a tube containing the cylinder-shaped tubular magnet. However, patients can be scanned in sitting, standing, or bending positions with an upright MRI.
  2. For cardiac MRI, EKG leads are applied (p. 359).
  3. The patient is instructed to remain very still during the procedure. The patient may be asked to stop breathing for short periods of time.

M

4. During the scan, the patient can talk to and hear the staff via microphone or earphones placed in the scanner.

5. A contrast medium called gadolinium is a paramagnetic enhancement agent that crosses the blood-brain barrier. It is especially useful for distinguishing hypermetabolic abnormalities such as tumors. If this is to be administered, approximately 10 to 15 mL is injected in the vein. Imaging can begin shortly after the injection. No dietary restrictions are necessary before using this agent.

- Note that a qualified radiologic technologist performs this procedure in approximately 30 to 90 minutes.

PT Tell the patient that the only discomfort associated with this procedure may be lying still on a hard surface and a possible tingling sensation in teeth containing metal fillings. Also, an injection may be needed for administration of the contrast medium.

After

PT Inform the patient that no special postprocedural care is needed.

Abnormal findings

Brain

Cerebral tumor
Cerebrovascular accident
Aneurysm
Arteriovenous malformation
Hemorrhage
Subdural hematoma
Multiple sclerosis
Atrophy of the brain

Heart

Myocardial ischemia/infarction
Ventricular dysfunction/enlargement
Valvular disease
Intracardiac thrombus
Pericarditis/effusion
Cardiac or pericardial masses
Ventricular dilatation or hypertrophy
Congenital heart defects (e.g., septal defects)
Diseases of the great vessels

Other

Tumor (primary or metastatic)
Abscess
Edema
Bone destructive lesion
Joint disorder
Degenerative vertebral discs
Kidney stones or gallstones

notes

mammography (Mammogram)

Type of test X-ray

Normal findings

Category 1: Negative
Category 2: Benign findings noted
Category 3: Probably benign findings: short-term follow-up is suggested
Category 4: Suspicious findings: further evaluation is indicated
Category 5: Cancer is highly suspected
Category 6: Known breast cancer
Category 0: Abnormality noted for which more imaging is recommended

Test explanation and related physiology

Mammography is an x-ray examination of the breast. Careful interpretation of these radiographs can identify cancers. In many cases, breast cancers can be detected before they become palpable. Early detection of breast cancer improves patient survival. Radiographic signs of breast cancer include fine, stippled, clustered calcifications (white specks on the breast radiographs); a poorly defined, spiculated mass; asymmetric density; and skin thickening.

Although mammography is not a substitute for breast biopsy, results are reliable and accurate when interpreted by a skilled radiologist. The detection rate for breast cancer with mammography is greater than 85%. This means that fewer than 15% of breast cancers are missed at mammography. Cancers that are missed are in areas of the breast that are not well imaged by the radiograph (e.g., the high axillary tail of the breast), are in women with very dense breast tissue, or are too small to identify. Mammography also can detect other diseases of the breast, such as acute suppurative mastitis, abscess, fibrocystic changes, cysts, benign tumors (e.g., fibroadenoma), and intraglandular lymph nodes.

Women younger than age 25 years are most susceptible to the neoplastic effects of ionizing radiation. Therefore, mammography is rarely recommended in young women. Most mammograms include two views of each breast (in the cranial to caudal dimension and in the medial to lateral dimension). It is important to inform the woman that "callbacks" are common if the radiologist sees something that should be more thoroughly evaluated with magnified views, deeper views, or breast ultrasonography (see page 189). Mammograms can be performed using analogue radiographs or digital technology *(digital mammography)*.

Mammography is performed by a certified radiologic technologist in approximately 10 minutes. The radiographs are interpreted by an accredited radiologist. Moderate discomfort is associated with mammography. This is caused by the pressure required to compress the breast tissue while the radiographs are obtained.

Mammography can also be used to locate a mammographically identified (i.e., not palpable) lesion for surgical or nonsurgical biopsy. Nonsurgical needle biopsy with a *stereotactic biopsy* device is the least invasive manner of obtaining tissue from a nonpalpable mammographic abnormality. For this procedure, the patient is placed prone on a specialized table (Figure 30). The mammogram is connected to a computer that can identify the exact location of the mammographic abnormality.

Breast tomography (three-dimensional mammography) through different thicknesses of the breast tissue increases sensitivity of the test. Unfortunately, this technique is too expensive for screening nonsymptomatic women.

M

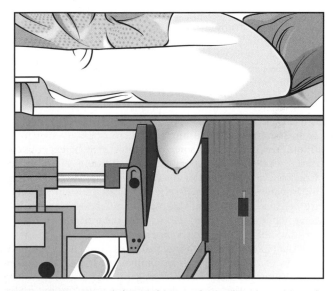

FIGURE 30 Stereotactic breast biopsy. The patient is positioned on the table with the breast pendulous through the aperture. The breast is compressed, with the target lesion centered in the biopsy window.

Mammography can be used for screening asymptomatic women for breast cancer. The frequency and ages of women that benefit most from screening mammography is presently debated. Various professional and government organizations have published guidelines for screening mammography. In general, women between the ages of 40 to 70 years would be considered good candidates for annual mammogram screening. Screening should be performed earlier for women who are at increased risk for breast cancer. Mammogram screening should be discontinued if a woman's projected duration of life is estimated to be less than 7 years. Diagnostic mammography, however, is indicated for any woman (older than the age of 25 years) who has breast symptom.

Contraindications

- Patients who are pregnant, unless the benefits outweigh the risks of fetal damage
- Women younger than age 25

Interfering factors

- Talc powder and deodorant can give the impression of calcification within the breast.
- Jewelry worn around the neck can preclude total visualization.
- Breast augmentation implants prevent total visualization of the breast. However, implants can be displaced so the native breast tissue can be imaged.
- Previous breast surgery can alter or distort the findings.

Procedure and patient care

Before

PT Explain the procedure to the patient.

PT Inform the patient that some discomfort may be experienced during breast compression. This compression allows better visualization of the breast tissue. Assure the patient that the breast will not be harmed by the compression. Premenopausal women with very sensitive breasts may choose to schedule their mammogram 1 to 2 weeks after their menses to reduce any discomfort caused by compression.

PT Tell the patient that no fasting is required.

PT Explain to the patient that a minimal radiation dose will be used during the test.

PT Instruct the patient to disrobe above the waist and put on an x-ray gown.

- Markers will be placed on any skin bump that may be interpreted as an abnormality on the x-ray image.

During

- Note the following procedural steps:
  1. The procedure takes place in the radiology department or in a breast center with a mammogram machine.
  2. One breast is placed on the x-ray plate.
  3. The x-ray cone is brought down on top of the breast to compress it gently between the broadened cone and the x-ray plate.
  4. The x-ray image is obtained. This is the craniocaudal view.
  5. The x-ray plate is turned about 45 degrees medially and placed on the inner aspect of the breast.
  6. The broadened cone is brought in medially and again gently compresses the breast. This creates the mediolateral view.
  7. Occasionally other views, such as *direct lateral* (90 degree) or *magnified spot views*, are obtained to visualize more clearly an area of suspicion.
- Note that mammography is performed by a radiologic technologist in approximately 10 minutes. The x-ray images are interpreted by a radiologist.
- **PT** Tell the patient that some discomfort may be caused by the pressure required to compress the breast tissue while the x-ray images are being taken.

M

After

PT Take this opportunity to instruct the patient in breast self-examination.

Abnormal findings

Breast cancer
Benign tumor (e.g., fibroadenoma)
Breast cyst
Fibrocystic changes
Breast abscess
Suppurative mastitis

notes

maternal screen testing (Maternal triple screen, Maternal quadruple screen)

Type of test Blood or urine

Normal findings Low probability of fetal defects

Test explanation and related physiology

These tests are provided to pregnant women early in pregnancy to identify potential birth defects or serious chromosomal/genetic abnormalities. These screening tests may indicate the potential for the presence of fetal defects (particularly trisomy 21 [Down syndrome] or trisomy 18). They may also indicate increased risk for neural tube defects (e.g., myelomeningocele, spina bifida) or abdominal wall defects (omphalocele or gastroschisis).

The incidence of these abnormalities is directly related to maternal age. In the United States, maternal screening is routinely offered to all pregnant women, usually in their second trimester of pregnancy. Patients must understand that this is a screening test, not a diagnostic test. If the screening tests are positive, more accurate definitive testing, such as chorionic villus sampling (CVS) in early pregnancy or amniocentesis in mid-pregnancy, is recommended. Most pregnant women over 35 years of age routinely have CVS or amniocentesis without maternal screening.

There are several variations of this test available:
- *Double test* measures two markers: hCG (p. 530) and alpha-fetoprotein (AFP, p. 39).
- *Triple test* (maternal triple screen test) measures three markers: human chorionic gonadotropic (hCG), AFP, and estriol (p. 405). AFP is produced in the yolk sac and fetal liver. Unconjugated estriol and hCG are produced by the placenta.
- *Quadruple test* measures four markers: hCG, AFP, estriol, and inhibin A.
- *Fully integrated screen test* measures AFP, estriol, fetal nuchal translucency (p. 697), beta and total hCG, and pregnancy-associated plasma protein-A (PAPP-A, p. 742).

The maternal triple screen test offers a 50% to 80% chance of detecting pregnancies with trisomy 21 as compared to AFP alone, which has only a 30% chance of detection. The quadruple screen is now routinely recommended and is combined with fetal nuchal translucency (FTN) (see pelvic ultrasonography, p. 697). These tests are most accurately performed during the second trimester of pregnancy, more specifically between the 14th and 24th weeks (ideal 16th and 18th weeks). The use of ultrasound to accurately indicate gestational age improves the sensitivity and specificity of maternal serum screening.

First trimester screening for genetic defects is an option for pregnant women. This testing would include fetal nuchal translucency (see pelvic ultrasonography, p. 697) combined with the beta subunit of hCG (beta hCG, p. 530), and pregnancy-associated plasma protein-A (PAPP-A, p. 742). A low level of PAPP-A may indicate an increased risk for having a stillborn baby. These tests have detection rates comparable to standard second-trimester triple screening.

First trimester (11 to 13 weeks) screening offers several potential advantages over second-trimester screening. When test results are negative, it may help reduce maternal anxiety earlier. If results are positive, it allows women to take advantage of first trimester prenatal diagnosis by CVS at 10 to 12 weeks or early pregnancy amniocentesis. Detecting problems earlier in the pregnancy may allow women to prepare for a child with health problems. It also affords women greater privacy and less health risk if they elect to terminate the pregnancy. In first trimester testing, open neural tube defects cannot be determined.

With trisomy 21, second trimester absolute maternal serum levels of AFP and unconjugated estriol are about 25% lower than normal levels, and maternal serum hCG is approximately two times higher than the normal hCG level. The results of the screening are expressed in *multiples of median (MoM)*. AFP and urinary estriol (E_3) values during pregnancies with trisomy 21 are lower than those associated with normal pregnancies, which means that values below the mean are below 1 MoM. The hCG value for trisomy 21 is above 1 MoM. The MoM, fetal age, and maternal weight are used to calculate the possible risk for chromosomal abnormalities (e.g., trisomy 21). All of the previously named maternal screening tests are discussed elsewhere in this book. For the sake of thoroughness, inhibin A is discussed here.

Inhibin A is normally secreted by the granulosa cells in the ovaries and inhibits the production of follicle-stimulating hormone (FSH) by the pituitary gland. Inhibin A is a glycoprotein of placental origin in pregnancy similar to hCG. Levels in maternal serum remain relatively constant through the 15th to 18th week of pregnancy. Inhibin A is important in the control of fetal development. Maternal serum levels of inhibin A are twice as high in

M

pregnancies affected by trisomy 21 as in unaffected pregnancies. The discovery of this fact led to the inclusion of inhibin A in the serum screening tests for trisomy 21. Inhibin A concentrations are significantly lower in women with normal pregnancies than in women with pregnancies that result in spontaneous abortions. Furthermore, circulating concentrations of inhibin A appear to reflect tumor mass for certain forms of ovarian cancer. More accurate diagnostic testing is required if screening tests are abnormal.

Procedure and patient care

Before

PT Explain the procedure to the patient.

- Allow the patient to express her concerns and fears regarding the potential for birth defects.

During

- Most of these tests can be done with a venous blood sample in a red-top tube. hCG and estriol can also be tested by collecting a urine sample.

After

- Provide the results to the patient (and other family members if the patient desires) during a personal consultation.
- Allow the patient to express her concerns if the results are positive.
- Assist the patient in scheduling and obtaining more accurate diagnostic testing if the results are positive.

Abnormal findings

Positive screening tests (trisomy 21, trisomy 18, neural tube defects, abdominal wall defects)

notes

measles rubeola antibody

Type of test Blood

Normal findings Negative

Test explanation and related physiology

The measles virus is an RNA paramyxovirus and is not the virus that causes the German measles; see rubella (p. 810). Although it is most usually a self-limiting disease, the virus can easily be spread (by respiratory droplets) to nonimmune pregnant women and cause preterm delivery or spontaneous abortion.

Testing for measles virus includes serologic identification of immunoglobulin G (IgG) and IgM antibodies. IgG elevation represents a previous infection or prior immunization. IgM indicates an acute infection or prior immunization. A fourfold rise in IgM indicates a current infection.

This test is used to diagnose measles in patients with a rash or viral syndrome when the diagnosis cannot be made clinically. Even more important, however, this test is used to establish and document immunity by previous measles infection or by previous vaccination. Populations commonly tested to document immunity include college students, health care workers, and pregnant women.

Procedure and patient care

- See inside front cover for Routine Blood Testing.
- Fasting: no.
- Blood tube commonly used: red.
- **PT** Inform the patient when to return for a follow-up rubeola titer if indicated.
- **PT** If the results are negative for immunity, recommend immunization. For women of childbearing age, vaccination should precede future pregnancy.

Abnormal findings

Active measles virus infection
Previous measles virus infection leading to immunity

notes

Meckel diverticulum nuclear scan

Type of test Nuclear medicine

Normal findings No increased uptake of radionuclide in the right lower quadrant of the abdomen

Test explanation and related physiology

Meckel diverticulum is the most common congenital abnormality of the intestinal tract. It is a persistent remnant of the omphalomesenteric tract. The diverticulum usually occurs in the ileum approximately 2 feet proximal to the ileocecal valve. Approximately 20% to 25% of Meckel diverticulum is lined internally by ectopic gastric mucosa. This gastric mucosa can secrete acid and cause ulceration of the intestinal mucosa nearby. Bleeding, inflammation, and intussusception are other potential complications of this congenital abnormality. The majority of these complications occur by 2 years of age.

Both normal gastric mucosa within the stomach and ectopic gastric mucosa in Meckel diverticulum concentrate ^{99m}Tc pertechnetate. When this radionuclide is injected intravenously, it is concentrated in the ectopic gastric mucosa of Meckel diverticulum. One can then expect to see a hot spot in the right lower quadrant of the abdomen at about the same time as the normal stomach mucosa is visualized. This is a very sensitive and specific test for this congenital abnormality.

It is possible that Meckel diverticulum is present but contains no ectopic gastric mucosa within. Usually these are not symptomatic. No concentration of radionuclide will occur within the diverticulum. This test is not helpful in these cases.

Other conditions can simulate a hot spot compatible with Meckel diverticulum containing ectopic gastric mucosa. Usually these are associated with inflammatory processes within the abdomen (e.g., appendicitis or ectopic pregnancy).

Procedure and patient care

Before

PT Explain the procedure to the patient.

PT Advise the patient to refrain from eating or drinking anything for 6 to 12 hours before the examination.

• A histamine H_2-receptor antagonist is usually given for 1 to 2 days before the scan. This blocks secretion of the radionuclide from the ectopic gastric mucosa and improves visualization of Meckel diverticulum.

During
- The patient lies in a supine position, and a large-view nuclear detector camera is placed over the patient's abdomen to identify concentration of nuclear material after intravenous injection.
- Images are taken at 5-minute intervals for 1 hour.
- Patients may be asked to lie on their left side to minimize the excretion of the radionuclide from the normal stomach, flooding the intestine with radionuclide and precluding visualization of Meckel diverticulum.
- Occasionally glucagon is provided to prolong intestinal transit time and avoid downstream contamination with the radionuclide.
- Occasionally gastrin is given to increase the uptake of the radionuclide by the ectopic gastric mucosa.
- There is no pain associated with this test.

After
- The patient is asked to void, and a repeat image is obtained. This is to ensure that Meckel diverticulum has not been hidden by a distended bladder.
- **PT** Because only tracer doses of radioisotopes are used, inform the patient that no precautions need to be taken by others against radiation.

Abnormal findings

Meckel diverticula

notes

M

mediastinoscopy

Type of test Endoscopy

Normal findings No abnormal mediastinal lymph node tissue

Test explanation and related physiology

Mediastinoscopy is a surgical procedure in which a rigid mediastinoscope (a lighted instrument scope) is inserted through a small incision made at the suprasternal notch. The scope is passed into the superior mediastinum to inspect the mediastinal lymph nodes and to remove biopsy specimens. Because these lymph nodes receive lymphatic drainage from the lungs, their assessment can provide information on intrathoracic diseases (e.g., carcinoma, granulomatous infections, and sarcoidosis). Therefore, mediastinoscopy is used in establishing the diagnosis of various intrathoracic diseases.

This procedure is also used to stage patients with lung cancer and to assess whether they are surgical candidates. Evidence of metastasis is usually a contraindication to thoracotomy because the tumor is considered inoperable. Tumors occurring in the mediastinum (e.g., thymoma or lymphoma) can also be biopsied through the mediastinoscope.

Potential complications

- Puncture of the esophagus, trachea, or blood vessels

Procedure and patient care

Before

PT Explain the procedure to the patient.

- Ensure that the physician has obtained the informed consent for this procedure.
- Check whether the patient's blood needs to be typed and crossmatched.
- Provide preoperative care as with any other surgical procedure.
- Keep the patient NPO after midnight on the day of the test.

During

- Note the following procedural steps:
  1. The patient is taken to the operating room for this surgical procedure.
  2. The patient is placed under general anesthesia.
  3. An incision is made in the suprasternal notch.
  4. The mediastinoscope is passed through this neck incision and into the superior mediastinum.

5. The lymph nodes are biopsied.
6. The scope is withdrawn, and the incision is sutured closed.
- Note that this procedure is performed by a surgeon in approximately 1 hour.
PT Inform the patient that he or she is asleep during the procedure.

After
- Provide postoperative care as with any other surgical procedure.
- Assess the patient for mediastinal crepitus on auscultation, which may indicate mediastinal air from pneumothorax or the bronchus or esophagus.
- Note that distended neck veins and pulsus paradoxus may indicate lack of cardiac filling due to a large mediastinal hematoma.
- Assess the patient for cough or shortness of breath, which may indicate a pneumothorax.
- Observe the patient for hypotension and tachycardia, which may indicate bleeding from the biopsy site or the great vessels.
- Evaluate the patient for hoarseness, which may indicate injury to the recurrent laryngeal nerve.
- Assess the patient for fever, chills, and sepsis, which may indicate mediastinitis from infection.

Abnormal findings

Lung cancer
Metastasis
Sarcoidosis
Thymoma
Tuberculosis
Hodgkin disease
Lymphoma
Infection

notes

M

metanephrine, plasma free (Fractionated metanephrines)

Type of test Blood

Normal findings

Normetanephrine: <0.5 nmol/L or 18-111 pg/mL by HPLC
Metanephrine: <0.9 nmol/L or 12-60 pg/mL by HPLC
(Results vary among laboratories.)

Test explanation and related physiology

Pheochromocytoma, although rarely a cause of hypertension, are potentially lethal tumors. They produce several catecholamines that can cause episodic or persistent hypertension that is unresponsive to conventional treatment. The current diagnosis of pheochromocytoma depends on biochemical evidence of catecholamine overproduction by the tumor.

Until recently, urinary vanillylmandelic acid (VMA) and catecholamine measurements (p. 973) were used. Urinary testing is not as sensitive as plasma testing. The development of high-performance liquid chromatography (HPLC) allowed for better sensitivity in measuring plasma free metanephrine levels. This is a blood test that measures the amount of metanephrine and normetanephrine, which are metabolites of epinephrine and norepinephrine, respectively.

The high sensitivity of plasma free metanephrine testing provides a high negative predictive value to the test. This means that if the concentrations of the free metanephrines are normal in the blood, then it is very unlikely that a patient has a pheochromocytoma. In about 80% of patients with pheochromocytoma, the magnitude of increase in plasma free metanephrines is so large that the tumor can be confirmed with close to 100% probability. Intermediate concentrations of normetanephrine and metanephrine are considered indeterminate. Urinary testing may clarify indeterminate findings. However, comparison of plasma metanephrines and urine metanephrines requires caution because different catecholamine metabolites are measured.

When interpreting results, the following may be helpful:

○ Any sample in which the concentrations of *both* normetanephrine and metanephrine are less than the upper reference range limit should be considered normal, and the presence of pheochromocytoma is highly unlikely.

○ Any sample where the concentrations of *either* normetanephrine or metanephrine exceed their respective upper reference range limits should be considered elevated.

○ Whenever the normetanephrine or metanephrine concentration exceeds the indeterminate range, the presence of pheochromocytoma is highly probable and should be located via imaging techniques. Pheochromocytoma suppression and provocative testing (page 704) may assist in identifying this tumor.

Interfering factors

- Increased levels of metanephrines may be caused by caffeine or alcohol.
- Vigorous exercise, stress, and starvation may cause increased metanephrine levels.
- ✘ Drugs that may cause *increased* metanephrine levels include epinephrine- or norepinephrine-containing drugs, levodopa, lithium, and nitroglycerin.
- ✘ Acetaminophen can interfere with HPLC testing of metanephrines and should be avoided for 48 hours prior to testing.

Procedure and patient care

Before

PT Explain the procedure to the patient.
PT Explain the dietary and medicinal restrictions.

During

- Identify and minimize factors contributing to patient stress.
- Physical and emotional stress may alter test results.
- The patient may be asked to lie down and rest quietly for 15 to 30 minutes prior to sample collection.
- The blood sample may be collected while supine.
- Collect a venous blood sample in a chilled lavender- or pink-top tube. Invert to mix with preservatives.

After

- Apply pressure to the venipuncture site.
- Send the specimen to the laboratory as soon as the test is completed.

Abnormal findings

▲ Increased levels
  Pheochromocytoma

notes

methemoglobin (Hemoglobin M)

Type of test Blood

Normal findings

0.06-0.24 g/dL or 9.3-37.2 μmol/L (SI units)
0.4%-1.5% of total hemoglobin

Possible critical values >40% of total hemoglobin

Test explanation and related physiology

Methemoglobin is formed during the production of normal adult hemoglobin. If oxygenation of the iron component in the protohemoglobin occurs without subsequent reduction of the heme iron back to its Fe^{+2} form as exists in normal hemoglobin, excess methemoglobin accumulates. The oxidized iron form in methemoglobin is unable to combine with oxygen to carry the oxygen to the peripheral tissues. Therefore, the oxyhemoglobin dissociation curve is shifted to the left, resulting in cyanosis and hypoxia.

Methemoglobinemia can be congenital or acquired. Hemoglobin M disease is a genetic defect that results in a group of abnormal hemoglobins that are methemoglobins. Another genetic mutation can cause a deficiency in reduced nicotinamide adenine dinucleotide (NADH) methemoglobin reductase enzyme that is required to deoxygenate methemoglobin to normal adult hemoglobin. These forms of methemoglobinemia occur in infants, are usually severe, are not amenable to treatment, and are often fatal.

Acquired methemoglobinemia is a result of ingestion of nitrates (e.g., from well water) or such drugs as phenacetin, sulfonamides, isoniazid, local anesthetics, and some antibiotics. This form of the disease commonly occurs in older individuals and results in an acute crisis that is treated effectively with ascorbic acid or methylene blue. Methylene blue, however, is contraindicated in G6PD deficiency.

Interfering factors

• Tobacco use and carbon monoxide poisoning are associated with increased methemoglobin levels.

✗ Drugs that may cause *increased* levels include some antibiotics, isoniazid, local anesthetics, and sulfonamides.

Procedure and patient care

- See inside front cover for Routine Blood Testing.
- Fasting: no.
- Blood tube commonly used: green.
- Methemoglobin is very unstable. Place the specimen in an ice slush immediately after collection.
- Be prepared to provide oxygen support and close monitoring in the event the patient becomes increasingly hypoxic.

Abnormal findings

Methemoglobinemia (hereditary or acquired)

notes

M

methylated septin 9 DNA (mSEPT9, ColoVantage)

Type of test Blood

Normal findings

0.0005-50 ng DNA

Test explanation and related physiology

Because of the inconvenience and discomfort associated with routine screening (see colonoscopy, p. 271; stool for occult blood testing, p. 864) for colorectal cancer, many choose not to undergo testing and thereby preclude the opportunity for the early detection of an intestinal cancer. Recently, a blood test for the detection of methylated septin 9 DNA (mSEPT9) has been developed that, when positive, is very sensitive for the presence of a colorectal cancer. Using real-time methylated PCR, septin can be isolated and quantified from extracted nucleic acid in the plasma. This test has been validated in several clinical studies; there is a strong association between detection of mSEPT9 in blood plasma with presence of colorectal cancer.

A positive test result means there is an increased likelihood for the presence of a colorectal cancer or polyp. Individuals with positive test results are encouraged to undergo a diagnostic colonoscopy. Not all individuals with colorectal cancer will have a positive test result. Therefore, individuals with a negative result should follow usual colorectal cancer screening guidelines. Accuracy data indicate that this test outperforms stool for occult blood testing.

Procedure and patient care

- See inside front cover for Routine Blood Testing.
- Fasting: no.
- Blood tube commonly used: lavender.

Abnormal findings

▲ **Increased levels**
- Colorectal cancer
- Colorectal polyps

notes

microalbumin (MA)

Type of test Urine

Normal findings

MA: <2 mg/dL
MA/creatinine ratio:
  Males: <17 mg/g creatinine
  Females: <25 mg/g creatinine

Test explanation and related physiology

Microalbuminuria refers to an albumin concentration in the urine that is greater than normal but not detectable with routine protein testing. Normally, only small amounts of albumin are filtered through the renal glomeruli, and that small quantity can be reabsorbed by the renal tubules. However, when the increased glomerular permeability of albumin overcomes tubular reabsorption capability, albumin is spilled in the urine. Preceding this stage of disease is a period of microalbuminuria that would normally go undetected. Therefore, MA is an early indication of renal disease.

For the diabetic patient, the amount of albumin in the urine is related to duration of the disease and the degree of glycemic control. MA is the earliest indicator for the development of diabetic complications (nephropathy, cardiovascular disease [CVD], and hypertension). MA can identify diabetic nephropathy 5 years before routine protein urine tests. Diabetics with elevated MA have a five- to tenfold increase in the occurrence of CVD mortality, retinopathy, and end-stage kidney disease.

It is recommended that all diabetics older than the age of 12 be screened annually for MA. This can be done through a spot urine specimen by using a semiquantitative Micral Urine Test Strip. If MA is present, the test should be repeated two more times. If two of three MA urine tests are positive, a quantitative measurement using a 24-hour urine specimen should be performed.

The presence of MA in nondiabetics is an early indicator of lower life expectancy due to CVD and hypertension. Nondiabetic nephropathies also may be associated with microalbuminuria. Life insurance underwriters are increasingly using MA testing to indicate life expectancy.

M

Interfering factors

- Urinary tract infection, blood, or acid/base abnormalities can cause elevated MA levels and falsely indicate a more serious prognosis.
- ✗ Oxytetracycline may interfere with test results.

Procedure and patient care

- See inside front cover for Routine Urine Testing.
- Ensure that the patient does not have any acute infection or urinary bleeding that could cause a false-positive result.
- If the urine specimen contains vaginal discharge or bleeding, a clean-catch or midstream specimen will be needed.
- Ensure that the urine sample is at room temperature for testing.
- If using a Micral Urine Test Strip:
  1. Dip the test strip into the urine for 5 seconds.
  2. Allow the strip to dry for 1 minute.
  3. Compare the strip with the color scale on the label.
- If a 24-hour urine collection is requested, the specimen should be refrigerated. However, it will be warmed to room temperature prior to testing.
- **PT** If the results are positive, inform the patient that the test should be repeated in 1 week.

Abnormal findings

▲ **Increased levels**
  Diabetes mellitus
  Hypertension
  Cardiovascular disease
  Nephropathy
  Urinary bleeding
  Hemoglobinuria
  Myoglobinuria

notes

microglobulin (Beta$_2$-microglobulin [β_2m], Alpha-1-microglobulin, Retinol binding protein)

Type of test Blood; urine; fluid analysis

Normal findings

Beta$_2$-microglobulin:
  Blood: 0.70-1.80 mcg/mL
  Urine: ≤300 ug/L
  CSF: 0-2.4 mg/L
Retinol binding protein:
  Urine: <163 mcg/24 hours
Alpha-1-microglobulin:
  Urine: <50 years: <13 mg/g creatinine
          ≥50 years: <20 mg/g creatinine

Test explanation and related physiology

Beta$_2$-microglobulin [β_2m] is a protein found on the surface of all cells. It is an HLA major histocompatibility antigen that exists in increased numbers on white blood cells and particularly on lymphatic cells. Production of this protein increases as these cells reproduce or are destroyed. β_2m is increased in patients with malignancies (especially B-cell lymphoma, leukemia, or multiple myeloma), chronic infections, and chronic severe inflammatory diseases. It is an accurate measurement of tumor disease activity, stage of disease, and prognosis and, as such, is an important tumor marker.

β_2m, alpha-1-microglobulin, and retinol binding proteins pass freely through glomerular membranes and are almost completely reabsorbed by renal proximal tubule cells. Due to extensive tubular reabsorption, under normal conditions very little of these proteins appear in the final excreted urine. Therefore, an increase in the urinary excretion of these proteins indicates proximal tubular disease or toxicity and/or impaired proximal tubular function. Therefore, these proteins are helpful in differentiating between various types of renal disease. In patients with aminoglycoside toxicity, heavy metal nephrotoxicity, or tubular disease, protein urine levels are elevated. Excretion is increased 100 to 1000 times normal levels in cadmium-exposed workers. This test is used to monitor these workers.

β_2m is particularly helpful in the differential diagnosis of renal disease. If blood and urine levels are obtained simultaneously, one can differentiate glomerular from tubular disease. In glomerular disease, because of poor glomerular filtration,

M

blood levels are high and urine levels are low. In tubular disease, because of poor tubular reabsorption, the blood levels are low and urine levels are high. Blood levels increase early in kidney transplant rejection.

Increased CSF levels of β_2m indicate central nervous system involvement with leukemia, lymphoma, HIV, or multiple sclerosis.

Interfering factors

- Results could be affected by recent nuclear imaging when β_2m testing is performed by radioimmunoassay.
- β_2m is unstable in acid urine.

Procedure and patient care

Before

PT Explain the procedure to the patient to minimize anxiety.

During

Blood
- Collect a venous blood sample in a red-top tube.

Urine
PT Instruct the patient to begin the 24-hour collection after voiding. Follow guidelines on inside front cover.
- A random urine level can also be used as a specimen when corrected for creatinine.

After

- Apply pressure to the venipuncture site.

Abnormal findings

▲ **Increased urine levels**
   Renal tubule disease
   Drug-induced renal toxicity
   Heavy metal–induced renal disease
   Lymphomas, leukemia, myeloma

▲ **Increased serum levels**
   Lymphomas, leukemia, myeloma
   Glomerular renal disease
   Renal transplant rejection
   Viral infections, especially HIV and cytomegalovirus
   Chronic inflammatory processes

notes

mononucleosis rapid test (Mononuclear heterophil test, Heterophil antibody test, Monospot test)

Type of test Blood

Normal findings Negative (<1:28 titer)

Test explanation and related physiology

The mononucleosis rapid test is performed to diagnose infectious mononucleosis (IM), a disease caused by the Epstein-Barr virus (EBV). Usually young adults are affected by IM. The clinical presentation is fever, pharyngitis, lymphadenopathy, and splenomegaly. Detectable levels of the IM heterophile antibody can usually be expected to occur between the 6th and 10th day following the onset of symptoms. The level usually increases through the 2nd or 3rd week of illness and, thereafter, can be expected to persist, gradually declining over a 12-month period. The IM heterophile antibody has been associated with several diseases other than IM. These include leukemia, Burkitt lymphoma, pancreatic carcinoma, viral hepatitis, cytomegalovirus infections, and others.

Several heterophil agglutination tests are available, but the most frequently performed is the rapid slide test for IM (previously called the *Monospot test*).

Procedure and patient care

- See inside front cover for Routine Blood Testing.
- Fasting: no.
- Blood tube commonly used: red.

Abnormal findings

Infectious mononucleosis
Chronic EBV infection
Chronic fatigue syndrome
Burkitt lymphoma
Some forms of chronic hepatitis

notes

M

Mycoplasma pneumoniae antibodies, IgG and IgM

Type of test blood

Normal findings

IgG

≤0.9 (negative)
0.91-1.09 (equivocal)
≥1.1 (positive)

IgM

≤0.90 (negative)
0.91-1.09 (equivocal)
≥1.1 (positive)

IgM by IFA

Negative (reported as positive or negative)

Test Explanation

Several diseases have been associated with the *Mycoplasma pneumoniae* infection, including pharyngitis, tracheobronchitis, pneumonia, and inflammation of the tympanic membrane. *Mycoplasma pneumoniae* accounts for approximately 20% of all cases of pneumonia. Classically, it causes a disease that has been described as primary atypical pneumonia. The disease is of insidious onset with fever, headache, and malaise for 2 to 4 days before the onset of respiratory symptoms. These infections may be associated with cold agglutinin syndrome (p. 267).

Positive IgM results are consistent with acute infection, although there may be some cross-reactivity associated with other *Mycoplasma* infections. A single positive IgG result only indicates previous immunologic exposure.

Procedure and patient care

- See inside front cover for Routine Blood Testing.
- Fasting: no.
- Blood tube commonly used: red.
- Transport the specimen immediately to the laboratory. Avoid undue cooling of the specimen that may lead to agglutination.

Abnormal findings

Mycoplasma infection

notes

myelography (Myelogram)

Type of test X-ray with contrast dye

Normal findings Normal spinal canal

Test explanation and related physiology

By placing radiopaque dye into the subarachnoid space of the spinal canal, the contents of the canal can be radiographically outlined. Cord tumors, meningeal tumors, metastatic spinal tumors, herniated intravertebral discs, and arthritic bone spurs can be readily detected by this study. These lesions appear as canal narrowing or as varying degrees of obstruction to the flow of the dye column within the canal. The entire canal (from lumbar to cervical areas) can be examined. This test is indicated in patients with severe back pain or localized neurologic signs that suggest the canal as the location of these injuries. Because this test is usually performed by lumbar puncture (LP, p. 596), all the potential complications of that procedure exist.

A *water-soluble* contrast material is now used for myelography. This contrast does not need to be removed at the end of the procedure, because it is water soluble and will be completely resorbed by the blood and excreted by the kidneys.

M

Contraindications

- Patients with multiple sclerosis, because exacerbation may be precipitated by myelography
- Patients with increased intracranial pressure, because LP may cause herniation of the brain
- Patients with infection near the LP site, because this may precipitate bacterial meningitis
- Patients who are allergic to shellfish or iodinated dye

Potential complications

- Headache
- Meningitis
- Herniation of the brain
- Seizures
- Allergic reaction to iodinated dye
- Hypoglycemia or acidosis may occur in patients who are taking metformin (Glucophage) and receive iodinated dye.

Procedure and patient care

Before

PT Explain the procedure to the patient.

- Ensure that the physician has obtained written and informed consent for this procedure.
- Assess the patient for allergies to iodinated contrast dye or shellfish.
- Ascertain whether the patient has recently taken phenothiazines, tricyclic antidepressants, CNS stimulants, or amphetamines if metrizamide will be used. These medications should be avoided, because they could decrease the seizure threshold.
- Have the patient empty the bladder and bowel before myelography if possible.

PT Explain to the patient that he or she must lie very still during the procedure.

- Note that food and fluid restrictions vary according to the type of dye used. Check with the radiology department for specific restrictions.

PT Inform the patient that he or she will be tilted into an up-and-down position on the table so that the dye can properly fill the spinal canal and provide adequate visualization in the desired area.

During

- Note the following procedural steps:
  1. A lumbar puncture (p. 596) is performed.
  2. Fifteen milliliters of cerebrospinal fluid (CSF) is withdrawn, and 15 mL or more of radiopaque dye is injected into the spinal canal.
  3. The patient is placed in the prone position on the tilt table with the head tilted down.
  4. Representative x-ray images are taken.
  5. After myelography is performed, the needle is removed and a dressing is applied.
- Note that this procedure is done by a radiologist in approximately 45 minutes.
- Keep in mind that patient response varies from mild discomfort to severe pain.

After

- Note that nursing interventions after the procedure depend on the type of contrast agent used.

PT Usually place the patient on bed rest with the head slightly elevated for several hours afterward, as indicated. Position the patient as specifically ordered by the physician in consultation with the radiologist.

- Monitor the patient's vital signs and ability to void.
- **PT** Encourage the patient to drink fluids to enhance excretion of the dye and to hasten replacement of CSF.
- See p. xviii for appropriate interventions concerning the care of patients with iodine allergy.

Abnormal findings

Cord tumor
Meningeal tumor
Metastatic spinal tumor
Meningioma
Cervical ankylosing spondylosis
Arthritic lumbar stenosis
Herniated intravertebral discs
Arthritic bone spurs
Neurofibroma
Avulsion of nerve roots
Cysts
Astrocytoma

notes

M

myoglobin

Type of test Blood

Normal findings <90 mcg/L or <90 mcg/L (SI units)

Test explanation and related physiology

Myoglobin is an oxygen-binding protein found in cardiac and skeletal muscle. Measurement of myoglobin provides an early index of damage to the myocardium in myocardial infarction (MI) or reinfarction. Increased levels, which indicate cardiac muscle injury or death, occur in about 3 hours. Although this test is more sensitive than creatine phosphokinase (CPK) isoenzymes (p. 308), it is not as specific. The benefit of myoglobin over CPK-MB is that it may become elevated earlier in some patients.

Disease or trauma of the skeletal muscle also causes elevations in myoglobin. Because myoglobin is excreted in the urine and is nephrotoxic, urine levels must be monitored in patients with high levels.

Interfering factors

• Recent administration of radioactive substances
• Increased myoglobin levels can occur after IM injections.

Procedure and patient care

• See inside front cover for Routine Blood Testing.
• Fasting: no.
• Blood tube commonly used: red.

Abnormal findings

▲ **Increased levels**
Myocardial infarction
Skeletal muscle inflammation (myositis)
Malignant hyperthermia
Muscular dystrophy
Skeletal muscle ischemia
Skeletal muscle trauma
Rhabdomyolysis

▼ **Decreased levels**
Polymyositis

notes

natriuretic peptides (Atrial natriuretic peptide [ANP], Brain natriuretic peptide [BNP], N-terminal fragment of pro–brain [B-type] natriuretic peptide [NT–pro-BNP], C-type natriuretic peptide [CNP], Ventricular natriuretic peptide, CHF peptides)

Type of test Blood

Normal findings

ANP: 22-77 pg/mL or 22-77 ng/L (SI units)

BNP: <100 pg/mL

CNP: Yet to be determined

Test explanation and related physiology

Natriuretic peptides (NPs) are used to identify and stratify patients with congestive heart failure (CHF). NPs are neuroendocrine peptides that oppose the activity of the renin-angiotensin system. There are three major NPs: ANP, BNP, and CNP. ANP is synthesized in the cardiac atrial muscle. The main source of BNP is the cardiac ventricle. CNP was first localized in the nervous system but later found to be produced by the endothelial cells. The cardiac peptides are continuously released by the heart muscle cells in low levels. But, the rate of release can be increased by a variety of neuroendocrine and physiologic factors, including hemodynamic load, to regulate cardiac preload and afterload. Because of these properties, BNP and ANP have been implicated in the pathophysiology of hypertension, CHF, and atherosclerosis. ANP and BNP are released in response to atrial and ventricular stretch, respectively. They cause vasorelaxation and inhibit the secretion of aldosterone from the adrenal gland and renin from the kidney, thereby increasing natriuresis and reducing blood volume.

BNP, in particular, correlates well to left ventricular pressures. As a result, BNP is a good marker for CHF. The higher the levels of BNP are, the more severe the CHF. This test is used in urgent care settings to aid in the differential diagnosis of shortness of breath (SOB). If BNP is elevated, the SOB is because of CHF. If BNP levels are normal, the SOB is pulmonary and not cardiac. This is particularly helpful in evaluating SOB in patients with cardiac and chronic lung disease.

Furthermore, BNP is a helpful prognosticator and is used in CHF risk stratification. CHF patients whose BNP levels do not rapidly return to normal with treatment experience a significantly higher risk for mortality in the ensuing months than do those whose BNP levels rapidly normalize with treatment. In early rejection of heart transplants, BNP levels can be elevated.

N

In some laboratories, BNP is measured as an *N-terminal fragment of pro–brain (B-type) natriuretic peptide (NT–pro-BNP).* The clinical information provided by either the BNP or the pro-BNP is about the same, and the tests are used interchangeably. Screening diabetics for BNP elevation to determine the risk for cardiac diseases is used because of the low cost of performing the test as compared to an echocardiogram. BNP is also elevated in patients with prolonged systemic hypertension and in patients with acute myocardial infarction (MI).

Interfering factors

- BNP levels are generally higher in healthy women than healthy men.
- BNP levels are higher in older patients.
- BNP levels are elevated for 1 month postoperatively in patients who have had cardiac surgery.
- There are several different methods of measuring BNP. Normal values vary whether or not the whole protein of a BNP fragment protein is measured.
- ✗ Natrecor (nesiritide), a recombination form of the endogenous human peptide used to treat CHF, will *increase* plasma BNP levels for several days.

Procedure and patient care

- See inside front cover for Routine Blood Testing.
- Fasting: no.
- Blood tube commonly used: lavender.

Abnormal findings

▲ Increased levels
   Congestive heart failure
   Myocardial infarction
   Systemic hypertension
   Cor pulmonale
   Heart transplant rejection

notes

neuron-specific enolase (NSE)

Type of test Blood

Normal findings <8.6 µg/L

Test explanation and related physiology

NSE is a glycolytic enzyme that catalyzes the conversion of phosphoglycerate to phosphoenol pyruvate. It is present in neuroendocrine cells and amine precursor uptake and decarboxylation (APUD) cells. Elevated NSE concentrations are observed in patients with neuroblastoma, pancreatic islet cell carcinoma, medullary thyroid carcinoma, pheochromocytoma, and other neuroendocrine tumors.

NSE levels are frequently increased in patients with small cell lung cancer (SCLC) and infrequently in patients with non-SCLC. NSE can be used to monitor disease progression and management in SCLC. Levels of NSE can occasionally be elevated in benign disorders such as pneumonia and benign hepatobiliary diseases.

Procedure and patient care

- See inside front cover for Routine Blood Testing.
- Fasting: no.
- Blood tube commonly used: red.

Abnormal findings

▲ Increased levels

Small cell lung cancer

Neuroblastoma

APUD tumors

notes

neutrophil antibody screen (Granulocyte antibodies, Polymorphonucleocyte antibodies [PMN ab], Antigranulocyte antibodies, Antineutrophil antibodies, Neutrophil antibodies, Leukoagglutinin)

Type of test Blood

Normal findings Negative for neutrophil antibodies

Test explanation and related physiology

Neutrophil antibodies are antibodies directed toward white blood cells (WBCs). They develop during blood transfusions or transplacental bleeds and sometimes in patients with autoimmune disorders. Patients who experience a transfusion reaction despite complete compatibility testing before blood administration should have a *neutrophil antibody screen* to see if WBC incompatibility is the source of the reaction. This test is most commonly a part of posttransfusion antibody screening, which is a battery of testing performed if a transfusion reaction is suspected. It is also used in infants in the evaluation of unexplained neutropenia and in patients with suspected or known autoimmune disease.

Most commonly, in blood transfusion reactions, the recipient has antibodies to the donor WBCs and experiences a fever during transfusion. More severe, however, is the reaction when the donor plasma contains antibodies to the recipient's WBCs. This nonhemolytic reaction can lead to severe transfusion reactions, including acute pulmonary failure *(transfusion-related acute lung injury [TRALI])* and multiorgan system failure.

Interfering factors

- Recent administration of dextran
- Recent administration of intravenous (IV) contrast media
- Blood transfusion in the past 3 months

Procedure and patient care

- See inside front cover for Routine Blood Testing.
- Fasting: no.
- Blood tube commonly used: red or lavender.

Abnormal findings

Transfusion-related acute lung injury (TRALI)
Alloimmune neonatal neutropenia
Autoimmune neutropenia

notes

neutrophil gelatinase–associated lipocalin (NGAL, Lipocalin-2)

Type of test Blood

Normal findings No rise in NGAL from baseline. (Results vary according to testing methods.)

Test explanation and related physiology

NGAL is a predictor for acute kidney injury (AKI), previously referred to as acute renal failure, and chronic kidney disease (CKD). There are no early markers for acute or chronic renal disease. Serum creatinine levels rise only after there has been significant renal impairment and injury. It is important to note that the earlier renal disease or injury is identified, the more successfully it can be treated. Early treatment also helps to lower the morbidity associated with the disease. This is particularly important in patients who have serious nonrenal disease (e.g., heart surgery, renal transplant, sepsis). In these patients, severe AKI increases morbidity and mortality of hospitalized patients.

NGAL is a member of the lipocalin family of proteins, which bind and transport small lipophilic molecules. NGAL is generally expressed in low concentrations from the renal tubules, but it increases greatly in the presence of epithelial injury and inflammation. A marked elevation in NGAL indicates that renal injury has occurred, and aggressive supportive treatment should be instituted. NGAL concentrations rise 48 hours before a rise in creatinine is noted. NGAL can be detected in both urine and blood within 2 hours of a renal insult.

NGAL can be measured in the urine, plasma, or serum samples with ELISA test kits. Results are available in less than 1 hour in a standard laboratory with conventional ELISA equipment. This is particularly helpful in an intensive care environment. By itself, the absolute baseline laboratory result is not as important as are the succeeding results. Normal values vary according to which laboratory method is used and the patient's baseline GFR. NGAL varies inversely with the GFR.

NGAL measurements are being used increasingly in a variety of clinical situations leading to AKI (e.g., during cardiac surgery, kidney transplantation, contrast nephropathy, and hemolytic uremic syndrome) and in the intensive care setting. They are also useful in conditions leading to CKD (e.g., lupus nephritis,

N

glomerulonephritis, obstruction, dysplasia, polycystic kidney disease, IgA nephropathy, renal dysplasia, obstructive uropathy, and glomerular and cystic diseases).

Procedure and patient care

- See inside front cover for Routine Blood Testing.
- Fasting: no.
- Blood tube commonly used: red.
- Collect urine specimens at the same time each day, for consecutive days.
- Results are compared to previous day's testing.

Abnormal findings

▲ **Increased levels**
  Primary or secondary renal disease

notes

newborn metabolic screening

Type of test Blood

Normal findings Negative

Possible critical values Positive for any one of the tests

Test explanation and related physiology

Newborn screening is the practice of testing every newborn for certain harmful or potentially fatal disorders that aren't otherwise apparent at birth. Newborn screening tests take place before the newborn leaves the hospital. If these diseases are not accurately diagnosed and treated, they can cause mental retardation, severe illness, and premature death in newborns. Many of these are metabolic disorders, often called *inborn errors of metabolism*. Other disorders that may be detected through screening are endocrine or hematologic. In most states, this testing is mandatory.

Within 48 hours of a child's birth, a sample of blood is obtained from a heel stick, and the blood is analyzed. The sample, called a *blood spot*, is tested at a reference laboratory. It is generally recommended that the sample be taken *after* the first 24 hours of life. Some tests, such as the one for phenylketonuria (PKU), may not be as sensitive until the newborn has ingested an ample amount of the amino acid phenylalanine, which is a constituent of both human and cow milk, and after the postnatal thyroid surge has subsided. This is generally after about 2 days.

Tandem mass spectrometry can detect the blood components that are elevated in certain disorders, and it is capable of screening for more than 20 inherited metabolic disorders with a single test. The following disorders are typically included in newborn screening programs:

- *PKU:* An inherited disease, PKU is characterized by deficiency of the enzyme phenylalanine hydroxylase, which converts phenylalanine to tyrosine. Phenylalanine is an essential amino acid necessary for growth; however, any excess must be degraded by conversion to tyrosine. An infant with PKU lacks the ability to make this necessary conversion. Thus, phenylalanine accumulates in the body and spills over into the urine. If the amount of phenylalanine is not restricted in infants with PKU, progressive mental retardation results. A low-phenylalanine diet will need to be followed throughout childhood and adolescence and perhaps into adult life. (Incidence: 1 in 10,000 to 25,000.)

N

- *Congenital hypothyroidism:* Affected babies without treatment experience retarded growth and brain development. If the disorder is detected early, a baby can be treated with oral doses of thyroid hormone to permit normal development. (Incidence: 1 in 4000.)

- *Galactosemia:* Babies with galactosemia lack the enzyme that converts galactose into glucose, a sugar the body is able to use. As a result, milk and other dairy products must be eliminated from the diet. Otherwise, galactose can build up and cause blindness, severe mental retardation, growth deficiency, and even death. (Incidence: 1 in 60,000 to 80,000.) There are several less severe forms of galactosemia that may be detected by newborn screening. These may not require any intervention.

- *Sickle cell anemia:* Sickle cell disease is an inherited blood disease in which red blood cells stretch into abnormal *sickle* shapes (p. 836). This can cause episodes of pain, damage to vital organs (e.g., the lungs and kidneys), and even death. Young children with sickle cell anemia are especially prone to certain dangerous bacterial infections. (Incidence: about 1 in 500 African American births, and 1 in 1000 to 1400 Hispanic American births.)

- *Biotinidase deficiency:* Babies with this condition don't have enough biotinidase, an enzyme that recycles biotin (one of the B vitamins) in the body. This deficiency may cause seizures, poor muscle control, immune system impairment, hearing loss, mental retardation, coma, and even death. If the deficiency is detected early, however, problems can be prevented by biotin administration. (Incidence: 1 in 126,000.)

- *Congenital adrenal hyperplasia:* This is actually a group of disorders resulting in a deficiency of adrenal hormones. It can affect the development of the genitals and may cause death. Lifelong treatment through hormone supplementation manages the condition. (Incidence: 1 in 12,000.)

- *Maple syrup urine disease (MSUD):* Babies with MSUD are missing an enzyme needed to process the amino acids leucine, isoleucine, and valine (present in protein-rich foods such as milk, meat, and eggs) that are essential for the body's normal growth. When these are not processed properly, they can build up in the body, causing urine to smell like maple syrup or sweet, burnt sugar. These babies usually have little appetite and are extremely irritable.

If not detected and treated early, MSUD can cause mental retardation, physical disability, and even death. A carefully controlled diet free of high-protein foods can prevent these outcomes. (Incidence: 1 in 250,000.)

- *Homocystinuria:* This metabolic disorder results from a deficiency in cystathionine β-synthase, responsible for the metabolism of methionine and homocysteine. If untreated, it can lead to dislocated lenses of the eyes, mental retardation, skeletal abnormalities, and hypercoagulability. However, a special diet combined with dietary supplements may help prevent most of these problems. (Incidence: 1 in 50,000 to 150,000.)
- *Tyrosinemia:* Babies with this disorder cannot metabolize tyrosine. If it accumulates in the body, it can cause mild retardation, language skill difficulties, liver problems, and even death from liver failure. A special diet and sometimes a liver transplant are needed to treat the condition. Early diagnosis and treatment seem to offset long-term problems. (Incidence: not yet determined.)
- *Cystic fibrosis:* This is an inherited disorder expressed in the lung and gastrointestinal tract that causes cells to release a thick mucus leading to chronic respiratory disease, problems with digestion, and poor growth. There is no known cure; treatment involves trying to prevent the serious lung infections associated with it and providing adequate nutrition. (Incidence: 1 in 2000 Caucasian births.)
- *Toxoplasmosis:* Toxoplasmosis is a parasitic infection that can be transmitted through the mother's placenta to an unborn child. The disease-causing organism, which is found in undercooked meat, can invade the brain, eye, and muscle, possibly resulting in blindness and mental retardation. (Incidence: 1 in 1000.)

These aren't the only metabolic disorders that can be detected through newborn screening. Certain other rare disorders can also be detected and may include Duchenne muscular dystrophy, HIV, and neuroblastoma. Hematologic disorders, such as glucose-6-phosphate dehydrogenase (G6PD) deficiency and thalassemia, can also be identified.

Most, but not all, states require newborns' hearing to be screened before they are discharged from the hospital. The hearing test involves placing a tiny earphone in the baby's ear and measuring his or her response to sound.

Interfering factors

- Premature infants may have false-positive results because of delayed development of liver enzymes.
- Infants tested before 24 hours of age may have false-negative results.
- Feeding problems may cause false-negative results.

Procedure and patient care

Before

PT Inform the parents about the purpose and method of the test.

- Assess the infant's feeding patterns before performing the test. An inadequate amount of protein ingested before performing the test can cause false-negative results.

During

- Place a few drops of blood from a heel stick in each circle on the filter paper.

After

PT Inform the parents that if test results are positive they will be notified by their health care provider, and further testing/treatment will be recommended.

Abnormal findings

Metabolic diseases
Endocrine diseases
Hematologic diseases

notes

nicotine and metabolites (Nicotine, Continine, 3-Hydroxy cotinine, Nornicotine, Anabasine)

Type of test Urine/blood

Normal findings

Urine:

	Unexposed nontobacco user (ng/mL)	Passive exposure (non-tobacco user) (ng/mL)	Abstinent user for >2 weeks (ng/mL)	Active tobacco product user (ng/mL)
Nicotine	<2	<20	<30	1000-5000
Cotinine	<5	<20	<50	1000-8000
3-OH-Cotinine	<50	<50	<120	3000-25,000
Nornicotine	<2	<2	<2	30-900
Anabasine	<3	<3	<3	3-500

Serum:

	Unexposed nontobacco user (ng/mL)	Passive exposure (non-tobacco user) (ng/mL)	Abstinent user for >2 weeks (ng/mL)	Active tobacco product user (ng/mL)
Nicotine	<2	<2	<2	30-50
Cotinine	<2	<8	<2	200-800
3-OH-Cotinine	<2	<2	<2	100-500

Test explanation and related physiology

Nicotine is metabolized into cotinine and 3-hydroxy cotinine, which are measurable in urine and serum. The word "cotinine" is actually an anagram of "nicotine"—the eight letters are rearranged. In addition to nicotine and metabolites, tobacco products also contain other alkaloids (anabasine and nornicotine). These tests are used to assess compliance with smoking cessation programs and to qualify for surgical procedures. They are also used by insurance companies to determine if the applicant is a smoker. These tests can differentiate patient tobacco use as the following:

- Active user
- Abstinent >2 weeks
- Passively exposed non-user
- Unexposed non-user

Cotinine and 3-hydroxy cotinine have an in vivo half-life of approximately 20 hours and are typically detectable for several days to up to 1 week after the use of tobacco. Because the level of these metabolites in the blood is proportionate to the amount of exposure to tobacco smoke, it is a valuable indicator of tobacco smoke exposure. Nicotine and its metabolites can be measured in the serum, urine, and other biofluids (most commonly the saliva). Cotinine is found in urine from 2 to 4 days after tobacco use. Serum or plasma testing is required when a valid urine specimen cannot be obtained or to detect recent use (within past 2 weeks). Blood cotinine will increase no matter how the tobacco is used (smoked, chew, dip, or snuff products). Nicotine levels have an in vivo half-life of approximately 2 hours, which is too short to be useful as a marker of smoking status.

Anabasine (only measured in the urine) is present in tobacco products but not nicotine replacement therapies. Nicotine, cotinine, 3-hydroxy cotinine, and nornicotine will also be elevated by the use of any of the nicotine replacement gum, patch, or pill products. The presence of anabasine >10 ng/mL or nornicotine >30 ng/mL in urine indicates current tobacco use, irrespective of whether the subject is on nicotine replacement therapy. The presence of nornicotine without anabasine is consistent with use of nicotine replacement products. Heavy tobacco users who abstain from tobacco for 2 weeks exhibit urine nicotine values <30 ng/mL, cotinine values <50 ng/mL, anabasine values <2 ng/mL, and nornicotine values <2 ng/mL. Passive exposure to tobacco smoke can cause accumulation of nicotine metabolites in nontobacco users. Urine cotinine has been observed to accumulate up to 20 ng/mL from passive exposure. Neither anabasine nor nornicotine accumulates from passive exposure. Because hydration status and renal function may affect urinary cotinine results, a spot urine cotinine test is accompanied by a spot urine creatinine.

For smokers, another method of determining tobacco use is *expired carbon monoxide testing*. Again, a relatively short half-life (≈4 hours) limits the reliability and accuracy. Furthermore, carbon monoxide testing is unable to detect the use of smokeless tobacco.

Interfering factors

- Menthol cigarettes may increase cotinine levels because the menthol retains cotinine in the blood for a longer period of time.
- Diluted or adulterated urine may alter results.

Procedure and patient care

Before

PT Explain the procedure to the patient and indicate the type of specimen needed.

- Obtain an accurate history of recent tobacco use.

During

Blood

- Collect venous blood in a red-top, lavender-top (EDTA), or pink-top (K_2EDTA) tube. See inside front cover for Routine Blood Testing.

Urine

- Obtain a random spot urine specimen of at least 5 mL. See inside front cover for Routine Urine Testing.
- Immediately transport the specimen to the laboratory.

Saliva

- Ask the patient to spit at least 1 mL of saliva into a spit container.
- Alternatively, dental gauze rolls can be placed in the mouth for 15 minutes and then placed in a storage container for transport.

After

- Keep the specimens in a cool place if they cannot be transported to the laboratory immediately.

Abnormal finding

Tobacco exposure

notes

5′-nucleotidase

Type of test Blood

Normal findings 0-1.6 units at 37° C or 0-1.6 units at 37° C (SI units)

Test explanation and related physiology

5′-Nucleotidase is an enzyme specific to the liver. The 5′-nucleotidase level is elevated in patients with liver diseases, especially those associated with cholestasis. It provides information similar to alkaline phosphatase (ALP, p. 29). However, ALP is not specific to the liver. When doubt as to the cause of an elevated ALP exists, 5′-nucleotidase is recommended. If that enzyme is elevated along with the ALP, the source of the pathology is certainly in the liver. If the 5′-nucleotidase is normal in the face of an elevated ALP, the source of pathology is outside the liver. Gamma-glutamyl transpeptidase (GGTP, see p. 452) is used similarly because it is also specific to the liver.

Interfering factors

- Drugs that may cause *increased* 5′-nucleotidase levels include hepatotoxic agents.

Procedure and patient care

- See inside front cover for Routine Blood Testing.
- Fasting: no.
- Blood tube commonly used: red.

Abnormal findings

▲ **Increased levels**
Bile duct obstruction
Cholestasis
Hepatitis
Cirrhosis
Hepatic necrosis, ischemia, tumor
Hepatotoxic drugs

notes

obstruction series

Type of test X-ray

Normal findings

No evidence of bowel obstruction
No abnormal calcifications
No free air

Test explanation and related physiology

The obstruction series is a group of x-ray images performed on the abdomen of patients with suspected bowel obstruction, paralytic ileus, perforated viscus, abdominal abscess, kidney stones, appendicitis, or foreign body ingestion. This series of images usually consists of at least two x-ray studies. The first is an *erect abdominal* image that should include visualization of both diaphragms. The image is examined for evidence of free air under either diaphragm, which is pathognomonic for a perforated viscus. This view is also used to detect air-fluid levels within the intestine; the presence of an air-fluid level is compatible with bowel obstruction or paralytic ileus. Occasionally patients are too ill to stand erect. In this case, an x-ray image can be taken with the patient in the left lateral decubitus position.

The second view in the obstruction series is usually a *supine abdominal* x-ray study. This x-ray is also called a *KUB (kidney, ureter, bladder)* film. A calcification within the course of the ureter could indicate a kidney or ureteral stone. An abdominal abscess may be seen as a cluster of tiny bubbles within one localized area. A small calcification in the right lower quadrant on the film of a patient complaining of pain in this quadrant may be an appendicolith. A gas-filled, distended bowel is compatible with bowel obstruction or paralytic ileus. The obstruction series can also be used to monitor the clinical course of patients with gastrointestinal (GI) disease.

Frequently, a *cross-table lateral* view of the abdomen is included in an obstruction series to detect abdominal aorta calcification, which often occurs in older patients.

Finally, the *supine abdominal* x-ray study can be used as a *scout image* before performing GI or abdominal x-ray studies that use contrast.

Contraindications

- Patients who are pregnant, unless the benefits outweigh the risk to the fetus

Interfering factors

- Previous GI barium contrast study

Procedure and patient care

Before

PT Explain the procedure to the patient.
- Ensure that all radiopaque clothing has been removed.

PT Remind the patient that no GI contrast will be used.

During

- Although the procedure varies from facility to facility, note that usually a supine abdominal x-ray image, erect abdominal image, and perhaps a lower erect chest image are taken. Often a cross-table lateral x-ray image is also included.
- Note that the obstruction series is performed in minutes in the radiology department by a radiologic technologist; however, it can be performed at the bedside with a portable x-ray machine. A radiologist interprets the images.

PT Tell the patient that no discomfort is associated with this study.

After

- Note that no special aftercare is needed.

Abnormal findings

Kidney stone	Abdominal aortic calcification
Bowel obstruction	Appendicolithiasis
Organomegaly	Paralytic ileus
Presence of a foreign body	Abdominal aortic aneurysm
Bladder distention	Peritoneal effusion/ascites
Abdominal abscess	Abnormal position of the kidneys
Perforated viscus	Soft tissue masses

notes

octreotide scan (Carcinoid nuclear scan, Neuroendocrine nuclear scan)

Type of test Nuclear scan

Normal findings No evidence of increased uptake throughout the body

Test explanation and related physiology

Octreotide scans are used to identify and localize neuroendocrine primary and metastatic tumors. These scans are indicated on patients with known neuroendocrine tumors.

Most neuroendocrine tumors have a somatostatin receptor on the cellular membrane. Octreotide is an analogue of somatostatin. When combined with a radiopharmaceutical (e.g., I^{123} or indium-111 DTPA), the radiolabeled octreotide will attach to the somatostatin receptors of the neuroendocrine tumor cells. With the use of a scintillator camera, the uptake can be identified. This test is used to identify primary and metastatic neuroendocrine tumors. It is also used to monitor the course of the disease.

The use of *single-photon emission computed tomography (SPECT)* imaging improves the sensitivity of this test. Many different types of hormone-producing tumors can be detected by this scan, most notably carcinoid, gastrinoma, insulinoma, glucagonoma, pheochromocytoma, and small cell lung cancer. Other abnormalities can pick up octreotide, including granulomatous infections, rheumatoid arthritis, and nonhormonal cancers (breast, lymphoma, and non–small cell lung cancers).

Contraindications

- Patients who are pregnant or lactating because of risk of damage to the fetus or infant

Interfering factors

- Barium in the gastrointestinal (GI) tract overlying the liver or spleen
  Barium produces defects that may be mistaken for masses.

Procedure and patient care

Before

PT Explain the procedure to the patient.

PT Tell the patient that no fasting is required.

PT Assure the patient that he or she will not be exposed to large amounts of radiation, because only tracer doses are used.

- If an iodinated radionuclide is to be used, ensure that the patient does not have an allergy to iodine.
- If an iodinated radionuclide is to be used, administer 5 drops of Lugol's solution (iodine) daily for 3 days. This will avoid uptake of the radionuclide by the thyroid gland.
- **PT** If the patient has been receiving octreotide as a form of antineoplastic treatment, this must be discontinued for 2 weeks before scanning. Inform the patient.

During

- Note the following procedural steps:
  1. The patient is taken to nuclear medicine, where the radionuclide is administered intravenously.
  2. One hour after injection, a gamma ray detector/camera is successively placed over the entire body.
  3. The patient is placed in supine, lateral, and prone positions.
  4. The radionuclide image is recorded. SPECT images may also be performed.
  5. After 4 hours, the patient is given a strong laxative to clear the octreotide from the bowel.
  6. Repeat scanning is performed at 2, 4, 24, and 48 hours after administration of the octreotide.
- Note that the imaging procedure is performed by a trained technologist in approximately ½ hour. A physician trained in nuclear medicine interprets the results.
- **PT** Inform the patient that the only discomfort associated with this procedure is the IV injection of the radionuclide.

After

- **PT** Because tracer doses of radioisotopes are used, inform the patient that no radiation precautions are needed.

Abnormal findings

Carcinoid tumors
Neuroendocrine tumors
Granulomatous infections (e.g., sarcoidosis and tuberculosis)

notes

osmolality, blood (Serum osmolality)

Type of test   Blood

Normal findings

Adult/elderly: 285-295 mOsm/kg H_2O or 285-295 mmol/kg (SI units)

Child: 275-290 mOsm/kg H_2O

Possible critical values

<265 mOsm/kg H_2O

>320 mOsm/kg H_2O

Test explanation and related physiology

Osmolality measures the number of dissolved particles in serum/plasma per unit volume. As the amount of free water in the blood increases or the number of particles decreases per unit volume of serum, osmolality decreases. As the amount of water in the blood decreases or the number of particles per unit volume increases, osmolality increases. Osmolality increases with dehydration and decreases with overhydration.

An elaborate feedback mechanism controls osmolality. Increased osmolality will stimulate secretion of antidiuretic hormone (ADH); this will result in increased water reabsorption in the kidneys, more concentrated urine, and less concentrated serum. A low serum osmolality will suppress the release of ADH, resulting in decreased water resorption and large amounts of dilute urine. The simultaneous use of urine osmolality (see p. 671) helps in the interpretation and evaluation of problems involving osmolality.

The serum osmolality test is useful in evaluating fluid and electrolyte imbalance. The test is very helpful in the evaluation of seizures, ascites, hydration status, acid/base balance, suspected ADH abnormalities, and suspected poisoning. Osmolality is also helpful in identifying the presence of organic acids, sugars, and ethanol.

Osmolality can be predicted based on calculations of serum sodium, glucose, and BUN—the three most important solutes in the blood. The equation is:

$$\text{Osmolality} = 2 \times \text{Na} + \frac{\text{Glu}}{18} + \frac{\text{BUN}}{2.8}$$

The measured osmolality should not exceed the predicted by more than 10 mOsm/kg. A difference of more than 10 mOsm/kg is considered an *osmolal gap* or *delta gap*. Causes for a serum osmolal gap include mannitol, ethanol, methanol, ethylene glycol, and other toxins in very high concentration. Another measure providing similar data is the ratio of serum sodium to osmolality. Normally, the ratio of serum sodium, in mEq/L, to serum osmolality, in mOsm/kg, is between 0.43 and 0.5. The ratio may be distorted in drug intoxication.

Osmolality may have a role in evaluation of coma patients. Values of >385 mOsm/kg H_2O are associated with stupor in patients with hyperglycemia. When values of 400 to 420 mOsm/kg are detected, grand mal seizures can occur. Values greater than 420 mOsm/kg can be lethal. The simultaneous use of urine osmolality (p. 671) helps in the interpretation and evaluation of problems with osmolality.

Interfering factors

- Such diseases as cerebrovascular accident (stroke) or brain tumors may interfere with test results through inappropriate secretion of ADH.

Procedure and patient care

- See inside front cover for Routine Blood Testing.
- Fasting: no.
- Blood tube commonly used: red.
- For pediatric patients, draw blood from a heel stick.

Abnormal findings

▲ **Increased levels**
Hypernatremia
Dehydration
Hyperglycemia
Mannitol therapy
Azotemia
Uremia
Ingestion of ethanol, methanol, or ethylene glycol
Hyperosmolar nonketotic hyperglycemia
Diabetes insipidus
Hypercalcemia
Renal tubular necrosis
Severe pyelonephritis
Ketosis
Shock

▼ **Decreased levels**
Hyponatremia
Overhydration
Syndrome of inappropriate antidiuretic hormone (SIADH) secretion
Paraneoplastic syndromes associated with lung carcinoma

notes

osmolality, urine (Urine osmolality)

Type of test Urine

Normal findings

12- to 14-hour fluid restriction: >850 mOsm/kg H_2O (SI units)

Random specimen: 50-1200 mOsm/kg H_2O, depending on fluid intake, or 50-1200 mmol/kg (SI units)

Test explanation and related physiology

Osmolality is the measurement of the number of dissolved particles in a solution. It is a more exact measurement of urine concentration than specific gravity, because specific gravity depends on the number and precise nature of the particles in the urine. Specific gravity also requires correction for the presence of glucose or protein, as well as for temperature; in contrast, osmolality depends only on the number of particles of solute in a unit of solution. Osmolality also can be measured over a wider range of urine concentrations than specific gravity and with greater accuracy.

Osmolality is used in the precise evaluation of the concentrating and diluting abilities of the kidney. With normal fluid intake and normal diet, a patient will produce a urine of about 500 to 850 mOsm/kg water. The normal kidney can concentrate a urine to 800 to 1400 mOsm/kg. With excess fluid intake, a minimal osmolality of 40 to 80 mOsm/kg can be obtained. With dehydration, the urine osmolality should be 3 to 4 times the plasma osmolality.

Osmolality is used in the evaluation of kidney function and the ability to excrete ammonium salts. Osmolality may be used as part of the urinalysis when the patient has glycosuria or proteinuria or has had tests that use radiopaque substances. In these situations, the *urine osmolar gap* increases because of other organic osmolar particles. The urine osmolar gap is the sum of all the particles predicted or calculated to be in the urine (electrolytes, urea, and glucose) compared with the actual measurement of the osmolality. The predicted/calculated urine osmolality can then be determined by urine levels of sodium, potassium, glucose, and urea nitrogen.

$$\text{Osmolality} = 2 \times ([Na + K]) + \frac{\text{urea nitrogen}}{2.8} + \frac{\text{glucose}}{18}$$

Normally, the osmolar gap is 80 to 100 mOsm/kg of H_2O. The urine osmolality is more easily interpreted when the serum osmolality (p. 669) is simultaneously performed. More information concerning the state of renal water handling or abnormalities of urine dilution or concentration can be obtained if urinary osmolality is compared to serum osmolality and if urine electrolyte studies are performed. Normally, the ratio of urine osmolality to serum osmolality is 1.0 to 3.0, reflecting a wide range of urine osmolality.

Procedure and patient care

- See inside front cover for Routine Urine Testing.
- **PT** Tell the patient that no special preparation is necessary for a random urine specimen.
- **PT** Inform the patient that preparation for a fasting urine specimen may require a high-protein diet for 3 days before the test.
- **PT** Instruct the patient to eat a dry supper the evening before the test and to drink no fluids until the test is completed the next morning.
- Preferably, collect a first-voided urine specimen for a random sample.
- Indicate on the laboratory slip the patient's fasting status.

Abnormal findings

▲ **Increased levels**
SIADH secretion
Acidosis
Shock
Hypernatremia
Hepatic cirrhosis
Congestive heart failure
Addison disease

▼ **Decreased levels**
Diabetes insipidus
Hypercalcemia
Excess fluid intake
Renal tubular necrosis
Aldosteronism
Hypokalemia
Severe pyelonephritis

notes

oximetry (Pulse oximetry, Oxygen saturation)

Type of test Photodiagnostic

Normal findings ≥95%

Possible critical values ≤75%

Test explanation and related physiology

Oximetry is a noninvasive method of monitoring arterial blood oxygen saturation (SaO_2). The SaO_2 is the ratio of oxygenated hemoglobin to the total amount of hemoglobin. The SaO_2 is expressed as a percentage; for example, a saturation of 95% indicates that 95% of the total hemoglobin attachments for oxygen have oxygen attached to them. The SaO_2 is an accurate approximation of oxygen saturation obtained from an arterial blood gas study (p. 109). By correlating the SaO_2 and the patient's physiologic status, a close estimate of the partial oxygen pressure (Po_2) can be obtained.

Oximetry is typically used for monitoring the patient's oxygenation status during the perioperative period (or any time of heavy sedation) and for patients receiving mechanical ventilation. This test is used in many clinical situations, such as pulmonary rehabilitation programs, stress testing, and sleep laboratories. Oximetry can be used to assess the body's response to various drugs, such as theophylline (which causes bronchodilation) and methacholine (which evokes bronchospasm in people with asthma). This test is commonly used to titrate levels of oxygen on hospitalized patients.

O_2 levels can also be measured in various body tissues. For example, monitors that continuously measure tissue O_2 partial pressures can be attached to a small catheter placed in the brain, heart, or peripheral muscle. *Brain tissue oxygen testing and monitoring* is the most common use of this technology. It is used to monitor the condition of the brain following severe head trauma by measuring cerebral blood flow and pulmonary oxygenation. It is more accurate than intracranial pressure for indicating brain injury.

Procedure and patient care

Before

PT Explain the procedure to the patient.

PT Tell the patient that no fasting is required.

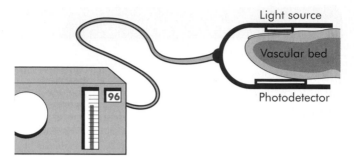

FIGURE 31 Oximetry. The pulse oximeter passes a beam of light through the tissue. The amount of light absorbed by the oxygen-saturated hemoglobin is measured by the sensor.

During

- Rub the patient's earlobe, pinna (upper part of the ear), or fingertip to increase blood flow.
- Clip the monitoring probe or sensor to the ear or finger. A beam of light passes through the tissue, and the sensor measures the amount of light the tissue absorbs (Figure 31).
- Note that this study is usually performed by a respiratory therapist or nurse at the patient's bedside in a few seconds.
- **PT** Tell the patient that no discomfort is associated with this study.

After

- Note that no special aftercare is needed.

Abnormal findings

▲ **Increased levels**
Increased inspired O_2
Hyperventilation

▼ **Decreased levels**
Inadequate O_2 in inspired air
Hypoxic lung diseases
Hypoxic cardiac diseases
Severe hypoventilation states

notes

pancreatic enzymes (Pancreatic secretory test, Amylase, Lipase, Trypsin, Chymotrypsin)

Type of test   Fluid analysis

Normal findings

Volume: 2-4 mL/kg body weight
HCO_3 (Bicarbonate): 90-130 mEq/L
Amylase: 6.6-35.2 units/kg
Trypsin-like immunoreactivity: 10-57 ng/mL
Trypsin: ≥ 1:96
Chymotrypsin: by report

Test explanation and related physiology

Cystic fibrosis (CF) is an inherited disease characterized by abnormal secretion by exocrine glands within the bronchi, small intestines, pancreatic ducts, bile ducts, and skin (sweat glands). Because of this abnormal exocrine secretion, children with CF develop mucus plugs that obstruct their pancreatic ducts and can lead to significant malabsorption, steatorrhea, and diarrhea. The pancreatic enzymes (e.g., amylase, lipase, trypsin, and chymotrypsin) cannot be expelled into the duodenum and therefore are either completely absent or present only in diminished quantities within the duodenal aspirate. For the same reasons, bicarbonate and other neutralizing fluids cannot be secreted from the pancreas.

In this test, secretin and pancreozymin are used to stimulate pancreatic secretion of these enzymes and bicarbonate into the duodenum. The duodenal contents are then aspirated and examined for pH, bicarbonate, and pancreatic enzyme levels. Amylase is the most frequently measured enzyme. Diminished values are suggestive of CF. Pancreatic enzyme testing is not diagnostic of CF but is an excellent screening test, especially in newborns with meconium ileus. Genetic testing is required for definitive diagnosis of cystic fibrosis.

Trypsinogen, another pancreatic exocrine enzyme, is measured in the serum as *trypsin-like immunoreactivity*. This test is used to support the diagnosis of chronic pancreatitis. Levels diminish as pancreatic exocrine function becomes increasingly impaired.

When any of these pancreatic enzymes are measured in the serum, they can reflect acute inflammation of the pancreas. Similar to amylase and lipase, trypsin, chymotrypsin, and trypsin-like immunoreactivity are increased with acute pancreatic inflammation. Likewise, in patients with burned-out chronic

P

pancreatitis, serum measurements of these pancreatic enzymes are low.

Trypsinogen has two isoenzymes that are excreted in the urine. *Trypsinogen-1* is rapidly reabsorbed in the kidneys. *Trypsinogen-2*, however, is not well reabsorbed by the kidneys, and concentrations increase in the urine during acute pancreatitis.

A physician obtains the duodenal contents in approximately 2 hours in the x-ray department. Discomfort and gagging may occur during placement of the Dreiling tube. The pancreatic enzymes are then measured and serially diluted for quantification.

Procedure and patient care

Before

PT Explain the procedure to the patient and/or parents.

PT Instruct the adult patient to fast for 12 hours before testing.

• Determine pediatric fasting times according to the patient's age.

During

• Note the following procedural steps:
  1. With the use of fluoroscopy, a Dreiling tube is passed through the patient's nose and into the stomach.
  2. The distal lumen of the tube is placed within the duodenum.
  3. The proximal lumen of the tube is placed within the stomach.
  4. Both lumens are aspirated. The gastric lumen is continually aspirated to avoid contamination of the gastric contents in the duodenum aspirate.
  5. A control specimen of the duodenal juices is collected for 20 minutes.
  6. The patient is tested for sensitivity to secretin and pancreozymin by low-dose intradermal injection.
  7. If no sensitivity is present, these hormones are administered intravenously. Secretin can be expected to stimulate pancreatic fluid and bicarbonate secretion. Pancreozymin can be expected to stimulate pancreatic enzyme (lipase, amylase, trypsin, chymotrypsin) secretion.
  8. Four duodenal aspirates are collected at 20-minute intervals and placed in the specimen container.
  9. Each specimen is analyzed for pH, volume, bicarbonate, and amylase levels.

• Note that a physician performs this test in approximately 2 hours in the laboratory or at the patient's bedside.

PT Tell the patient that he or she may have discomfort and gagging during placement of the Dreiling tube.

After

- Place the aspirated specimens on ice. Send them to the chemistry laboratory as soon as the test is completed.
- Remove the Dreiling tube after completion of the test. Give appropriate nose and mouth care.
- Allow the patient to resume a normal diet.

Abnormal findings

▲ **Increased levels**
  Acute pancreatitis

▼ **Decreased levels**
  Cystic fibrosis
  Sprue
  Chronic pancreatitis

notes

P

pancreatobiliary FISH testing

Type of test Microscopic examination

Normal findings No chromosomal ploidy abnormalities

Test explanation and related physiology

It is sometimes difficult to differentiate benign bile duct strictures from early pancreatobiliary cancer. When a stricture is identified on an endoscopic retrograde cholangiopancreatography (ERCP, p. 384), cancer must be considered as a possible cause. If an obvious cancer is not seen at the time of ERCP, a brush is repeatedly swept along the bile duct to obtain duct surface cells for conventional cytology to identify cancer cells. In conventional cytology, the brushing specimens are placed on a slide and stained with a PAP stain. Slides are then interpreted by a cytopathologist to determine whether they show features that are positive for malignancy, suspicious for malignancy, atypical (meaning there are cells that are not normal but cannot be definitely ascribed to a neoplastic process), or negative for malignancy.

With the use of fluorescence in situ hybridization (FISH) testing, three chromosome enumeration probes and a gene-specific probe to P16 tumor suppressor gene are able to determine if more than one pair of chromosomes or P16 genes exists in the cells obtained from the brushings of the bile duct during ERCP. If extra copies of two or more of the chromosomes or P16 genes are evident, the cells are considered to be *polysomic*, which indicates a high chance of malignancy. Based on conventional cytology, FISH testing, and other clinical data, the likelihood of cancer can be calculated.

Contraindications

• See ERCP.

Potential complications

• See ERCP.

Interfering factors

• Errors in obtaining a good specimen can influence results.
• Cytologic examination is always affected by physician interpretation.

Procedure and patient care

Before

PT Explain the procedure to the patient.
- Obtain informed consent from the patient.
- Keep the patient NPO as of midnight the day of the test.
- Follow the procedure for ERCP.

During

- During ERCP, a rounded brush is placed through the accessory lumen of the endoscope and passed repeatedly through the stricture.
- The brush is then swished in a cytology solution for FISH or directly smeared on a slide and preserved for conventional cytology.

After

- Follow the procedure for ERCP.

Abnormal findings

Sclerosing cholangitis

Biliary sclerosis

Tumor or strictures of the pancreatobiliary duct

notes

P

Papanicolaou smear (Pap smear, Pap test, Cytologic test for cancer, Liquid-based cervical cytology [LBCC], ThinPrep)

Type of test Microscopic examination

Normal findings No abnormal or atypical cells

Test explanation and related physiology

A Pap smear can detect neoplastic cells in cervical and vaginal secretions. This test is based on the fact that normal cells and abnormal cervical and endometrial neoplastic cells are shed into the cervical and vaginal secretions. By examining these secretions microscopically, one can detect early cellular changes associated with premalignant conditions or an existing malignant condition. The Pap smear is 95% accurate in detecting cervical carcinoma; however, its accuracy in the detection of endometrial carcinoma is only approximately 40%.

The Bethesda System for reporting cervical and vaginal cytologic diagnoses was developed and revised by the National Cancer Institute (NCI) to minimize discrepancy in result reporting and to create a standardized framework for reporting results that were clinically useful. This system was updated in 2001 and includes evaluation of the following five components:

- Adequacy of specimen
- General categorization (optional)
- Interpretation/Result
    a. Negative for intraepithelial lesion or malignancy
    b. Epithelial cell abnormalities
- Automated review and ancillary testing (such as HPV, see page 534)
- Educational notes (optional)

A common method of Pap smear specimen collection is *liquid-based cervical cytology (LBCC)*. With this technique, the specimen obtained from the cervix is placed into a preservative solution instead of smearing it onto a slide as is done during conventional Pap smear testing (CPT). Any blood cells and debris are then isolated by centrifuge, leaving only cervical cells. A thin film of the residuum is then placed on a slide to be evaluated. The specimen can be split into two parts. The first is evaluated for cytopathology. In the event that cytologic abnormalities of undetermined significance are found that could be better elucidated with further testing, the cells in the second split specimen are used for that testing (to avoid having to obtain another cervical sample). For example, if cellular changes are found that may be related to HPV, the second split specimen is tested by real-time PCR for HPV DNA (p. 534). HPV has been implicated as the cause of more than 95% of cervical cancers. When compared with CPT, LBCC has a significantly greater percentage of satisfactory specimens for Pap testing and better detection of pathology.

Automated Pap smear readings are increasingly being used because the volume of screening Pap smears exceeds the ability of the cytopathologists to spend enough time to accurately interpret the slides. Automation is especially accurate when performed on LBCC specimens. The ThinPrep Imaging System, for example, integrates automated imaging with screening by cytotechnologists to identify fields that contain potentially relevant cellular abnormalities. If the cytotechnologist identifies significant abnormalities, the slide is examined by the cytopathologist. LBCC may eventually replace CPT. A slightly different and less expensive technique called the *PapSpin* uses a special brush placed in a collection device and centrifuged to provide a cellular concentrate for microscopic examination.

Similar to screening for all cancers, as more studies become available, guidelines change. Furthermore, different medical professional societies may differ on certain aspects of appropriate Pap smear guidelines. Not only did the U.S. Preventive Services Task Force (USPSTF) recommend that the HPV test (page 534) is appropriate for some women as part of routine cervical cancer screening, but it also changed its recommendations as follows.

- Women age 21 to 65 years should get Pap tests no more than every 3 years; previous guidelines, issued in 2003, recommended that women be screened "at least" every 3 years, allowing for annual screens.
- Women age 30 to 65 years may extend the interval between screens to 5 years if they use HPV tests in conjunction with the Pap test; the HPV test should not be used in younger women because many of them will have HPV infection that they will naturally clear without treatment.
- Women younger than age 21 years should not be screened for cervical cancer, regardless of sexual history; previous advice recommended that women begin cervical cancer screening within 3 years of becoming sexually active.
- Women older than age 65 years should not be screened as long as they have had consistently normal Pap test results and are not at high risk for cervical cancer.

P

The guidelines apply to healthy women who do not have abnormal Pap test results. They do not apply to women who have a history of cervical cancer.

Contraindications

- Patients currently having routine, normal menses, because this can alter test interpretation
- Patients with vaginal infections
  Cellular changes that may be misinterpreted as dysplastic may transiently occur during these infections.

Interfering factors

- A delay in fixing a specimen allows the cells to dry, destroys the effectiveness of the stain, and makes interpretation difficult.
- Using lubricating jelly on the speculum can alter the specimen.
- Douching and tub bathing may wash away cellular deposits.
- Menstrual flow may alter test results.
- Infections may interfere with hormonal cytology.
- ✗ Such drugs as digitalis and tetracycline may alter the test results by affecting the squamous epithelium.

Procedure and patient care

Before

- **PT** Explain the procedure to the patient.
- **PT** Instruct the patient not to douche or tub bathe during the 24 hours before the Pap smear. (Some physicians prefer that patients refrain from sexual intercourse for 24 to 48 hours.)
- **PT** Instruct the patient to empty her bladder.
- **PT** Tell the patient that no fasting or sedation is required.

During

- Note the following procedural steps:
  1. The patient is placed in the lithotomy position.
  2. A vaginal speculum is inserted to expose the cervix.
  3. Material is collected from the cervical canal by rotating a moist saline cotton swab or spatula within the cervical canal and in the squamocolumnar junction (Figure 32).
  4. The cells are immediately wiped across a clean glass slide and fixed either by immersing the slide in equal parts of 95% alcohol and ether or by using a commercial spray (e.g., Aqua Net hair spray). The secretions must be fixed before drying because drying will distort the cells and make interpretation difficult.

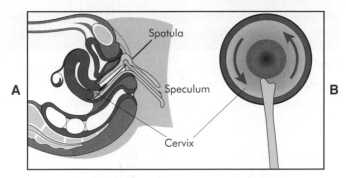

FIGURE 32 Papanicolaou (Pap) smear. **A,** The vaginal speculum is shown in position to allow direct visualization of the cervix. **B,** The cervix is scraped with the bifid end of a wooden spatula.

  5. If *liquid-based cervical cytology* is performed, the cervical specimen is placed in the fixative preservative solution. After being placed in this solution, cells can be evaluated any time within the next 3 weeks if kept frozen.
  6. The slide is labeled with the patient's name, age, and parity and with the date of her last menstrual period.
• Note that a Pap smear is obtained by a nurse or a physician in approximately 10 minutes.
PT Tell the patient that no discomfort, except for insertion of the speculum, is associated with this procedure.

After
PT Inform the patient that usually she will not be notified unless further evaluation is necessary.

Abnormal findings

Cancer	Reactive inflammatory changes
Infertility	Fungal infection
Sexually transmitted disease	Parasitic infection
HPV infection	Herpes infection

notes

paracentesis (Peritoneal fluid analysis, Ascitic fluid cytology, Peritoneal tap)

Type of test   Fluid analysis

Normal findings

Gross appearance: clear, serous, light yellow, <50 mL
Red blood cells (RBCs): none
White blood cells (WBCs): <300/μl
Protein: <4.1 g/dL
Glucose: 70-100 mg/dL
Amylase: 138-404 units/L
Ammonia: <50 mcg/dL
Alkaline phosphatase
    Adult male: 90-240 units/L
    Female <45 years: 76-196 units/L
    Female >45 years: 87-250 units/L
Lactic dehydrogenase (LDH): similar to serum LDH
Cytology: no malignant cells
Bacteria: none
Fungi: none
Carcinoembryonic antigen (CEA): negative

Test explanation and related physiology

Paracentesis is an invasive procedure entailing the insertion of a needle or catheter into the peritoneal cavity (Figure 33) for removal of ascitic fluid for diagnostic and therapeutic purposes.

Diagnostically, paracentesis is performed to obtain and analyze fluid to determine the etiology of the peritoneal effusion. Peritoneal fluid is classified as to whether it is a transudate or exudate. This is an important differentiation and is very helpful in determining the etiology of the effusion. *Transudates* are most frequently caused by congestive heart failure, cirrhosis, nephrotic syndrome, myxedema, peritoneal dialysis, and hypoproteinemia. *Exudates* are most often found in infectious or neoplastic conditions. However, collagen vascular disease, gastrointestinal diseases, trauma, and drug hypersensitivity also may cause an exudative effusion.

Therapeutically, this procedure is done to remove large amounts of fluid from the abdominal cavity. Usually these patients experience transient relief of symptoms (shortness of breath, distention, and early satiety) because of the removal of fluid within the abdominal cavity.

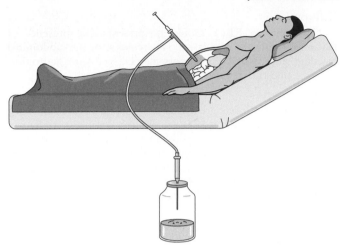

FIGURE 33 Paracentesis. A catheter is placed through the skin and abdominal muscle wall and into the peritoneal cavity containing free fluid.

The peritoneal fluid is usually evaluated for gross appearance, RBCs, WBCs, protein, glucose, amylase, ammonia, alkaline phosphatase, LDH, cytology, bacteria, fungi, and other tests (e.g., CEA levels). Each is discussed separately. Urea and creatinine may be measured if there is a question that the fluid may represent urine from a perforated bladder.

Gross appearance

Transudative peritoneal fluid may be clear, serous, or light yellow, especially in patients with hepatic cirrhosis. Milk-colored peritoneal fluid may result from the escape of chyle from blocked abdominal or thoracic lymphatic ducts. Conditions that may cause lymphatic blockage include lymphoma, carcinoma, and tuberculosis involving the abdominal or thoracic lymph nodes.

Exudative fluid is cloudy or turbid. Bloody fluid may be the result of a traumatic tap, intraabdominal bleeding, tumor, or hemorrhagic pancreatitis. Bile-stained green fluid may result from a ruptured gallbladder, acute pancreatitis, or perforated intestines.

Cell counts

Normally, no RBCs should be present. The presence of RBCs may indicate neoplasms, tuberculosis, or intraabdominal bleeding. Increased WBC counts may be seen with peritonitis, cirrhosis, and tuberculosis.

Protein count

Total protein levels greater than 3 g/dL are characteristic of exudates, whereas transudates usually have a protein content of less than 3 g/dL. It is now thought that the *albumin gradient* between serum and ascitic fluid can differentiate better between the transudate and exudate nature of ascites than can the total protein content. Values of 1.1 g/dL or more suggest a transudate, and values less than 1.1 g/dL suggest an exudate. The total protein ratio (fluid/serum) has been used to differentiate exudate from transudate. A total protein ratio of fluid to serum of greater than 0.5 is considered to be an exudate.

Glucose

Usually peritoneal glucose levels approximate serum glucose levels. Decreased levels may indicate tuberculous/bacterial peritonitis or peritoneal carcinomatosis.

Amylase

Increased amylase levels may be seen in patients with pancreatic trauma; pancreatic pseudocyst; acute pancreatitis; and intestinal necrosis, perforation, or strangulation. In these diseases, the amylase level is usually more than 1.5 times higher than serum levels.

Ammonia

High ammonia levels occur in ruptured or strangulated intestines and with a ruptured appendix or ulcer.

Alkaline phosphatase

Levels of alkaline phosphatase are greatly increased in infarcted or strangulated intestines.

Lactic dehydrogenase

A peritoneal fluid/serum LDH ratio of greater than 0.6 is typical of an exudate. An exudate is identified with a higher degree of accuracy if the peritoneal fluid/serum protein ratio is greater than 0.5 and the peritoneal fluid/serum LDH ratio is greater than 0.6.

Cytology

A cytologic study is performed to detect tumors. It can be difficult to differentiate malignancy from severe inflammatory mesothelial cells. Cytology examination of the fluid is improved by spinning down a large volume of fluid and examining the sediment.

Bacteria

Usually the fluid is cultured, and the antibiotic sensitivities are determined. Gram stains are often performed.

Gram stain and bacteriologic culture

The presence of bacteria may indicate intraabdominal infection. Culture and Gram stains identify the organisms.

Fungi

Fungi may indicate infections with histoplasmosis, candidiasis, or coccidioidomycosis.

Carcinoembryonic antigen

Peritoneal fluid levels for CEA are associated with abdominal malignancy, usually arising from the gastrointestinal tract.

Contraindications

- Patients with coagulation or bleeding abnormalities
- Patients with only a small amount of fluid and extensive previous abdominal surgery

Potential complications

- Hypovolemia if a large volume of peritoneal fluid is removed
- Peritonitis

Procedure and patient care

Before

PT Explain the procedure to the patient.
- Obtain informed consent for this procedure.
PT Tell the patient that no fasting or sedation is necessary.
PT Have the patient empty the bladder before the test.
- Measure abdominal girth.
- Obtain the patient's weight.
- Obtain baseline vital signs.

During

- Note the following procedural steps:
  1. Place the patient in a high Fowler position in bed.
  2. Paracentesis is performed under a strict sterile technique.
  3. The needle insertion site is aseptically cleansed and anesthetized locally.
  4. A scalpel may be used to make a stab wound in the skin to allow the cannula or needle to enter.

5. A trocar, cannula, or needle is threaded through the incision.
6. Tubing is attached to the cannula. The other end of the tubing is placed in the collection receptacle (usually a container with a pressurized vacuum).

- Note that this procedure is performed by a physician at the patient's bedside, in a procedure room, or in the physician's office in less than 30 minutes. Usually the volume removed is limited to about 4 L at any one time to avoid hypovolemia if the ascites is rapidly reaccumulated.

PT Although local anesthetics eliminate pain at the insertion site, tell the patient that he or she will feel a pressure-like pain as the needle is inserted.

After

- All tests on peritoneal fluid should be performed immediately to avoid false results due to chemical or cellular deterioration.
- Place a small bandage over the needle site.
- Send the specimen promptly to the laboratory.
- Observe the puncture site for bleeding, continued drainage, or signs of inflammation.
- Measure the abdominal girth and weight of the patient; compare with baseline values.
- Monitor vital signs for evidence of hemodynamic changes.
- Because of the high protein content of ascitic fluid, albumin infusions may be ordered after paracentesis to compensate for protein loss.
- Occasionally ascitic fluid will continue to leak out of the needle tract after removal of the needle. A suture can stop that. If unsuccessful, a collection bag should be used.

Abnormal findings

Exudate	Transudate
Lymphoma	Hepatic cirrhosis
Carcinoma	Portal hypertension
Tuberculosis	Nephrotic syndrome
Peritonitis	Hypoproteinemia
Pancreatitis	Congestive heart failure
Ruptured viscus	Abdominal trauma
	Peritoneal bleeding

notes

parathyroid hormone (PTH, Parathormone)

Type of test Blood

Normal findings

Intact (whole): 10-65 pg/mL or 10-65 ng/L (SI units)
N terminal: 8-24 pg/mL
C terminal: 50-330 pg/mL

Test explanation and related physiology

PTH is secreted by the parathyroid gland in response to hypocalcemia. This test is useful in establishing a diagnosis of hyperparathyroidism and distinguishing nonparathyroid from parathyroid causes of hypercalcemia. Increased PTH levels are seen in patients with hyperparathyroidism (primary, secondary, or tertiary); in patients with nonparathyroid, ectopic PTH-producing tumors (pseudohyperparathyroidism); or as a normal compensatory response to hypocalcemia in patients with malabsorption or vitamin D deficiency.

It is important to measure serum calcium simultaneous with the measurement of PTH. Most laboratories have a PTH/calcium nomogram already made up, indicating what PTH level is considered normal for each calcium level.

Decreased PTH levels are seen in patients with hypoparathyroidism or as a compensatory response to hypercalcemia in patients with metastatic bone tumors, sarcoidosis, vitamin D intoxication, or milk-alkali syndrome. Of course, surgical ablation of the parathyroids is another cause of hypoparathyroidism.

Whole (intact) PTH is metabolized to several different fragments, including an N terminal, a midregion (or midmolecule), and a C terminal. Intact PTH and all fragments generally provide accurate information concerning the level of PTH in the blood. Intact PTH is probably the most often tested because it is the most reliable.

Interfering factors

- Recent injection of radioisotopes
- Drugs that *increase* PTH include anticonvulsants, isoniazid, lithium, rifampin, and steroids.
- Drugs that *decrease* PTH include cimetidine and propranolol.

Procedure and patient care

- See inside front cover for Routine Blood Testing.
- Fasting: yes.
- Blood tube commonly used: red.
- Obtain a morning blood specimen, because diurnal rhythm affects PTH levels. (Check with the laboratory if the patient works at night.)
- Note that some laboratories require blood in an iced plastic syringe.
- Obtain a serum calcium level determination at the same time if ordered. Serum PTH and serum calcium levels are important in the differential diagnosis.
- Indicate the time the blood was drawn on the laboratory slip, because a diurnal rhythm affects test results.

Abnormal findings

▲ **Increased levels**
Hyperparathyroidism secondary to adenoma or carcinoma of the parathyroid gland
Non–PTH-producing tumors (paraneoplastic syndrome)
Lung carcinoma
Kidney carcinoma
Hypocalcemia
Chronic renal failure
Malabsorption syndrome
Vitamin D deficiency
Rickets
Osteomalacia
Congenital renal defect

▼ **Decreased levels**
Hypoparathyroidism
Hypercalcemia
Metastatic bone tumor
Sarcoidosis
Autoimmune destruction of the parathyroid glands
Vitamin D intoxication
Milk-alkali syndrome
Graves disease
Hypomagnesemia
DiGeorge syndrome

notes

parathyroid scan (Parathyroid scintigraphy)

Type of test Nuclear medicine

Normal findings No increased parathyroid uptake

Test explanation and related physiology

Hypercalcemia can be caused by hyperparathyroidism. Parathyroid hyperplasia, adenoma, or cancer can cause hyperparathyroidism. It is important for the surgeon planning resection of the parathyroid abnormality to know how many parathyroid glands are involved and their locations. Preoperative parathyroid scanning is the most accurate method of providing this information. Parathyroid hyperplasia causes enlargement of all four parathyroid glands. A parathyroid adenoma or cancer, however, causes enlargement of only one parathyroid gland and suppression of the other three glands.

Parathyroids are located most commonly on the lateral borders of the thyroid lobes—two on each side. However, parathyroid anatomic location varies considerably, and they may be located anywhere from the upper neck to the lower mediastinum. Parathyroid scanning is also done immediately prior to surgery to help the surgeon identify the parathyroid glands and particularly the pathologic glands. In this test, the scan is performed on the parathyroid glands as described previously. In the operating room, if the preoperative scan result is abnormal, the surgeon scans the suspect area of the neck with a gamma ray detector probe. Increased counts are noted in the regions where the parathyroid abnormalities are located. Noniodinated technetium MIBI (methoxyisobutylisonitrite) is now most commonly used for parathyroid scans. Scans are performed using planar images and using single-photon emission computed tomography/computed tomography (SPECT/CT) images for three-dimensional image reconstruction.

Contraindications

• Patients who are pregnant

Procedure and patient care

Before

PT Explain the procedure to the patient.

PT Tell the patient that fasting is usually not required.

During

- Note the following procedural step for the single tracer double phase (STDP) method.
  1. Technetium-99m sestamibi is injected intravenously.
  2. At 15 minutes and 3 hours, the patient is placed in a supine position. For planar images, the detector is passed over the neck and upper chest area, and the radioactive counts are recorded and displayed.
  3. For SPECT/CT screening, the patient is placed in the appropriate unit in the supine position.
  4. Initially, the tracer lights up both the thyroid and parathyroid glands. At 3 hours, the tracer remains only in the pathologic parathyroid tissue.
- Note that this study is performed by a nuclear technologist and interpreted by a physician in the nuclear medicine department.

PT Tell the patient that no discomfort is associated with this study.

After

PT Assure the patient that the dose of radioactive technetium used in this test is minute and therefore harmless.

Abnormal findings

Parathyroid adenoma, carcinoma, or hyperplasia

Aberrantly placed parathyroid tissue in the upper neck, thyroid gland, or mediastinum

notes

partial thromboplastin time, activated (APTT, Partial thromboplastin time [PTT])

Type of test Blood

Normal findings

APTT: 30-40 seconds
PTT: 60-70 seconds
Patients receiving anticoagulant therapy: 1.5-2.5 times the control value in seconds

Possible critical values

APTT: >70 seconds
PTT: >100 seconds

Test explanation and related physiology

The PTT test is used to assess the intrinsic system and the common pathway of clot formation. PTT evaluates factors I (fibrinogen), II (prothrombin), V, VIII, IX, X, XI, and XII. When any of these factors exist in inadequate quantities, such as in hemophilia A and B or consumptive coagulopathy, PTT is prolonged. Because factors II, IX, and X are vitamin K–dependent factors, biliary obstruction, which precludes gastrointestinal absorption of fat and fat-soluble vitamins (e.g., vitamin K), can reduce their concentration and thus prolong PTT. Because coagulation factors are made in the liver, hepatocellular diseases will also prolong PTT.

Heparin has been found to inactivate prothrombin (factor II) and prevent the formation of thromboplastin. These actions prolong the intrinsic clotting pathway for approximately 4 to 6 hours after each dose of heparin. Thus, heparin is capable of providing therapeutic anticoagulation. The appropriate dose of heparin can be monitored by PTT. Test results are given in seconds, along with a control value. The control value may vary slightly from day to day because of the reagents used.

Recently activators have been added to PTT test reagents to shorten normal clotting time and provide a narrow normal range. This shortened time is called the *activated* PTT (APTT). Normal APTT is 30 to 40 seconds. Desired ranges for therapeutic anticoagulation are 1.5 to 2.5 times normal (e.g., 70 seconds). The APTT specimen should be drawn 30 to 60 minutes before the patient's next heparin dose is given. If the APTT is less than 50 seconds, the patient may not be receiving therapeutic anticoagulation and need more heparin. An APTT greater than

P

100 seconds indicates that too much heparin is being given; the risk of serious spontaneous bleeding exists when the APTT is this high. The effects of heparin can be reversed immediately by the administration of 1 mg of protamine sulfate for every 100 units of the heparin dose.

Heparin's effect, unlike that of warfarin, is immediate and short-lived. When a thromboembolic episode (e.g., pulmonary embolism, arterial embolism, thrombophlebitis) occurs, immediate and complete anticoagulation is most rapidly and safely achieved by heparin administration. This drug is often given during cardiac and vascular surgery to prevent intravascular clotting during clamping of the vessels. Often, small doses of heparin (5000 units subcutaneously every 12 hours) are given to prevent thromboembolism in high-risk patients. This dose alters the PTT very little, and the risk of spontaneous bleeding is minimal.

APTT is also used to determine *activated protein C (APC) resistance* (p. 417). APC resistance testing is performed in the evaluation of thrombotic patients. A standard APTT test is performed first in the absence of, and then in the presence of, commercially available APC. The APTT is normally prolonged in the presence of APC due to APC's anticoagulant action. An abnormality is detected if the APTT is not prolonged. This results from a resistance to APC, most commonly caused by an abnormal factor V Leiden.

Normal pregnancy has been associated with prolonged APTT times. Factor XI deficiency and antiphospholipid antibody are two major abnormalities identified in pregnant patients with prolonged APTT. These coagulopathies are not usually associated with excessive bleeding or thromboembolism. At the same time, pregnancy or oral contraceptive (OC) use is also associated with prolonged APTT. This is due, in large part, to a factor V mutation (factor V Leiden), which potentiates the prothrombotic effect of OC.

Interfering factors

☒ Drugs that may prolong PTT test values include antihistamines, ascorbic acid, chlorpromazine, heparin, and salicylates.

Procedure and patient care

- See inside front cover for Routine Blood Testing.
- Fasting: no.
- Blood tube commonly used: blue.

- If the patient is receiving heparin by intermittent injection, plan to draw the blood specimen for the APTT 30 minutes to 1 hour before the next dose of heparin.
- If the patient is receiving continuous heparin, draw the blood at any time.
- Apply pressure to the venipuncture site. Remember, if the patient is receiving anticoagulants or has coagulopathies, the bleeding time will be increased.
- Assess the patient to detect possible bleeding. Check for blood in the urine and all other excretions and assess the patient for bruises, petechiae, and low back pain.
- If severe bleeding occurs, note that the anticoagulant effect of heparin can be reversed by parenteral administration of protamine sulfate.

Abnormal findings

▲ **Increased levels**
Acquired or congenital
    clotting factor deficiencies
    (e.g., hypofibrinogenemia,
    von Willebrand disease,
    and hemophilia)
Cirrhosis of the liver
Vitamin K deficiency
Disseminated intravascular
    coagulation
Heparin administration

▼ **Decreased levels**
Early stages
    of disseminated
    intravascular
    coagulation
Extensive cancer

notes

parvovirus B19 antibody

Type of test Blood

Normal findings Negative for immunoglobulin M (IgM)- and IgG-specific antibodies to parvovirus B19

Test explanation and related physiology

The parvovirus B19 is known to be a human pathogen. Many of the severe manifestations of B19 viremia relate to the ability of the virus to infect and lyse red blood cell precursors in the bone marrow.

Erythema infectiosum is the most common manifestation of B19 infection and occurs predominantly in children. This pathogen is also referred to as *fifth disease* or *academy rash*. Parvovirus B19 has also been associated with a number of other clinical problems, including joint inflammation, purpura, hydrops fetalis, and aplastic anemia.

Because of the recently discovered spectrum of disease caused by parvovirus B19, laboratory diagnosis has come into great demand. Serologic testing for parvovirus B19–specific IgM and IgG antibodies can be done. Acute infections can be determined by B19-compatible symptoms and the presence of IgM antibodies that remain detectable up to a few months. Past infection or immunity is documented by IgG antibodies that persist with IgM antibodies. Fetal infection may be recognized by hydrops fetalis and the presence of B19 DNA in amniotic fluid or fetal blood.

Procedure and patient care

- See inside front cover for Routine Blood Testing.
- Fasting: no.
- Blood tube commonly used: verify with lab.
- **PT** Inform the patient that it normally requires approximately 2 to 3 days to get test results.

Abnormal findings

▲ **Increased levels**

Erythema infectiosum (fifth disease)

Joint arthralgia and arthritis

Hydrops fetalis

Fetal loss

Transient aplastic anemia

Chronic anemia in immunodeficient patients

Bone marrow failure

notes

pelvic ultrasonography (Pelvic ultrasonography in pregnancy, Obstetric ultrasonography, Vaginal ultrasound)

Type of test Ultrasound

Normal findings Normal fetal and placental size and position

Test explanation and related physiology

Ultrasound examination of the female patient is a harmless, noninvasive method of evaluating the female genital tract and fetus. It should be noted that pelvic ultrasonography can be performed with the transducer placed on the anterior abdomen (see Figure 1, p. 2) or in the vagina with a specially designed vaginal probe. Vaginal ultrasound adds significant accuracy in identifying paracervical, endometrial, and ovarian pathology that otherwise may not be detected with the anterior abdominal probe.

Pelvic ultrasonography may be useful in the *obstetric patient* in the following circumstances:

- Making an early diagnosis of normal pregnancy and abnormal pregnancy (e.g., tubal pregnancy)
- Identifying multiple pregnancies
- Differentiating a tumor (e.g., hydatidiform mole) from a normal pregnancy
- Determining the age of the fetus by the diameter of the head
- Measuring the rate of fetal growth
- Identifying placental abnormalities (e.g., abruptio placentae and placenta previa)
- Diagnosing ectopic pregnancy
- Providing a realistic image of the fetus using three- or four-dimensional imaging
- Evaluating the kidneys and upper collecting system
- Localizing the placenta before amniocentesis
- Making a differential diagnosis of various uterine and ovarian enlargements (e.g., polyhydramnios)

Ultrasound is a very accurate and easily performed screening test to recognize risks of fetal abnormalities (see amniotic fluid index, p. 424). *Fetal nuchal translucency (FNT)* is an ultrasound measurement of subcutaneous edema in the neck region of the fetus. It is performed at 10 to 14 weeks of gestation. Major heart defects, trisomy 21, and other genetic defects are associated with increased edema in this location at this age of gestation. Screening for chromosomal defects by measurement of FNT identifies 80% of fetuses with trisomy 21 for a false-positive rate

P

of 5%. With FNT, these abnormalities can be identified earlier in the pregnancy, when abortion is still possible.

Pelvic ultrasound is used in the *nonpregnant woman* to monitor the endometrium in patients who take tamoxifen and to aid in the diagnosis of:

- Ovarian cyst or tumor
- Tubo-ovarian abscess
- Uterine fibroids or cancer
- Pelvic inflammatory disease (PID)
- Thickened uterine endometrium (stripe) (caused by cancer, hyperplasia, etc.)

When a woman is unable to visualize or palpate the string of an intrauterine device (IUD), ultrasound is indicated to determine whether the IUD has perforated the uterus, been expulsed, or been incorporated with an intrauterine pregnancy.

Contraindications

- Patients with latex allergy
  Vaginal ultrasound requires placement of the probe in a latex condom–like sac.

Interfering factors

- Patients who have had recent gastrointestinal (GI) contrast studies, because barium creates severe distortion of reflective sound waves
- Patients with air-filled bowels, because gas does not transmit the sound waves well
- Failure to fill the bladder may make the image uninterpretable.

Procedure and patient care

Before

- **PT** Explain the procedure to the patient.
- **PT** Tell the patient that no fasting or sedation is required.
- **PT** Assure the patient that this study has no known deleterious effects on maternal or fetal tissues.
- **PT** Give the patient three to four glasses (200 to 350 mL) of water or another liquid 1 hour before the examination, and instruct the patient *not* to void until after the procedure is completed. This will permit visualization of the bladder, which is used as a reference point in pelvic anatomy.
- No water is required for vaginal ultrasound.
- If a transabdominal ultrasound is required urgently and there is not time to fill the bladder by ingestion of fluids, a bladder catheter is inserted and the bladder is filled with water.

During

- Note the following procedural steps:
  1. The patient is taken to the ultrasound room and placed in the supine position on the examining table.
  2. The ultrasonographer applies a greasy conductive paste to the abdomen to enhance sound transmission and reception.
  3. A transducer is passed over the skin.
  4. If a vaginal probe is used, it is inserted via the vagina and angled to identify the various parts of the pelvis.
  5. Pictures are taken of the reflections.
  6. During the examination, fetal structures are usually pointed out to the mother.
- Note that this procedure is performed in approximately 20 minutes.
- **PT** Inform the patient that no discomfort is associated with this study other than having a full bladder and the urge to void.

After

- Remove the lubricant from the patient's skin.

Abnormal findings

Tubal pregnancy
Abdominal pregnancy
Hydatidiform mole of the uterus
Intrauterine growth retardation
Multiple pregnancy
Fetal death
Abruptio placentae
Abnormal fetal position
Fetal anomalies
Placenta previa
Polyhydramnios
Neoplasm of the ovaries, uterus, or fallopian tubes
Cysts
Abscesses
Hydrocephalus of the fetus

notes

P

pepsinogen

Type of test   Blood/urine

Normal findings

Pepsinogen I: 28-100 ng/ml
Pepsinogen II: <22 ng/mL

Test explanation and related physiology

Pepsinogens are secreted in the stomach and are made in the oxyntic gland mucosa of the proximal stomach. When exposed to gastric acid, pepsinogen is converted to pepsin, an active enzyme that is proteolytic and promotes digestion. Patients with gastric atrophy or pernicious anemia (PA) or those who have had a gastrectomy have low levels of pepsinogen I. Pepsinogen I levels are elevated in patients with ulcer disease. Pepsinogen I has been used as a subclinical marker of increased risk for stomach cancer. Pepsinogen I can also be measured in the urine.

Pepsinogen II is made by oxyntic gland mucosa cells that are in the distal stomach and proximal duodenum. Because PA generally affects the proximal stomach, diminished levels of pepsinogen I with normal levels of pepsinogen II are strongly supportive of PA.

Procedure and patient care

- See inside front cover for Routine Blood Testing.
- Fasting: yes.
- Blood tube commonly used: red.
- **PT** Tell the patient that antacids or other medications affecting stomach acidity or gastrointestinal motility should be discontinued, if possible, for at least 48 hours before collection. Verify with the laboratory or health care provider.
- The specimen is usually frozen because most testing is performed in a central laboratory.

Abnormal findings

▼ **Decreased values**
  Pernicious anemia
  Gastric atrophy
  Chronic gastritis
  Peptic ulcer disease

notes

pericardiocentesis

Type of test Fluid analysis

Normal findings Less than 50 mL of clear, straw-colored fluid without evidence of any bacteria, blood, or malignant cells

Test explanation and related physiology

Pericardiocentesis, which involves the aspiration of fluid from the pericardial sac with a needle, may be performed for therapeutic and diagnostic purposes. Therapeutically, the test is performed to relieve cardiac tamponade by removing fluid and improving diastolic filling. Diagnostically, pericardiocentesis is performed to remove a sample of pericardial fluid for laboratory examination to determine the cause of the fluid. This is similar to the evaluation described for peritoneal and pleural fluid (p. 684 and p. 883, respectively).

Contraindications

- Patients who are uncooperative because of the risk of lacerations to the epicardium or coronary artery
- Patients with a bleeding disorder
  Inadvertent puncture of the myocardium may create uncontrollable bleeding, leading to tamponade.

Potential complications

- Laceration of the coronary artery or myocardium
- Needle-induced ventricular arrhythmias
- Myocardial infarction
- Pneumothorax caused by inadvertent puncture of the lung
- Liver laceration caused by inadvertent puncture
- Pleural infection
- Vasovagal arrest

Procedure and patient care

Before

PT Explain the procedure to the patient.
- Obtain informed consent for this procedure.
- Restrict fluid and food intake for 4 hours (if possible).
- Obtain IV access for infusion of fluids and cardiac medications if required.
- Administer pretest medication. Atropine may be given to prevent the vasovagal reflex of bradycardia and hypotension.

P

During

- Note the following procedural steps:
  1. The patient is placed in the supine position.
  2. An area in the fifth to sixth intercostal space at the left sternal margin (or subxyphoid) is prepared and draped.
  3. After skin anesthesia is performed, a large-bore pericardiocentesis needle is placed on a 50-mL syringe and introduced into the pericardial sac (Figure 34).
  4. An electrocardiographic lead is often attached by a clip to the needle to identify any ST-segment elevations.
  5. Pericardial fluid is aspirated.
  6. Some patients who have recurring cardiac tamponade may require placement of an indwelling pericardial catheter.

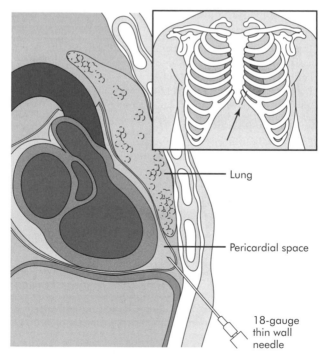

FIGURE 34 Pericardiocentesis using subxyphoid route for aspiration of pericardial fluid. The 18-gauge needle is introduced at a 30- to 40-degree angle.

7. With certain types of pericarditis, medications (e.g., antibiotics, antineoplastic drugs, corticosteroids) may be instilled during pericardiocentesis.

• Note that a physician usually performs this procedure in the cardiac catheterization laboratory, operating room, or emergency room in approximately 10 to 20 minutes.

PT Tell the patient that this procedure is associated with very little discomfort.

After

• Closely monitor the patient's vital signs. An increased temperature may indicate infection. Pericardial bleeding would be marked by hypotension or pulsus paradoxus.

• Check the dressing frequently for drainage.

• Label and number the specimen tubes that contain the pericardial fluid, and deliver them to the appropriate laboratories for examination. Note the following possibilities:

   ○ Usually the fluid is taken to the chemistry laboratory, where the color, turbidity, glucose, albumin, protein, and lactic dehydrogenase levels are obtained.

   ○ A tube of blood often goes to the hematology laboratory, where red and white blood cells are evaluated.

   ○ The bacteriology laboratory performs routine cultures, Gram stains, fungal studies, acid-fast bacilli smears, and so on.

   ○ When malignancy is suspected, the fluid should be sent for cytology.

• Apply a sterile dressing to the catheter if one has been left for continuing pericardial drainage.

• Establish a closed system if continued pericardial drainage is required.

• Note that to minimize infection, pericardial catheters, if used, are usually removed after 2 days.

Abnormal findings

Pericarditis	Metastatic cancer
Uremia	Blunt or penetrating cardiac trauma
Hypoproteinemia	Rupture of ventricular aneurysm
Congestive heart failure	Collagen vascular diseases

notes

pheochromocytoma suppression and provocative testing (Clonidine suppression test [CST], Glucagon stimulation test)

Type of test Blood

Normal findings

Glucagon stimulation

Norepinephrine: <3 times basal levels

Clonidine suppression

Norepinephrine: >50% reduction in basal levels or <500 pg/mL
Epinephrine: >50% reduction in basal levels or <275 pg/mL

Test explanation and related physiology

In patients with significantly high blood pressure refractory to treatment, the diagnosis of pheochromocytoma is often considered. When catecholamine levels are excessive (norepinephrine >2000 pg/mL), the diagnosis is easily made. However, when basal levels are not significantly elevated, it is difficult to differentiate essential hypertension from a functioning pheochromocytoma. Suppression and provocative tests may be necessary. Glucagon is used as the provocative agent. In patients with pheochromocytoma, the response is accentuated. Clonidine is normally a potent suppressor of catecholamine production, yet it has little to no effect on catecholamines in patients with pheochromocytoma. Testing of metanephrines (see page 636) provides higher diagnostic sensitivity than catecholamine assays in screening for pheochromocytoma.

Contraindications

- Hypovolemic/dehydrated patients
  These patients should not have suppression testing because they could experience a precipitous drop in blood pressure.

Potential complications

- Drowsiness during CST
- Hypotension during CST, especially in patients treated aggressively for hypertension
- Extremely high blood pressure during provocative testing

Interfering factors

- False suppression with CST may occur in patients with low basal catecholamine levels.

Procedure and patient care

Before

PT Explain the procedure to the patient.

- Identify the medications being administered prior to testing.
- The patient must be reclining calmly for 30 minutes prior to testing.

During

- Collect a venous blood sample from an antecubital vein in a heparinized tube for determination of basal catecholamine levels.
- Monitor vital signs closely throughout the testing period.

Glucagon provocative test

- Administer a prescribed dose of glucagon intravenously.
- Two minutes later, obtain a blood specimen as described above.

Clonidine suppression test

- Administer a prescribed dose of clonidine orally.
- Three hours later, obtain a blood specimen as described above.

After

- Monitor vital signs for at least 1 hour after conclusion of the procedure.

Abnormal findings

Pheochromocytoma

notes

P

phosphate (PO₄, Phosphorus [P])

Type of test Blood

Normal findings

Adult: 3.0-4.5 mg/dL or 0.97-1.45 mmol/L (SI units)
Elderly: values slightly lower than adult
Child: 4.5-6.5 mg/dL or 1.45-2.1 mmol/L (SI units)
Newborn: 4.3-9.3 mg/dL or 1.4-3.0 mmol/L (SI units)

Possible critical values <1 mg/dL

Test explanation and related physiology

Phosphorus in the body exists in the form of a phosphate. The terms phosphorus and phosphate are used interchangeably throughout this and other discussions. Most of the phosphate in the body is a part of organic compounds. Only a small part of total body phosphate is inorganic phosphate (i.e., not part of another organic compound). It is the *inorganic* phosphate that is measured when one requests a phosphate, phosphorus, inorganic phosphorus, or inorganic phosphate. Most of the body's inorganic phosphorus is intracellular and combined with calcium within the skeleton; however, approximately 15% of the phosphorus exists in the blood as a phosphate salt.

Dietary phosphorus is absorbed in the small bowel. The absorption is very efficient, and only rarely is hypophosphatemia caused by gastrointestinal malabsorption. Phosphorus levels are determined by calcium metabolism, parathormone (parathyroid hormone [PTH]), renal excretion, and, to a lesser degree, intestinal absorption. Because an inverse relationship exists between calcium and phosphorus, a decrease of one mineral results in an increase in the other. The regulation of phosphate by PTH is such that PTH tends to decrease phosphate resorption in the kidney. PTH and vitamin D, however, tend to stimulate phosphate absorption weakly within the gut. Hypophosphatemia may have four general causes: shift of phosphate from extracellular to intracellular, renal phosphate wasting, loss from the gastrointestinal tract, and loss from intracellular stores. Hyperphosphatemia is usually secondary to increased intake or an inability of the kidneys to excrete phosphate.

Interfering factors

- Laxatives or enemas containing sodium phosphate can increase phosphorus levels.

- Recent carbohydrate ingestion, including IV glucose administration, causes decreased phosphorus levels because phosphorus enters the cell with glucose.
- ✔ Drugs that may cause *increased* levels include methicillin and vitamin D (excessive).
- ✔ Drugs that may cause *decreased* levels include albuterol, anesthesia agents, antacids, estrogens, insulin, mannitol, and oral contraceptives.

Procedure and patient care
- See inside front cover for Routine Blood Testing.
- Fasting: yes.
- Blood tube commonly used: red.
- If indicated, discontinue IV fluids with glucose for several hours before the test.
- Avoid hemolysis. Handle the tube carefully.
- Use a heel stick to draw blood from infants.

Abnormal findings

▲ **Increased levels (hyperphosphatemia)**
Renal failure
Increased dietary or IV intake of phosphorus
Acromegaly
Hypoparathyroidism
Bone metastasis
Sarcoidosis
Hypocalcemia
Liver disease
Acidosis
Rhabdomyolysis
Advanced lymphoma or myeloma
Hemolytic anemia

▼ **Decreased levels (hypophosphatemia)**
Inadequate dietary ingestion of phosphorus
Chronic antacid ingestion
Hyperparathyroidism
Hypercalcemia
Chronic alcoholism
Vitamin D deficiency
Diabetic acidosis
Hyperinsulinism
Rickets (childhood)
Osteomalacia (adult)
Malnutrition
Alkalosis
Sepsis (gram-negative)

P

notes

PI-linked antigen (Phosphatidylinositol antigen)

Type of test Blood

Normal findings

RBCs

Type I (normal expression): 99%-100%

Type II (partial deficient): 0.00%-0.99%

Type III (deficient): 0.00%-0.01%

Granulocytes: 0.00%-0.01%

Monocytes: 0.00%-0.05%

Test explanation and related physiology

Paroxysmal nocturnal hemoglobinuria (PNH) is an acquired hematologic disorder characterized by nocturnal hemoglobinuria, chronic hemolytic anemia, thrombosis, pancytopenia, and, in some patients, acute or chronic myeloid malignancies. PNH appears to be a hematopoietic stem cell disorder that affects erythroid, granulocytic, and megakaryocytic cell lines. The abnormal cells in PNH have been shown to lack glycosylphosphatidylinositol (GPI)-linked proteins in RBCs and WBCs. Mutations in the *phosphatidylinositol glycan A (PIGA)* gene have been identified consistently in patients with PNH, thus confirming the biological defect in this disorder.

Flow cytometric immunophenotyping of peripheral blood (WBC and RBC) is performed to evaluate the presence or absence of PI-linked antigens (CD14, FLAER, and/or CD59 antigens), using monoclonal antibodies directed against them. These proteins are absent on the blood cells of patients with PNH. Determination of PI-linked antigens is not only useful in the diagnosis of PNH but also in monitoring of the disease.

Procedure and patient care

- See inside front cover for Routine Blood Testing.
- Fasting: no.
- Blood tube commonly used: yellow.

Abnormal findings

▼ Decreased levels

PNH

notes

placental growth factor (PGF)

Type of test Blood

Normal findings

Nonpregnant women: <50 pg/mL
Pregnant women at 22 weeks' gestation: >200 pg/mL

Test explanation and related physiology

Preeclampsia is one of the most common medical complications of pregnancy and is associated with considerable maternal and neonatal morbidity and mortality. Normally, PGF rises steadily throughout pregnancy to levels exceeding 500 pg/mL. When PGF is tested at 13 to 16 weeks of gestation and it is found to be significantly decreased, the patient is at considerable risk for preeclampsia. Likewise, patients with markedly increased levels of soluble fms-like tyrosine kinase-1 (sFlt-1), which is a known inhibitor of PGF, are also at risk for preeclampsia. PGF is a protein that is produced during pregnancy by the placental trophoblast.

Preeclampsia can be predicted by a combination of factors in the maternal history, including black racial origin, high body mass index, family history of preeclampsia, and personal history of preeclampsia. Screening at risk women with PGF, sFlt-1, PAPP-A (page 742), and uterine artery Doppler would identify women who would develop early and late preeclampsia. Intensive maternal and fetal monitoring could improve pregnancy outcomes.

Procedure and patient care

- See inside front cover for Routine Blood Testing.
- Fasting: no.
- Blood tube commonly used: red.

Abnormal findings

▼ Decreased blood levels
Hypertension
Preeclampsia

notes

plasminogen (Fibrinolysin)

Type of test Blood

Normal findings 2.4-4.4 Committee on Thrombolytic Agents (CTA) units/mL

Test explanation and related physiology

This test is used to diagnose suspected plasminogen deficiency in patients who have multiple thromboembolic episodes. Plasminogen is a protein involved in the fibrinolytic process of intravascular blood clot dissolution (see Figure 10, p. 264). Plasminogen is converted to plasmin by proteolytic cleavage. This reaction can be catalyzed by urokinase, streptokinase, or tissue plasminogen activator (t-PA). Plasmin can destroy fibrin and dissolve clots. This fibrinolytic system is a normal part of the balance between coagulation and fibrinolysis.

Plasminogen levels are occasionally measured during fibrinolytic therapy (for coronary and peripheral arterial occlusion) and are diminished with full fibrinolysis. Decreased levels of plasminogen are also found in hyperfibrinolytic states (e.g., disseminated intravascular coagulation [DIC], primary fibrinolysis). Because plasminogen is made in the liver, patients with cirrhosis or other severe liver diseases can be expected to have decreased levels. There are rare cases of hereditary deficiencies of this protein. Inflammatory conditions may have mild elevations of plasminogens, which are acute-phase reactant proteins.

Interfering factors

- Pregnancy and especially eclampsia are associated with increased values.

Procedure and patient care

- See inside front cover for Routine Blood Testing.
- Fasting: no.
- Blood tube commonly used: blue.

Abnormal findings

▲ **Increased levels**
Pregnancy
Inflammatory conditions

▼ **Decreased levels**
Hyperfibrinolytic state
(e.g., DIC, fibrinolysis)
Primary liver disease
Syndrome associated
with hypercoagulation
(e.g., venous and
arterial clotting)
Rare congenital
deficiencies
Malnutrition

notes

P

plasminogen activator inhibitor 1 (PAI-1)

Type of test Blood

Normal findings

Antigen assay: 2-46 ng/mL
Activity: < 31.1 IU/mL

Test explanation and related physiology

PAI-1 is a protein that inhibits plasminogen activators. During fibrinolysis, tissue plasminogen activator (tPA) converts plasminogen into plasmin. Plasmin plays a critical role in fibrinolysis by degrading fibrin (see Figure 10, p. 264). PAI-1 is the primary inhibitor of tPA and urokinase plasminogen activator (uPA) in the blood. PAI-1 limits the production of plasmin and keeps fibrinolysis in check.

Elevated levels of PAI-1 are associated with a predisposition to thrombosis, including veno-occlusive disease after bone marrow transplantation or high dose chemotherapy. Familial thrombosis has been associated with inherited elevation of plasma PAI-1 activity. Increased levels of PAI-1 have also been reported in a number of conditions, including malignancy, liver disease, the postoperative period, septic shock, the second and third trimesters of pregnancy, obesity, coronary heart disease, and restenosis after coronary angioplasty. Increased levels may reduce the effectiveness of antithrombolytic therapy. Patients with insulin resistance syndrome and diabetes mellitus tend to have increased PAI-1 levels.

Low plasma levels of the active form of PAI-1 have been associated with abnormal, clinically significant bleeding. Complete deficiency of PAI-1, either congenital or acquired, is associated with bleeding manifestations that include hemarthroses, hematomas, menorrhagia, easy bruising, and postoperative hemorrhage.

PAI-1 antigen can be measured directly by ELISA or by PCR genotyping. PAI-1 activity can be measured by bio-immunoassay. Results vary by methodology.

Interfering factors

- Because PAI-1 is an acute-phase reactant, it can become transiently elevated by infection, inflammation, or trauma.
- Levels increase during pregnancy.

- PAI-1 has a circadian rhythm, with the highest concentrations occurring in the morning and the lowest concentrations in the afternoon and evening.

Procedure and patient care

- See inside front cover for Routine Blood Testing.
- Fasting: no.
- Blood tube commonly used: light blue.

Discard the first several milliliters of blood if PAI-1 is the only test being drawn. If multiple tests are being drawn, fill the light blue–top tube after any red-top tube.

- Gently invert the blood tube several times after collection.

Abnormal findings

▲ **Increased levels**
Acute coronary syndrome
Coronary artery disease
Restenosis after coronary
   angioplasty
Infection
Inflammation
Trauma
Diabetes mellitus
Insulin resistance syndrome
Pregnancy

▼ **Decreased levels**
Bleeding disorders

notes

P

platelet aggregation test

Type of test Blood

Normal findings Dependent on the platelet agonist used

Test explanation and related physiology

Platelet aggregation is an important part of hemostasis. Surrounding an area of acute blood vessel endothelial injury is a clump of platelets. Normal platelets adhere to this area of injury, and through a series of chemical reactions, they attract other platelets to the area. This is platelet aggregation, the first step of hemostasis. After this step, the normal coagulation factor waterfall occurs (see Figure 10, p. 264). Certain diseases that affect either platelet number or function can inhibit platelet aggregation and thereby prolong bleeding times. Congenital syndromes, uremia, myeloproliferative disorders, and certain drugs are associated with abnormal platelet aggregation. If blood is passed through a heart-lung or dialysis pump, platelet injury can occur and aggregation can be reduced.

Interfering factors

- Factors that may cause increased platelet aggregation include blood storage temperature, hyperbilirubinemia, hemoglobinemia, hyperlipidemia, and platelet count.
- ✘ Drugs that may cause *decreased* platelet aggregation include antibiotics, aspirin, nonsteroidal antiinflammatory agents, and thienopyridine antiplatelet drugs (e.g., ticlopidine, clopidogrel).

Procedure and patient care

- See inside front cover for Routine Blood Testing.
- Fasting: no.
- Blood tube commonly used: blue.
- Remember that abnormalities in platelet aggregation can prolong bleeding time, and a significant hematoma at the venipuncture site may occur.

Abnormal findings

▲ **Prolonged platelet aggregation**

Various congenital disorders (e.g., Wiskott-Aldrich syndrome, Bernard-Soulier syndrome, glycogen storage, von Willebrand disease)

Connective tissue disorder (e.g., lupus erythematosus)

Recent cardiopulmonary or dialysis bypass

Various myeloproliferative diseases

Primary protein disease

Uremia

notes

platelet antibody detection (Antiplatelet antibody detection)

Type of test Blood

Normal findings No antiplatelet antibodies identified

Test explanation and related physiology

Immune-mediated destruction of platelets may be caused either by autoantibodies directed against antigens located on the same person's platelets or by alloantibodies that develop after exposure to transfused platelets received from a donor. These antibodies are usually directed to an antigen on the platelet membrane, such as *human lymphocyte antigen (HLA)* (p. 533) or *platelet-specific antigens,* such as *PLA1* and *PLA2.*

Antibodies directed to platelets cause early destruction of the platelets and subsequent thrombocytopenia. Immunologic thrombocytopenia includes the following:

- *Idiopathic thrombocytopenia purpura (ITP)*
  Platelet-associated IgG antibodies are detected in 90% of these patients.
- *Posttransfusion purpura*
  This is usually associated with an antibody to ABO, HLA, or PLA antigens on the RBC.
- *Maternal-fetal platelet antigen incompatibility (neonatal thrombocytopenia)*
  This occurs when the fetal platelet contains a PLA1 antigen that is absent in the mother. Neonatal thrombocytopenia can also occur if the mother has ITP autoantibodies that are passed through the placenta and destroy the fetal platelets.
- *Drug-induced thrombocytopenia*
  Although a host of drugs are known to induce autoimmune-mediated thrombocytopenia, heparin is the most common and causes heparin-induced thrombocytopenia (HIT). There are two types of HIT, type I and type II, that may develop. Type I HIT is generally considered a benign condition and is not antibody mediated. In type II HIT, thrombocytopenia is usually more severe and is antibody-mediated. Type II HIT is caused by an IgG antibody and usually occurs after 6 to 8 days of intravenous heparin therapy. Although platelet counts may be low, bleeding is unusual. Rather, paradoxical thromboembolism is the most worrisome complication and may be attributable to

platelet activation caused by the antiheparin-PF4 antibody complex instigating platelet aggregation.

HIT occurs in about 1% to 5% of patients taking heparin for 5 to 10 days, and heparin-induced thrombosis occurs in one third to one half of these patients. Cessation of heparin is mandatory, and alternative anticoagulation is initiated. The diagnosis is suspected based on clinical symptoms, recent heparin administration, and low platelet counts. The diagnosis is confirmed by identifying *heparin-induced thrombocytopenia antibodies (HITAs)*. This test uses an enzyme-linked immunosorbent assay to detect HIT-specific antibodies to heparin-PF4 complex.

Other drugs known to cause antiplatelet antibodies include analgesics (salicylates), antibiotics (cephalosporins), cimetidine, diuretics, heavy metals (e.g., gold), hypnotics, oral hypoglycemic agents, quinidine-like drugs, and many others (e.g., digoxin).

Interfering factors

- Blood transfusion may cause the development of isoantibodies to HLA antigens on the platelets or red blood cells.

Procedure and patient care

- See inside front cover for Routine Blood Testing.
- Fasting: no.
- Blood tube commonly used: red.

Abnormal findings

▲ Increased levels

Idiopathic thrombocytopenia purpura
Neonatal thrombocytopenia
Posttransfusion purpura
Heparin-induced thrombocytopenia
Drug-induced thrombocytopenia
Paroxysmal hemoglobinuria

notes

platelet count (Thrombocyte count)

Type of test Blood

Normal findings

Adult/elderly: 150,000-400,000/mm³ or 150-400 × 10⁹/L (SI units)

Premature infant: 100,000-300,000/mm³

Newborn: 150,000-300,000/mm³

Infant: 200,000-475,000/mm³

Child: 150,000-400,000/mm³

Possible critical vaues <50,000 or >1 million/mm³

Test explanation and related physiology

The platelet count is a count of the number of platelets (thrombocytes) per cubic milliliter of blood. It is performed on patients who develop petechiae (small hemorrhages in the skin), spontaneous bleeding, or increasingly heavy menses. It is also used to monitor the course of the disease or therapy for thrombocytopenia or bone marrow failure.

Platelet activity is essential to blood clotting. Counts of 150,000 to 400,000/mm³ are considered normal. Counts of less than 100,000/mm³ are generally considered to indicate *thrombocytopenia*; *thrombocytosis (thrombocythemia)* is generally said to exist when counts are greater than 400,000/mm³. Common associative diseases with thrombocytosis are iron deficiency anemia and malignancy (leukemia, lymphoma, or solid tumors, such as those involving the colon). Thrombocytosis may also occur with polycythemia vera, postsplenectomy syndromes, and a variety of acute/chronic infections or inflammatory processes.

Spontaneous hemorrhage may occur with thrombocytopenia. Spontaneous bleeding is a serious danger when platelet counts fall below 20,000/mm³. Petechiae and ecchymosis also occur at that level of thrombocytopenia. With counts above 40,000/mm³, spontaneous bleeding rarely occurs, but prolonged bleeding from trauma or surgery may occur at this level. Causes of thrombocytopenia (decreased number of platelets) include the following:

- Reduced production of platelets (secondary to bone marrow failure or infiltration of fibrosis, tumor, etc.)
- Sequestration of platelets (secondary to hypersplenism)

- Accelerated destruction of platelets (secondary to antibodies [see antiplatelet antibodies, p. 716], infections, drugs, prosthetic heart valves)
- Consumption of platelets (secondary to disseminated intravascular coagulation)
- Platelet loss from hemorrhage
- Dilution with large volumes of blood transfusions that contain very few, if any, platelets

Interfering factors

- Living at high altitudes may cause increased platelet levels.
- Because platelets can clump together, automated counting is subject to at least a 10% to 15% error.
- Strenuous exercise may cause increased levels.
- Decreased levels may be seen before menstruation.
- ✘ Drugs that may cause *increased* levels include oral contraceptives.
- ✘ Drugs that may cause *decreased* levels include chemotherapeutic agents, chloramphenicol, colchicine, H_2-blocking agents (cimetidine, ranitidine), hydralazine, indomethacin, isoniazid, levofloxacin, quinidine, streptomycin, sulfonamides, thiazide diuretics, and tolbutamide.

Procedure and patient care

- See inside front cover for Routine Blood Testing.
- Fasting: no.
- Blood tube commonly used: lavender.
- If the results indicate that the patient has a serious platelet deficiency, perform the following steps:
  - Observe the patient for signs and symptoms of bleeding.
  - Check for blood in the urine and all excretions.
  - Assess the patient for bruises, petechiae, bleeding from the gums, epistaxis, and low back pain.
  - Reassess all venipuncture sites for signs of hematoma formation.

P

Abnormal findings

▲ Increased levels
(thrombocytosis)
Malignant disorder
Polycythemia vera
Postsplenectomy syndrome
Rheumatoid arthritis
Iron deficiency anemia

▼ Decreased levels
(thrombocytopenia)
Hypersplenism
Hemorrhage
Immune
thrombocytopenia
Leukemia and other
myelofibrosis
disorders
Thrombotic
thrombocytopenia
Inherited
thrombocytopenia
disorders (e.g.,
Wiskott-Aldrich,
Bernard-Soulier, or
Zieve syndromes)
Disseminated
intravascular
coagulation
Systemic lupus
erythematosus
Pernicious anemia
Some hemolytic anemias
Cancer chemotherapy
Acute/chronic infection

notes

platelet function assay (Platelet closure time, PCT, Aspirin resistance tests, Bleeding time [BT], 11-Dehydro-thromboxane B2)

Type of test Blood, urine

Normal findings

Platelet closure time (blood)
    CADP: 64-120 seconds
    CEPI: 89-193 seconds
11-Dehydro-thromboxane B2 (urine)
    Males: 0-1089 pg/mg of creatinine
    Females: 0-1811 pg/mg of creatinine
Bleeding time (blood)
    1-9 minutes (Ivy method)

Test explanation and related physiology

Platelet dysfunction may be acquired, inherited, or induced by platelet-inhibiting agents. It is clinically important to assess platelet function as a potential cause of a bleeding diathesis (epistaxis, menorrhagia, postoperative bleeding, or easy bruising). The most common causes of platelet dysfunction are related to uremia, liver disease, von Willebrand disease (vWD), and exposure to such agents as acetyl salicylic acid (ASA, aspirin). Several tests are used to evaluate platelet function. Compared with other alternatives, bleeding time (BT) is a bit more labor intensive, and its accuracy is heavily dependent on operator skills. Furthermore, its results are not easily reproduced and quantified. The platelet aggregation study (page 714) may also have similar problems. With the development of an automated platelet function analyzer device, clinical laboratories can easily measure *platelet closure time (PCT)* to quantify platelet function. Furthermore, PCT can differentiate aspirin affects from other causes of platelet dysfunction.

In a platelet function analyzer, anticoagulated whole blood is passed over membranes at a standardized flow rate, creating high shear rates that result in platelet attachment, activation, and aggregation on the membrane. A hole in the membrane is occluded when a stable platelet plug develops. The time required to obtain full occlusion of the aperture is reported as the PCT in seconds. The test is sensitive to platelet adherence and aggregation abnormalities and may allow the discrimination of aspirin-like defects and intrinsic platelet disorder. If a collagen/epinephrine (CEPI) membrane is used during testing, intrinsic platelet dysfunction can be identified.

If a collagen/adenosine-5'-diphosphate (CADP) membrane is used during testing, a combination of both results may be able to demonstrate the impact of aspirin on platelets. This test can also be used to determine resistance of aspirin's therapeutic anticoagulation effects on platelets. This is one of several *aspirin resistance tests* that are performed to determine the effectiveness of aspirin on inhibiting platelet aggregation and thereby protecting the patient from vascular thromboembolic disease (Table 28).

To measure *bleeding time,* a small standard superficial incision is made in the forearm, and the time required for the bleeding to stop is recorded. If a larger skin vessel is lacerated during the test, the bleeding time will be artificially prolonged. A repeat test is required.

Aspirin resistance can be determined by platelet closure time or by measurement of *11-dehydro-thromboxane B2 (11-dTXB2)* in the urine. Thromboxane A2 is produced by the enzyme cyclo-oxygenase-1 (COX1) by activated platelets and still further stimulates platelet activation, platelet aggregation, and vasoconstriction. 11-dTXB2 is the stable, inactive metabolite of thromboxane A2. Urinary 11-dTXB2, therefore, is an indication of platelet activation and aggregation. Elevated values are associated with an increased risk of acute ischemic stroke and myocardial infarction. Effective aspirin therapy should reduce the level of this metabolite in the urine. If not, the patient may be aspirin resistant and may be more safely treated with an alternative therapy such as increasing the dosage of aspirin or placing the patient on another antiplatelet medication.

Urinary 11-dTXB2 offers an advantage over blood aspirin resistance tests because it is not subject to interference from in vitro platelet activation caused by local vein trauma or insufficient anticoagulation during blood sample collection.

TABLE 28   Platelet closure time

	Normal	ASA effect	Intrinsic platelet disorders
CEPI membrane*	Normal	Abnormal	Abnormal
CADP membrane**	Normal	Normal	Abnormal

*CEPI: collagen/epinephrine
**CADP: collagen/adenosine-5'-diphosphate

Interfering factors

- Low hematocrit or platelet count can prolong PCT and BT.
- Aspirin and nonsteroidal antiinflammatory drugs (NSAIDs) can *prolong* PCT and DT test results or decrease urinary 11-dTXB2 levels.
- Thienopyridines can *prolong* test PCT.

Procedure and patient care

- See inside front cover for Routine Blood Testing.
- Fasting: no.
- Blood tube commonly used: light blue.
- Obtain a drug history to determine whether the patient has recently had aspirin or any other medications that may affect test results. Patient should not have taken NSAIDs within 72 hours or aspirin within 2 weeks before collection of a specimen for baseline analysis.
- For urinary 11-dTXB2, randomly collect 10 mL of urine. No preservative is necessary.

Abnormal findings

▲ **Prolonged times or increased values**

Intrinsic platelet defects
Some myelodysplastic syndromes
Some myeloid leukemias
Some myeloproliferative neoplasms
Bernard-Soulier syndrome
Glanzmann thromboasthenia
Hermansky-Pudlak syndrome
Hereditary telangiectasia

Platelet/blood vessel interaction defects
von Willebrand disease
Cushing syndrome
Henoch-Schönlein syndrome
Uremia

Elevated B2 (11-dTXB2) (on aspirin therapy)
Increased risk of thromboembolic disease

notes

P

platelet volume, mean (Mean platelet volume [MPV])

Type of test Blood

Normal findings 7.4-10.4 fL

Test explanation and related physiology

The MPV is a measure of the volume of a large number of platelets determined by an automated analyzer. MPV is to platelets as mean corpuscular volume (p. 788) is to the red blood cell.

The MPV varies with total platelet production. In cases of thrombocytopenia, despite normal reactive bone marrow (e.g., hypersplenism), the normal bone marrow releases immature platelets to attempt to maintain a normal platelet count. These immature platelets are larger, and the MPV is elevated. When bone marrow production of platelets is inadequate, the platelets that are released are small. This is reflected as a low MPV; in this way, the MPV is useful in the differential diagnosis of thrombocytopenic disorders.

Procedure and patient care

- See inside front cover for Routine Blood Testing.
- Fasting: no.
- Blood tube commonly used: lavender.
- If the patient is known to have a low platelet count, perform the following steps:
    - Observe the patient for signs and symptoms of bleeding.
    - Check for blood in the urine and all excretions.
    - Assess the patient for bruises, petechiae, bleeding of the gums, epistaxis, and low back pain.

Abnormal findings

▲ **Increased levels**
Valvular heart disease
Immune thrombocytopenia
Massive hemorrhage
B_{12} or folate deficiency
Myelogenous leukemia

▼ **Decreased levels**
Aplastic anemia
Chemotherapy-induced
  myelosuppression
Wiskott-Aldrich syndrome

notes

plethysmography, arterial (Ankle-brachial index [ABI])

Type of test   Manometric

Normal findings

<20 mm Hg difference in systolic blood pressure of the lower extremity compared with the upper extremity

Normal pulse wave amplitude showing a steep upswing; an acute, narrow peak; and a more gentle downslope containing a dicrotic notch (normal arterial pulse wave)

Ankle/brachial ratio: 0.9-1.3

Test explanation and related physiology

Plethysmography is usually performed to rule out occlusive disease of the lower extremities; however, it also can identify arteriosclerotic disease in the upper extremities. This test requires one normal extremity against which the other extremities may be compared.

Arterial plethysmography is performed by applying three blood pressure cuffs to the proximal, middle, and distal parts of an extremity. Pressure readings are also taken in the upper arm (brachial) artery. These are then attached to a pulse volume recorder (plethysmograph), and each pulse wave can be displayed. A reduction in amplitude of a pulse wave in any of the three cuffs indicates arterial occlusion immediately proximal to the area where the decreased amplitude is noted. Also, measurements of arterial pressures are performed at each cuff site. A difference in pressure of greater than 20 mm Hg indicates a degree of arterial occlusion in the extremity. A positive result is reliable evidence of arteriosclerotic peripheral vascular occlusion. However, a negative result does not definitely exclude this diagnosis because extensive vascular collateralization can compensate for even a complete arterial occlusion.

An ankle/brachial ratio of <0.9 indicates peripheral vascular disease in the lower extremity. Arterial plethysmography can also be performed immediately after exercise to determine whether symptoms of claudication are caused by peripheral vascular occlusive disease.

Although it is not as accurate as arteriography (p. 117), plethysmography is performed without serious complications and can be done for extremely ill patients who cannot be transported to the arteriography laboratory.

P

Interfering factors

- Arterial occlusion proximal to the extremity
- Cigarette smoking can cause transient arterial constriction.

Procedure and patient care

Before

PT Explain the procedure to the patient.

PT Tell the patient that no fasting is required.

PT Inform the patient that this test is painless.

PT Tell the patient that he or she must lie still during the testing procedure.

- Remove all clothing from the patient's extremities.

PT Instruct the patient to avoid smoking for at least 30 minutes before the test. Nicotine creates constriction of the peripheral arteries and alters the test results.

During

- Note the following procedural steps:
  1. The patient is placed in the semirecumbent position.
  2. The cuffs are applied to the extremities and then inflated to 65 mm Hg to increase their sensitivity to pulse waves.
  3. The pulse waves are recorded on plethysmographic paper.
  4. The amplitudes and form of the pulse wave of each cuff are measured and compared. A marked reduction in wave amplitude indicates arterial occlusive disease.
- This noninvasive test is usually performed in the vascular laboratory or at the patient's bedside by a vascular technologist in approximately 30 minutes.

PT Inform the patient that results are usually interpreted by a physician and are available in a few hours.

PT Remind the patient that no discomfort is associated with this test.

After

- Encourage the patient to verbalize any concerns regarding the test results.

Abnormal findings

Arterial occlusive disease
Arterial trauma
Small vessel diabetic changes
Vascular diseases (e.g., Raynaud phenomenon)
Arterial embolization

notes

pleural biopsy

Type of test Microscopic examination of tissue

Normal findings No evidence of pathology

Test explanation and related physiology

This test may be indicated when the pleural fluid obtained by thoracentesis (p. 883) is exudative fluid, which suggests infection, neoplasm, or tuberculosis. The pleural biopsy can distinguish among these disease processes. It is also performed when chest imaging indicates a pleural-based tumor, reaction, or thickening.

Pleural biopsy is the removal of pleural tissue for histologic examination. It is usually performed by a percutaneous needle biopsy. It also can be performed via thoracoscopy (p. 889), which is done by inserting a scope into the pleural space for inspection and biopsy of the pleura. Pleural tissue also may be obtained by an *open pleural biopsy*, which involves a limited thoracotomy and requires general anesthesia. For this procedure, a small intercostal incision is made, and the biopsy of the pleura is done under direct observation. The advantage of an open procedure is that a larger piece of pleura can be obtained.

Contraindications

- Patients with prolonged bleeding or clotting times

Potential complications

- Bleeding or injury to the lung
- Pneumothorax

Procedure and patient care

Before

PT Explain the procedure to the patient.

- Obtain informed consent for this procedure.

PT Tell the patient that no fasting or sedation is required.

PT Instruct the patient to remain very still during the procedure. Any movement may cause inadvertent needle damage.

During

- Note the following procedural steps for percutaneous needle biopsy:
  1. This procedure is usually performed with the patient in a sitting position with his or her shoulders and arms elevated and supported by a padded overbed table.

2. After the presence of fluid has been determined by the thoracentesis technique, the skin overlying the biopsy site is anesthetized and pierced with a scalpel blade.

3. A needle is inserted with a cannula until fluid is removed. (Some fluid is left in the pleural space after the thoracentesis to make the biopsy easier.)

4. The inner needle is removed, and a blunt-tipped, hooked biopsy trocar attached to a three-way stopcock is inserted into the cannula.

5. The patient is instructed to expire all air and then perform the Valsalva maneuver to prevent air from entering the pleural space.

6. The cannula and biopsy trocar are withdrawn while the hook catches the parietal wall and takes a specimen with its cutting edge.

7. Usually three biopsy specimens are taken from different sites during the same session.

8. The specimens are placed in a fixative solution and sent to the laboratory immediately.

9. After the specimens are taken, additional parietal fluid can be removed.

- Note that this procedure is performed by a physician at the patient's bedside, in a special procedure room, or in the physician's office in approximately 30 minutes.
- **PT** Tell the patient that because of the local anesthetic little discomfort is associated with this procedure.

After

- Apply an adhesive bandage to the biopsy site.
- Note that a chest x-ray image is usually taken to detect the potential complication of pneumothorax.
- Observe the patient for signs of respiratory distress (e.g., shortness of breath, diminished breath sounds) on the side of the biopsy.
- **PT** Instruct the patient to report any shortness of breath.
- Observe the patient's vital signs frequently for evidence of bleeding (increased pulse, decreased blood pressure).
- Ensure that the biopsy specimen is sent immediately to the laboratory.

Abnormal findings

Neoplasm
Tuberculosis

notes

porphyrins and porphobilinogens

Type of test Urine (fresh and 24-hour)

Normal findings

	Male (mcg/24 hr)	Female (mcg/24 hr)
Total porphyrins	8-149	3-78
Uroporphyrin	4-46	3-22
Coproporphyrin	<96	<60

Porphobilinogens: 0-2 mg/24 hr or 0-8.8 μmol/day (SI units)

Test explanation and related physiology

This test is a quantitative measurement of porphyrins and porphobilinogens. Along with measurement of aminolevulinic acid (p. 337), the various forms of porphyria can be identified.

Porphyria is a group of genetic disorders associated with enzyme deficiencies involved with porphyrin synthesis or metabolism. Porphyrins (e.g., uroporphyrin and coproporphyrin) and porphobilinogens are important building blocks in the synthesis of heme. Heme is incorporated into hemoglobin in the erythroid cells. In most forms of porphyria, increased levels of porphyrins and porphobilinogens are found in the urine. Heavy metal (lead) intoxication is also associated with increased porphyrins in the urine.

Urine tests for porphyrins are not as accurate as plasma measurements and pattern identification for the various forms of porphyria. They are accurate, however, in screening for porphyria, especially the intermittent variety. Porphyrin fractionation of erythrocytes and plasma provides specific assays for primary red blood cell porphyrins. These assays are predominantly used to differentiate the various forms of congenital porphyrias. Plasma measurement of *free erythrocyte protoporphyrin (FEP)* is helpful in the diagnosis of iron deficiency anemia or lead intoxication.

Interfering factors

✂ Drugs that may alter test results include aminosalicylic acid, barbiturates, chloral hydrate, chlorpropamide, ethyl alcohol, griseofulvin, morphine, oral contraceptives, phenazopyridine, procaine, and sulfonamides.

P

Procedure and patient care

- See inside front cover for Routine Urine Testing for random and 24-hour collection.
- Protect the specimen from light.
- **PT** Instruct the patient to avoid alcohol during the collection period.
- Keep the 24-hour urine in a light-resistant specimen bottle with a preservative to prevent degradation of the light-sensitive porphyrin.
- **PT** Encourage the patient to drink fluids during the 24 hours unless contraindicated for medical purposes.

Abnormal findings

▲ **Increased levels**
Porphyrias
Liver disease
Lead poisoning
Pellagra

notes

positron emission tomography (PET scan)

Type of test Nuclear scan, x-ray

Normal findings No abnormal areas of increased or decreased uptake

Test explanation and related physiology

PET scanning is used in many areas of medicine, most commonly for evaluation of the heart and brain. It is also commonly used in many aspects of oncology. In PET scanning, radioactive chemicals are administered to the patient. These chemicals are used in the normal metabolic process of the cells of the particular organ being imaged. Positrons emitted from the radioactive chemicals in the organ are sensed by a series of detectors positioned around the patient. The positron emissions are recorded and reconstructed by computer analysis into a high-resolution three-dimensional image indicating a particular metabolic process in a specific anatomic site. A computed tomography (CT) x-ray scan is performed on the patient at the same time to assist in the development and interpretation of the images created. PET/CT scans provide images representing not only anatomy but also physiology.

Depending on the particular radionuclide used, PET can demonstrate the glucose metabolism, oxygenation, blood flow, and tissue perfusion of any specific area. Pathologic conditions are recognized and diagnosed by alterations in the normal metabolic process.

Certain radioactive chemical compounds provide specific information depending on the information required and the organ being evaluated. A cyclotron is used to create the radioactive chemical. Radioactive oxygen is used to make radioactive water ($H_2^{15}O$). This is used to evaluate blood flow and tissue perfusion of an organ.

Radioactive fluorine is applied to a glucose analogue and called *fluorodeoxyglucose (FDG)*. Because most cells use glucose as an energy source, FDG is particularly useful in concentrating in regions of high metabolic activity of a particular organ. The greatest use of PET scan has been in the fields of neurology, cardiology, and oncology.

With most PET units, PET/CT imaging can be performed by the same machine. This is called *PET/CT image fusion* or *PET/CT co-registration*. These composite views, which allow the information from two different studies to be digitally correlated and superimposed onto one image, lead to more precise

P

information and accurate diagnoses. The CT images are acquired with the use of iodine contrast. In less than 60 minutes after the FDG is administered, the PET scan is performed in the same unit. The images are imposed on each other. The combined PET/CT scans provide images that pinpoint the location of abnormal metabolic activity within the body.

Neurology

Most brain imaging is performed with FDG. The brain uses glucose as its sole metabolic fuel. Pathologic areas of the brain that are more metabolically active (e.g., cancers) more avidly take up FDG than do normal areas. Because of the high physiologic rate at which glucose is metabolized by normal brain tissue, the detectability of tumors with only modest increases in glucose metabolism, such as low-grade tumors and, in some cases, recurrent tumors, is difficult with FDG. Another radioactive marker that is being used is 3,4-dihydroxy-6-18 F-fluoro-L-phenylalanine (18 F-FDOPA). This seems to improve visibility of low-grade brain tumors.

Epilepsy, Parkinson disease, and Huntington disease are identified as localized areas of increased metabolic activity indicating rapid nerve firing. Brain trauma resulting in a hematoma or bleeding is evident as decreased metabolic activity in the area of trauma. Stroke can also be identified and its extent determined. With the use of radioactive water ($H_2^{15}O$), brain blood flow can be determined. Areas of decreased blood flow take up less $H_2^{15}O$ than normal areas and represent areas at risk for stroke.

Alzheimer disease can be recognized by identifying hypometabolism in multiple areas of the brain (temporal and parietal lobe). PET scanning with amyloid imaging using radioactive markers such as Pittsburgh agent compound B (PiB), flutemetamol, or fluorine-18 has been very helpful in identifying amyloid protein precursors (page 58) in the brain. These agents bind to the beta-amyloid plaques that are increased in patients with Alzheimer disease. A negative PET scan with amyloid imaging eliminates the possibility of Alzheimer disease in a patient with cognitive impairment. Because other neurologic conditions (especially in elderly people) are also associated with amyloid neuritic plaques, a positive scan does not establish the diagnosis of Alzheimer disease with certainty.

Cardiology

PET scans of the heart can show decreased blood flow, indicating coronary artery occlusive disease. PET scans are also used when cardiac muscle function is reduced. A PET scan can indicate whether the dysfunction arises from reversible ischemic muscle that would benefit from revascularization or from muscle tissue that is no longer viable. In the former case, surgical revascularization should be considered. In the latter case, revascularization would not be beneficial.

Oncology

The most commonly used agent in oncology is FDG because increased glucose metabolism is so prevalent in malignant tumors compared with normal or benign pathologic tissue. PET can be used to visualize rapidly growing tumors and indicate their anatomic location. It is used to determine tumor response to therapy, identify recurrence of tumor after surgical removal, and differentiate tumor from other pathologic conditions (e.g., infection). PET is particularly helpful in identifying regional and metastatic spread for a particular tumor. PET is more accurate in oncologic staging than CT scan. Its sensitivity exceeds 95% with a specificity of more than 80%. In lung cancer, for example, if the FDG fails to concentrate in any area other than the primary tumor, no spread is suspected and the patient is considered an ideal candidate for surgery. PET has also been particularly useful for identifying metastasis from lung, melanoma, breast, pancreas, colon, lymphoma, and brain cancers.

Rapidly growing tumors are associated with a high metabolic rate and therefore concentrate FDG particularly well. The amount of uptake of FDG is measured by the standardized uptake value (SUV)—the amount of uptake of FDG in tumor compared with the normal tissue in that same area. SUV helps to distinguish between benign and malignant lesions—the higher the SUV, the more likely the tumor is malignant.

When the SUV is greater than the "cutoff value" (as determined by each institution), cancer rather than a benign pathologic condition is suspected. PET scanning is particularly helpful in the evaluation of solitary pulmonary nodules. CT scans and chest radiographs are inadequate to distinguish benign from malignant lesions. PET scanning can accurately provide that information more than 75% of the time.

Bone

A PET/CT scan with a sodium fluoride F18 injection (^{18}F NaF) scans the entire skeletal system and produces high-resolution images of the bones. These images are used to detect areas of abnormal bone growth associated with tumors. This

P

test is more accurate than conventional nuclear bone scans. The PET/CT scan of the bone is particularly helpful for patients with prostate or breast cancer. The uptake of ^{18}F NaF in the skeleton reflects sites of increased blood flow and bone remodeling associated with bone injury or metastatic disease. A bone PET/CT scan's high-resolution images and its ability to scan the entire skeleton make it very helpful in detecting bone disease.

Small parts PET scans are being used with increasing frequency for foot inflammatory pathology. *PET mammography or positron emission mammography (PEM)* is seeing growing use as a tool for diagnostic breast imaging. PEM holds the promise of improving the sensitivity and specificity of routine mammography (see page 624)

Interfering factors

- Recent use (within 24 hours) of caffeine, alcohol, or tobacco may affect test results.
- Ingestion of a small- to moderate-sized meal can cause a marked uptake of FDG in the gut and muscles, thereby leaving little or no radionuclide to be taken up by tumor. This can cause a false-negative result.
- Anxiety can cause increased uptake in multiple areas (e.g., neck, upper mediastinum) of the body. If the patient is anxious, sedatives can be administered 30 minutes before testing. However, these could interfere with PET scanning of the brain if cognitive activities will be used to measure changes in brain activity.
- Mild to moderate exercise can instigate marked uptake of FDG in the muscles, thereby leaving little or no radionuclide to be taken up by tumor. This causes a false-negative result.
- The liver and spleen avidly take up FDG. Therefore, those organs are difficult to evaluate on PET imaging.
- FDG is excreted by the urinary system. As a result, the bladder may obscure areas of increased uptake in the pelvis.
- Uptake of FDG can occur in the lymph node basin draining the site of the FDG injection. If PET is being done to stage tumors that could metastasize to those lymph nodes, the FDG should be injected on the contralateral side.

Procedure and patient care

Before

PT Explain the procedure to the patient.

- Obtain informed consent if required by the institution.

PT Inform the patient that he or she may have an intravenous (IV) line inserted.

PT Inform the patient that he or she may need to restrict food or fluids for 4 hours on the day of the test. The patient should refrain from alcohol, caffeine, and tobacco for 24 hours.

PT Instruct patients with diabetes to take their pretest dose of insulin at a meal 3 to 4 hours before the test.

PT Tell the patient that no sedatives or tranquilizers should be taken, because he or she may need to perform certain mental activities during the brain PET scan.

PT Tell the patient to empty the bladder before the test for comfort. A Foley catheter may be inserted for PET scanning of the pelvic region.

PT Tell the patient that the only discomfort associated with this study is insertion of the IV line.

• Depending on the organ being evaluated, specific protocols may exist for the examination.

During

• Note the following procedural steps:
  1. The patient is positioned in a comfortable, reclining chair.
  2. The radioactive material can be infused through an IV line.
  3. The gamma rays that penetrate the tissues are recorded outside the body by a circular array of detectors and are displayed by a computer.
  4. Extraneous auditory and visual stimuli are minimized by a blindfold and ear plugs.
  5. If the chest is being scanned, instruct the patient to breathe in a shallow manner until the middle of the chest is reached. Then ask the patient to hold the breath after expiration until the middle of the abdomen is reached. This will improve visibility of the chest anatomy.

• Note that a physician performs this procedure with a trained technologist in approximately 40 to 90 minutes.

After

PT Instruct the patient to change position slowly from lying to standing to avoid postural hypotension.

PT Encourage the patient to drink fluids and urinate frequently to aid in removal of the radioisotope from the bladder.

Abnormal findings

Myocardial infarction	Huntington disease
Coronary artery disease	Dementia
Cerebrovascular accident	Alzheimer disease
Epilepsy	Malignant tumor
Parkinson disease	

notes

potassium, blood (K)

Type of test Blood

Normal findings

Adult/elderly: 3.5-5.0 mEq/L or 3.5-5.0 mmol/L (SI units)
Child: 3.4-4.7 mEq/L
Infant: 4.1-5.3 mEq/L
Newborn: 3.9-5.9 mEq/L

Possible critical values

Adult: <2.5 or >6.5 mEq/L
Newborn: <2.5 or >8 mEq/L

Test explanation and related physiology

Potassium (K) is the major cation within the cell. Intracellular K concentration is approximately 150 mEq/L, whereas normal serum K concentration is approximately 4 mEq/L. Because the serum concentration of K is so small, minor changes in concentration have significant consequences. K is excreted by the kidneys, and there is no resorption of K from the kidneys. Therefore, if K is not adequately supplied in the diet (or by IV administration in patients who are unable to eat), serum K levels can drop rapidly.

Serum K concentration depends on many factors, including the following:

- *Aldosterone* (and, to a lesser extent, the glucocorticosteroids). This hormone tends to increase renal losses of K.
- *Sodium resorption.* As sodium is resorbed, K is lost.
- *Acid/base balance.* Alkalotic states tend to lower serum K levels by causing a shift of K into the cell. Acidotic states tend to raise serum K levels by reversing that shift.

Symptoms of hyperkalemia include irritability, nausea, vomiting, intestinal colic, and diarrhea. An electrocardiogram may demonstrate peaked T waves, a widened QRS complex, and depressed ST segment. Signs of hypokalemia are related to decreases in contractility of smooth, skeletal, and cardiac muscles, which result in weakness, paralysis, hyporeflexia, ileus, increased cardiac sensitivity to digoxin, cardiac arrhythmias, flattened T waves, and prominent U waves. This electrolyte has profound effects on the heart rate and contractility. The K level should be followed carefully in patients with uremia, Addison disease, vomiting, or diarrhea; in patients on steroid therapy; and in patients taking K-depleting diuretics. K must be closely monitored in patients taking digitalis-like drugs because cardiac arrhythmias may be induced by hypokalemia and digoxin.

Interfering factors

- Movement of the forearm with a tourniquet in place may increase K levels.
- Hemolysis during venipuncture causes increased levels.
- ✗ Drugs that may cause *increased* K levels include aminocaproic acid, antibiotics, antineoplastic drugs, captopril, epinephrine, heparin, histamine, isoniazid, lithium, mannitol, potassium-sparing diuretics, potassium supplements, and succinylcholine.
- ✗ Drugs that may cause *decreased* levels include acetazolamide, aminosalicylic acid, amphotericin B, carbenicillin, cisplatin, diuretics (potassium wasting), glucose infusions, insulin, laxatives, lithium carbonate, penicillin G sodium (high doses), phenothiazines, salicylates, and sodium polystyrene sulfonate (Kayexalate).

Procedure and patient care

- See inside front cover for Routine Blood Testing.
- Fasting: no.
- Blood tube commonly used: red or green.
- **PT** Instruct the patient to avoid opening and closing the hand after a tourniquet is applied.
- Avoid hemolysis.
- Evaluate patients with increased or decreased K levels for cardiac arrhythmias.
- Monitor patients taking digoxin and diuretics for hypokalemia.
- If indicated, administer resin exchanges (e.g., Kayexalate enema) to correct hyperkalemia.

P

Abnormal findings

▲ **Increased levels (hyperkalemia)**
Excessive dietary intake
Excessive IV intake
Acute or chronic renal failure
Hypoaldosteronism
Aldosterone-inhibiting diuretics
Crush injury to tissues
Hemolysis
Transfusion of hemolyzed blood
Infection
Acidosis
Dehydration

▼ **Decreased levels (hypokalemia)**
Deficient dietary intake
Deficient IV intake
Burns
Gastrointestinal disorders (e.g., diarrhea, vomiting)
Diuretics
Hyperaldosteronism
Cushing syndrome
Renal tubular acidosis
Licorice ingestion
Insulin administration
Glucose administration
Ascites
Renal artery stenosis
Cystic fibrosis
Trauma
Surgery

notes

potassium, urine (K)

Type of test Urine (24-hour)

Normal findings

25-100 mEq/L/day or 25-100 mmol/day (SI units)
(Values vary greatly with diet.)

Test explanation and related physiology

Potassium (K) is the major cation within the cell (p. 736). K can be measured in both a spot collection and a 24-hour urine collection. K concentration in the urine depends on many factors. Aldosterone and, to a lesser extent, glucocorticosteroids tend to increase the renal losses of K. Acid/base balance is dependent on K excretion to a small degree. In alkalotic states, hydrogen can be resorbed in exchange for K. The kidneys cannot resorb K. Therefore, the intake of K is balanced by kidney excretion.

Interfering factors

- Dietary intake affects K levels.
- Excessive intake of licorice may cause increased levels.
- Drugs that may cause *increased* levels include diuretics, glucocorticoids, and salicylates.

Procedure and patient care

- See inside front cover for Routine Urine Testing.

Abnormal findings

▲ **Increased levels**
Chronic renal failure
Renal tubular acidosis
Cushing syndrome
Hyperaldosteronism
Excessive intake of licorice
Alkalosis
Diuretic therapy

▼ **Decreased levels**
Dehydration
Addison disease
Malnutrition
Vomiting
Diarrhea
Malabsorption
Acute renal failure

notes

prealbumin (PAB, Thyroxine-binding prealbumin [TBPA], Thyretin, Transthyretin)

Type of test Blood; urine (24-hour); cerebrospinal fluid (CSF) analysis

Normal findings

Serum

Adult/elderly: 15-36 mg/dL or 150-360 mg/L (SI units)
Child
    <5 days: 6-21 mg/dL
    1-5 years: 14-30 mg/dL
    6-9 years: 15-33 mg/dL
    10-13 years: 22-36 mg/dL
    14-19 years: 22-45 mg/dL

Urine (24-hour)
0.017-0.047 mg/day

Cerebrospinal fluid
Approximately 2% of total CSF protein

Possible critical values Serum prealbumin levels <10.7 mg/dL indicate severe nutritional deficiency.

Test explanation and related physiology

Prealbumin is one of the major plasma proteins. Because prealbumin can bind thyroxine, it is also called *thyroxine-binding prealbumin (TBA)*. However, prealbumin is secondary to thyroxine-binding globulin in the transportation of triiodothyronine (T_3) and thyroxine (T_4). Prealbumin also plays a role in the transport and metabolism of vitamin A.

Because prealbumin levels in serum fluctuate more rapidly in response to alterations in synthetic rate than do those of other serum proteins, clinical interest in the quantification of serum prealbumin has centered on its usefulness as a marker of nutritional status. Its half-life of 1.9 days is much less than the 21-day half-life of albumin (p. 771). Because prealbumin has a short half-life, it is a sensitive indicator of any change affecting protein synthesis and catabolism. For this reason, prealbumin is frequently ordered to monitor the effectiveness of total parenteral nutrition (TPN).

Prealbumin is significantly reduced in hepatobiliary disease because of impaired synthesis. Prealbumin is also a negative acute-phase reactant protein; serum levels decrease in inflammation, malignancy, and protein-wasting diseases of the intestines or kidneys. Because zinc is required for synthesis of prealbumin, low levels occur with a zinc deficiency. Increased levels of prealbumin occur in Hodgkin disease and chronic kidney disease.

Interfering factors

- Coexistent inflammation may make the interpretation of test results impossible.
- ☛ Drugs that may cause *increased* levels include anabolic steroids, androgens, and prednisolone.
- ☛ Drugs that may cause *decreased* levels include amiodarone, estrogens, and oral contraceptives.

Procedure and patient care

- See inside front cover for Routine Blood Testing.
- Fasting: no.
- Blood tube commonly used: red.
- If the patient is going to collect a 24-hour urine specimen, provide a collection bottle. (See guidelines in inside front cover.)

Abnormal findings

▲ Increased levels
Some cases of nephrotic
  syndrome
Hodgkin disease
Chronic kidney disease
Pregnancy

▼ Decreased levels
Malnutrition
Liver damage
Burns
Salicylate poisoning
Inflammation
Infection

notes

pregnancy-associated plasma protein-A (PAPP-A)

Type of test   Blood

Normal findings

Normal values vary by laboratory and duration of pregnancy

Test explanation and related physiology

Pregnancy-associated plasma protein-A (PAPP-A) is made by the trophoblasts and released into the maternal circulation during pregnancy. Women with low blood levels of PAPP-A at 8 to 14 weeks of gestation have an increased risk of intrauterine growth restriction, trisomy 21, premature delivery, preeclampsia, and stillbirth. This protein rapidly rises in the first trimester of normal pregnancy. However, in Down-affected pregnancy, serum levels are half that of unaffected pregnancies. Furthermore, low levels of PAPP-A in maternal serum in the first trimester are associated with adverse fetal outcomes, including fetal death in utero and intrauterine growth retardation. This test is commonly used in conjunction with other pregnancy and maternal screening tests (p. 628).

PAPP-A is present in unstable atherosclerotic plaques, and circulating levels are elevated in acute coronary syndromes, which may reflect the instability of the plaques. PAPP-A is an independent marker of unstable angina and acute myocardial infarction. It is also a risk factor in predicting death after an acute myocardial event.

PAPP-A exists in a bound form (to eosinophil major basic protein [proMBP]) and in a free form. In general, the bound form most accurately predicts pregnancy outcome, whereas the free form most accurately predicts coronary atherosclerotic disease.

Interfering factors

- Levels increase with increased maternal body weight and longer duration of pregnancy.

Procedure and patient care

- See inside front cover for Routine Blood Testing.
- Fasting: no.
- Blood tube commonly used: red.
- Allow the patient to express her concerns and fears regarding the potential for birth defects.
- hCG and estriol can also be tested by collecting a urine sample.

- Provide the results to the patient (and other family members if the patient desires) during a personal consultation.
PT Assist the patient in scheduling and obtaining more accurate diagnostic testing if the results are positive.

Abnormal findings

Positive screening tests (trisomy 21, trisomy 18, neural tube defects, abdominal wall defects)
Coronary atherosclerotic disease

notes

P

pregnanediol

Type of test   Urine (24-hour)

Normal findings

<2 years: <0.1 mg/day
<9 years: <0.5 mg/day
10-15 years: 0.1-1.2 mg/day
Adult male: 0-1.9 mg/day
Adult female
    Follicular phase: <2.6 mg/day
    Luteal: 2.6-10.6 mg/day
Pregnancy
    First trimester: 10-35 mg/day
    Second trimester: 35-70 mg/day
    Third trimester: 70-100 mg/day

Test explanation and related physiology

Urinary pregnanediol is measured to evaluate progesterone production by the ovaries and placenta. The main effect of progesterone is on the endometrium. It initiates the endometrial secretory phase in anticipation of implantation of a fertilized ovum. Normally, progesterone is secreted by the ovarian corpus luteum after ovulation. Both serum progesterone levels and the urine concentration of progesterone metabolites (pregnanediol and others) are significantly increased during the latter half of an ovulatory cycle. Pregnanediol is the most easily measured metabolite of progesterone.

Because pregnanediol levels rise rapidly after ovulation, this study is useful in documenting whether ovulation has occurred and, if so, its exact time. During pregnancy, pregnanediol levels normally rise because of the placental production of progesterone. Repeated assays can be used to monitor the status of the placenta in women who are having difficulty becoming pregnant or maintaining a pregnancy. This study is also used to monitor high-risk pregnancies.

Hormone assays for urinary pregnanediol are primarily used today to monitor progesterone supplementation in patients with an inadequate luteal phase. Urinary assays may be supplemented by plasma assays (progesterone assay, p. 746), which are quicker and more accurate.

Interfering factors

- Drugs that may cause *increased* levels include adrenocorticotropic hormone.
- Drugs that may cause *decreased* levels include oral contraceptives and progesterones.

Procedure and patient care

- See inside front cover for Routine Urine Testing.
- Record on the laboratory slip the date of the last menstrual period or the week of gestation during pregnancy.

Abnormal findings

▲ **Increased levels**
Ovulation
Pregnancy
Luteal cysts of ovary
Arrhenoblastoma of ovary
Hyperadrenocorticalism
Choriocarcinoma of ovary
Adrenocortical hyperplasia

▼ **Decreased levels**
Threatened abortion
Fetal death
Toxemia of pregnancy
Amenorrhea
Ovarian hypofunction
Placental failure
Preeclampsia
Ovarian neoplasm
Breast neoplasm

notes

progesterone assay

Type of test   Blood

Normal findings

<9 years: <20 ng/dL
10-15 years: <20 ng/dL
Adult male: 10-50 ng/dL
Adult female
    Follicular phase: <50 ng/dL
    Luteal: 300-2500 ng/dL
    Postmenopausal: <40 ng/dL
Pregnancy
    First trimester: 725-4400 ng/dL
    Second trimester: 1950-8250 ng/dL
    Third trimester: 6500-22,900 ng/dL

Test explanation and related physiology

The major effect of progesterone is to induce the development of the secretory phase of the endometrium in anticipation of implantation of a fertilized ovum. Normally, progesterone is secreted by the ovarian corpus luteum following ovulation. Serum progesterone level is significantly increased during the second half of the ovulatory cycle. Normally, blood samples drawn at days 8 and 21 of the menstrual cycle show a large increase in progesterone levels in the latter specimen, indicating that ovulation has occurred. Therefore, this study is useful in documenting whether ovulation has occurred and, if so, its exact time. This is very useful information for a woman who has difficulty becoming pregnant. A series of measurements can help define the day of ovulation.

In pregnancy, progesterone is produced by the corpus luteum for the first few weeks. After that, the placenta begins to make progesterone. Progesterone levels should progressively rise during pregnancy because of placental production. Repeated assays can be used to monitor the status of the placenta in cases of high-risk pregnancy. Progesterone assay is also used today to monitor progesterone supplementation in patients with an inadequate luteal phase to maintain an early pregnancy.

Interfering factors

- Recent use of radioisotopes may affect test results.
- Hemolysis caused by rough handling of the sample may affect test results.

✼ Drugs that may interfere with test results include clomiphene, estrogen, and progesterone.

Procedure and patient care

- See inside front cover for Routine Blood Testing.
- Fasting: no.
- Blood tube commonly used: red.
- Indicate the date of the last menstrual period on the laboratory slip.

Abnormal findings

▲ **Increased levels**
Ovulation
Pregnancy
Luteal cysts of ovary
Hyperadrenocorticalism
Adrenocortical hyperplasia
Choriocarcinoma of ovary
Hydatidiform mole
  of the uterus

▼ **Decreased levels**
Preeclampsia
Toxemia of pregnancy
Threatened abortion
Placental failure
Fetal death
Ovarian neoplasm
Amenorrhea
Ovarian hypofunction

notes

P

progesterone receptor assay (PR assay, PRA, PgR)

Type of test Tumor-specimen analysis

Normal findings

Immunochemistry
Negative: <5% of the cells stain for receptors
Positive: >5% of the cells stain for receptors
Reverse-transcriptase polymerase chain reaction (RT-PCR)
Negative: <5.5 units
Positive: >5.5 units

Test explanation and related physiology

The PR assay is used in determination of the prognosis and treatment of breast cancer and, to a lesser degree, other cancers. This assay helps determine whether a tumor is likely to respond to endocrine medical or surgical therapy. The test is done on breast cancer specimens when a primary or recurrent cancer is identified; it is usually done in conjunction with an estrogen receptor (ER) assay (p. 408) to increase the predictability of a tumor response to hormone therapy. Breast tumors in postmenopausal women tend to be PR positive more often than in premenopausal women. PR-positive tumors are suspected to be associated with a better prognosis than PR-negative tumors. Tumor response rates to medical or surgical hormonal manipulation are potentiated if the ER assay is positive. Response rates are as follows:

- ER positive, PR positive: 75%
- ER negative, PR positive: 60%
- ER positive, PR negative: 35%
- ER negative, PR negative: 25%

The most commonly used laboratory method provides accurate information on paraffin-embedded tissue using immunohistochemical staining for PR proteins. Positive reactivity by immunohistochemistry is observed in the nuclei of the tumor cells. Results are usually available in less than 1 week. Only the cancerous tissue is evaluated for PR receptors.

Other tumors (e.g., ovarian, melanoma, uterine, pancreatic) are occasionally studied for ER and PR assay. This is done mostly within clinical trials.

Interfering factors

✘ The use of such hormones as progesterone or estrogen may cause false-negative results.

Procedure and patient care

Before

PT Explain the procedure to the patient.

- Prepare the patient for breast biopsy per routine protocol.
- Record the menstrual status of the patient.
- Record any exogenous hormone the patient may have used during the last 2 months.

PT Instruct the patient to discontinue exogenous hormones before breast biopsy. This is done in consultation with the physician.

During

- The surgeon obtains tissue.
- This tissue should be placed on ice or in formalin.
- Part of the tissue is used for routine histology. A portion of the paraffin block is sent to a reference laboratory.
- Results are usually available in 1 week.

After

- Provide routine postoperative care.

Abnormal findings

▲ **Increased levels**
  Hormonally dependent cancer

notes

P

prolactin levels (PRLs)

Type of test Blood

Normal findings

Adult male: 3-13 ng/mL
Adult female: 3-27 ng/mL
Pregnant female: 20-400 ng/mL

Test explanation and related physiology

Prolactin is a hormone secreted by the anterior pituitary gland (adenohypophysis). In females, prolactin promotes lactation. Its role in males is not clear. During sleep, prolactin levels increase twofold to threefold to circulating levels equaling those of pregnant women. With breast stimulation, pregnancy, nursing, stress, or exercise, a surge of this hormone occurs. It is elevated in patients with prolactin-secreting pituitary acidophilic or chromophobic adenomas. To a lesser extent, moderately high prolactin levels have been observed in women with secondary amenorrhea (i.e., postpubertal) and galactorrhea. Paraneoplastic tumors (e.g., lung cancer) may cause ectopic secretion of prolactin as well. In general, very high prolactin levels are more likely to be caused by pituitary adenoma than other causes.

The prolactin level is helpful for monitoring the disease activity of pituitary adenomas. Several *prolactin stimulation tests* (with TRH or chlorpromazine) and *prolactin suppression tests* (with levodopa) have been designed to help differentiate pituitary adenoma from other causes of prolactin overproduction.

Interfering factors

- Stress from illness, trauma, surgery, or even the fear of a blood test can elevate levels.
- Prolactin levels are transiently elevated after seizures.
- Drugs that may cause *increased* values include anticonvulsants, antihistamines, antinausea/antiemetic drugs, antipsychotic drugs, anti-tuberculosis medications, ergot derivatives, estrogens/progesterone, histamine antagonists, monoamine oxidase inhibitors, opiates, oral contraceptives, reserpine, serotonin reuptake inhibitors, several antihypertensive drugs, and some illegal drugs.
- Drugs that may cause *decreased* values are clonidine, dopamine, ergot alkaloid derivatives, and levodopa.

Procedure and patient care

- See inside front cover for Routine Blood Testing.
- Fasting: no.
- Blood tube commonly used: red.
- **PT** Inform the patient that blood should be drawn in the morning.
- Transfer the specimen to the laboratory as soon as possible. If a delay occurs, the specimen should be placed on ice.

Abnormal findings

▲ **Increased levels**

Galactorrhea

Amenorrhea

Prolactin-secreting pituitary tumor

Infiltrative diseases of the hypothalamus and pituitary stalk

Hypothyroidism

Renal failure

Anorexia nervosa

Perineoplastic ectopic production of prolactin

Metastatic cancer to the pituitary gland

Polycystic ovary syndrome

Stress

Empty sella syndrome

▼ **Decreased levels**

Pituitary apoplexy

Pituitary destruction from tumor (craniopharyngioma)

notes

ProstaScint scan (Radioimmunoscintigraphy [RIS])

Type of test Nuclear scan

Normal findings No increased uptake outside the prostate gland

Test explanation and related physiology

By using a radionuclide that is able to attach to prostate cancer cells only, metastatic prostate cancer outside the prostate gland can be easily identified. Disease outside the prostate (e.g., retroperitoneum, liver, lung, or bone) indicates metastatic prostate cancer.

This scan is helpful in staging newly diagnosed prostate cancer patients who are at high risk for metastatic disease to the lymph nodes or other organs. This test can also be used to identify recurrent or metastatic disease after curative therapy. This test can document completeness of anti–prostate cancer therapy.

Contraindications

- Patients who are unable to be immobile for 1 hour

Interfering factors

- Prior bone scans confound image interpretation.
- Areas of inflammation (e.g., degenerative joint disease, inflammatory bowel disease, or recent trauma) can confound interpretation.

Procedure and patient care

Before

- **PT** Explain the procedure to the patient.
- **PT** Explain that no fasting is required before the test.
- **PT** Instruct the patient to use a mild laxative the evening before imaging. A cleansing enema may be administered 1 hour before imaging. Early in the scanning, radionuclide accumulates in the bowel.
- **PT** Tell the patient to void before each image.

During

- After proper identification, the patient is injected with the radiolabeled monoclonal antibody.
- Initial images are obtained 30 minutes after injection. Images are repeated over as many as 5 days.
- Little or no discomfort is associated with this procedure.

- The procedure takes approximately 1 hour each day over a period of 1 to 5 days.
- This procedure is performed in the nuclear medicine department.

After

PT Inform the patient that no precautions need to be taken by others against radiation exposure because only tracer doses of radioisotopes are used.

- Encourage the patient to increase oral fluid intake on testing days.

Abnormal findings

Primary or recurrent prostate cancer

notes

P

prostate/rectal sonogram (Ultrasound prostate)

Type of test Ultrasound

Normal findings Normal size, contour, and consistency of the prostate gland

Test explanation and related physiology

Rectal ultrasound of the prostate is a very valuable tool in the early diagnosis of prostate cancer. When combined with rectal digital examination and prostate-specific antigen (p. 756), very small prostate cancers can be identified. Prostate/rectal sonography is also helpful in evaluating the seminal vessels and other perirectal tissue. Ultrasound is very helpful in guiding the direction of a prostate biopsy (Figure 35) and in quantitating the volume of prostate cancer. When radiation therapy implantation is required for treatment, ultrasound is used to map the exact location of the prostate cancer. Rectal ultrasound is very helpful in staging rectal cancers as well. The depth of transmural involvement and presence of extrarectal extension can be accurately assessed.

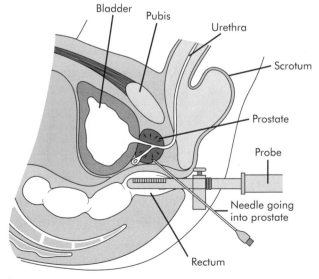

FIGURE 35 Rectal ultrasonography. Diagram demonstrating transrectal biopsy of the prostate.

Real-time ultrasonography requires the emission of high-frequency sound waves from a special transducer placed in the rectum. The sound waves are bounced back to the transducer and are electronically converted into a pictorial image.

Contraindications

- Patients with latex allergy
  Rectal ultrasound requires placement of the probe in a latex condom–like sac.

Interfering factors

- Stool within the rectum

Procedure and patient care

Before

PT Explain the procedure to the patient.

PT Instruct the patient that a small-volume rectal enema may be required approximately 1 hour before the ultrasound examination.

During

- The patient is placed in the left lateral decubitus position.
- A digital rectal examination may be performed to assess the prostate gland or rectal tumor.
- A draped and lubricated ultrasound probe is placed in the rectum.
- Scans are performed in various spatial planes.

After

- Provide the patient with tissue material to cleanse the perianal area.

Abnormal findings

Prostate cancer
Benign prostatic hypertrophy
Prostatitis
Seminal vesicle tumor
Prostate abscess
Perirectal abscess
Intrarectal or perirectal tumor

notes

prostate-specific antigen (PSA)

Type of test   Blood

Normal findings

0-2.5 ng/mL is low
2.6-10 ng/mL is slightly to moderately elevated
10-19.9 ng/mL is moderately elevated
≥20 ng/mL is significantly elevated

Test explanation and related physiology

PSA is a glycoprotein found in high concentrations in the prostatic lumen. Significant barriers, such as prostate glandular tissue and vascular structure, are interposed between the prostatic lumen and the bloodstream. These protective barriers can be broached when disease exists (e.g., cancer, infection, and benign hypertrophy). PSA can be detected in all males; however, levels are greatly increased in patients with prostate cancer.

Elevated PSA levels are associated with prostate cancer. Levels greater than 4 ng/mL have been found in more than 80% of men with prostate cancer. The higher the levels, the greater the tumor burden. The PSA assay is also a sensitive test for monitoring response to therapy. Successful surgery, radiation, or hormone therapy is associated with a marked reduction in the PSA blood level. Significant elevation in PSA subsequently indicates the recurrence of prostatic cancer.

There is considerable controversy regarding the use of PSA screening among asymptomatic men. The US Preventative Services Task Force (USPSTF) and other professional societies have indicated that mortality from prostate cancer is not significantly reduced by annual PSA screening. Furthermore, most believe that "PSA screening–identified" prostate cancer is not an aggressive cancer and is not associated with a significant increase in mortality. Approximately 80% of PSA screening testing is falsely positive. A positive screening test often triggers a biopsy and even potential life-threatening surgery with very little benefit. However, high-risk men such as those of African American descent or with a genetic predisposition (e.g., *BRCA* genetic mutation) or a strong family history should be offered annual PSA testing and digital rectal examinations (DREs).

It is important to be aware that some patients with early prostate cancer will not have elevated levels of PSA. It is equally important to recognize that PSA levels greater then

4 ng/mL are not always associated with cancer. The PSA is limited by a lack of specificity within the diagnostic gray zone of 4 to 10 ng/mL. PSA levels also may be minimally elevated in patients with benign prostatic hypertrophy (BPH) and prostatitis. In an effort to increase the accuracy of PSA testing, other measures of PSA have been proposed including the following:

- *PSA velocity*: PSA velocity is the change in PSA levels over time. A sharp rise in the PSA level raises the suspicion of cancer and may indicate a fast growing cancer.
- *Age-adjusted PSA*: Age is an important factor in increasing PSA levels. Men younger than 50 should have a PSA level less than 2.4 ng/mL, whereas a PSA level up to 6.5 ng/mL would be considered normal for men in their 70s.
- *PSA density*: PSA density considers the relationship of the PSA level to the size of the prostate. The use of PSA density to interpret PSA results is controversial because cancer might be overlooked in a man with an enlarged prostate.
- *Free versus bound PSA*: PSA circulates in the blood in two forms: free or bound to a protein molecule. With benign prostate conditions (e.g., BPH), there is more free PSA (FPSA); cancer produces more of the bound form. When the FPSA is less than 25%, there is a high likelihood of cancer.
- *Alteration of PSA cutoff level*: Some researchers have suggested lowering the cutoff levels that determine whether a PSA measurement is normal or elevated. For example, a number of studies have used cutoff levels of 2.5 or 3.0 ng/mL (rather than 4.0 ng/mL).
- *Prostate-specific proteins*: Patterns of prostate proteins are being studied to determine whether a biopsy is necessary when a person has a slightly elevated PSA level or an abnormal DRE. *Prostatic-specific membrane antigen* may, with further study, represent an excellent marker for prostate cancer. Another protein of interest is *early prostate cancer antigen (EPCA)*. Unlike PSA, this protein isn't found in normal prostate cells. Instead, EPCA occurs in relatively large amounts only in prostate cancer cells. Furthermore, EPCA levels are significantly higher in patients whose cancers spread outside the prostate compared to those with disease confined to the gland.
- *Prostate cancer–specific biomarkers*: These biomarkers are made up of RNA that is present in prostate cancer cells at very high levels due to overexpression of particular genes.

P

These biomarkers can be detected in the urine of prostate cancer patients after a short period of professional prostate massage. The most commonly tested marker is prostate cancer gene 3 (PCA3). Other genetic markers tested include GOLPH2, SPINK1, and TMPRSS2-ERG. These biomarkers are not elevated in noncancerous prostate disease. Furthermore these biomarkers are not influenced by patient age or prostate volume.

PSA is used in the staging of men with known prostate cancer. For example, men with PSA levels less than 10 ng/mL are most likely to have localized disease and respond well to local therapy (radical prostatectomy or radiation therapy).

PSA is used to follow up men after treatment for prostate cancer. Periodic PSA testing should follow any form of treatment for prostate cancer, because PSA levels can indicate the need for further treatment. Following curative radical prostatectomy or radiation therapy, PSA levels should probably be 0 to 0.5 ng/mL. The pattern of PSA rise after local therapy for prostate cancer can help distinguish between local recurrence and distant spread. Patients with elevated PSA levels more than 24 months after local treatment and with a PSA doubling time after 12 months are likely to have recurrence.

Interfering factors

- Rectal examinations may elevate PSA levels.
  The PSA specimen should be drawn before rectal examination of the prostate or several hours afterward.
- Prostatic manipulation by biopsy or transurethral resection of the prostate (TURP) may elevate PSA levels.
  The test should be done before surgery or 6 weeks afterward.
- Ejaculation within 24 hours of blood testing is associated with elevated PSA levels.
- Recent urinary tract infection or prostatitis can cause elevations of PSA for as long as 6 weeks.
- Diethylstilbestrol (DES) and finasteride (Propecia, Proscar) cause *decreased* levels of PSA by about 50%.

Procedure and patient care

- See inside front cover for Routine Blood Testing.
- Fasting: no.
- Blood tube commonly used: red.
- The use of the percent-free PSA demands strict sample handling that is not required with the total PSA. Check for specific guidelines.

Abnormal findings

▲ **Increased levels**
 Prostate cancer
 Benign prostatic hypertrophy
 Prostatitis

notes

P

> **protein** (Protein electrophoresis, Immunofixation electrophoresis [IFE], Serum protein electrophoresis [SPEP], Albumin, Globulin, Total protein)

Type of test   Blood; urine

Normal findings

Adult/elderly
  Total protein: 6.4-8.3 g/dL or 64-83 g/L (SI units)
  Albumin: 3.5-5 g/dL or 35-50 g/L (SI units)
  Globulin: 2.3-3.4 g/dL
    Alpha$_1$ globulin: 0.1-0.3 g/dL or 1-3 g/L (SI units)
    Alpha$_2$ globulin: 0.6-1 g/dL or 6-10 g/L (SI units)
    Beta globulin: 0.7-1.1 g/dL or 7-11 g/L (SI units)
Children
  Total protein
    Premature infant: 4.2-7.6 g/dL
    Newborn: 4.6-7.4 g/dL
    Infant: 6-6.7 g/dL
    Child: 6.2-8 g/dL
  Albumin
    Premature infant: 3-4.2 g/dL
    Newborn: 3.5-5.4 g/dL
    Infant: 4.4-5.4 g/dL
    Child: 4-5.9 g/dL
No protein abnormality on electrophoresis

Test explanation and related physiology

Proteins are constituents of muscles, enzymes, hormones, transport vehicles, hemoglobin, and several other key functional and structural entities in the body. They are the most significant component contributing to the osmotic pressure in the vascular space. This osmotic pressure keeps fluid in the vascular space, minimizing extravasation of fluid. Albumin and globulin constitute most of the protein in the body and are measured together as the total protein.

Albumin is a protein that is formed in the liver. It makes up approximately 60% of the total protein. The major effect of albumin in the blood is to maintain colloidal osmotic pressure. Furthermore, albumin transports important blood constituents, such as drugs, hormones, and enzymes. Albumin is synthesized in the liver and is therefore a measure of hepatic function. When disease affects the liver cell, the hepatocyte loses its ability to synthesize albumin. The serum albumin level is greatly decreased.

However, because the half-life of albumin is 12 to 18 days, severe impairment of hepatic albumin synthesis may not be recognized until after that period.

Globulins represent all non-albumin proteins. Their role in maintaining osmotic pressure is far less than that of albumin. Alpha$_1$ globulins are mostly alpha$_1$ antitrypsin. Some transporting proteins, such as thyroid and cortisol-binding globulin, also contribute to this electrophoretic zone. Alpha$_2$ globulins include serum haptoglobins (which bind hemoglobin during hemolysis), ceruloplasmin (which is a carrier for copper), prothrombin, and cholinesterase (which is an enzyme used in the catabolism of acetylcholine). Beta$_1$ globulins include lipoproteins, transferrin, plasminogen, and complement proteins; beta$_2$ globulins include fibrinogen. Gamma globulins are the immunoglobulins (antibodies) (p. 541). To a lesser degree, globulins also act as transport vehicles.

Serum albumin and some globulins are measures of nutrition. Malnourished patients, especially after surgery, have a greatly decreased level of serum proteins. Burn patients and patients who have protein-losing enteropathies and uropathies have low levels of protein despite normal synthesis.

In some diseases, albumin is selectively diminished, and globulins are normal or increased to maintain a normal total protein level. For example, in collagen vascular diseases (e.g., lupus erythematosus), capillary permeability is increased. Albumin, a molecule that is generally smaller than globulin, is selectively lost into the extravascular space. Another group of diseases similarly associated with low albumin, high globulin, and normal total protein levels is chronic liver diseases. In these diseases, the liver cannot produce albumin, but globulin is adequately made in the reticuloendothelial system. In both of these types of diseases, the albumin level is low but the total protein level is normal because of increased globulin levels. These changes, however, can be detected if one measures the *albumin/globulin ratio*. Normally this ratio exceeds 1.0. The diseases just described that selectively affect albumin levels are associated with lesser ratios. Increased total protein levels, particularly the globulin fraction, occur with multiple myeloma and other gammopathies. It is important to note that proteins can be factitiously elevated in dehydrated patients.

Serum protein electrophoresis (SPEP) can separate the various components of blood protein into bands or zones according to their electrical charge. Several well-established electrophoretic patterns have been identified and can be associated with specific diseases (Table 29).

P

TABLE 29 Protein electrophoresis patterns in specific diseases

Pattern	Electrophoresis	Disease
Acute reaction	↓ Albumin ↑ Alpha$_2$ globulin	Acute infections, tissue necrosis, burns, surgery, stress, myocardial infarction
Chronic inflammatory	sl. ↓ Albumin sl. ↑ Gamma globulin N Alpha$_2$ globulin	Chronic infection, granulomatous diseases, cirrhosis, rheumatoid-collagen diseases
Nephrotic syndrome	↓↓ Albumin ↑↑ Alpha$_2$ globulin N ↑ Beta globulin	Nephrotic syndrome
Far-advanced cirrhosis	↓ Albumin ↑ Gamma globulin Incorporation of beta and gamma peaks	Far-advanced cirrhosis
Polyclonal gamma globulin elevation	↑↑ Gamma globulin with a broad peak	Cirrhosis, chronic infection, sarcoidosis, tuberculosis, endocarditis, rheumatoid-collagen diseases
Hypogamma-globulinemia	↓ Gamma globulin with normal other globulin levels	Light-chain multiple myeloma
Monoclonal gammopathy	Thin spikes in the beta (IgA, IgM) and gamma globulins	Myeloma, Waldenström macroglobulinemia, gammopathies

↓, Decreased; ↑, increased; sl. ↓, slightly decreased; sl. ↑, slightly increased; N, normal; ↓↓, greatly decreased; ↑↑, greatly increased.

If a spike is detected, immunofixation electrophoresis (IFE) can be done. In general, polyclonal spikes are associated with infectious or inflammatory diseases, whereas monoclonal-specific spikes are often neoplastic. IFE is used to indicate deficiencies or excesses as seen with macroglobulinemia, monoclonal gammopathy of undetermined significance (MGUS), and multiple myeloma.

Immunofixation is also able to determine whether a monoclonal spike is caused by light-chain or other protein abnormalities. Specific monoclonal protein studies can be performed on the urine or the blood. Monoclonal immunoglobulin heavy chain (gamma, aplha, mu, delta, or epsilon) and/or light chains (kappa or lambda) can be identified.

This test is also used to follow the course of the disease or treatment in patients with known monoclonal immunoglobulinopathies. For example, with successful treatment for neoplastic gammopathies, IFE, upon repetition, can demonstrate reduction in the specific immunoglobulin. Finally, this test is helpful in defining more clearly the immune status of a patient whose immune system may be compromised.

Protein electrophoresis is also used to evaluate the major protein fractions found in urine. Normally only a small amount of albumin is seen. Urinary protein electrophoresis is useful in classifying the type of renal damage, if present. IFE is useful in characterizing M-components observed in the protein electrophoresis and in identifying light-chain disease. These electrophoresis techniques can be applied to the CSF or any body fluid.

Interfering factors

- Prolonged application of a tourniquet can increase both fractions of total proteins.
- Sampling of peripheral venous blood proximal to an IV administration site can result in an inaccurately low protein level. Likewise, massive IV infusion of crystalloid fluid can result in acute hypoproteinemia.
- ✗ Drugs that may cause *increased* protein levels include anabolic steroids, androgens, corticosteroids, dextran, growth hormone, insulin, phenazopyridine, and progesterone.
- ✗ Drugs that may cause *decreased* protein levels include ammonium ions, estrogens, hepatotoxic drugs, and oral contraceptives.

Procedure and patient care

Before

PT Explain the procedure to the patient.

PT Tell the patient that no fasting or special preparation is required.

During

Blood

- Collect a venous blood sample in a gold-top tube. The blood used for immunoglobulin electrophoresis can be reused.
- Indicate on the laboratory slip if the patient has received any vaccinations or immunizations within the past 6 months. Also, list any drugs that may affect test results.

Urine

PT Instruct the patient to begin the 24-hour collection after voiding. Follow guidelines on inside front cover.

After

- Apply pressure to the venipuncture site.

Abnormal findings

▲ **Increased blood monoclonal immunoglobulins**
Multiple myeloma
Waldenström macroglobulinemia

▲ **Increased blood polyclonal immunoglobulins**
Amyloidosis
Autoimmune diseases
Chronic infection/inflammation
Chronic liver disease

▲ **Increased urine monoclonal immunoglobulins**
Multiple myeloma
Waldenström macroglobulinemia

See also Table 29.

notes

protein C, protein S

Type of test Blood

Normal findings

Protein S: 60%-130% of normal activity

Protein C: 70%-150% of normal activity

Protein C levels are lower in females and decrease with age in both males and females.

Test explanation and related physiology

The plasma coagulation system is tightly regulated between thrombosis and fibrinolysis. This precise regulation is important. The protein C–protein S system is an important regulator of coagulation. Protein C inhibits the regulation of activated factor VIII and factor V (see Figure 10, p. 264). This function of protein C is enhanced by protein S. Congenital deficiencies of these vitamin K–dependent proteins may cause spontaneous intravascular thrombosis. Furthermore, dysfunctional forms of the proteins result in a hypercoagulable state. In addition, nearly 50% of hypercoagulable states are caused by the presence of a factor V (factor V Leiden, p. 416) that is resistant to protein C inhibition. Acquired deficiencies are less commonly symptomatic.

These proteins are vitamin K dependent and are decreased in patients who are taking Coumadin, in liver diseases, and in severe malnutrition. Of the total plasma protein S, approximately 60% circulates bound to C4bBP complement protein, whereas the remaining 40% circulates as free protein S. Only free protein S has anticoagulant function. Because complement regulatory proteins are acute phase reactants, autoimmune diseases and other inflammatory diseases are associated with increased binding of protein S causing an acquired protein S deficiency. Affected patients may experience hypercoagulable events. Measurement of plasma free protein S antigen is performed as the initial testing for protein S deficiency.

Interfering factors

- Decreased protein C may occur in the postoperative state.
- Pregnancy or the use of exogenous sex hormones is associated with decreases in proteins C and S.
- Active clotting states, such as DVT, can lower levels of proteins S and C.
- ✔ Drugs that can *decrease* levels include vitamin K inhibitors (e.g., Coumadin).

Procedure and patient care

- See inside front cover for Routine Blood Testing.
- Fasting: no.
- Blood tube commonly used: blue.

If more than one blood test is to be obtained, draw the blood for protein C or S second to avoid contamination with tissue thromboplastin that may occur in the first tube. If only blood for protein C or S is being drawn, draw a red-top tube first (and throw it away), and then draw the blood for this study in a blue-top tube (two-tube method of blood draw).

PT If the patient is found to be deficient in either protein, encourage the patient's family members to be tested, because they may be similarly affected.

Abnormal findings

▼ **Decreased levels**
  Congenital deficiency of protein C or protein S
  Disseminated intravascular coagulation (DIC)
  Hypercoagulable states
  Pulmonary emboli
  Arterial or venous thrombosis
  Vitamin K deficiency due to drugs or malnutrition
  Malignancy
  Autoimmune diseases
  Inflammation
  Warfarin

notes

prothrombin time (PT, Pro-time, International normalized ratio [INR])

Type of test Blood

Normal findings (depend on reagents used for PT)

11.0-12.5 seconds; 85%-100%
Full anticoagulant therapy: >1.5-2 times control value; 20% to 30%
INR: 0.8-1.1

Possible critical values
>20 seconds
INR: >5.5

Test explanation and related physiology

The PT is used to evaluate the adequacy of the extrinsic system and common pathway in the clotting mechanism. The PT measures the clotting ability of factors I (fibrinogen), II (prothrombin), V, VII, and X. When these clotting factors exist in deficient quantities, PT is prolonged. Many diseases and drugs are associated with decreased levels of these factors. These include the following:

- *Hepatocellular liver disease* (e.g., cirrhosis, hepatitis, and neoplastic invasive processes)

    Factors I, II, V, VII, IX, and X are produced in the liver. With severe hepatocellular dysfunction, synthesis of these factors will not occur.

- *Obstructive biliary disease* (e.g., bile duct obstruction secondary to tumor or gallstones or intrahepatic cholestasis secondary to sepsis or drugs)

    As a result of the biliary obstruction, the bile necessary for fat absorption fails to enter the gut, and fat malabsorption results. Vitamins A, D, E, and K are fat soluble and also are not absorbed. Because the synthesis of factors II, VII, IX, and X depends on vitamin K, these factors will not be adequately produced and serum concentrations will fall.

    Parenchymal (hepatocellular) liver disease can be differentiated from obstructive biliary disease by determination of the patient's response to parenteral vitamin K administration. If PT returns to normal after 1 to 3 days of vitamin K administration (10 mg IM twice a day), one can safely assume that the patient has obstructive biliary disease that is causing vitamin K malabsorption. If, on the other hand, PT does not return to normal with the vitamin

P

K injections, one can assume that severe hepatocellular disease exists and that the liver cells are incapable of synthesizing the clotting factors no matter how much vitamin K is available.

- *Oral anticoagulant administration*

    The coumarin derivatives dicumarol and warfarin (Coumadin, Panwarfin) are used to prevent coagulation in patients with thromboembolic disease. These drugs interfere with the production of vitamin K–dependent clotting factors, which results in a prolongation of PT, as previously described. The adequacy of coumarin therapy can be monitored by following the patient's PT. For anticoagulation, the INR typically should be between 2.0 and 3.0 for patients with atrial fibrillation, and between 3.0 and 4.0 for patients with mechanical heart valves. However, the ideal INR must be individualized for each patient (Table 30).

PT test results are usually given in seconds, along with a control value. The control value usually varies somewhat from day to day because the reagents used may vary. The patient's PT should be approximately equal to the control value. Some laboratories report PT values as percentages of normal activity, because the patient's results are compared with a curve representing normal clotting time. Normally, the patient's PT is 85% to 100%.

To have uniform PT results for physicians in different parts of the country and the world, the World Health Organization has recommended that PT results include the use of the *international normalized ratio (INR)* value. The reported INR results are independent of the reagents or methods used. Most hospitals are now reporting PT times in both absolute and INR numbers.

TABLE 30   Preferred INR according to indication for anticoagulation

Indication	Preferred INR
Deep-vein thrombosis prophylaxis	1.5-2.0
Orthopedic surgery	2.0-3.0
Deep-vein thrombosis	2.0-3.0
Atrial fibrillation	2.0-3.0
Pulmonary embolism	2.5-3.5
Prosthetic valve prophylaxis	3.0-4.0

Such factors as weight, body mass index, age, diet, and concurrent medications are known to affect warfarin dose requirements during anticoagulation therapy. Warfarin interferes with the regeneration of reduced vitamin K from oxidized vitamin K in the vitamin K oxidoreductase (VKOR) complex. A recently identified gene for the major subunit of VKOR, called VKORC1, has been identified and may explain up to 44% of the variance in warfarin dose requirements. Furthermore, warfarin is metabolized in part by the cytochrome P-450 enzyme CYP2C9. The CYP2C9*2 and CYP2C9*3 genetic mutations have been shown to decrease the enzyme activity of these metabolizing enzymes, which has led to warfarin sensitivity and, in serious cases, bleeding complications. A *warfarin pharmacogenomic test panel* is available that can identify any mutations in the VKORC1 -1639, CYP2C9*2, or CYP2C9*3 genes. The warfarin pharmacogenomic test can be used as part of an algorithm to determine the best initial warfarin dose and does not replace the need for routine PT testing for the calculation of the INR.

Point-of-care home testing is now available for patients who require long-term anticoagulation with warfarin. Like glucose monitoring, a finger stick is performed. A drop of blood is placed on the testing strip and inserted into the handheld testing device. The PT and INR are provided in a few minutes. The treating physician is notified by phone and any therapeutic changes can be instigated the same day.

Interfering factors

- Alcohol intake can increase PT levels.
- A high-fat diet may decrease PT levels.
- ✘ Drugs that may cause *increased* levels include allopurinol, aminosalicylic acid, barbiturates, beta-lactam antibiotics, cephalosporins, cholestyramine, chloral hydrate, chlorproma-zine, cimetidine, clofibrate, colestipol, ethyl alcohol, gluca-gon, heparin, methyldopa, neomycin, oral anticoagulants, propylthiouracil, quinidine, quinine, salicylates, and sulfonamides.
- ✘ Drugs that may cause *decreased* levels include anabolic steroids, barbiturates, chloral hydrate, digitalis, diphenhydramine, estrogens, griseofulvin, oral contraceptives, and vitamin K.

Procedure and patient care

- See inside front cover for Routine Blood Testing.
- Fasting: no.
- Blood tube commonly used: light blue.

- Obtain the blood specimen before the patient is given the daily dose of warfarin.
- Remember, hemostasis will be delayed if the patient is taking warfarin or if the patient has any coagulopathies.
- Patients taking warfarin will have their doses regulated by PT and INR values.
- If the PT is greatly prolonged, evaluate the patient for bleeding tendencies.

PT Teach patients on warfarin to check themselves for bleeding.

- The anticoagulant effect of warfarin can be reversed by the slow parenteral administration of vitamin K.

PT Instruct patients on warfarin therapy not to take any other medications unless approved by their physician.

Abnormal findings

▲ **Increased levels**

Cirrhosis

Hepatitis

Vitamin K deficiency

Salicylate intoxication

Bile duct obstruction

Coumarin ingestion

Disseminated intravascular coagulation

Massive blood transfusion

Hereditary factor deficiency

notes

pulmonary angiography (Pulmonary arteriography)

Type of test X-ray with contrast dye

Normal findings Normal pulmonary vasculature

Test explanation and related physiology

Through an injection of a radiographic contrast material into the pulmonary arteries, pulmonary angiography permits visualization of the pulmonary vasculature. Angiography is used to detect pulmonary embolism when the lung scan yields inconclusive results. This study has mostly been replaced by CT of the chest (p. 290).

Bronchial angiography can be done to identify bleeding sites in the lungs. For this procedure, catheters are placed transarterially into the orifice of bronchial arteries. Radiopaque material is then injected, and the arteries are visualized. If a bleeding site is identified, the site can be injected with a sclerosing agent to prevent further bleeding.

Contraindications

- Patients with allergies to shellfish or iodinated dye
- Patients who are pregnant, unless the benefits outweigh the risks
- Patients with bleeding disorders

Potential complications

- Allergic reaction to iodinated dye
- Hypoglycemia or acidosis may occur in patients who are taking metformin and receive iodine dye.
- Cardiac arrhythmia
  Premature ventricular contractions during right-sided heart catheterization may lead to ventricular tachycardia and ventricular fibrillation.

Procedure and patient care

Before

PT Explain the procedure to the patient.
- Ensure that written and informed consent for this procedure is obtained.
PT Inform the patient that a warm flush will be felt when the dye is injected.
- Check the patient for allergies to iodinated dyes and shellfish.
- Determine whether the patient has ventricular arrhythmias.
- Keep the patient NPO after midnight on the day of the test.

P

- Administer preprocedural medications as ordered. Atropine may be given to decrease secretions. Meperidine may be used for sedation and relaxation.

During

- Note the following procedural steps:
  1. The patient is placed on an x-ray table in the supine position.
  2. A catheter is placed into the femoral vein and passed into the inferior vena cava.
  3. With fluoroscopic visualization, the catheter is advanced into the main pulmonary artery, where the dye is injected.
  4. X-ray images of the chest are immediately taken in timed sequence. This allows all vessels visualized by the injection to be photographed. If filling defects are seen in the contrast-filled vessels, pulmonary emboli are present.
  5. If *bronchial angiography* is performed, the femoral artery is cannulated instead of the vein.
- Note that this test is performed by a physician in approximately 1 hour.
- **PT** During injection of dye, inform the patient that he or she will feel a burning sensation and flush throughout the body.

After

- Observe the catheter insertion site for inflammation, hemorrhage, and hematoma.
- Assess the patient's vital signs for evidence of bleeding.
- Apply cold compresses to the puncture site if needed to reduce swelling or discomfort.

Abnormal findings

Pulmonary embolism
Congenital and acquired lesions of the pulmonary vessels (e.g., pulmonary hypertension)
Tumor

notes

pulmonary function tests (PFTs)

Type of test Airflow assessment

Normal findings Vary with the patient's age, sex, height, and weight

Test explanation and related physiology

PFTs are performed to detect abnormalities in respiratory function and to determine the extent of any pulmonary abnormality. The main reasons for pulmonary function tests include:

- Preoperative evaluation of the lungs and pulmonary reserve
- Evaluation of the response to bronchodilator therapy
- Differentiation between restrictive and obstructive forms of chronic pulmonary disease. *Restrictive* defects occur when ventilation is disturbed by a limitation in chest expansion. Inspiration is primarily affected. *Obstructive* defects occur when ventilation is disturbed by an increase in airway resistance. Expiration is primarily affected.
- Determination of the diffusing capacity of the lungs (D_L). Rates are based on the difference in concentration of gases in inspired and expired air.
- Performance of inhalation tests in patients with allergies

PFTs include spirometry, measurement of airflow rates, and calculation of lung volumes and capacities. Exercise pulmonary stress testing can also be performed to provide data concerning the patient's pulmonary reserve.

Spirometry is performed first. On the basis of age, height, weight, race, and sex, normal values for the volumes and flow rates can be predicted. If the actual values are greater than 80% of predicted values, the person is considered normal. Spirometry provides information about obstruction or restriction of airflow. If airflow rates are significantly diminished (<60% of normal), spirometry can be repeated after bronchodilators are administered by nebulizer.

PFTs include determination of the following:

- *Forced vital capacity.* FVC is the amount of air that can be forcefully expelled from a maximally inflated lung position. This volume is decreased below the expected value in obstructive and restrictive pulmonary diseases.
- *Forced expiratory volume in 1 second.* FEV_1 is the volume of air expelled during the first second of the FVC. In patients with obstructive disease, airways are narrowed and resistance to flow is high. Therefore, not as much air can be expelled in

P

1 second, and FEV$_1$ will be reduced below the predicted value. In restrictive lung disease, FEV$_1$ is decreased not because of airway resistance but because the amount of air originally inhaled is less. One should therefore measure the FEV$_1$/FVC ratio. A normal value of 80% is found in patients with restrictive lung disease. In obstructive lung disease, this ratio is considerably less than 80%.

- *Maximal midexpiratory flow.* MMEF is the maximal rate of airflow through the pulmonary tree during forced expiration. This is also called *forced midexpiratory flow.* MMEF is reduced below expected values in obstructive diseases and normal in restrictive diseases.

- *Maximal volume ventilation.* MVV, formerly called *maximal breathing capacity,* is the maximal volume of air that the patient can breathe in and out during 1 minute. MVV is decreased below the expected value in both restrictive and obstructive pulmonary disease.

A comprehensive pulmonary function study also may include evaluation of the following lung volumes and lung capacities, many of which are illustrated in Figure 36.

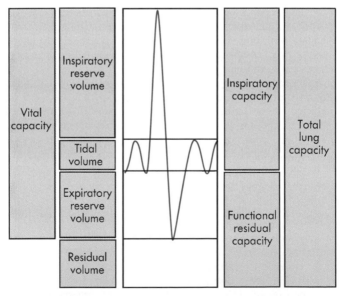

FIGURE 36 Relationship of lung volumes and capacities.

- *Tidal volume.* TV or V_t is the volume of air inspired and expired with each normal respiration.
- *Inspiratory reserve volume.* IRV is the maximal volume of air that can be inspired from the end of a normal inspiration. It represents forced inspiration over and beyond the tidal volume.
- *Expiratory reserve volume.* ERV is the maximal volume of air that can be exhaled after a normal expiration.
- *Residual volume.* RV is the volume of air remaining in the lungs following forced expiration.
- *Inspiratory capacity.* IC is the maximal amount of air that can be inspired after a normal expiration (IC = TV + IRV).
- *Functional residual capacity.* FRC is the amount of air left in the lungs after a normal expiration (FRC = ERV + RV).
- *Vital capacity.* VC is the maximal amount of air that can be expired after a maximal inspiration (VC = TV + IRV + ERV).
- *Total lung capacity.* TLC is the volume to which the lungs can be expanded with the greatest inspiratory effort (TLC = TV + IRV + ERV + RV).
- *Minute volume.* MV, sometimes called *minute ventilation*, is the volume of air inhaled and exhaled per minute.
- *Dead space.* Dead space is the part of the tidal volume that does not participate in alveolar gas exchange. This would include the air in the trachea.
- *Forced expiratory flow$_{200-1200}$.* $FEF_{200-1200}$ is the airflow rate of expired air between 200 mL and 1200 mL during the FVC. This is the portion of the airflow curve that is the most affected by airway obstruction.
- *Forced expiratory flow$_{25-75}$.* FEF_{25-75} is the airflow rate of expired air between 25% and 75% of the flow during the FVC. This is the part of the airflow curve that is the most affected by airway obstruction.
- *Peak inspiratory flow rate.* PIFR is the flow rate of inspired air during maximum inspiration. This is used to indicate large (trachea and bronchi) airway disease.
- *Peak expiratory flow rate.* PEFR is the maximum airflow rate during forced expiration.

Spirometry is the standard method for measuring most relative lung volumes; however, it is incapable of providing information about absolute volumes of air in the lung. Thus, a different approach is required to measure RV, FRC, and TLC. Two of the most common methods of obtaining information about these volumes are *body plethysmography* and *gas dilution tests*.

In *body plethysmography*, the patient sits inside an airtight box and inhales or exhales to a particular volume (usually FRC), and then a shutter drops across the breathing tube. The patient makes respiratory efforts against the closed shutter. Changes in total lung volumes can be easily measured instead of calculated. From those values, assuming pressures in the box are stable, airway resistance and lung compliance can be measured.

Gas dilution or *gas exchange* studies measure the D_L (i.e., the amount of gas exchanged across the alveolar-capillary membrane per minute). Gases, like helium, have densities lower than air. These gases are not affected by turbulent airflow. As a result, the use of helium provides an extremely accurate method of measuring even the most minimal airway resistance existing in the small airways. This is used to test *volume of isoflow (VisoV)*, which is helpful in identifying early obstructive changes.

Contraindications

- Patients who are in pain, because of the inability for deep inspiration and expiration
- Patients who are unable to cooperate

Procedure and patient care

Before

PT Explain the test to the patient.

PT Inform the patient that cooperation is necessary.

PT Instruct the patient not to use bronchodilators (if requested by health care provider) or smoke for 6 hours before this test.

PT Tell the patient the use of small-dose meter inhalers and aerosol therapy may be withheld before this study. Verify with health care provider.

- Measure and record the patient's height and weight before this study to determine the predicted values.

During

- Note the following procedural steps:

Spirometry and airflow rates

1. The patient is taken to the pulmonary function laboratory.
2. The patient breathes through a sterile mouthpiece and into a spirometer to measure and record the values.
3. The patient is asked to inhale as deeply as possible and then forcibly exhale as much air as possible. This is repeated several times (usually two to three times). The two best are used for calculations.
4. From this, the machine computes FVC, FEV_1, $FEV_1/$ FVC, PIFR, PEFR, and MMEF.

5. The patient is asked to breathe in and out as deeply and frequently as possible for 15 seconds. The total volume breathed is recorded and multiplied by 4 to obtain the MVV.

6. The patient is asked to breathe in and out normally into the spirometer and then exhale forcibly from the end tidal volume expiration point. This provides the ERV.

7. The patient is asked to breathe in and out normally into the spirometer and then inhale forcibly from the end tidal volume expiration point. This provides the IC.

8. The patient is asked to breathe in and out maximally. This is a measure of VC and the calculated TLC.

Gas exchange/diffusing capacity of the lung (D_L)

1. The D_L of CO is usually measured by having the patient inhale a CO mixture.

2. D_LCO is calculated with an analysis of the amount of CO exhaled compared with the amount inhaled.

Inhalation tests (bronchial provocation studies)

1. These tests also may be performed during pulmonary function studies to establish a cause-and-effect relationship in some patients with inhalant allergies.

2. The *provocholine challenge* test is typically used to detect the presence of hyperactive airway diseases. This test would not be indicated for a patient with asthma.

3. Care is taken during this challenge test to reverse any severe bronchospasm with prompt administration of an inhalant bronchodilator.

After

- Note that patients with severe respiratory problems are occasionally exhausted after the testing and will need rest.

Abnormal findings

Pulmonary fibrosis	Inhalation pneumonitis
Interstitial lung diseases	Postpneumonectomy
Tumor	Bronchiectasis
Chest wall trauma	Airway infection
Emphysema	Pneumonia
Chronic bronchitis	Neuromuscular disease
Asthma	Hypersensitivity bronchospasm

notes

> **pyelography** (Intravenous pyelography [IVP], Excretory urography [EUG], Intravenous urography [IUG, IVU], Retrograde pyelography, Antegrade pyelography)

Type of test X-ray with contrast dye

Normal findings

Normal size, shape, and position of the kidneys, renal pelvis, ureters, and bladder

Normal kidney excretory function as evidenced by the length of time for passage of contrast material through the kidneys

Test explanation and related physiology

Pyelography is an x-ray study that uses radiopaque contrast material to visualize the kidneys, renal pelvis, ureters, and bladder. The contrast can be injected intravenously, through a catheter placed into the ureter (retrograde), or through a catheter placed into the proximal renal collecting system (antegrade).

IVP is indicated for patients with:
- Pain compatible with urinary stones
- Blood in the urine
- Proposed pelvic surgery to locate the ureters
- Trauma to the urinary system
- Urinary outlet obstruction
- A suspected kidney tumor

For IVP, dye is injected intravenously, filtered out at the kidney by the glomeruli, and then passed through the renal tubules. X-ray images taken at set intervals over the next 30 minutes will show passage of the dye material through the kidneys and ureters and into the bladder.

If the artery leading to one of the kidneys is blocked, the dye cannot enter that part of the renal system, and that kidney or part thereof will not be visualized. If the artery is partially blocked, the length of time required for the appearance of the contrast material will be prolonged.

With primary glomerular disease (e.g., glomerulonephritis), the glomerular filtrate is reduced, which causes a reduction in the quantity of dye filtered. Therefore, it requires more time for enough dye to enter the kidney filtrate and allow for renal opacification. As a result, kidney visualization is delayed. This indicates an estimate of renal function.

Defects in dye filling of the kidney can indicate renal tumors or cysts. Often intrinsic tumors, stones, extrinsic tumors, and scarring can partially or completely obstruct the flow of dye through the collecting system (pelvis, ureters, bladder). CT scanning (p. 281), however, is the method of choice for diagnosing urolithiasis.

If the obstruction has been of sufficient duration, the collecting system proximal to the obstruction will be dilated (hydronephrosis). Retroperitoneal and pelvic tumors, aneurysms, and enlarged lymph nodes also can produce extrinsic compression and distortions of the opacified collecting system.

IVP is also used to assess the effect of trauma on the urinary system. Renal hematomas distort the renal contour. Renal artery laceration is suggested by nonopacification of one kidney. Laceration of the kidneys, pelvis, ureters, or bladder often causes urine leaks, which are identified by dye extravasation from the urinary system. Furthermore, IVP is used to assess a patient for congenital absence or malposition of the kidneys. Horseshoe kidneys (connection of the two kidneys), double ureters, and pelvic kidneys are typical congenital abnormalities.

Retrograde pyelography refers to radiographic visualization of the urinary tract through ureteral catheterization and the injection of contrast material. The ureters are catheterized during cystoscopy. A radiopaque material is injected into the ureters, and x-ray images are taken. This test can be performed even if the patient has an allergy to IV contrast dye, because none of the dye injected into the ureters is absorbed.

Retrograde pyelography is helpful in radiographically examining the ureters in patients when visualization with intravenous pyelography is inadequate or contraindicated. When a ureter is obstructed, IVP will visualize only the ureter proximal to the obstruction, if at all. To visualize the distal part of the ureter, retrograde pyelography is necessary. Also, in patients with unilateral renal disease, the involved kidney and collecting system are not visualized because renal function is so poor. As a result, no dye will be filtered into the collecting system (during IVP) by the nonfunctioning kidney. To rule out ureteral obstruction as a cause of the unilateral kidney disease, retrograde pyelography must be done.

Antegrade pyelography provides visualization of the renal pelvis for accurate placement of nephrostomy tubes. This study is used to identify the upper collecting system in an obstructed kidney to be used as a map for accurate percutaneous placement of a nephrostomy tube. This is performed on patients who have an obstruction of the ureter and hydronephrosis. With this procedure, the renal pelvis is identified with CT imaging or ultrasound. A needle is placed into the pelvis. Radiopaque dye is then injected and the entire upper renal collecting system is demonstrated by obtaining x-ray images in rapid succession. Proper positioning for the nephrostomy is then decided based on these images.

Contraindications

- Patients who are allergic to shellfish or iodinated dyes
- Patients who are severely dehydrated, because this can cause renal shutdown and failure (Geriatric patients are particularly vulnerable.)
- Patients with renal insufficiency, as evidenced by a blood urea nitrogen value greater than 40 mg/dL, because the iodinated nephrotoxic dye can worsen kidney function
- Patients with multiple myeloma, because the iodinated nephrotoxic dye can worsen renal function
- Patients who are pregnant, unless the benefits outweigh the risks of radiation exposure to the fetus

Potential complications

- Allergy to iodine dye
- Infiltration of contrast dye
- Renal failure
  This occurs most often in elderly patients who are chronically dehydrated before the dye injection.
- Hypoglycemia or acidosis may occur in patients who are taking metformin (Glucophage) and receive iodine dye.
- Hemorrhage at the needle puncture site during antegrade pyelography, because the kidney is highly vascular
- Complications associated with *retrograde pyelography* include:
  - Urinary tract infection
  - Sepsis by seeding the bloodstream with bacteria from infected urine
  - Perforation of the bladder or ureter
  - Hematuria
  - Temporary obstruction to ureter caused by ureteral edema

Interfering factors

- Fecal material, gas, or barium in the bowel may obscure visualization of the renal system.
- Abnormal renal function studies may prevent adequate visualization of the urinary tract.
- Retained barium from previous studies may obscure visualization. Studies using barium (e.g., barium enema) should be scheduled after an IVP.

Procedure and patient care

Before

PT Explain the procedure to the patient. Inform the patient that several x-ray images will be taken over 30 minutes.

- Obtain informed consent if required by the institution.
- Check the patient for allergies to iodinated dye and shellfish.
- Give the patient a laxative or a cathartic, if ordered, the evening before the test.

PT Inform the patient of the required food and fluid restrictions. Some institutions prefer abstinence from solid foods for 8 hours before testing. Some allow a clear-liquid breakfast on the test day.

- Ensure adequate hydration for the patient (IV or oral) before and after the test to avoid dye-induced renal failure.
- Note that pediatric patients will have decreased fasting times, as ordered on an individual basis.
- Note that elderly and debilitated patients should have fasting times indicated specifically for them.
- Note that patients receiving high rates of IV fluids may have infusion rates decreased for several hours before the study to increase the concentration of the dye within the urinary system.
- Assess the patient's blood urea nitrogen and creatinine levels. Renal function could deteriorate as a result of the dye injection.
- Give the patient an enema or suppository on the morning of the study, if ordered.
- If the antegrade or retrograde pyelography will be performed with the patient under general anesthesia, follow routine general anesthesia precautions. Keep the patient NPO after midnight on the day of the test. Fluids may be given intravenously.

During

- Note the following procedural steps for *IVP*:
  1. The patient is taken to the radiology department and placed in the supine position.
  2. A plain image of the abdomen (KUB) is taken to ensure that no residual stool obscures visualization of the renal system. This also screens for calculi in the renal collecting system.
  3. Skin testing for iodine allergy is often done.
  4. A peripheral IV line is started (if not in place), and a contrast dye (e.g., Hypaque, Renografin) is given.
  5. X-ray images are taken at specific times, usually at 1, 5, 10, 15, 20, and 30 minutes and sometimes longer, to follow

the course of the dye from the cortex of the kidney to the bladder.

6. The patient is taken to the bathroom and asked to void.
7. A postvoiding image is taken to visualize the empty bladder.

PT Inform the patient that the dye injection often causes a transitory flushing of the face, a feeling of warmth, a salty taste in the mouth, or even transient nausea. Initial IV needle placement and lying on a hard x-ray table are the only other discomforts associated with IVP.

- Note the following procedural steps for *retrograde pyelography*:
  1. The ureteral catheters are passed into the ureters by means of cystoscopy (p. 326).
  2. Radiopaque contrast material (e.g., Hypaque, Renografin) is injected into the ureteral catheters, and x-ray images are taken.
  3. The entire ureter and renal pelvis are demonstrated.
  4. As the catheters are withdrawn, more dye is injected, and more x-ray images are taken to visualize the complete outline of the ureters.
  5. A delayed image is often performed to assess the emptying capabilities of the ureter. This is usually done about 5 minutes after the last injection.
  6. If obstruction is noted, a stent may be left in the ureter so that the ureter can drain.

- Note the following procedural steps for *antegrade pyelography*:
  1. The renal pelvis is localized by means of ultrasound.
  2. Under local anesthesia, a thin-walled needle is advanced into the lumen of the renal pelvis.
  3. Contrast material is injected and x-ray images in posteroanterior (PA), oblique, and anteroposterior (AP) views are obtained.
  4. The nephrostomy tube is placed over guidewires and its position is affirmed by repeating the x-rays.

PT Inform the patient that antegrade or retrograde pyelography is uncomfortable. If awake, the patient will feel pressure and an urge to void.

After

PT Maintain adequate oral or IV hydration for several hours after the IVP to counteract fluid depletion caused by the test preparation. Encourage fluid intake.

PT Assess the patient's urinary output. A decreased output may be an indication of renal failure.

PT Evaluate elderly and debilitated patients for weakness because of the combination of fasting and catharsis necessary for test preparation. Instruct these patients to ambulate only with assistance.

• Note the color of the urine; a pink tinge is typically present. Report bright red blood or clots to the physician.

• See p. xviii for appropriate interventions concerning care for patients with iodine allergy.

Abnormal findings

Pyelonephritis
Glomerulonephritis
Kidney tumor
Renal hematoma
Renal laceration
Cyst or polycystic disease of the kidney
Congenital abnormality of the urologic tract
Renal or ureteral calculi
Trauma to the kidneys, ureters, or bladder
Tumor of the collecting system
Hydronephrosis
Extrinsic compression of the collecting system (e.g., caused by tumor, aneurysm)
Bladder tumor
Prostate enlargement (male)

notes

P

rabies-neutralizing antibody test

Type of test Blood

Normal findings <1:5

Test explanation and related physiology

Identification and documentation of the presence of rabies virus–neutralizing antibody are important for veterinary health care workers and others who may be or may have been exposed to the rabies virus. This test may be performed on patients who are at great risk for animal bites and have received the human diploid cell rabies vaccine (HDCV). A rabies titer of greater than 1:5 is considered to be protective.

The rabies virus antibody test is also used in making the diagnosis of rabies in a patient suspected of having been exposed to the virus. A fourfold rise in antibody titer over several weeks in a person not previously exposed to the HDCV indicates rabies exposure.

Procedure and patient care

- See inside front cover for Routine Blood Testing.
- Fasting: no.
- Blood tube commonly used: red.

Abnormal findings

Exposure to rabies vaccine
Recent bite exposure to rabies virus
Active rabies in a patient or animal

notes

red blood cell count (RBC count, Erythrocyte count)

Type of test Blood

Normal findings (RBC × 10^6/μl or RBC × 10^{12}/L [SI units])

Adult/elderly
   Male: 4.7-6.1
   Female: 4.2-5.4
Children
   Newborn: 4.8-7.1
   2-8 weeks: 4.0-6.0
   2-6 months: 3.5-5.5
   6 months-1 year: 3.5-5.2
   1-6 years: 4.0-5.5
   6-18 years: 4.0-5.5

Test explanation and related physiology

This test is a count of the number of circulating red blood cells (RBCs) in 1 mm³ of peripheral venous blood. The RBC count is routinely performed as part of a complete blood count. Within each RBC are molecules of hemoglobin that permit the transport and exchange of oxygen to the tissues and carbon dioxide from the tissues. RBCs are produced by the erythroid elements in the bone marrow. Under the stimulation of erythropoietin, RBC production is increased.

Normally, RBCs survive in the peripheral blood for approximately 120 days. During that time, RBCs are transported through the bloodstream. In the smallest of capillaries, the RBCs must fold and bend to conform to the size of these tiny vessels. Toward the end of the life of an RBC, the cell membrane becomes less pliable; the aged RBC is then lysed and extracted from circulation by the spleen. Abnormal RBCs have a shorter life span and are extracted earlier. Intravascular RBC trauma, such as that caused by artificial heart valves or peripheral vascular atherosclerotic plaques, also shortens the life of the RBC. An enlarged spleen, such as that caused by portal hypertension or leukemia, may inappropriately destroy and remove normal RBCs from circulation.

Normal RBC values vary according to gender and age. Women tend to have lower values than men, and RBC counts tend to decrease with age. When the value is decreased below the range of the expected normal value, the patient is said to be anemic. Low RBC values are caused by decreased bone marrow

R

production (e.g., myelofibrosis, leukemia, renal disease, or dietary deficiencies), increased blood loss (e.g., bleeding), or increased RBC destruction (hemolysis).

RBC counts greater than normal can be physiologically induced as a result of the body's requirements for greater oxygen-carrying capacity (e.g., at high altitudes). Diseases that produce chronic hypoxia (e.g., congenital heart disease) also provoke this physiologic increase in RBCs. Polycythemia vera is a neoplastic condition causing uncontrolled production of RBCs.

Interfering factors

- Normal decreases are seen in RBCs during pregnancy because of normal body fluid increases and dilution of the RBCs.
- Persons living at high altitudes have increased RBCs.
- Hydration status: Dehydration factitiously increases the RBC count, and overhydration decreases the RBC count.
- ✗ Drugs that may cause *increased* RBC levels include erythro-poietin and gentamicin.
- ✗ Drugs that *decrease* RBC levels are many, including those that decrease marrow production or those that cause hemolysis.

Procedure and patient care

- See inside front cover for Routine Blood Testing.
- Fasting: no.
- Blood tube commonly used: lavender.
- Thoroughly mix the blood with the anticoagulant by tilting the tube.
- Avoid hemolysis.

Abnormal findings

▲ **Increased levels**
 High altitude
 Congenital heart disease
 Polycythemia vera
 Dehydration/
  hemoconcentration
 Cor pulmonale
 Pulmonary fibrosis
 Thalassemia trait
 Severe COPD

▼ **Decreased levels**
 Hemorrhage
 Hemolysis
 Anemia
 Hemoglobinopathy
 Advanced cancer
 Bone marrow failure
 Leukemia
 Lymphoma
 Antineoplastic chemotherapy
 Chronic illness
 Renal disease
 Overhydration
 Multiple myeloma
 Pernicious anemia
 Rheumatoid disease
 Subacute endocarditis
 Pregnancy
 Dietary deficiency
 Prosthetic valves

notes

R

red blood cell indices (RBC indices, Blood indices)

Type of test Blood

Normal findings

Mean corpuscular volume (MCV)
Adult/elderly/child: 80-95 fL
Newborn: 96-108 fL

Mean corpuscular hemoglobin (MCH)
Adult/elderly/child: 27-31 pg
Newborn: 32-34 pg

Mean corpuscular hemoglobin concentration (MCHC)
Adult/elderly/child: 32-36 g/dL (or 32%-36%)
Newborn: 32-33 g/dL (or 32%-33%)

Red blood cell distribution width (RDW)
Adult: 11%-14.5%

Test explanation and related physiology

The RBC indices provide information about the size (MCV and RDW), hemoglobin content (MCH), and hemoglobin concentration (MCHC) of RBCs. This test is routinely performed as part of a complete blood count (CBC). The results of the RBC, hematocrit, and hemoglobin tests are necessary to calculate the RBC indices. When investigating anemia, it is helpful to categorize the anemia according to the RBC indices, as shown in Table 31. Cell size is indicated by the terms *normocytic*, *microcytic*, and *macrocytic*. Hemoglobin content is indicated by the terms *normochromic*, *hypochromic*, and *hyperchromic*. Additional information about RBC size, shape, color, and intracellular structure is described in the blood smear study (p. 156).

Mean corpuscular volume

The MCV is a measure of the average volume, or size, of a single RBC and is therefore used in classifying anemias. When the MCV value is increased, the RBC is said to be abnormally large, or *macrocytic*. This is most frequently seen in megaloblastic anemias (e.g., vitamin B_{12} or folic acid deficiency). When the MCV value is decreased, the RBC is said to be abnormally small, or *microcytic*. This is associated with iron deficiency anemia or thalassemia.

TABLE 31   Categorization of anemia according to RBC indices

Normocytic,[1] normochromic[2] anemia
Iron deficiency (detected early)
Chronic illness (e.g., sepsis, tumor)
Acute blood loss
Aplastic anemia (e.g., total body therapeutic irradiation)
Acquired hemolytic anemias (e.g., from a prosthetic cardiac valve)
Renal disease (because of the loss of erythropoietin)

Microcytic,[3] hypochromic[4] anemia
Iron deficiency (detected late)
Thalassemia
Lead poisoning

Microcytic, normochromic anemia
Chronic illnesses

Macrocytic,[5] normochromic anemia
Vitamin B_{12} or folic acid deficiency
Phenytoin ingestion
Chemotherapy
Some myelodysplastic syndromes
Myeloid leukemia
Ethanol toxicity
Thyroid dysfunction

[1]Normocytic—normal RBC size
[2]Normochromic—normal color (normal hemoglobin content)
[3]Microcytic—smaller than normal RBC size
[4]Hypochromic—less than normal color (decreased hemoglobin content)
[5]Macrocytic—larger than normal RBC size

R

Mean corpuscular hemoglobin

The MCH is a measure of the average amount of hemoglobin in an RBC. MCH is calculated as follows:

$$MCH = \frac{Hemoglobin\ (g/dL) \times 10}{RBC\ (million/mm^3)}$$

Because macrocytic cells generally have more hemoglobin and microcytic cells have less hemoglobin, the causes for these values closely resemble those for the MCV value.

Mean corpuscular hemoglobin concentration

The MCHC is a measure of the average concentration or percentage of hemoglobin in a single RBC. MCHC is calculated as follows:

$$MCHC = \frac{Hemoglobin\,(g/dL) \times 100}{Hematocrit\,(\%)}$$

When values are decreased, the cell has a deficiency of hemoglobin and is said to be *hypochromic* (frequently seen in iron deficiency anemia and thalassemia). When values are normal, the anemia is said to be *normochromic* (e.g., hemolytic anemia). RBCs cannot be considered *hyperchromic*. Only 37 g/dL of hemoglobin can fit into the RBC. Alterations in RBC shape (spherocytosis), RBC agglutination, and a hemolyzed specimen may cause automated counting machines to indicate MCHC levels above normal.

Red blood cell distribution width

The RDW is an indication of the variation in RBC size. It is calculated with a machine by using the MCV and RBC values. Variations in the width of RBCs may be helpful when classifying certain types of anemia. The RDW is essentially an indicator of the degree of *anisocytosis*, a blood condition characterized by RBCs of variable and abnormal size.

Interfering factors

- Abnormal RBC size may affect indices.
- Extremely elevated white blood cell counts may affect RBC indices.
- Large RBC precursors (e.g., reticulocytes [p. 805]) cause an abnormally high MCV.
- Marked elevation in lipid levels (>2000 mg/dL) causes automated cell counters to indicate high hemoglobin levels. MCHC and MCH will be calculated falsely high.
- The presence of cold agglutinins also falsely elevates MCHC, MCH, and MCV.
- ✗ Drugs that may *increase* MCV results include azathioprine, phenytoin, and zidovudine.

Procedure and patient care

- See inside front cover for Routine Blood Testing.
- Fasting: no.
- Blood tube commonly used: lavender.

Abnormal findings

▲ **Increased MCV**
Liver disease
Antimetabolite therapy
Alcoholism
Pernicious anemia
   (vitamin B_{12} deficiency)
Folic acid deficiency

▲ **Increased MCH**
Macrocytic anemia

▲ **Increased MCHC**
Spherocytosis
Intravascular hemolysis
Cold agglutinins

▲ **Increased RDW**
Iron deficiency anemia
B_{12} or folate deficiency anemia
Hemoglobinopathies
   (e.g., sickle cell disease)
Hemolytic anemias
Posthemorrhagic anemias

▼ **Decreased MCV**
Iron deficiency anemia
Thalassemia
Anemia caused by
   chronic illness

▼ **Decreased MCH**
Microcytic anemia
Hypochromic anemia

▼ **Decreased MCHC**
Iron deficiency anemia
Thalassemia

notes

R

renal biopsy (Kidney biopsy)

Type of test　Microscopic examination of tissue

Normal findings　No pathologic conditions

Test explanation and related physiology

Biopsy of the kidney affords microscopic examination of renal tissue. Renal biopsy is performed for the following purposes:

- To diagnose the cause of renal disease (e.g., poststrepto-coccal glomerulonephritis, Goodpasture syndrome, lupus nephritis)
- To detect primary and metastatic malignancy of the kidney in patients who may not be candidates for surgery
- To evaluate the degree of rejection that occurs after kidney transplantation, which enables the physician to determine the appropriate dose of immunosuppressive agents

Renal biopsy is most often obtained percutaneously (Figure 37). During this procedure, a needle is inserted through the skin and into the kidney to obtain a sample of kidney tissue. The biopsy needle is more accurately placed when guided by CT scanning, ultrasonography, or fluoroscopy. These techniques allow more precise localization of the desired kidney tissue.

Occasionally, open renal biopsy is performed. This involves an incision through the flank and dissection to expose the kidney surgically.

Contraindications

- Patients with coagulation disorders because of the risk of excessive bleeding
- Patients with operable kidney tumors, because tumor cells may be disseminated during the procedure
- Patients with hydronephrosis, because the enlarged renal pelvis can be easily entered and cause a persistent urine leak requiring surgical repair
- Patients with urinary tract infections, because the needle insertion may disseminate the active infection throughout the retroperitoneum

Potential complications

- Hemorrhage from the highly vascular renal tissue
- Inadvertent puncture of the liver, lung, bowel, aorta, and inferior vena cava
- Infection when an open biopsy is performed

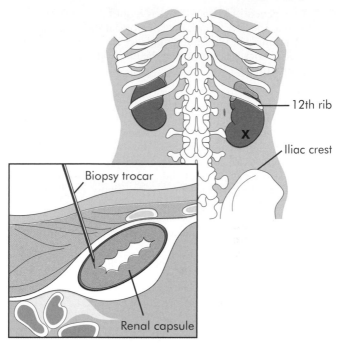

FIGURE 37 Renal biopsy. A biopsy needle is placed through the posterior lower chest wall and into the renal parenchyma, from which tissue is extracted.

Procedure and patient care

Before

PT Explain the procedure to the patient.
- Ensure that written and informed consent for this procedure is obtained by the physician.
- Keep the patient NPO after midnight on the day of the test in the event that bleeding or inadvertent puncture of an abdominal organ may necessitate surgical intervention.
- Assess the patient's coagulation studies (prothrombin time, partial thromboplastin time).
- Check the patient's hemoglobin and hematocrit values.
- Note that the patient may need to be typed and crossmatched for blood in the event of severe hemorrhage requiring transfusions.

PT Tell the patient that no sedative is required.

- Note that the needle stick may be done at the bedside.
- If CT scanning or ultrasound guidance is to be used, note that the needle stick is performed in the radiology or ultrasonography department.

During

- Note the following procedural steps:
  1. The patient is placed in a prone position with a sandbag or pillow under the abdomen to straighten the spine.
  2. Under sterile conditions, the skin overlying the kidneys is infiltrated with a local anesthetic (lidocaine).
  3. While the patient holds his or her breath to stop kidney motion, the physician inserts the biopsy needle into the kidney and takes a specimen.
  4. After this procedure is completed, the needle is removed, and pressure is applied to the site for approximately 20 minutes.
- Note that this procedure is performed by a physician in approximately 10 minutes.

PT Tell the patient that this procedure is uncomfortable but only minimally if enough lidocaine is used.

After

- After the test, apply a pressure dressing.
- Turn the patient onto his or her back and keep him or her on bed rest for approximately 24 hours.
- Check the patient's vital signs, puncture site, and hematocrit values frequently during the 24-hour period.

PT Instruct the patient to avoid any activity that increases abdominal venous pressure (e.g., coughing).

- Assess the patient for signs and symptoms of hemorrhage (e.g., decrease in blood pressure, increase in pulse, pallor, backache, flank pain, shoulder pain, lightheadedness).
- Evaluate the patient's abdomen for signs of bowel or liver penetration (e.g., abdominal pain and tenderness, abdominal muscle guarding and rigidity, decreased bowel sounds).

PT Instruct the patient to avoid strenuous exercise (e.g., heavy lifting, contact sports, horseback riding), or any activity that could cause jolting of the kidney, for at least 2 weeks.

PT Instruct the patient to report burning during urination or development of a fever. Either could indicate a urinary tract infection.

- Inspect all urine specimens for gross hematuria. Usually the patient's urine will contain blood initially, but this generally will not continue after the first 24 hours. Urine samples may be placed in consecutive chronologic order to facilitate comparison for evaluation of hematuria. This is referred to as *rack* or *serial* urine samples.

PT Encourage the patient to drink large amounts of fluid to prevent clot formation and urine retention.

• Frequently obtain blood for hemoglobin and hematocrit determination after the biopsy specimen to assess the patient for active bleeding. One purple-top tube of blood is needed.

Abnormal findings

Renal disease (e.g., poststreptococcal conditions, glomerulone-phritis, lupus nephritis)

Primary and metastatic malignancy of the kidney

Rejection of kidney transplant

notes

R

> **renal scanning** (Kidney scan, Radiorenography, Radionuclide renal imaging, Nuclear imaging of the kidney, DSMA renal scan, DTPA renal scan, Captopril renal scan)

Type of test Nuclear scan

Normal findings Normal size, shape, and function of the kidney

Test explanation and related physiology

Renal scans are used to indicate the perfusion, function, and structure of the kidneys. They are also used to indicate the presence of ureteral obstruction or renovascular hypertension. Because this study uses no iodinated dyes, it is safe to perform on patients who have iodine allergies or compromised renal function. Renal scans are used to monitor renal function in patients with known renal disease. This scan also plays a large part in the diagnosis of renal transplant rejection.

This nuclear procedure provides visualization of the urinary tract after IV administration of a radioisotope. The radioactive material is detected by a scintillator camera, which can detect the gamma rays emitted by the radionuclide in the kidney. Scans do not interfere with the normal physiologic process of the kidney. The resultant image (scan) indicates distribution of the radionuclide within the kidney and ureters.

There are several kinds of renal scans, depending on what information is needed to be obtained. Different isotopes may be more suitable for different scans, based on the manner in which the kidney handles the radioisotope.

Renal blood flow (perfusion) scan

This type of renal scan is used to evaluate the blood flow to each kidney. It is used to identify renal artery stenosis, renovascular hypertension, and rejection of renal transplant. Also, it is used to demonstrate hypervascular lesions (renal cell carcinoma) in the kidney.

Decreased gamma activity is noted in a kidney with arterial stenosis or renovascular hypertension. Decreased activity relative to the aorta is noted in a transplanted kidney that is experiencing rejection. Localized increased gamma activity is noted in a kidney that contains a hypervascular tumor (cancer).

Renal structural scan

This type of renal scan is performed to outline the structure of the kidney to identify pathology that may alter normal anatomic structure (e.g., tumor, cyst, abscess). Congenital disorders (e.g., hypoplasia or aplasia of the kidney, malposition of the kidney) can also be detected. A filling defect in the renal parenchyma may indicate a tumor, cyst, abscess, or infarction. A horseshoe-shaped kidney, pelvic kidney, or absence of a kidney may be evident. Also, information concerning postrenal transplants can be obtained with this scan. Anatomic alterations in the parenchymal distribution of tracer may indicate transplant rejection. Tc-DTPA (Technetium diethylenetriamine pentaacetic acid) or Tc-disodium monomethane arsonate (DSMA) can be used for this scan.

Renal function scan (renogram)

Renal function can be determined by documenting the capability of the kidney to take up and excrete a particular radioisotope. A well-functioning kidney can be expected to rapidly assimilate the isotope and then excrete it. A poorly functioning kidney will not be able to take up the isotope rapidly or excrete it in a timely manner. Renal function can be monitored by serially repeating this test and comparing results. Each radioactive tracer is handled by the kidney in a different manner. Different renal functions can be tested according to which isotope is used:

- Technetium-99 m diethylenetriamine pentaacetic acid (^{99}mTc-DTPA) measures glomerular filtration.
- Technetium-99 m mercaptoacetyl triglycine (^{99}mTc-MAG3) measures both glomerular filtration and tubular cell secretion.

Renal hypertension scan

This scan is used to identify the presence and location of renovascular hypertension. It usually uses angiotensin-converting enzyme (ACE) inhibitors, such as captopril. The *captopril scan* (captopril renography/scintigraphy) determines the functional significance of a renal artery or arteriole stenosis. These scans may predict the response of the blood pressure to medical treatment, angioplasty, or surgery.

Renal obstruction scan

This scan is performed to identify obstruction of the outflow tract of the kidney caused by obstruction of the renal pelvis, ureter, or bladder outlet. Ultrasound, CT scanning, or MRI are preferable and more accurate for anatomic abnormalities, tumors, and cysts.

Often several of these scans are combined to obtain the maximum possible information about the renal system. A *triple renal study* may use all of these techniques to evaluate renal blood perfusion, structure, and excretion. Radionuclear scans are also helpful in the evaluation of arterial trauma.

Contraindications

- Patients who are pregnant, unless the benefits outweigh the risks of fetal damage

Procedure and patient care

Before

PT Explain the procedure to the patient.

- Do not schedule a renal scan within 24 hours after an intravenous pyelogram.

PT Assure the patient that he or she will not be exposed to large amounts of radioactivity because only tracer doses of isotopes are used.

PT Remind the patient to void before the scan.

PT Tell the patient that no sedation or fasting is required but that good hydration is essential.

PT Instruct the patient to drink two to three glasses of water before the scan.

During

- Note the following procedural steps:
  1. The unsedated, nonfasting patient is taken to the nuclear medicine department.
  2. A peripheral IV injection of radionuclide is given. It takes only minutes for the radioisotopes to be concentrated in the kidneys.
  3. While the patient assumes a supine or sitting position, a gamma ray scintigraphy camera is passed over the kidney area and records the radioactive uptake on film.
  4. Scans may be repeated at different intervals after the initial isotope injection.
  5. Unique features of the various scans:
     a. For a *furosemide (Lasix) renal scan* or a *diuretic renal scan*, images are obtained for 10 to 20 minutes; then furosemide is administered through an IV, and another 20 minutes of images is obtained.
     b. For the *captopril renal scan*, the patient is scanned after the administration of captopril.
     c. For the *renal blood flow* and the *renal function scans*, scanning is started immediately after the injection.
     d. For *structural renal scans*, the patient is asked to lie still for the entire time of the scan (30 minutes).
- Note that the duration of this test varies from 1 to 4 hours, depending on the specific information required. Perfusion scans are done in approximately 20 minutes and functional

scans in less than 1 hour. Static structure scans require 20 minutes to 4 hours for completion.

- Note that this study is performed by a nuclear medicine technologist or physician.

PT Tell the patient that no pain or discomfort is associated with this procedure.

PT Inform the patient that he or she must lie still during this study.

After

PT Because only tracer doses of radioisotopes are used, inform the patient that no precautions need to be taken against radioactive exposure.

PT Tell the patient that the radioactive substance is usually excreted from the body within 6 to 24 hours. Encourage the patient to drink fluids.

Abnormal findings

Urinary obstruction
Pyelonephritis
Renovascular hypertension
Absence of kidney function
Renal infarction
Renal arterial atherosclerosis
Glomerulonephritis
Renal tumor
Congenital abnormalities
Renal trauma
Transplant rejection
Acute tubular necrosis
Renal abscess
Renal cyst

notes

renin assay, plasma (Plasma renin activity [PRA], Plasma renin concentration [PRC])

Type of test Blood

Normal findings

Plasma renin assay

Adult/elderly

Upright position, *sodium-depleted* (sodium-restricted diet)
Ages 20-39 years: 2.9-24 ng/mL/hr
>40 years: 2.9-10.8 ng/mL/hr

Upright position, *sodium-repleted* (normal sodium diet)
Ages 20-39 years: 0.6-4.3 ng/mL/hr
>40 years: 0.6-3 ng/mL/hr

Child

0-3 years: <16.6 ng/mL/hr
3-6 years: <6.7 ng/mL/hr
6-9 years: <4.4 ng/mL/hr
9-12 years: <5.9 ng/mL/hr
12-15 years: <4.2 ng/mL/hr
15-18 years: <4.3 ng/mL/hr

Renal vein

Renin ratio of involved kidney to uninvolved kidney <1.4

Test explanation and related physiology

Renin is an enzyme released by the juxtaglomerular apparatus of the kidney into the renal veins in response to hyperkalemia, sodium depletion, decreased renal blood perfusion, or hypovolemia. Renin activates the renin-angiotensin system, which produces angiotensins I, II, and III (see page 59), powerful vasoconstrictors that also stimulate aldosterone production from the adrenal cortex. Angiotensin and aldosterone increase blood volume, blood pressure, and sodium retention by the kidney (Figure 38). After release of renin from the kidney into the bloodstream, angiotensinogen, an alpha$_2$ globulin that is made in the liver, is converted into angiotensin I. This is then converted into angiotensin II in the lung.

Renin is not actually measured in this test. Plasma renin activity (PRA) measures enzyme ability to convert angiotensinogen to angiotensin I and is limited by the availability of angiotensinogen. The PRA test actually measures, by radioimmunoassay, the rate of angiotensin I generation per unit time. This is a commonly used renin assay. The specimen must be drawn under ideal

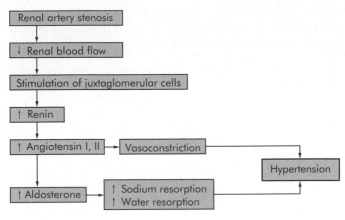

FIGURE 38 Physiology of renovascular hypertension.

circumstances, handled by the local laboratory correctly, and transferred to the central laboratory in a timely manner. Even then, results may vary significantly.

The PRA test is a screening procedure for the detection of renal-based or renovascular hypertension. The PRA may be supplemented by other tests, such as the renal vein renin assay. A determination of the PRA and a simultaneous measurement of the plasma aldosterone (page 25) level are used in the differential diagnosis of primary versus secondary hyperaldosteronism. Patients with primary hyperaldosteronism (adrenal adenoma overproducing aldosterone or Conn syndrome) will have increased aldosterone production associated with suppressed renin activity. The aldosterone/renin ratio is ≥20. Patients with secondary hyperaldosteronism (caused by renovascular occlusive disease or primary renal disease) will have increased levels of aldosterone and plasma renin.

Renal vein assays for renin are used to diagnose and lateralize renovascular hypertension, that is, hypertension that is related to inappropriately high renin levels from a diseased kidney or a hypoperfused kidney. The renal veins can be identified using injection of a radiopaque dye into the inferior vena cava. A catheter is placed into each renal vein, and blood is withdrawn from each vein. PRA is determined in each sample. If hypertension is caused by renal artery stenosis or renal pathology, the renal vein renin level of the affected kidney should be 1.5 or more times greater than that of the unaffected kidney or peripheral venous sample. If the levels are the same, the hypertension is

R

not caused by a renovascular source. This is very helpful in determining whether a stenosis seen on a renal angiogram is significantly contributing to hypertension. Any stenosis identified on an arteriogram would not be considered severe enough to cause renin-related hypertension if renin levels from the renal vein were not at least 1.4 times those of the opposite kidney. Another cause for the patient's elevated blood pressure should be considered.

The *renin stimulation test* can be performed to more clearly diagnose and distinguish primary and secondary hyperaldosteronism. In this test, PRA is obtained while the patient is in the recumbent position and on a low-salt diet. The PRA is then repeated with the patient on the same diet while the patient is standing erect. In primary hyperaldosteronism the blood volume is greatly expanded. A change in position or reduced salt intake will not result in decreased renal perfusion or sodium level. Therefore, renin levels do not increase. In secondary hyperaldosteronism (or normal persons with essential hypertension), the renal perfusion decreases while in the upright position and sodium levels do decrease with decreased intake. Therefore, renin levels increase.

The PRA is assessed as part of the *captopril test* (a screening test for renovascular hypertension). Patients with renovascular hypertension have greater falls in blood pressure and increases in PRA after administration of angiotensin-converting enzyme (ACE) inhibitors than do those with essential hypertension. For the captopril test, the patient receives an oral dose of captopril (ACE inhibitor) after a baseline PRA test, and blood pressure measurements are then taken. Subsequent blood pressure measurements and a repeat PRA test at 60 minutes are used for test interpretation. This is an excellent screening procedure to determine the need for a more invasive radiographic evaluation (e.g., digital subtraction renal arteriography or bilateral renal arteriography).

Contraindications

- Patients who are allergic to shellfish or iodinated dye

Potential complications

- Allergic reaction to iodinated dye

Interfering factors

- Renin levels are affected by pregnancy, salt intake, and licorice ingestion.

- Values are higher in patients on low-salt diets and when the patient is in an upright position.
- Posture: renin is increased in the erect position and decreased in the recumbent position.
- Values are higher early in the day. There is a diurnal variation in renin production.
- ☙ Spironolactone interferes with renin testing and should be discontinued 4 to 6 weeks prior to renin testing.
- ☙ Drugs that *increase* levels of renin include ACE inhibitors, antihypertensives, diuretics, estrogens, oral contraceptives, and vasodilators.
- ☙ Drugs that *decrease* renin levels include beta-blockers, clonidine, licorice, nonsteroidal antiinflammatory agents, potassium, and reserpine.

Procedure and patient care

Before
- **PT** Explain the procedure to the patient.
- **PT** Instruct the patient to maintain a normal diet with a restricted amount of sodium (approximately 3 g/day) for 3 days before the test. A high-sodium diet causes a decrease in renin.
- A urine sodium (p. 862) may be obtained to normalize PRA to salt intake.
- **PT** Instruct the patient to discontinue medications that may interfere with results for 2 to 4 weeks before the test as ordered by the physician.
- Usually draw a fasting blood sample because renin values are higher in the morning.
- **PT** For stimulation tests, instruct the patient to significantly reduce sodium intake for 3 days before testing.
- Ensure that the patient stands or sits upright for 2 hours before the blood is drawn.
- If a recumbent sample is ordered, have the patient remain in bed in the morning until the blood has been obtained.

During
- The test is usually performed with the patient in an upright position.
- For the stimulation tests, the blood is drawn in the recumbent and upright positions.
- Release the tourniquet immediately prior to obtaining the blood specimen because stasis can lower renin levels.
- Collect a venous blood sample and place it in a chilled lavender-top tube.

R

- Gently invert the blood tube to allow adequate mixing of the blood sample and the anticoagulant.
- Record the patient's position and dietary status and time of day on the laboratory slip.
- Place the tube of blood on ice and immediately send it to the laboratory.

After

- Apply pressure to the venipuncture site.
- **PT** Tell the patient that usually a normal diet may be resumed.

Abnormal findings

▲ **Increased levels**
Essential hypertension
Malignant hypertension
Renovascular hypertension
Chronic renal failure
Salt-losing gastrointestinal disease (e.g., diarrhea)
Addison disease
Renin-producing renal tumor
Bartter syndrome
Cirrhosis
Hyperkalemia
Hemorrhage
Hypovolemia

▼ **Decreased levels**
Primary hyperaldosteronism
Steroid therapy
Congenital adrenal hyperplasia
Chronic renal impairment
Hypervolemia
Ectopic ACTH syndrome

notes

reticulocyte count (Retic count)

Type of test Blood

Normal findings

Reticulocyte count:
   Adult/elderly/child: 0.5%-2%
   Infant: 0.5%-3.1%
   Newborn: 2.5%-6.5%
Reticulocyte index: 1.0

Test explanation and related physiology

The reticulocyte count is a test for determining bone marrow function and evaluating erythropoietic activity. This test is also useful in classifying anemias. A reticulocyte is an immature red blood cell (RBC) that can be readily identified under a microscope. Normally there are a small number of reticulocytes in the bloodstream.

The reticulocyte count gives an indication of RBC production by the bone marrow. Increased reticulocyte counts indicate that the marrow is putting an increased number of RBCs into the bloodstream, usually in response to anemia. A normal or low reticulocyte count in a patient with anemia indicates that the marrow response to the anemia by way of production of RBCs is inadequate and perhaps contributing to or the cause of the anemia (as in aplastic anemia, iron deficiency, vitamin B_{12} deficiency, or depletion of iron stores). An elevated reticulocyte count found in patients with a normal hemogram indicates increased RBC production compensating for an ongoing loss of RBCs (hemolysis or hemorrhage).

Because the reticulocyte count is a percentage of the total number of RBCs, a normal to low number of reticulocytes can appear high in the anemic patient, because the total number of mature RBCs is low. To determine whether a reticulocyte count indicates an appropriate erythropoietic (RBC marrow) response in patients with anemia and a decreased hematocrit, one should calculate the *reticulocyte index*:

Reticulocyte index =

$$\text{Reticulocyte count (in\%)} \times \frac{\text{Patient's hematocrit}}{\text{Normal hematocrit}}$$

The reticulocyte index in a patient with a good marrow response to the anemia should be 1.0. If it is below 1.0, even though the reticulocyte count is elevated, the bone marrow response is inadequate in its ability to compensate.

Interfering factors

- Pregnancy may cause an increased reticulocyte count.
- RBCs containing Howell-Jolly bodies look like reticulocytes and can be miscounted by some automated counter machines to be reticulocytes and give a falsely high number of reticulocytes.

Procedure and patient care

- See inside front cover for Routine Blood Testing.
- Fasting: no.
- Blood tube commonly used: lavender.

Abnormal findings

▲ Increased levels
  Hemolytic anemia
  Sickle cell anemia
  Hemorrhage (3 to 4 days
    later)
  Postsplenectomy
  Hemolytic disease of the
    newborn
  Pregnancy
  Leukemias
  Recovery from nutritional
    anemias

▼ Decreased levels
  Pernicious anemia
  Folic acid deficiency
  Iron deficiency anemia
  Adrenocortical hypofunction
  Aplastic anemia
  Radiation therapy
  Marrow failure
  Anterior pituitary
    hypofunction
  Chronic infection
  Cirrhosis
  Malignancy

notes

rheumatoid factor (RF)

Type of test Blood

Normal findings

Negative (<60 units/mL by nephelometric testing)
(Elderly patients may have slightly increased values.)

Test explanation and related physiology

Rheumatoid arthritis (RA) is a chronic inflammatory disease that affects most joints, especially the metacarpal and phalangeal joints, the proximal interphalangeal joints, and the wrists; however, any synovial joint can be involved.

In this disease, abnormal immunoglobulin G (IgG) antibodies produced by lymphocytes in the synovial membranes act as antigens. Other IgG and IgM antibodies in the patient's serum react with the fc component of the abnormal synovial antigenic IgG to produce immune complexes. These immune complexes activate the complement system and other inflammatory systems to cause joint damage. The reactive IgM is called *RF*. Tissues other than the joints, including those of the blood vessels, lungs, nerves, and heart, may also be involved in the autoimmune inflammation.

Tests for RF are directed toward identification of the IgM antibodies. The exact role, if any, that RF plays in the pathophysiology of the disease is not well known. Approximately 80% of patients with RA have positive RF titers. To be considered positive, RF must be found in a dilution of greater than 1:80; when RF is found in titers less than 1:80, such diseases as systemic lupus erythematosus, scleroderma, and other autoimmune conditions should be considered. Although the normal value is "no rheumatoid factor identifiable at low titers," a small number of normal patients will have RF present at a very low titer. Furthermore, a negative RF does not exclude the diagnosis of RA. RF is not a useful disease marker because its presence does not disappear in patients who are experiencing a remission from the disease symptoms.

Other autoimmune diseases (see Table 1, p. 87), such as systemic lupus erythematosus and Sjögren syndrome, also may cause a positive RF test. RF is occasionally seen in patients with tuberculosis, chronic hepatitis, infectious mononucleosis, and subacute bacterial endocarditis as well.

R

Interfering factors

- Elderly patients often have false-positive results.
- Hemolysis or lipemia may be associated with false-positive results.

Procedure and patient care

- See inside front cover for Routine Blood Testing.
- Fasting: no.
- Blood tube commonly used: red.

Abnormal findings

▲ **Increased levels**

Rheumatoid arthritis

Other autoimmune diseases (e.g., systemic lupus erythematosus)

Chronic viral infection

Subacute bacterial endocarditis

Tuberculosis

Chronic hepatitis

Dermatomyositis

Scleroderma

Infectious mononucleosis

Leukemia

Cirrhosis

Syphilis

Renal disease

notes

ribosome P antibodies (Ribosomal P Ab, Anti–ribosome P antibodies)

Type of test Blood

Normal findings Negative

Test explanation and related physiology

This antibody test should not be confused with the anti-extractable nuclear antibodies (antiribonucleoprotein antibody, p. 75). Ribosome P antibodies are used as an adjunct in the evaluation of patients with lupus erythematosus (LE). Antibodies to ribosome P proteins are considered highly specific for LE and have been reported in patients with central nervous system (CNS) involvement (i.e., lupus psychosis). This antibody is therefore an aid in the differential diagnosis of neuropsychiatric symptoms in patients with LE. Because patients with LE may manifest signs and symptoms of CNS diseases, including neuropsychiatric symptoms, the presence of antibodies to ribosome P protein may be useful in the differential diagnosis of such patients. Most patients with LE do not have detectable levels of antibodies to ribosome P protein. But when they do, CNS involvement should be considered possible.

Procedure and patient care

- See inside front cover for Routine Blood Testing.
- Fasting: no.
- Blood tube commonly used: red.
- Check the venipuncture site for infection. Patients with autoimmune disease have compromised immune systems.

Abnormal findings

▲ **Increased levels**

Lupus erythematosus

notes

R

rubella antibody test (German measles test)

Type of test Blood

Normal findings

Method	Result	Interpretation
HAI titer	<1:8	No immunity to rubella
HAI titer	>1:20	Immune to rubella
LA	Negative	No immunity to rubella
ELISA IgM	<0.9 IU/mL	No infection
ELISA IgM	>1.1 IU/mL	Active infection
ELISA IgG	<7 IU/mL	No immunity to rubella
ELISA IgG	>10 IU/mL	Immune to rubella

LA, Latex agglutination; *ELISA*, enzyme-linked immunosorbent assay; *HAI*, hemagglutination inhibition.

Possible critical values Evidence of susceptibility in pregnant women with recent exposure to rubella

Test explanation and related physiology

Screening for rubella antibodies is done to detect immunity to rubella. These tests detect the presence of immunoglobulin G (IgG) and/or IgM antibodies to rubella (the causative agent for German measles). They become elevated a few days to a few weeks after the onset of the rash, depending on what method of testing is used. IgM tends to disappear after about 6 weeks. IgG, however, persists at low but detectable levels for years. These antibodies become elevated in patients with active rubella infection or with past infections.

In the past decade, children have been vaccinated with rubella to prevent the effects of the disease and to minimize infection. Rubella testing documents immunity to rubella. Rubella immunity testing is suggested for all health care workers. Most importantly, however, it is done to verify the presence or absence of rubella immunity in pregnant women, because congenital rubella infection in the first trimester of pregnancy is associated with congenital abnormalities of the fetus (heart defects, brain damage, deafness), abortion, or stillbirth. The term TORCH (toxoplasmosis, other, rubella, cytomegalovirus, herpes) has been applied to infections with recognized detrimental effects on the fetus. The effects on the fetus may be direct or indirect (e.g., precipitating abortion or premature labor). All of these tests are discussed separately (see separate listings).

If the woman's titer is greater than 1:10 to 1:20, she is not susceptible to rubella. If the woman's titer is 1:8 or less, she has little or no immunity to rubella. A fourfold increase in HAI rubella titer from the acute to the convalescent titer indicates that the rash was caused by an active rubella infection. Alternatively, an IgM antibody titer could be done. If the titer is positive, recent infection has occurred. IgM titers appear 1 to 2 days after onset of the rash and disappear 5 to 6 weeks after infection.

Antirubella antibody testing is also used to diagnose rubella in infants (congenital rubella). IgM antirubella antibodies cannot pass through the placenta. If an infant has IgM antibodies, acute congenital or newborn rubella is suspected. Antibody testing is often used in children with congenital abnormalities that may have come from congenital rubella infection.

Procedure and patient care

- See inside front cover for Routine Blood Testing.
- Fasting: no.
- Blood tube commonly used: red.
- **PT** Inform the patient when to return for a follow-up HAI titer if indicated.

Abnormal findings

Active rubella infection
Previous rubella infection leading to immunity

notes

R

salivary gland nuclear imaging (Parotid gland nuclear imaging)

Type of test Nuclear medicine

Normal findings Normal function of the salivary gland. No tumor or duct obstruction.

Test explanation and related physiology

The ability of the epithelial cells of the salivary glands to transport large pertechnetate ions from the blood and to secrete them into the saliva provides the principle for imaging the salivary glands. The functional capabilities, structural integrity, and location of the glands can be assessed. Usually, the parotid gland alone is visualized. Occasionally, the submandibular glands can be seen.

Indications for salivary gland nuclear imaging include patients with the following:

- Xerostomia (dry mouth)
- Pain
- Tumors
- Possible parotid duct obstruction

By following the radionuclide immediately after injection, blood flow can be evaluated. In about 10 minutes after injection, gland function becomes obvious by uptake of the radionuclide into the gland. Five to 10 minutes later, one should see secretion of nuclear material into the mouth. Washout demonstrates complete salivary gland excretion. Usually the patient is asked to suck on a lemon to encourage rapid washout. This test can indicate inflammation; hypofunction; location and character of tumors; and duct obstruction.

Contraindications

- Patients who are pregnant, unless the benefits outweigh the risks

Interfering factors

- Rinsing the mouth prior to study may reduce excretion.

Procedure and patient care

Before

PT Explain the procedure to the patient.

PT Tell the patient that no specific preparation is necessary.

- Make certain that the patient does not receive any thyroid-blocking agents within 48 hours of testing.

During

- Tc-99m pertechnetate is injected into the antecubital vein.
- Dynamic planar images are obtained immediately.
- Repeat images are obtained every 3 to 5 minutes for a total of 15 to 20 minutes.
- Three-dimensional images are often obtained by using SPECT/CT imaging.
- Administer a salivary gland stimulant after completion of static images. Either lemon juice or a lemon slice should be swished in the mouth and then expectorated.
- Washout images are obtained 5 to 10 minutes after the salivary gland stimulant. The thyroid gland is included for reference/comparison.

After

PT Assure the patient that the dose of radioactive technetium used in this test is minute and therefore harmless. No isolation or special urine precautions are needed.

Abnormal findings

Sjögren syndrome

Benign mixed tumors/pleomorphic adenomas

Malignant lesions (e.g., adenocarcinomas, squamous cell carcinomas, undifferentiated and mixed carcinomas)

Salivary duct obstruction

notes

S

SARS viral testing

Type of test Blood; fluid analysis

Normal findings No SARS virus

Test explanation and related physiology

Severe acute respiratory syndrome, or SARS, is caused by a coronavirus (CoV). China's southern Guangdong province, which includes Hong Kong, was believed to be the source of the virus. The incubation period is about 8 to 10 days. Symptoms are similar to any pneumonia (fever, chills, and cough). The diagnosis should be suspected in a symptomatic patient who lives in or has traveled to an area having documented transmission of the illness. Routine testing for the SARS virus is not conducted unless a cluster of cases develops and health officials are able to rule out all other infectious agents.

The diagnosis can only be made with positive test results in the following situations with:

- One specimen tested on two occasions using the original clinical specimen on each occasion,
- Two clinical specimens from different sources (e.g., nasopharyngeal and stool), and
- Two clinical specimens collected from the same source on two different days (e.g., two nasopharyngeal aspirates).

Eight types of respiratory specimens may be collected for viral and/or bacterial diagnostics: (1) nasopharyngeal wash/aspirates, (2) nasopharyngeal swabs, (3) oropharyngeal swabs, (4) bronchoalveolar lavage, (5) tracheal aspirate, (6) pleural fluid tap, (7) sputum, and (8) postmortem tissue. A nasopharyngeal wash/aspirate is the specimen of choice for detection of most respiratory viruses.

Serum and blood (plasma) should be collected early in the illness. Both acute and convalescent serum specimens should be collected for antibody testing. To confirm or rule out SARS-CoV infection, it is important to collect convalescent serum specimens more than 28 days after the onset of illness.

Procedure and patient care

Before

PT Explain the procedure to the patient.

- Observe all universal precautions in handling the specimen.
- Observe strict isolation technique. This disease is contagious.

During

- To obtain a *nasopharyngeal wash/aspirate*, have the patient sit with the head tilted slightly backward. Instill 1 mL to 1.5 mL of nonbacteriostatic saline (pH 7.0) into one nostril. Flush a plastic catheter or tubing with 2 mL to 3 mL of saline. Insert the tubing into the nostril. Aspirate nasopharyngeal secretions. Repeat this procedure for the other nostril. Collect the specimens in sterile vials.
- To obtain a *nasopharyngeal* or *oropharyngeal swab*, use only sterile Dacron or rayon swabs with plastic shafts. Do not use a cotton swab or swabs with wooden sticks, as they may contain substances that inactivate some viruses and inhibit PCR testing. Insert the swab into the nostril. Leave the swab in place for a few seconds to absorb secretions. Swab both nostrils. (For *oropharyngeal culture*, swab the posterior pharynx and tonsillar areas, avoiding the tongue.)
- To collect *sputum*, educate the patient about the difference between sputum and oral secretions. Have the patient rinse the mouth with water and then expectorate deep-cough sputum directly into a sterile screw-cap sputum collection cup or sterile, dry container.
- To collect *blood*, collect whole blood in a serum separator tube for serum RT-PCR testing or for ELISA antibody testing. Collect blood in an EDTA (purple-top) tube for plasma testing.

After

- Provide acute care for respiratory illness.
- If shipping the specimen domestically, use cold packs to keep the sample at 4° C. If shipping internationally, pack in dry ice.

Abnormal findings

SARS

S

notes

scrotal ultrasound (Ultrasound of testes)

Type of test   Ultrasound

Normal findings   Normal size, shape, and configuration of the testicles

Test explanation and related physiology

Scrotal ultrasound is a noninvasive, nonionizing, rapid method for scrotal examination. Through the use of reflected sound waves, ultrasonography provides accurate visualization of the scrotum and its contents. Ultrasonography requires the emission of high-frequency sound waves from the transducer to penetrate the organ being studied. The sound waves are bounced back to the transducer and electronically converted into a pictorial image.

Present uses for scrotal ultrasound include:

- Evaluation of scrotal masses
- Measurement of testicular size
- Evaluation of scrotal trauma
- Evaluation of scrotal pain and identification of torsion of the testicle
- Evaluation of occult testicular neoplasm
- Surveillance of patients with prior primary or metastatic testicular neoplasms
- Follow-up for testicular infections
- Location of undescended testicles

The testicle and extratesticular intrascrotal tissues are examined. The accuracy of scrotal ultrasound is 90% to 95%. Both benign and malignant tumors can be identified with ultrasound. Benign abnormalities, such as testicular abscess, orchitis, testicular infarction, and testicular torsion, also can be identified. Extratesticular lesions, such as hydrocele (fluid in the scrotum), hematocele (blood in the scrotum), and pyocele (pus in the scrotum), can be identified. Scrotal and groin ultrasound has been very helpful in locating cryptorchid (undescended) testicles.

Ultrasonography of the scrotum is now the preferred method to identify torsion of the testicle. Ultrasonography is a very accurate method of identifying microlithiasis in the testicles. When identified, microcalcifications in the testicle indicate a marked increased risk for testicular cancer. Calcifications can also occur after orchitis or trauma. In most cases, both testicles are routinely imaged during the ultrasound exam.

The use of color Doppler is very helpful in determining blood flow to the testicle. If there is torsion of the testicle, color

Doppler will indicate markedly reduced blood flow; immediate surgical exploration would be required. Scrotal ultrasound has replaced scrotal nuclear imaging for the diagnosis of testicular torsion because results can be obtained immediately.

There is very little discomfort associated with testicular ultrasound. It is usually performed by an ultrasound technologist and interpreted by an ultrasound physician.

Procedure and patient care

Before

PT Explain the procedure to the patient.

PT Tell the patient that no fasting is required.

During

- Note the following procedural steps:
  1. Careful examination of the scrotum is performed by the physician. Usually a short history is obtained.
  2. The scrotum is supported by a towel or cradled by the examiner's gloved hand.
  3. A greasy, conductive paste is applied to the scrotum. This paste enhances sound wave transmission and reception.
  4. Thorough scanning in the sagittal, transverse, and oblique projections is performed.
- The test takes approximately 20 to 30 minutes.

After

- Remove the coupling agent from the patient's scrotum.

Abnormal findings

Benign testicular tumor
Malignant testicular tumor
Occult testicular tumor
Testicular infection (orchitis)
Hydrocele
Hematocele
Pyocele
Varicocele
Epididymitis
Spermatocele
Scrotal hernia
Cryptorchidism
Hematoma
Testicular torsion

S

notes

semen analysis (Sperm count, Sperm examination)

Type of test Fluid analysis

Normal findings

Volume: 2-5 mL
Liquefaction time: 20-30 minutes after collection
Appearance: Normal
Motile/mL: ≥10×10⁶
Sperm/mL: ≥20×10⁶
Viscosity: ≥3
Agglutination: ≥3
Supravital: ≥75% live
Fructose: Positive
pH: 7.12-8
Sperm count (density): ≥20 million/mL
Sperm motility: ≥50% at 1 hour
Sperm morphology: >30% (Kruger criteria >14%) normally shaped

Test explanation and related physiology

Semen analysis is one of the most important aspects of the fertility workup because the cause of a woman's inability to conceive often lies with the man. The freshly collected semen is first measured for volume. After liquefaction of the white, gelatinous ejaculate, a sperm count is done. Men with very low or very high counts likely are infertile. The motility of the sperm is then evaluated; at least 50% should show progressive motility. Morphology is studied by staining a semen preparation and calculating the number of normal versus abnormal sperm forms. The sperm specimen is considered abnormal if greater than 70% of the sperm have abnormal forms. A semen analysis should be done at least twice, and possibly a third time, 3 weeks apart.

More exhaustive semen analysis for male infertility may include a *sperm penetration assay (SPA)*, a multi-step laboratory test that offers a biological assessment of several aspects of human sperm fertilizing ability. *Hyaluronan binding assay (HBA)* is a qualitative assay used to determine the maturity of sperm in a fresh semen sample. The assay is based on the ability of mature, but not immature, sperm to bind to hyaluronan, the main mucopolysaccharide of the egg matrix and a component of human follicular fluid. A low level of sperm binding to hyaluronan suggests that there is a low proportion of mature sperm in the sample. Similar to the sperm penetration assay, it has been suggested that the HBA assay may be used to determine the need for an intracytoplasmic sperm injection procedure as part of an assisted reproductive technique.

Aside from the conventional parameters of sperm quality, such as concentration, motility, and morphology, sperm DNA integrity is a potential cause of idiopathic male infertility. Although sperm with fragmented DNA may be able to fertilize oocytes, subsequent embryo and fetal development may be impaired. DNA fragmentation in sperm increases with age. Flow cytometry tests of DNA integrity that are available include the *sperm chromatin structure assay test* and the *sperm DNA fragmentation assay (SDFA) test.*

Semen analysis is a measure of testicular function. Inadequate sperm production can be the result of primary gonadal failure (Klinefelter syndrome, infection, radiation, or surgical orchidectomy) or secondary gonadal failure (caused by pituitary diseases). Men with aspermia (no sperm) or oligospermia (less than 20 million/mL) should be evaluated endocrinologically for pituitary, thyroid, or testicular aberrations.

A normal semen analysis alone does not accurately assess the male factor unless the effect of the partner's cervical secretion on sperm survival is also determined (see Sims-Huhner test, p. 840). In addition to its value in infertility workups, semen analysis is also helpful in documenting adequate sterilization after a vasectomy. It is usually performed 6 weeks after the surgery.

Interfering factors

- ☑ Drugs that may cause *decreased* semen levels include antineoplastic agents (e.g., methotrexate), cimetidine, estrogens, and methyltestosterone.

Procedure and patient care

Before

- PT Explain the procedure to the patient.
- PT Instruct the patient to abstain from sexual activity for 2 to 3 days before collecting the specimen. Prolonged abstinence before the collection should be discouraged because the quality of the sperm cells, especially their motility, may diminish.
- • Give the patient the proper container for the sperm collection.
- PT Instruct the patient to avoid alcoholic beverages for several days before the collection.
- • For evaluation of the adequacy of vasectomy, the patient should ejaculate once or twice before the day of examination.

During

- Note that semen is best collected by ejaculation into a clean container. For the best results, the specimen should be collected in the physician's office or laboratory by masturbation.
- **PT** Note that less satisfactory specimens can be obtained in the patient's home by coitus interruptus or masturbation. Note the following procedural steps:
  1. Instruct the patient to deliver these home specimens to the laboratory within 1 hour after collection.
  2. Tell the patient to avoid excessive heat and cold during transportation of the specimen.

After

- Record the date of the previous semen emission along with the collection time and date of the fresh specimen.
- **PT** Tell the patient when and how to obtain the test results. Remember that abnormal results may have a devastating effect on the patient's sexuality.

Abnormal findings

Infertility
Vasectomy
Orchitis
Testicular atrophy
Testicular failure
Hyperpyrexia

notes

sentinel lymph node biopsy (SLNB, Lymphoscintigraphy)

Type of test   Nuclear scan

Normal findings   Uptake is noted in one or more lymph nodes. No tumor in the sentinel node.

Test explanation and related physiology

Lymphoscintigraphy is used to identify the sentinel lymph node, which is the first lymph node in line to catch metastasis from a nearby primary tumor. It is primarily used in breast cancer and melanoma. With this procedure, the sentinel node is identified and biopsied. This test is an important part of the standard treatment for breast and melanoma cancer surgery.

Contraindications

- Patients who have a large cancer in which lymph node metastasis is very likely
- Patients in early pregnancy unless the benefit outweighs the risk of damage to the fetus

Potential complications

- Anaphylaxis with injection of isosulfan blue dye

Procedure and patient care

Before

PT Explain the procedure to the patient.

- Because this is an operative procedure, routine preoperative nursing processes should be carried out, including obtaining operative consent, keeping the patient NPO, and surgical site preparation as ordered.

During

Note the following procedural steps:

1. After the injection of technetium, the lymph node drainage basin is then scanned immediately and 1 to 24 hours later.
2. In the operating room, a handheld gamma detector locates hot areas of radionuclide uptake in the lymph node–bearing area. The most proximal hot node is excised as the sentinel node.
3. When using isosulfan blue, 4 to 5 mL of dye is injected around the tumor. Several minutes later, the lymphatics are stained blue and can be identified for biopsy.

S

After

PT Inform the patient that no precautions are required if technetium is used because the radionuclide dose is minimal.

PT If isosulfan blue dye is used, the patient's skin may develop a transient blue hue (looking almost like severe cyanosis). This will dissipate over the next 6 hours.

PT Warn the patient that the urine will have a blue tinge as a result of the isosulfan blue dye injection.

• Observe the patient for signs of allergy (rare) caused by the blue dye injection.

Abnormal findings

Metastatic tumor to lymph node

notes

serotonin (5-hydroxytryptamine, 5-HT) and chromogranin A

Type of test   Blood

Normal findings

Chromogranin A: ≤225 ng/mL
Serotonin: ≤230 ng/mL

Test explanation and related physiology

Serotonin is synthesized from the essential amino acid tryptophan chiefly in the gastrointestinal enterochromaffin cells (EC-cells). Many different stimuli can release serotonin from EC-cells. After it is secreted, in concert with other gut hormones, serotonin increases GI blood flow, motility, and fluid secretion. On the first pass through the liver, 30% to 80% of serotonin is metabolized, predominately to 5-hydroxyindoleacetic acid (5-HIAA) (p. 543), which is then excreted by the kidneys.

The main diseases that may be associated with measurable increases in serotonin are neuroectodermal tumors, in particular tumors arising from EC-cells. These tumors are collectively referred to as *carcinoids*. They are divided into *foregut* carcinoids, arising from the respiratory tract, stomach, pancreas, or duodenum (approximately 15% of cases); *midgut* carcinoids, occurring in the jejunum, ileum, or appendix (approximately 70% of cases); and *hindgut* carcinoids, which are found in the colon or rectum (approximately 15% of cases).

Carcinoids display a spectrum of aggressiveness with no clear distinguishing line between benign and malignant. The majority of carcinoid tumors do not cause significant clinical symptoms. Most symptoms are caused by elevated serotonins (carcinoid syndrome). The carcinoid syndrome consists of flushing, diarrhea, right-sided valvular heart lesions, and bronchoconstriction. The carcinoid syndrome is usually caused by midgut tumors. Because midgut tumors drain into the liver, nearly all of the serotonin is metabolized on first pass. Carcinoid symptoms, therefore, do not usually occur until liver or other distant metastases have developed, which bypass the hepatic metabolism.

Diagnosis of carcinoid tumors with symptoms suggestive of carcinoid syndrome rests on measurements of serum serotonin, urinary 5-HIAA (p. 543), and serum chromogranin A (a peptide that is cosecreted alongside serotonin by the neuroectodermal cells). Metastasizing midgut carcinoid tumors usually produce blood or serum serotonin concentrations greater than 1000 ng/mL.

S

It is usually impossible to diagnose small carcinoid tumors (>95% of cases) without any symptoms suggestive of carcinoid syndrome by measurement of serotonin, 5-HIAA, or chromogranin A. It is only after carcinoid tumors metastasize that serotonin becomes detectable.

Disease progression can be monitored in patients with serotonin-producing carcinoid tumors by measurement of serotonin or chromogranin A in blood. However, at levels above approximately 5000 ng/mL, there is no longer a linear relationship between tumor burden and blood serotonin levels. Urinary 5-HIAA and serum chromogranin A continue to increase in proportion to the tumor burden.

Chromogranin A also acts as a useful diagnostic marker for other neuroendocrine neoplasms, including the following: carcinoids; pheochromocytomas; neuroblastomas; medullary thyroid carcinomas; some pituitary tumors; functioning and nonfunctioning islet-cell tumors; and other amine precursor uptake and decarboxylation (APUD) tumors. It can also serve as a sensitive means for detecting residual or recurrent disease in treated patients. Carcinoid tumors, in particular colon and rectal carcinoids, almost always secrete chromogranin A.

Interfering factors

- Drugs that may cause *increased* serotonin levels include lithium, MAO inhibitors, methyldopa, morphine, and reserpine.
- Drugs that *decrease* serotonin levels include selective serotonin reuptake inhibitors (e.g., fluoxetine).

Procedure and patient care

- See inside front cover for Routine Blood Testing.
- Fasting: no.
- Blood tube commonly used: red.

Abnormal findings

▲ **Increased levels**
  Carcinoid tumors
  Neuroendocrine tumors
  Pheochromocytoma
  Small cell lung cancer

notes

sexual assault testing

Type of test Blood; fluid analysis

Normal findings No physical evidence of sexual assault

Test explanation and related physiology

The sexual assault victim needs to have psycho-emotional support, treatment of any physical injuries, and accurate and reliable evidentiary testing. Acute care centers have protocols in place that provide care to victims of sexual assault. Furthermore, in most circumstances, there are nurses specifically trained in obtaining the appropriate specimens. This person knows the importance of following the chain of evidence protocols to ensure that evidence is admissible in court.

The patient is first interviewed in a nonjudgmental manner. A thorough gynecologic history is obtained. A brief summary of the assault (if there was vaginal, oral, or anal penetration during the assault) and timing of the assault are important. After 72 hours, very little evidence still exists. It is important to ascertain whether the victim changed clothing, showered, or used a douche before coming to the hospital. These will affect the presence of evidence. The general demeanor of the patient, status of the clothing, and physical maturation assessment are documented.

The victim's clothes are removed and separately placed in a paper bag for possible DNA sources from the victim's or assailant's body parts. Plastic bags are not used because bacteria can grow in them and can destroy DNA. Photographs of all injuries should be obtained if possible. The victim is then examined for signs of external and internal injuries, and a pelvic exam performed. A *sexual assault evidence collection kit* is used to obtain all the needed specimens. The directions must be carefully followed to ensure all evidence is obtained and is useful toward identification and conviction of the perpetrator.

Vaginal secretions are obtained for sperm (p. 818) or other cells from the assailant. Acid phosphatase (p. 7) or PSA (p. 756) are also obtained using this specimen. Cervical secretions are obtained for sexually transmitted disease (STD) testing (p. 828). These anatomic areas, along with the anorectal area, are swabbed. In the male victim, penile and anorectal areas are swabbed. Pubic hair is obtained by combing or plucking. STD testing would include syphilis (p. 877), trichomoniasis (p. 825), gonorrhea (p. 825), and chlamydia (p. 243). Later, blood testing for human immunodeficiency virus (HIV, p. 521) and pregnancy (p. 530) is obtained.

S

Next, blood specimens are obtained for DNA testing per the testing kit directions, usually in an EDTA-containing tube (lavender top). More blood or urine also may be collected for evidence of mind-altering drugs/alcohol or STDs. After this testing, a more detailed examination of the vagina, cervix, and rectum is performed using a Wood lamp to more easily identify saliva or sperm from the assailant. These areas are examined for subtle injuries from forced penetration. Two methods used to identify these injuries are the *toluidine blue dye test* and a colposcope (p. 274). The toluidine blue dye test also can be used to identify recent or healed genital or anorectal injuries. A 1% aqueous solution is applied to the area of concern and washed off with a lubricant (e.g., K-Y jelly) or a 1% acetic acid solution. Injured mucosa will retain the dye and become more apparent to the naked eye. Finally, the fingernails are scraped underneath, which may potentially contain tissue from the assailant. Upon completion of the exam, the victim is usually interviewed by the police.

Unless medically contraindicated, all victims should be offered antimicrobial therapy to prevent STDs. The use of antiretroviral drugs in the prevention of HIV transmission may be recommended, and the current guideline for postexposure prophylaxis after needlestick injuries should be used. It may also be advisable to offer victims a hepatitis B vaccination or hepatitis B immunoglobulin.

A pregnancy test should be done. If there is a risk of pregnancy, the victim should be offered postcoital contraception if the rape occurred less than 72 hours before examination. If it occurred more than 72 hours but less than 7 days before the examination, an intrauterine contraceptive device may be used to prevent pregnancy. Pregnancy testing may be repeated during the week after the rape.

Contraindications

• The patient is emotionally unable to undergo testing.

Interfering factors

• Delays in examination after the alleged attack diminish the possibility of identifying meaningful evidence.

Procedure and patient care

Before

PT Explain the procedure and provide emotional support.

• Obtain consent to treat the patient.

- Assess the patient's emotional condition and determine if the victim is able to undergo sexual assault testing.

During

- Use the SAPS sexual assault evidence collection kit (SAECK) or similar test kit exactly as described to maintain the chain of evidence. See Box 6 below.
- Properly handle specimens to maintain the chain of custody.
- Refrigerate all blood and urine samples containing biological evidentiary material, such as DNA, to prevent putrefaction.
- It is important to examine carefully all areas of the body to help corroborate the victim's version of the alleged events.

After

- Notify police of the alleged assault.
- Assess the patient's need for urgent counseling support and make arrangements as needed.

BOX 6   DNA evidence collection: special precautions

To avoid contamination of evidence that may contain DNA, the special sexual assault kit should be used and the following precautions taken:
- Wear gloves and change them often.
- Use disposable instruments or clean them thoroughly before and after handling each sample.
- Avoid touching any area where you believe DNA may be present.
- Avoid talking, sneezing, or coughing over evidence.
- Avoid touching your face, nose, and mouth when collecting and packaging evidence.
- Keep evidence such as clothing and underwear dry, and transport it at room temperature.
- Ensure that the chain of custody is maintained at all times.

Abnormal findings

Rape
Sexual assault

notes

sexually transmitted disease testing (STD testing)

Type of test Microscopic examination

Normal findings No evidence of STD

Test explanation and related physiology

In the United States, common sexually transmitted diseases (STDs) include *Chlamydia*, genital herpes (herpes simplex virus), human papilloma virus (HPV), syphilis, human immunodeficiency virus (HIV), trichomonas, and gonorrhea (Table 32). In this test discussion, we will concentrate on *Trichomonas vaginalis* and *Neisseria gonorrhoeae*, as all others are discussed elsewhere in this reference book. Early identification of STDs enables sexual partners to obtain treatment as soon as possible and thereby reduce the risk of disease spread. Furthermore, prompt treatment reduces the risk of infertility in women. If the STD result is positive, sexual partners should be evaluated and treated. Performing STD testing is also part of the prenatal workup.

TABLE 32 Sexually transmitted diseases (STDs) and methods of diagnosis

Disease	Method of diagnosis
Gonorrhea	Cervical, urethral, anal, oropharyngeal cultures
Chlamydia Lymphogranuloma venereum *C. trachomatis*	Cervical and urethral cultures, serology, DNA probe testing (p. 243)
Herpes genitalis	Culture from lesion, serology (p. 510)
Syphilis	Serology, fluid cultures (CNS), darkfield slide (p. 877)
Hepatitis	Serology, nucleic acid testing (p. 505)
HIV	Serologic, virologic, nucleic acid testing (pp. 521, 517)
Trichomonas vaginalis	Cervical and urethral cultures, urine, ThinPrep PAP, serology, nucleic amplification tests
Candida	Wet mount, fungal culture
Gardnerella vaginalis	Cervical, urethral, anal cultures

T. vaginalis is a protozoan parasite that commonly infects the genital tract of men and women. Although 70% of infected individuals are asymptomatic, *Trichomonas* can cause urethritis, vaginitis, endometritis, pelvic inflammatory disease, pharyngitis, proctitis, epididymitis, prostatitis, and salpingitis. Children born of infected mothers may develop conjunctivitis, pneumonia, neonatal blindness, or neonatal neurologic injury and may even die. The most commonly used method for detection is microscopic examination of a wet-mount preparation of vaginal secretions. However, this method has only a 35% to 80% sensitivity. Culture of urethral or vaginal secretions also suffers from relatively low sensitivity. Culture is technically challenging and takes 5 to 7 days to complete. Molecular methods of testing urethral and vaginal secretions offer high sensitivity and specificity for detection of trichomoniasis.

Gonorrhea is caused by the bacterium *N. gonorrhoeae*. Many infections in women are asymptomatic. This organism causes genitourinary infections in women and men and may be associated with dysuria and vaginal, urethral, or rectal discharge. Complications include pelvic inflammatory disease in women and gonococcal epididymitis and prostatitis in men. Because infection in men is commonly associated with symptoms, screening of asymptomatic patients is not indicated. However, in light of the risk for asymptomatic infection in women, screening is recommended for women at high risk for infection. High-risk women include women with previous gonorrhea or other STD, inconsistent condom use, and new or multiple sex partners and women in certain demographic groups such as those in communities with high STD prevalence.

Culture was previously considered to be the gold standard test for diagnosis of *N. gonorrhoeae* infection. Yet successful culture methods are difficult. Molecular laboratory methods, such as polymerase chain reaction and nucleic acid amplification testing (NAAT), performed on urethral, rectal, vaginal, or oropharyngeal secretions provide superior sensitivity and specificity.

To obtain an appropriate specimen for women, swabs (that are sometimes specific to the particular laboratory) are obtained from the endocervix, vagina, urethra, urine, or a Pap ThinPrep. For men, a swab of the urethra or a urine specimen is used for testing. Rectal and throat swabs are performed in persons who have engaged in anal and oral intercourse. Because rectal gonorrhea accompanies genital gonorrhea in a high percentage of women, rectal cultures are recommended in all women with suspected gonorrhea. If the STD culture result is positive, treatment during pregnancy can prevent possible fetal complications (e.g., ophthalmia neonatorum) and maternal complications. Rectal and orogastric specimens should be performed on the neonates of infected mothers.

STD cultures and smears are obtained by a physician or nurse in several minutes during a pelvic examination. Very little discomfort is associated with these procedures.

Interfering factors

- *N. gonorrhoeae* is very sensitive to lubricants and disinfectants.
- Menses may alter test results.
- In women, douching within 24 hours before a cervical culture makes fewer organisms available for culture.
- In men, voiding within 1 hour before a urethral culture washes secretions out of the urethra.
- Fecal material may contaminate an anal culture.
- Blood, lubricants, and spermicides do not significantly interfere with test results.

Procedure and patient care

Before

PT Explain the purpose and procedure to the patient. Use a matter-of-fact, nonjudgmental approach.

PT Tell the patient that no fasting or sedation is required.

During

Cervical culture

1. The female patient is told to refrain from douching and tub bathing before the cervical culture.
2. The patient is placed in the lithotomy position, and a moistened, unlubricated vaginal speculum is inserted to expose the cervix (see Figure 32, p. 683).
3. Excess cervical mucus is removed with a cotton ball held in a ring forceps.
4. A sterile cotton-tipped swab is inserted into the endocervical canal and moved from side to side to obtain the specimen.
5. The swab is placed in sterile saline or a transporting fluid obtained from the laboratory. The specimen should be plated as soon as possible. The specimen should not be refrigerated.

Anal canal culture

1. An anal culture of the female or male patient is taken by inserting a sterile, cotton-tipped swab approximately 1 inch into the anal canal (Figure 39).
2. If stool contaminates the swab, a repeat swab is taken.

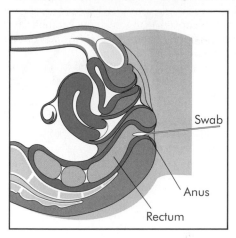

FIGURE 39 Rectal culture of the female. Method for obtaining an anorectal culture for sexually transmitted diseases in a female patient.

Oropharyngeal culture
1. This culture should be obtained in male and female patients who have engaged in oral intercourse.
2. A throat culture is best obtained by depressing the patient's tongue with a wooden tongue blade and touching the posterior wall of the throat with a sterile cotton-tipped swab.

Urethral culture
1. The urethral specimen should be obtained from the male patient before he voids. Voiding within 1 hour before collection washes secretions out of the urethra, making fewer organisms available for culture. The best time to obtain the specimen is before the first morning micturition.
2. A culture is taken by inserting a sterile swab gently into the anterior urethra (Figure 40).
3. It is advisable to place the male patient in the supine position to prevent falling if vasovagal syncope occurs during introduction of the cotton swab or wire loop into the urethra.
4. The patient is observed for hypotension, bradycardia, pallor, sweating, nausea, and weakness.
5. In a male patient, prostatic massage may increase the chances of obtaining positive cultures.

S

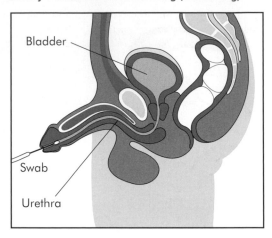

FIGURE 40 Urethral culture of the male. Method for obtaining a urethral culture for sexually transmitted diseases in a male patient.

Urine culture

Obtain the first catch voided specimen in the female patient. (Urine cultures for STD are not helpful in male patients.) A small quantity of urine is placed in the transporting fluid or sterile empty container obtained from the laboratory.

Pap smear ThinPrep (see page 680)

After

- Place the swabs for gonorrhea in a Thayer-Martin medium and roll them from side to side.
- Label and send the culture bottle to the microbiology laboratory.
- Transport the specimen to the laboratory as soon as possible.
- Handle all specimens as though they were capable of transmitting disease.
- Do not refrigerate the specimen.
- Mark the laboratory slip with the collection time, date, source of specimen, patient's age, current antibiotic therapy, and clinical diagnosis.
- **PT** Advise the patient to avoid intercourse and all sexual contact until test results are available.

PT If the culture results are positive, tell the patient to receive treatment and to have sexual partners evaluated.

• Note that repeat cultures should be taken after completion of treatment to evaluate therapy.

Abnormal findings

Sexually transmitted diseases

notes

S

sialography

Type of test X-ray

Normal findings No evidence of pathology in the salivary ducts and related structures

Test explanation and related physiology

Sialography is an x-ray procedure used to examine the salivary ducts (parotid, submaxillary, submandibular, and sublingual) and related glandular structures after injection of a contrast medium into the desired duct. This procedure is used to detect calculi, strictures, tumors, or inflammatory disease in patients who complain of pain, tenderness, or swelling in these areas.

Contraindications

- Patients with mouth infections

Potential complications

- Allergic reaction to the iodinated dye
  This rarely occurs because the dye is not administered intravenously.

Procedure and patient care

Before

- **PT** Explain the procedure to the patient. The thought of a dye injection in the mouth is frightening to many patients. Provide emotional support.
- Obtain informed consent if required by the institution.
- **PT** Instruct the patient to remove jewelry, hairpins, and dentures, which could obscure x-ray visualization.
- **PT** Instruct the patient to rinse his or her mouth with an antiseptic solution before the procedure to reduce the possibility of introducing bacteria into the ductal structures.

During

- Note the following procedural steps:
  1. X-ray studies are taken before the dye injection to ensure that stones are not present, which could prevent the contrast material from entering the ducts.
  2. The patient is placed in a supine position on an x-ray table.
  3. The contrast medium is injected directly into the desired orifice via a cannula or a special catheter.
  4. X-ray images are taken with the patient in various positions.

5. The patient is given a sour substance (e.g., lemon juice) orally to stimulate salivary excretion.
6. Another of x-ray studies is taken to evaluate ductal drainage.

- Note that a radiologist performs this procedure in the radiology department in less than 30 minutes.

PT Tell the patient that he or she may feel a little pressure as the contrast medium is injected into the ducts.

After

PT Encourage the patient to drink fluids to eliminate the dye.

Abnormal findings

Calculi
Strictures
Tumor
Inflammatory disease

notes

S

sickle cell screen (Sickledex, Hemoglobin [Hgb] S test)

Type of test Blood

Normal findings No sickle cells present or no Hgb S identified

Test explanation and related physiology

Both sickle cell disease (homozygous for Hgb S) and sickle cell trait (heterozygous for Hgb S) can be detected by this screening study. Sickle cell anemia results from a genetic homozygous defect and is caused by the presence of Hgb S instead of Hgb A. When Hgb S becomes deoxygenated, it tends to bend in a way that causes the red blood cell (RBC) to assume a sickle shape. These sickled RBCs cannot freely pass through the capillaries, and thus they cause plugging of the microvascular tree. This may compromise the blood supply to various organs. Hgb S is found in varying quantities in 8% to 10% of the black population.

The *Sickledex test* is a blood test that is positive if greater than 10% of the hemoglobin is Hgb S. This test is only a screening test, and its sensitivity varies according to the method used by the laboratory. Double heterozygosity for sickle trait when combined with another hemoglobinopathy (e.g., Hgb C disease) can cause a sickling disease. The definitive diagnosis of sickle cell disease or trait is made by Hgb electrophoresis (p. 502) or high-pressure liquid chromatography, in which Hgb S can be identified and quantified. Immunoassay methods using monoclonal antibodies are also being used to quantify Hgb S.

Interfering factors

- Any blood transfusions within 3 to 4 months before the sickle cell test may cause false-negative results because the donor's normal hemoglobin may dilute the recipient's abnormal Hgb S.
- Polycythemia or paraproteinemias may cause false-positive solubility results.
- Infants younger than 3 months may have false-negative results.
- ☑ Phenothiazines may cause false-negative results.

Procedure and patient care

- See inside front cover for Routine Blood Testing.
- Fasting: no.
- Blood tube commonly used: lavender.
- If the test is positive, further definitive testing should be performed.

PT Inform patients with sickle cell anemia that they should avoid situations in which hypoxia may occur (e.g., strenuous exercise, air travel in unpressurized aircraft, travel to high-altitude regions).

Abnormal findings

Sickle cell trait
Sickle cell anemia

notes

S

sigmoidoscopy (Proctoscopy, Anoscopy)

Type of test Endoscopy

Normal findings Normal anus, rectum, and sigmoid colon

Test explanation and related physiology

Endoscopy of the lower gastrointestinal (GI) tract is used to visualize and perform biopsies of tumors, polyps, hemorrhoids, or ulcers of the anus, rectum, and sigmoid colon. *Anoscopy* refers to examination of the anus; *proctoscopy* to examination of the anus and rectum; and *sigmoidoscopy* (the most frequent procedure) to examination of the anus, rectum, and sigmoid colon. This test can be performed with a rigid or flexible sigmoidoscope.

Furthermore, sigmoidoscopy, as with colonoscopy, can be therapeutic. Reduction of sigmoid volvulus, removal of polyps, and obliteration of hemorrhoids can be performed through the sigmoidoscope.

Contraindications

- Patients with diverticulitis
- Patients with painful anorectal conditions
- Patients with severe bleeding
- Patients suspected of having perforated colon lesions

Potential complications

- Perforation of the colon
- Bleeding from biopsy sites

Interfering factors

- Poor bowel preparation may obscure visualization.
- Rectal bleeding may preclude adequate visualization.

Procedure and patient care

Before

PT Explain the procedure to the patient.
- Obtain informed consent for this procedure.
- Assist the patient with bowel preparation. In most cases, two Fleet enemas are sufficient.
PT Instruct the patient to ingest only a light breakfast on the morning of the endoscopy.

During

- Note the following procedural steps:
    1. The patient is placed on the endoscopy table or bed in the left lateral decubitus position. Physicians often prefer the

knee-chest position. This procedure also can be performed with the patient in the lithotomy position.

2. Usually no sedation is required.
3. The anus is mildly dilated with a well-lubricated finger.
4. The rigid or flexible sigmoidoscope is placed into the rectum and advanced to the point of maximal penetration.
5. Air is insufflated during the procedure to distend more fully the lower intestinal tract.
6. The sigmoid, rectum, and anus are visualized.
7. Biopsies can be obtained and polypectomy performed.

- Note that a physician trained in GI endoscopy usually performs this procedure in the GI laboratory, operating room, patient's bedside, or outpatient clinic setting in approximately 15 to 20 minutes.

PT Tell the patient that he or she probably will feel discomfort and the urge to defecate as the sigmoidoscope is inserted.

After

PT Inform the patient that because air has been insufflated into the bowel during the procedure, he or she may have flatulence or gas pains. Ambulation may help.

- Observe the patient for signs of abdominal distention, increased tenderness, or rectal bleeding.
- Note that fever, chills, and increasing abdominal pain may indicate a bowel perforation.

PT Inform the patient that frequent, bloody bowel movements or rectal bleeding may indicate poor hemostasis if biopsy or polypectomy was performed.

Abnormal findings

Tumor (benign or malignant)
Polyps
Ulcerative colitis
Pseudomembranous colitis
Crohn disease
Intestinal ischemia
Irritable bowel syndrome

notes

Sims-Huhner test (Postcoital test, Postcoital cervical mucus test, Cervical mucus sperm penetration test)

Type of test   Fluid analysis

Normal findings

Cervical mucus adequate for sperm transmission, survival, and penetration

6 to 20 active sperm per high-power field

Test explanation and related physiology

The Sims-Huhner test consists of a postcoital examination of the cervical mucus to measure the ability of the sperm to penetrate the mucus and maintain motility. This test is used in the evaluation of infertile couples. It evaluates interaction between the sperm and the cervical mucus. It also measures the quality of the cervical mucus. This test can determine the effect of vaginal and cervical secretions on the activity of the sperm. It is performed only after a previously performed semen analysis has been determined to be normal.

This test is performed during the middle of the ovulatory cycle, because at this time the secretions should be optimal for sperm penetration and survival. During ovulation, the quantity of cervical mucus is maximal, whereas the viscosity is minimal, thus facilitating sperm penetration. The *endocervical mucus sample* is examined for color, viscosity, and tenacity *(spinnbarkeit)*. The fresh specimen is then spread on a clean glass slide and examined for the presence of sperm. Estimates of the total number of sperm and of the number of motile sperm per high-power field are reported. Normally 6 to 20 active sperm cells should be seen in each microscopic high-power field; if sperm are present but not active, the cervical environment is unsuitable (e.g., abnormal pH) for their survival.

After the specimen has dried on the glass slide, the mucus can be examined for *ferning*. This pattern is correlated with estrogen activity and is therefore present in all ovulatory women at midcycle. When the cervical mucus is checked again immediately before menstruation, no ferning is found because of progesterone activity. The Sims-Huhner study is invaluable in fertility examinations; however, it is not a substitute for the semen analysis. If the results of the Sims-Huhner test are less than optimal, the test is usually repeated during the same or next ovulatory cycle.

Procedure and patient care

Before

PT Explain the procedure to the patient.

PT Inform the patient that basal body temperature recordings should be used to indicate ovulation.

PT Tell the patient that no vaginal lubrication, douching, or bathing is permitted until after the vaginal cervical examination, because these factors will alter the cervical mucus.

PT Inform the patient that this study should be performed after 3 days of sexual abstinence.

PT Instruct the patient to remain in bed for 10 to 15 minutes after coitus to ensure cervical exposure to the semen. After resting, the patient should report to her physician for examination of her cervical mucus within 2 hours after coitus.

During

- Note that with the patient in the lithotomy position, the cervix is exposed by an unlubricated speculum. The specimen is aspirated from the endocervix and delivered to the laboratory for analysis.
- Note that this procedure is performed by a physician in approximately 5 minutes.

PT Tell the patient that the only discomfort associated with this study is insertion of the speculum.

After

PT Tell the patient how and when she may obtain the test results.

Abnormal findings

Infertility
Suspected rape

notes

S

> **skin biopsy** (Cutaneous immunofluorescence biopsy, Skin biopsy
> antibodies, Skin immunohistopathology, Direct immunofluorescence
> antibody test)

Type of test Microscopic examination

Normal findings

Normal skin histology
No evidence of IgG, IgA, or IgM antibody; complement C3; or
  fibrinogen

Test explanation and related physiology

Autoimmune skin diseases are associated with autoantibodies
in the skin and serum. Either can be tested (see antiscleroderma
antibody, page 91, and indirect immunofluorescence antibody).
Direct (testing for antibodies in the skin) immunofluorescence
antibody (IFA) is most specific and diagnostic. For this study,
a tissue specimen in or around the skin or mucosal lesion is
obtained and evaluated by routine histology and by IFA methods
for deposition of human immunoglobulins (IgG, IgA, or IgM),
complement C3, or fibrinogen components. This test is used to
evaluate, diagnose, and monitor treatment of immunologically
mediated dermatitis, such as pemphigoid, pemphigus, bullosa
acquisita, and bullous lupus erythematosus.

Procedure and patient care

Before

PT Explain the procedure to the patient.
• Obtain an informed consent.

During

• The skin area used for biopsy is surgically biopsied by usual
  technique.
• A 4-mm punch biopsy or elliptical tissue excision is obtained.

After

• Apply a dry, sterile dressing over the biopsy site.
PT Tell the patient that results may not be available for several
  days.
• Deliver the specimen (in a container preferred by the reference laboratory) to the laboratory immediately after the
  biopsy is taken.

Abnormal findings

Systemic lupus erythematosus
Discoid lupus erythematosus
Pemphigus
Bullous pemphigoid
Dermatitis herpetiformis

notes

S

skull x-ray

Type of test   X-ray

Normal findings   Normal skull and surrounding structures

Test explanation and related physiology

An x-ray image of the skull allows for visualization of the bones making up the skull, the nasal sinuses, and any cerebral calcification. Skull x-rays are rarely indicated today because of the availability of CT scanning of the brain (p. 287). However, skull x-rays are still used for determining skull bone suture lines in the evaluation of children with abnormal head shape or size.

Procedure and patient care

Before

PT Explain the procedure to the patient.

PT Instruct the patient to remove all objects above the neck because metal objects and dentures prevent x-ray visualization of the structures they cover.

• Avoid hyperextension and manipulation of the head if surgical injuries are suspected.

PT Tell the patient that no sedation or fasting is required.

During

• Note that the patient is taken to the radiology department and placed on an x-ray table. Axial, half-axial, posteroanterior, and lateral views of the skull are usually taken.

• Note that a radiologic technologist takes skull x-rays in a few minutes.

PT Tell the patient that this test is painless.

After

• If a prosthetic eye is present, note this on the x-ray examination request, because it can present a confusing shadow on x-ray image.

Abnormal findings

Skull fracture
Metastatic tumor
Sinusitis
Hemorrhage
Tumor
Hematoma
Congenital anomaly
Paget disease of bone

notes

sleep studies (Polysomnography [PSG])

Type of test   Electrodiagnostic; various

Normal findings

Respiratory disturbance index (RDI): <5 episodes of apnea per hour
Normal progress through sleep stages
No interruption in nasal or oral airflow
End-tidal CO_2: 30-45 mm Hg
Oximetry: ≥90%; no oxygen desaturation of >5%
Minimal snoring sounds
ECG: no disturbances in rate or rhythm
No evidence of restlessness
No apnea
MSLT: onset of sleep >9 minutes

Test explanation and related physiology

There are many types of sleep disorders. Most, however, are associated with impaired nighttime sleep and excessive daytime drowsiness. Sleep disorders can be caused by alterations in sleep times (e.g., night-shift workers), medications (stimulants), or psychiatric problems (e.g., depression, mania).

Sleep studies can identify the cause of the sleep disorders and indicate appropriate treatment. Sleep studies include polysomnography (PSG) and testing for wakefulness and sleepiness. A full PSG would include:

- *Electroencephalography:* This is limited to two or more channels (p. 365).
- *Electrooculography:* This documents eye movements (see electronystagmography, p. 376).
- *Electromyography:* This demonstrates muscle movement, usually of the chin and legs (p. 368).
- *Electrocardiography:* This determines heart rate and rhythm (p. 359).
- *Chest impedance:* This monitors chest wall movement and respirations.
- *Airflow monitors:* This measures the amount of airflow in and out of the mouth and nose.
- *CO_2 monitor:* This measures expiratory CO_2 levels.
- *Pulse oximetry:* This monitors tissue oxygen levels (p. 673).
- *Sound sensors:* These are used to document snoring sounds.
- *Audiovisual recordings:* These are used to document restless motion and fitfulness.

S

- *Esophageal pH probe:* This is used only if gastroesophageal reflux is considered to be a cause of paroxysmal nocturnal dyspnea and coughing (p. 397).

On occasions when sleep apnea alone is suspected, a four-channel PSG is performed. This more simplified test includes the ECG, chest impedance, airflow monitor, and O_2 oximetry. Audiovisual recordings are also performed.

A sleep screening study is often performed to see whether full sleep studies are indicated. This is done during sleep using pulse oximetry. If no hypoxia occurs, significant sleep apnea would be rare, and full studies are not indicated.

Sleep apnea can be obstructive or central. Obstructive apnea is by far the most common and is caused by muscle relaxation of the posterior pharyngeal muscles. Breathing stops for 10 to 40 seconds. Central sleep apnea is highlighted by simple cessation of breathing not due to an obstructed airway. Primary cardiac events that lead to significant and transient reduction in cardiac output can also cause apnea. Apnea from either cause is associated with an increase in heart rate, decreased oxygen levels, change in brain waves, and increased expiratory CO_2. Obstructive apnea is also associated with progressively diminished airflow.

During a sleep study, electrodes for the ECG, EEG, electrooculography, and electromyography are applied. The chest impedance belt monitors are also placed. Under audiovisual monitoring, the patient is placed in a comfortable room and sleeps. During sleep, information is synchronously gathered. The EEG determines the various stages of sleep, and the physiologic changes during each stage are documented.

Testing for obstructive sleep apnea is performed in a specially constructed sleep laboratory. This is a well-insulated room in which external sounds are blocked and room temperature is easily controlled. It is performed by a certified sleep technologist and interpreted by a physician trained in sleep disorders. The study is usually completed in one night, although occasionally two nights are required. A second day is often required to administer the *multiple sleep latency test (MSLT)* or the *multiple wake test (MWT)*. The MSLT is a measure of the patient's ability to sleep during a series of structured naps. The MSLT is typically done in the morning. The MWT is a measure of the patient's ability to not fall asleep during a period of what should be wakefulness. These tests are used to diagnose narcolepsy that follows a night of inadequate sleep.

These tests can also be used to determine the success of therapy for sleep disorders. The sleep study will be repeated after the patient has started using CPAP or a dental fixture for therapy. While on therapy, no sleep apnea should be noted. If the sleep apnea is significant on the initial sleep study, a *split study* can be performed, in which sleep is evaluated while the patient uses a CPAP machine for the next 4 hours. During that time, appropriate CPAP settings are calibrated to reduce apneic episodes while minimizing uncomfortable side effects.

Because of the expense and the psycho-emotional difficulties associated with testing in a sleep laboratory, there has been significant growth in unattended *home sleep studies*. The patient is attached to a multichannel monitor by a sleep technician as previously described. The technician does not remain in attendance. The monitoring device records all key data so that a sleep disorder can be identified.

Actigraphy can be used to determine sleep patterns and circadian rhythms. A sleep actigraph is a simple device that is worn like a wrist watch. It can be used during normal activities (except swimming or bathing) for several days and nights. It does not require an overnight stay at a sleep center. Doctors can use actigraphy to help diagnose sleep disorders, including circadian rhythm disorders, such as jet lag and shift work disorders. This test can also detect how well sleep treatments are working. Actigraphy can be used with PSG or alone.

Interfering factors

- Psychologically induced insomnia associated with being in a sleep center
- Environmental noises, temperature changes, or other sensations may affect the sleep pattern.
- Times for sleep testing that are different from usual times may affect sleep patterns and should be avoided.

Procedure and patient care

Before

PT Explain the procedure to the patient.

PT Instruct the patient to avoid caffeine for several days before testing.

PT Reassure the patient that monitoring equipment will not interrupt the patient's sleep pattern.

- Allow the patient to express concerns about videotaping and other forms of monitoring.
- Several sleep rating questionnaires are completed by both the patient and his or her sleeping partner.
- Age, weight, and medical history are recorded.

During

- Electrodes for ECG, EEG, and electromyography are applied to the patient. Excess hair may need to be shaved on male patients.
- Airflow, oximetry, and impedance monitors are also applied.
- When the patient is comfortable, he or she is allowed to sleep.
- The lights are turned off, and monitoring begins.
- For PSG, the patient is asked to sleep per normal routine.

Multiple sleep latency testing

- The patient is asked to nap about every 2 hours throughout the testing period.
- The nap is terminated after 20 minutes.
- Between naps, the patient must stay awake.

Multiple wake testing

- The patient is asked to stay awake and not nap.
- Monitoring is similar to that described for PSG except for impedance, sound, and airflow monitors.

After

- On completion of the sleep cycle, the monitors and electrodes are removed.
- Test results take several days to collate and interpret.

Abnormal findings

Obstructive sleep apnea
Central sleep apnea
Cardiac sleep apnea
Insomnia
Narcolepsy
Restless legs syndrome
Parasomnia
REM disorder

notes

small bowel follow-through (SBF, Small bowel enema)

Type of test X-ray with contrast dye

Normal findings

Normal positioning, motility, and patency of the small intestine
No evidence of intrinsic obstruction or extrinsic compression

Test explanation and related physiology

The SBF study is performed to identify abnormalities in the small bowel. Usually the patient is asked to drink barium; in patients who cannot drink, barium can be injected through a nasogastric tube. X-ray images are then taken at timed intervals (usually 30 minutes) to follow the progression of barium through the small intestine. Significant delays in transit time of the barium may occur with both benign and malignant forms of obstruction or diminished intestinal motility (ileus). On the other hand, the flow of barium is faster in patients who have hypermotility states of the small bowel (malabsorption syndromes). Failure of the progression through the small bowel can be seen in patients with partial mechanical small bowel obstruction or diminished intestinal motility, as seen in patients with diabetes. Furthermore, SBF series are helpful in identifying and defining the anatomy of small bowel fistulas.

A more accurate radiographic evaluation of the small intestine is provided by the *small bowel enema*. Unlike the SBF, in which the barium is swallowed by the patient, during the small bowel enema the barium is injected into a tube previously passed to the small bowel. This small bowel enema provides better visualization of the entire small bowel, because the barium is not diluted by gastric and duodenal juices. Tumors, ulcers, and small bowel fistulas are more easily identified and defined with the enema.

Contraindications

- Patients with a complete small bowel obstruction
- Patients suspected of having a perforated viscus
  Barium should not be used in these patients because it may cause prolonged and recurrent abscesses if it leaks out of the bowel. Gastrografin, a water-soluble contrast medium, can be used if perforation is suspected.
- Patients with unstable vital signs

Potential complications

- Barium-induced small bowel obstruction

S

Interfering factors

- Barium in the intestinal tract from a previous barium x-ray image may obstruct adequate visualization of the small bowel.
- Food or fluid in the gastrointestinal tract

Procedure and patient care

Before

PT Explain the procedure to the patient.

PT Instruct the patient not to eat anything for at least 8 hours before the test.

PT Inform the patient that the SBF series may take several hours. Suggest that the patient bring reading material or some paperwork to occupy his or her time.

During

- Note the following procedural steps:
  1. A specially prepared drink containing barium sulfate is mixed as a milkshake, which the patient drinks through a straw.
  2. Usually, an upper GI series is performed concomitantly (p. 941).
  3. The barium flow is followed through the upper GI tract fluoroscopically.
  4. At frequent intervals (15 to 60 minutes), repeat x-ray images are taken to follow the flow of barium through the small intestine. These images are repeated until barium is seen flowing into the right colon. This usually takes 60 to 120 minutes, but in patients with delayed progression of the barium, the test may take as long as 24 hours to complete.

Small bowel enema
  1. This is usually performed by placing a long weighted tube transorally; however, a tube also can be placed into the upper small bowel endoscopically.
  2. After the tube is in place, a thickened barium mixture is injected through the tube, and x-ray images are serially performed as described for the SBF.

- Note that this procedure is performed by a radiologist in the radiology department in approximately 30 minutes.

PT Tell the patient that this test is not uncomfortable.

After

PT Inform the patient of the need to evacuate adequately all the barium. Cathartics (e.g., magnesium citrate) are recommended. Initially, stools will be white and should return to normal color with complete evacuation.

Abnormal findings

Small bowel tumor

Small bowel obstruction from intrinsic tumors

Small bowel obstruction from adhesions, extrinsic tumors, or hernia

Inflammatory small bowel disease (e.g., Crohn disease)

Malabsorption syndromes (e.g., Whipple disease, sprue)

Congenital anatomic anomaly (e.g., malrotation)

Congenital abnormalities (e.g., small bowel atresia, duplication, Meckel diverticulum)

Small bowel intussusception

Small bowel perforation

notes

S

sodium (Na), blood

Type of test Blood

Normal findings

Adult/elderly: 136-145 mEq/L or 136-145 mmol/L (SI units)
Child: 136-145 mEq/L
Infant: 134-150 mEq/L
Newborn: 134-144 mEq/L

Possible critical values <120 or >160 mEq/L

Test explanation and related physiology

Sodium is the major cation in the extracellular space, where serum levels of approximately 140 mEq/L exist. The concentration of sodium intracellularly is only 5 mEq/L. Therefore, sodium salts are the major determinants of extracellular osmolality. The sodium content of the blood is a result of a balance between dietary sodium intake and renal excretion.

Many factors regulate homeostatic sodium balance. Aldosterone causes conservation of sodium by decreasing renal losses. Natriuretic hormone, or third factor, increases renal losses of sodium. Antidiuretic hormone (ADH), which controls the resorption of water at the distal tubules of the kidney, also affects serum sodium levels.

Physiologically, water and sodium are very closely interrelated. As free body water is increased, serum sodium is diluted, and the concentration may decrease. The kidney compensates by conserving sodium and excreting water. If free body water were to decrease, the serum sodium concentration would rise; the kidney would then respond by conserving free water.

Interfering factors

- Recent trauma, surgery, or shock may cause increased levels.
- ✘ Drugs that may cause *increased* levels include anabolic steroids, antibiotics, carbenicillin, clonidine, corticosteroids, cough medicines, estrogens, laxatives, methyldopa, and oral contraceptives.
- ✘ Drugs that may cause *decreased* levels include ACE inhibitors, captopril, carbamazepine, diuretics, haloperidol, heparin, nonsteroidal antiinflammatory drugs, IV fluids, sulfonylureas, triamterene, tricyclic antidepressants, and vasopressin.

Procedure and patient care
- See inside front cover for Routine Blood Testing.
- Fasting: no.
- Blood tube commonly used: red or green.

Abnormal findings

▲ Increased levels
(hypernatremia)
Increased sodium intake
Excessive dietary intake
Excessive sodium in
  IV fluids

Decreased sodium loss
Cushing syndrome
Hyperaldosteronism

*Excessive free body water
  loss*
Excessive sweating
Extensive thermal burns
Diabetes insipidus
Osmotic diuresis
GI loss

▼ Decreased levels
(hyponatremia)
Decreased sodium intake
Deficient dietary intake
Deficient sodium in IV
  fluids

Increased sodium loss
Addison disease
Diarrhea
Vomiting or nasogastric
  aspiration
Diuretic administration
Chronic renal insufficiency

Increased free body water
Excessive oral water
  intake
Excessive IV water
  intake
Congestive heart failure
Syndrome of inappropriate
  ADH (SIADH)
  secretion
Osmotic dilution

*Third-space losses
  of sodium*
Ascites
Peripheral edema
Pleural effusion
Intraluminal bowel loss
  (ileus or mechanical
  obstruction)

S

notes

sodium (Na), urine

Type of test   Urine (24-hour)

Normal findings

40-220 mEq/day or 40-220 mmol/day (SI units)
Spot urine: >20 mEq/L
Fractional excretion (FE_{Na}): 1-2%

Test explanation and related physiology

This test evaluates sodium balance in the body by determining the amount of sodium excreted in urine over 24 hours. Sodium is the major cation in the extracellular space. Measuring the amount of sodium in the urine is useful for evaluating patients with volume depletion, acute renal failure, adrenal disturbances, and acid/base imbalances. In the setting of acute renal failure, an increased value will indicate acute tubular necrosis, whereas a low value would be typical of prerenal azotemia.

This test is also useful when the serum sodium concentration is low. For example, in patients with hyponatremia caused by inadequate sodium intake, urine sodium will be low. In patients with hyponatremia caused by chronic renal failure, however, urine sodium concentration will be high.

Urine sodium excretions are helpful when the urine output is low (<500 mL/24 hr). However, a more accurate test to determine the cause of reduced urine output is the *fractional excretion of sodium* (FE_{Na}). FE_{Na} is the fraction of sodium actually excreted relative to the amount filtered by the kidney. FE_{Na} is a calculation based on the concentrations of sodium (Na) and creatinine (Cr) in the blood and the urine as follows:

Fractional excretion of sodium $(FE_{Na}) = (U_{Na} \times P_{Cr}) / (P_{Na} \times U_{Cr}) \times 100$

FE_{Na} is usually greater than 3% with acute tubular necrosis and severe obstruction of the urinary drainage of both kidneys. It is generally less than 1% in patients with acute glomerulonephritis, hepatorenal syndrome, and states of prerenal azotemia (e.g., congestive heart failure and dehydration). FE_{Na} may also be less than 1% with acute partial urinary tract obstruction.

Interfering factors

- Dietary salt intake may increase sodium levels.
- Altered kidney function may affect levels.
- ✶ Drugs that may cause *increased* levels include antibiotics, cough medicines, laxatives, and steroids.

☡ Drugs that may cause *decreased* levels include diuretics (e.g., furosemide) and steroids.

Procedure and patient care

- See inside front cover for Routine Urine Testing.
- If FE_{Na} is ordered, collect a venous blood sample in a gold-top tube for serum creatinine and sodium measurements.

Abnormal findings

▲ **Increased levels**
  Dehydration
  Starvation
  Adrenocortical insufficiency
  Diuretic therapy
  Hypothyroidism
  Syndrome of inappropriate
    ADH (SIADH) secretion
  Diabetic ketoacidosis
  Toxemia of pregnancy

▼ **Decreased levels**
  Congestive heart failure
  Malabsorption
  Diarrhea
  Renal failure
  Cushing syndrome
  Aldosteronism
  Diaphoresis
  Pulmonary emphysema
  Inadequate sodium intake

notes

S

spinal x-ray (Cervical, thoracic, lumbar, sacral, and coccygeal x-ray studies)

Type of test X-ray

Normal findings Normal spinal vertebrae

Test explanation and related physiology

Spinal x-ray studies may be performed to evaluate any area of the spine. They usually include anteroposterior, lateral, and oblique views of these structures. These x-ray images are often done to assess back or neck pain, degenerative arthritic changes, traumatic fractures, tumor metastasis, spondylosis (stress fracture of the vertebrae), and spondylolisthesis (slipping of one vertebral disc on the other). Cervical spinal x-ray studies are performed in cases of multiple trauma to ensure that there is no fracture before the patient is moved or the neck is manipulated. However, CT scanning of the cervical vertebrae is increasingly becoming the standard of practice to ensure that there is no cervical fracture. Spinal x-rays are very helpful in evaluating children and adults for spinal alignment abnormalities (e.g., kyphosis, scoliosis). MRI is another very accurate method of evaluating the spine.

Contraindications

- Patients who are pregnant, unless the benefits outweigh the risks

Procedure and patient care

Before

PT Explain the procedure to the patient.

PT Instruct the patient to remove any metal objects covering the area to be visualized.

- Immobilize the patient if a spinal fracture is suspected. Apply a neck brace if a cervical spine fracture is suspected.

PT Tell the patient that no fasting or sedation is required; however, if a fracture is suspected, the patient may be kept NPO.

During

- Note that the patient is placed on an x-ray table. Anterior, posterior, lateral, and oblique x-ray images are taken of the desired area on the spinal cord. These same views can also be obtained with the patient in the standing position.
- Note that a radiologic technologist takes spinal x-ray images in a few minutes.

PT Tell the patient that no discomfort is associated with this study.

After

- Note that positioning and patient activity depend on test results.

Abnormal findings

Degenerative arthritis changes
Traumatic or pathologic fracture
Spondylosis
Spondylolisthesis
Metastatic tumor invasion
Scoliosis
Suspected spinal osteomyelitis

notes

sputum culture and sensitivity (C&S, Culture and Gram stain)

Type of test Sputum

Normal findings Normal upper respiratory tract

Test explanation and related physiology

Sputum cultures are obtained to determine the presence of pathogenic bacteria in patients with respiratory infections (e.g., pneumonia). A *Gram stain* is the first step in the microbiologic analysis of sputum. Staining of sputum provides an opportunity to classify bacteria as gram-positive or gram-negative. This may be used to guide drug therapy until the C&S report is complete. The sputum sample is then applied to a series of bacterial culture plates. The bacteria that grow on those plates 1 to 3 days later are then identified. Determinations of bacterial sensitivity to various antibiotics are done to identify the most appropriate antimicrobial drug therapy. This is done by observing a ring of growth inhibition around an antibiotic plug in the culture medium.

Sputum for C&S should be collected before antimicrobial therapy is initiated, unless the test is being performed to evaluate the effectiveness of medications already being given. Preliminary reports are usually available in 24 hours. Cultures require at least 48 hours for completion. Sputum cultures for fungus and *Mycobacterium tuberculosis* may take 6 to 8 weeks.

Procedure and patient care

Before

PT Explain the procedure for sputum collection to the patient.

PT Remind the patient that sputum must be coughed up from the lungs and that saliva is not sputum.

• Hold antibiotics until after the sputum has been collected.

• If an elective specimen is to be obtained, give the patient a sterile sputum container on the night before the sputum is to be collected so that the morning specimen may be obtained on arising.

PT Instruct the patient to rinse out his or her mouth with water before the sputum collection to decrease contamination of the sputum by particles in the oropharynx.

During

• Note that sputum specimens are best when the patient first awakens in the morning and before eating or drinking.

- Collect at least 1 teaspoon of sputum in a sterile sputum container.
- Usually obtain sputum by having the patient cough after taking several deep breaths.
- If the patient is unable to produce a sputum specimen, stimulate coughing by lowering the head of the patient's bed or giving the patient an aerosol administration of a warm hypertonic solution.
- Note that other methods to collect sputum include endotracheal aspiration, fiberoptic bronchoscopy, and transtracheal aspiration.

After

PT Inform the patient to notify the nurse as soon as the sputum is collected.
- Label the sputum, and send it to the laboratory as soon as possible.
- Note any current antibiotic therapy on the laboratory slip.

Abnormal findings

Bacterial infection (e.g., pneumonia)
Viral infection
Atypical bacterial infection (e.g., tuberculosis)

notes

sputum cytology

Type of test   Sputum

Normal findings   Normal epithelial cells

Test explanation and related physiology

Tumors in the pulmonary system frequently slough cells into the sputum. When the sputum is gathered, the cells are examined. If the cytologic test is positive, malignant cells are seen, indicating a lung tumor. If only normal epithelial cells are seen, either no malignancy exists or any existing tumor is not shedding cells. Therefore, a positive test indicates malignancy; a negative test means nothing.

Bronchoscopy and percutaneous lung biopsy have supplanted the need for sputum cytology to a large degree. Now its greatest use is in patients who have an abnormal chest x-ray, productive cough, and nothing visible on bronchoscopy.

Procedure and patient care

Before

PT Explain the procedure for sputum collection to the patient.

PT Remind the patient that sputum must be coughed up from the lungs and that saliva is not sputum.

- Give the patient a sterile sputum container on the night before the sputum is to be collected so that the morning specimen may be obtained on arising.

During

- Sputum specimens are collected as described on p. 858.
- Usually collect sputum for cytology on three separate occasions.

After

PT Instruct the patient to notify the nurse as soon as the sputum is collected.

- Label the specimen, and send it to the laboratory as soon as possible.

Abnormal findings

Malignancies

notes

squamous cell carcinoma antigen (SCC antigen)

Type of test Blood

Normal findings ≤2.2 ng/mL

Test explanation

Squamous cell carcinoma (SCC) antigen is a glycoprotein that is expressed in normal epithelium and epithelial tissues. Although the neutral forms of SCC normally remain inside the cell, acidic SCC antigen is released and often elevated in patients who have SCCs or other nonmalignant squamous cell lesions. It can occur in several cancers (e.g., uterine, cervical, oral cavity, esophageal, lung, anal canal, and skin). SCC antigen may be involved in the malignant behavior of squamous cell cancers. Consequently, serum concentrations of SCC antigen can be used to monitor various SCCs after surgical removal. Concentrations that remain persistently elevated or begin to increase after tumor removal suggest persistent or recurrent disease. There may be an association between serum SCC antigen concentrations and tumor stage, size, and tumor aggressiveness.

Common sites for SCC include the skin, esophagus, lung, and head and neck cancers. A variety of nonmalignant benign diseases of the skin (e.g., eczema, erythrodermic epidermitis, pemphigus, and psoriasis), lungs (e.g., TB, adult respiratory distress syndrome, sarcoidosis, and the presence of pleural effusion), and other common conditions may result in increased serum concentrations of SCC antigen. Thus, SCC antigen results alone should not be interpreted as evidence of the presence or absence of malignant disease.

Procedure and patient care

- See inside front cover for Routine Blood Testing.
- Fasting: no.
- Blood tube commonly used: red.
- The blood sample may be sent to a central diagnostic laboratory, and results may not be available for 7 to 10 days.

Abnormal findings

Squamous cell carcinoma
Dermatitis
Pulmonary disease

notes

stool culture (Stool for culture and sensitivity [C&S], Stool for ova and parasites [O&P])

Type of test   Stool

Normal findings   Normal intestinal flora

Test explanation and related physiology

Normally, stool contains many bacteria and fungi. The more common organisms include *Enterococcus, Escherichia coli, Proteus, Pseudomonas, Staphylococcus aureus, Candida albicans, Bacteroides*, and *Clostridium*. Bacteria are indigenous to the bowel. Sometimes normal stool flora can become pathogenic if overgrowth of the bacteria occurs as a result of antibiotics (e.g., *Clostridium difficile*), immunosuppression, or overaggressive catharsis. *Salmonella, Shigella, Campylobacter, Yersinia*, pathogenic *E. coli, Clostridium*, and *Staphylococcus* are acquired bacteria that can infect the bowel. Parasites also may affect the stool. Common parasites are *Ascaris* (hookworm), *Strongyloides* (tapeworm), and *Giardia* (protozoans). Identification of any of these pathogens in the stool incriminates that parasite as the etiology of the infectious enteritis.

Infections of the bowel from bacteria, virus, or parasites usually present as diarrhea, excessive flatus, and abdominal discomfort. Patients who have been drinking well water, have been on prolonged antibiotics, or have traveled outside of the United States are especially susceptible.

Interfering factors

- Urine may inhibit the growth of bacteria. Therefore, urine should not be mixed with the feces during collection of a stool sample.
- Recent barium studies may obscure the detection of parasites.
- ☒ Drugs that may affect test results include antibiotics, bismuth, and mineral oil.

Procedure and patient care

Before

PT Explain the method of stool collection to the patient. Be matter of fact to avoid any embarrassment to the patient.

PT Instruct the patient not to mix urine or toilet paper with the stool specimen.

PT Instruct the patient to use an appropriate collection container.

During

PT Instruct the patient to defecate into a clean bedpan.

- Place a small amount of stool in a sterile collection container.
- Send mucus and blood streaks with the specimen.
- If a rectal swab is to be used, wear gloves and insert the cotton-tipped swab at least 1 inch into the anal canal. Then rotate the swab for 30 seconds and place it into the clean container.

Tape test

- Use this test when pinworms *(Enterobius)* are suspected.
- Place clear tape in the patient's perianal region. (This is especially helpful in children.)
- Because the female worm lays her eggs at night around the perianal area, apply the tape before bedtime and remove it in the morning before the patient gets out of bed.
- Press the sticky surface of the tape directly to a glass slide and examine microscopically for pinworm ova.

After

- Handle the stool specimen carefully as though it were capable of causing infection.
- Indicate on the laboratory slip any antibiotics that the patient may be taking.
- Promptly send the stool specimen to the laboratory. Delays in transfer of the specimen may affect viability of the organism.
- Note that some enteric pathogens occasionally take as long as 6 weeks to isolate.
- When pathogens are detected, maintain isolation of the patient's stool until therapy is completed.

Abnormal findings

Bacterial enterocolitis
Protozoan enterocolitis
Parasitic enterocolitis

notes

stool for occult blood (Stool for OB, Fecal occult blood test [FOBT], Fecal immunotest [FIT], DNA stool sample)

Type of test Stool

Normal findings No occult blood within stool

Test explanation and related physiology

This test is used for colorectal cancer screening of asymptomatic individuals. Normally only minimal quantities (2 mL to 2.5 mL) of blood are passed into the gastrointestinal (GI) tract. Usually this bleeding is not significant enough to cause a positive result in stool for occult blood (OB) testing. This test can detect OB when as little as 5 mL of blood is lost per day.

Tumors of the intestine grow into the lumen and are subjected to repeated trauma by the fecal stream. Eventually the friable neovascular tumor ulcerates and bleeding occurs. Most often, bleeding is so slight that gross blood is not seen in the stool. The blood can be detected by chemical assay or by immunohistochemistry. Guaiac is the most commonly performed chemical assay.

OB can also be detected by immunochemical methods that detect the human globin portion of hemoglobin using monoclonal antibodies. These tests are called *fecal immunochemical test (FIT)* or *immunochemical fecal occult blood test (iFOBT)*. These methods are as sensitive as guaiac testing but are not affected by red meats or plant oxidizers as described in the Interfering factors section. Immunochemical methods may fail to recognize OB from the upper GI tract because the globin is digested by the time it gets in the stool.

The *DNA stool sample test* is more sensitive than guaiac testing in the detection of significant colorectal precancerous, benign, and malignant tumors. Because most precancerous polyps do not bleed, they can be missed by FOBT. In contrast, all precancerous polyps shed cells that contain abnormal DNA. So, a stool-based DNA test designed to detect this DNA promises to be more accurate in the detection of precancerous polyps, which, when detected, can be removed before they turn into cancer.

Benign and malignant GI tumors, ulcers, inflammatory bowel disease, arteriovenous malformations, diverticulosis, and hematobilia (hemobilia) can all cause OB in the stool. Other more common abnormalities (e.g., hemorrhoids, swallowed blood from oral or nasopharyngeal bleeding) may also cause OB in the stool.

When OB testing is properly performed, a positive result obtained on multiple specimens collected on successive days warrants a thorough GI evaluation, usually with EGD (p. 401) and colonoscopy (p. 271). Regular screening, beginning at age 50, can reduce the number of people who die of colorectal cancer by as much as 60%.

Reducing or oxidizing agents (such as iron, radish, cantaloupe, cauliflower, vitamin C) can affect the results of guaiac or FIT. Furthermore, neither FIT nor guaiac testing detects slow upper GI bleeding because globin and heme are degraded during intestinal transit. To evaluate occult GI bleeding in these patients, a fluorometric method detects any hemoglobin or heme-derived porphyrins in the stool, is very sensitive, and provides quantitative results.

Interfering factors

- Vigorous exercise
- Bleeding gums following a dental procedure
- Ingestion of red meat within 3 days before testing
- Ingestion of peroxidase-rich fruits and vegetables (turnips, artichokes, mushrooms, radishes, horseradishes, broccoli, bean sprouts, cauliflower, oranges, bananas, cantaloupes, and grapes) may affect results.
- ✆ Drugs that may cause GI bleeding include anticoagulants, aspirin, colchicine, iron preparations (large doses), nonsteroidal antiarthritics, and steroids.
- ✆ Drugs that may cause false-positive results include colchicine, iron, oxidizing drugs (e.g., iodine, bromides, boric acid), and rauwolfia derivatives.
- ✆ Drugs that may cause false-negative results include vitamin C.

Procedure and patient care

Before

- PT Explain the procedure to the patient.
- PT Instruct the patient to refrain from eating any red meat for at least 3 days before the test.
- PT Instruct the patient to refrain from drugs known to interfere with OB testing.
- PT Instruct the patient as to the method of obtaining appropriate stool specimens. Many procedures are available (e.g., specimen cards, tissue wipes, test paper). Tests may be done at home with specimen cards (Hemoccult) and mailed.
- PT Instruct the patient not to mix urine with the stool specimen.

PT Inform the patient as to the need for multiple specimens obtained on separate days to increase the test's accuracy.

- Note that in some centers a high-residue diet is recommended to increase the abrasive effect of the stool.
- Be gentle in obtaining stool by digital rectal examination. A traumatic digital examination can cause a false-positive stool, especially in patients with prior anorectal disease, such as hemorrhoids.

During

Hemoccult slide test

- Place a stool sample on one side of guaiac paper.
- Place two drops of developer on the other side.
- Note that bluish discoloration indicates OB in the stool.

Tablet test

- Place a stool sample on the developer paper.
- Place a tablet on top of the stool specimen.
- Put two or three drops of tap water on the tablet and allow it to flow onto the paper.
- Note that bluish discoloration indicates OB in the stool.

After

PT Inform the patient of the results.

- If the tests are positive, inquire whether the patient violated any of the preparation recommendations.

Abnormal findings

GI tumor
Polyps
Ulcer
Varices
Inflammatory bowel disease
Diverticulosis
Ischemic bowel disease
GI trauma
Recent GI surgery
Hemorrhoids
Esophagitis
Gastritis

notes

Streptococcus serologic testing (Antistreptolysin O titer [ASO], Antideoxyribonuclease-B titer, [Anti-DNase-B, ADNase-B, ADB], *Streptococcus* group B antigen detection, Streptozyme)

Type of test Blood; CSF

Normal findings

Antistreptolysin O titer
 Adult/elderly: ≤160 Todd units/mL
 Child:
  Newborn: similar to mother's value
  6 months-2 years: ≤50 Todd units/mL
  2-4 years: ≤160 Todd units/mL
  5-12 years: 170-330 Todd units/mL

Antideoxyribonuclease-B titer
 Adult: ≤85 Todd units/mL or titer≤1:85
 Child:
  Preschool age: ≤60 Todd units/mL or titer≤1:60
  School age: ≤170 Todd units/mL or titer≤1:170

Streptozyme
 Titer<1:100

Streptococcus **group B antigen**
 none detected

Test explanation and related physiology

Infection by group A *Streptococcus* is unique because it can be followed by a serious nonpurulent complication (e.g., rheumatic fever, scarlet fever, glomerulonephritis). Serologic tests are used primarily to determine whether a previous group A *Streptococcus* infection (pharyngitis, pyodermia, pneumonia) has caused a poststreptococcal disease. These poststreptococcal diseases occur following the infection and after a period of latency during which the patient is asymptomatic.

These antibodies are directed against streptococcal extracellular products that are primarily enzymatic proteins. Serial rising titers of these antibodies over several weeks, followed by a slow fall in titers, are more supportive of the diagnosis of a previous streptococcal infection than is a single titer.

One such extracellular enzyme produced by streptococcus is called *streptolysin O*, which has the ability to destroy (lyse) red blood corpuscles. The streptolysin O is antigenic stimulating the immunologic production of a neutralizing *ASO antibody*. ASO appears in the serum 1 week to 1 month after the onset of a streptococcal infection. A high ASO titer is not specific for

S

a certain type of poststreptococcal disease (i.e., rheumatic fever versus glomerulonephritis), but merely indicates that a streptococcal infection is or has been present.

Like the ASO titer, *ADB* is used to detect previous streptococcal infections. Although this test may be more sensitive than the ASO titer, it is not used alone in the evaluation of streptococcal infections because its results are too variable.

The *Streptozyme* assay detects antibodies to multiple extracellular antigens of group A *Streptococcus*, including antistreptolysin O, antistreptokinase, and antihyaluronidase. Approximately 80% of specimens positive by Streptozyme have antistreptolysin O, and 10% have antistreptokinase and/or antihyaluronidase. The remaining 10% of positive samples are apparently due to ADB antibodies or other streptococcal extracellular antigens.

Streptococcus group B antigens accumulate in CSF, serum, or urine and provide a direct qualitative detection of bacterial antigens. These antigens indicate acute infection and are not related to poststreptococcal sequelae as described above. Confirmatory diagnosis of streptococcal infection is done by cultures (p. 891).

Interfering factors

- Increased beta-lipoprotein levels inhibit streptolysin O and give a falsely high ASO titer.
- ☑ Drugs that may cause *decreased* ASO levels include adrenocorticosteroids and antibiotics.

Procedure and patient care

- See inside front cover for Routine Blood Testing.
- Fasting: no.
- Blood tube commonly used: red.

Abnormal findings

▲ **Increased levels**
   Streptococcal infection
   Acute rheumatic fever
   Acute glomerulonephritis
   Bacterial endocarditis
   Scarlet fever
   Streptococcal pyoderma

notes

substance abuse testing (Urine drug testing, Drug screening, Toxicology screening)

Type of test Urine; blood; various

Normal findings Negative

Test explanation and related physiology

Substance abuse testing is used mostly by employers and law enforcement agencies. Employers use drug testing to promote and protect the safety, health, and well-being of their employees. Because many industrial fatalities are attributable to substance abuse, drug testing programs are common in the workplace. Furthermore, drug use is responsible for decreased productivity and increased absenteeism. Industrial testing is used at the time of preemployment, prepromotion, annual physical, after an accident, when there is reasonable suspicion, or for random testing or follow-up treatment surveillance.

Most commonly, a drug screen is performed to detect small amounts of any number of metabolites of commonly used drugs. If the screen result is positive, a more accurate and quantitative test is performed on the same specimen. Drug screens are available for a variety of drug categories. The most common are amphetamines, barbiturates, benzodiazepines, cannabinoids (marijuana [THC]), cocaine, methamphetamine, opiates (morphine and heroin), phencyclidine (PCP), carisoprodol, meprobamate, and propoxyphene (see Table 33). Alcohol testing is most commonly used by law enforcement (see ethanol, p. 410). Not only is drug testing helpful in identifying users, it also acts as a deterrent. Athletes can be tested for anabolic hormones, stimulants, diuretics, beta-blockers, street drugs, anti-estrogens, erythropoietin, and beta-2 agonists that may unfairly improve their performance. Health and life insurance companies routinely test for illicit drugs.

Until recently, substance abuse testing has used urine exclusively as the sample of choice. Urine drug testing is generally inexpensive. Urine is easily obtained, and it contains a large amount of drug metabolites. More important, urine can identify drug usage for several days after the last usage, whereas blood testing reflects drug usage only during the past few hours.

The absence of expected drug(s) and/or drug metabolite(s) may indicate non-compliance, inappropriate timing of specimen collection relative to drug administration, poor drug absorption, diluted/adulterated urine, or limitations of testing. The concentration at

S

TABLE 33 Typical multipanel drug screen

Drugs/Drug classes	Screen	Confirmation*
Marijuana	20 ng/mL	5 ng/mL
Cocaine	150 ng/mL	50 ng/mL
Opiates	300 ng/mL	5 ng/mL
Oxycodone	100 ng/mL	5 ng/mL
Phencyclidine	25 ng/mL	10 ng/mL
Amphetamines	300 ng/mL	200 ng/mL
MDMA (Ecstasy)	500 ng/mL	200 ng/mL
Barbiturates	200 ng/mL	50 ng/mL
Benzodiazepines	200 ng/mL	20 ng/mL
Methadone	150 ng/mL	10 ng/mL
Propoxyphene	300 ng/mL	10 g/mL

*Confirmatory tests are more sensitive and can detect metabolites at lower levels.

which the screening test can detect a drug or metabolite varies within a drug class.

Saliva, breath, hair, and sweat are becoming increasingly important and accurate specimens for specific drug testing. These testing methods are very expensive, however. Hair samples detect the presence of drugs used during the past 3 months. In addition, hair and nail samples may be used to detect or document exposure to arsenic and mercury. Nevertheless, urine testing remains the mainstay for drug testing.

Because a positive result can have a profound effect on a person's life, job, and accountability, it is not uncommon for a drug abuser to attempt to alter the urine specimen. Therefore, the urine sample is tested for odor, color, temperature, creatinine, pH, and specific gravity to ensure that it is a proper specimen. If the specimen does not meet these assessment standards, it is rejected and a second specimen is requested.

Toxicology screening tests for drug overdose and poisoning (e.g., lead and carbon monoxide) are best performed on blood. Results indicate current drug levels, which are used to determine or alter therapy. Toxicology studies are used to incriminate drugs as a cause or factor in the death of a person. They are also used to assess patients when poisoning contributes to an illness.

Interfering factors

- Poppy seeds can cause positive opiate results.
- Secondhand marijuana smoke can cause positive THC results.

- Detergents, bicarbonates, salt tablets, and blood can all foil accurate drug testing in a urine specimen.
- ✘ Ibuprofen can cause a false-positive THC result in some assay systems.
- ✘ Cold remedies can cause false-positive amphetamine results in some assay systems but not with the monoclonal antibody test.
- ✘ Antibiotics (e.g., amoxicillin) can cause false-positive results for heroin and/or cocaine.
- ✘ Aggressive use of diuretics can *decrease* urine drug levels.

Procedure and patient care

Before

- **PT** Explain the procedure to the patient or significant others based on standard guidelines.
- If the specimen is obtained for medicolegal testing, ensure that the patient or family member has signed a consent form.
- Obtain a list of prescription medicines that the patient is taking that may alter or confuse screening results. Obtain as much information as possible about the drug type, amount, and ingestion time.
- Carefully assess the patient for respiratory distress (a common adverse reaction of drug overdose).

During

- Collect blood and urine samples as designated by the laboratory.
- Ensure that patients provide their own urine. Urine specimens for substance abuse testing are usually collected in the presence of a health care provider.
- Be sure that the patient does not alter the urine specimen.
- For hair testing, cut 50 strands of hair from the scalp.
- A second confirmatory specimen may be obtained (and is used if results are positive).
- Collect gastric contents as indicated by the specific institution. An NG tube is required.

After

- Apply pressure to the venipuncture site.
- Refer the patient for appropriate drug and psychiatric counseling.
- Follow the chain of custody for the specimen as provided by standard guidelines of the institution.
- Place the specimen in the required container for delivery.

S

- Check the temperature of urine specimens within 3 minutes after voiding. The temperature should be between 97° and 99° F.
- The specimen may be sent to a nationally certified laboratory for federal workers or workplace testing. Local hospital laboratories are often able to test for many drugs.

Abnormal findings

Positive drug level

notes

swallowing examination (Videofluoroscopy swallowing examination)

Type of test X-ray with contrast dye

Normal findings Normal swallowing function and complete clearing of radiographic material through the upper digestive tract

Test explanation and related physiology

This test is performed to identify problems that exist in a patient who is unable to swallow. Problems in swallowing may result from local structural diseases, such as tumors, upper esophageal diverticula, inflammation, extrinsic compression of the upper gastrointestinal (GI) tract, or surgery on the oropharyngeal tract. Motility disorders of the upper GI tract (e.g., Zenker diverticulum) and neurologic disorders (e.g., stroke syndrome), Parkinson disease, and neuropathies also may cause difficulty in swallowing. Videofluoroscopy of the swallowing function allows a speech pathologist to delineate more clearly the exact pathology in the swallowing mechanism. This procedure then can be used to determine the most appropriate treatment and teach the patient the proper swallowing technique.

This test is performed by asking the patient to swallow barium or a barium-containing meal. With the use of videofluoroscopy, the swallowing function is visualized and documented. Morphologic abnormalities and functional impairment can be identified easily using the slow-frame progression and reversal that is available with videofluoroscopy. Although this test is similar to the barium swallow (p. 136), finer details of swallowing can be evaluated with the use of videofluoroscopy.

Contraindications

- Patients who aspirate their saliva are not candidates for this swallowing examination, because they will require nonswallowing methods of alimentation.

Procedure and patient care

Before

PT Explain the procedure to the patient.

PT Explain to the patient that no preparation is required.

During

- In the radiology department, the patient is asked to swallow a barium-containing meal. The consistency of the meal will be determined by the speech therapist and radiologist. The food may be liquid, semisoft (e.g., applesauce), or solid (e.g., a tea biscuit). While the patient is swallowing, videofluoroscopy is recorded in both the lateral and the anterior positions.
- The video is then repeatedly examined and reexamined by the radiologist and speech pathologist.

After

- No catharsis is required.

Abnormal findings

Oral pharyngeal inflammation
Cancer
Extrinsic compression
Neuromuscular disorder
Achalasia
Upper GI motility disorder (e.g., stroke syndrome, Parkinson disease, peripheral neuropathy)
Diffuse esophageal spasms
Zenker diverticulum

notes

sweat electrolytes test (Iontophoretic sweat test)

Type of test Fluid analysis

Normal findings

Sodium values in children

Normal: <70 mEq/L
Abnormal: >90 mEq/L
Equivocal: 70-90 mEq/L

Chloride values in children

Normal: <50 mEq/L
Abnormal: >60 mEq/L
Equivocal: 50-60 mEq/L

Test explanation and related physiology

Patients with cystic fibrosis have increased sodium and chloride contents in their sweat. This forms the basis of this test, which is both sensitive and specific for cystic fibrosis. Cystic fibrosis is an inherited disease characterized by abnormal secretion by exocrine glands in the bronchi, small intestines, pancreatic ducts, bile ducts, and skin (sweat glands). Sweat induced by electrical current *(pilocarpine iontophoresis)* is collected, and its sodium and chloride contents are measured. The degree of abnormality is no indication of the severity of cystic fibrosis; it merely indicates that the patient has the disease.

In children with recurrent respiratory tract infections, malabsorption syndromes, or failure to thrive, this test may be indicated to diagnose cystic fibrosis. This test is also used to screen children or siblings of cystic fibrosis patients for the disease. Almost all patients with cystic fibrosis have sweat sodium and chloride contents two to five times greater than normal values. In patients with suspicious clinical manifestations, these levels are diagnostic of cystic fibrosis.

Procedure and patient care

Before

PT Explain the procedure to the patient and/or parents.
PT Tell the patient and/or parents that no fasting is required.

During

- Note the following procedural steps:
  1. For iontophoresis, a low-level electrical current is applied to the test area (the thigh in infants and the forearm in older children).

2. The positive electrode is covered by gauze and saturated with pilocarpine hydrochloride, a stimulating drug that induces sweating.

3. The negative electrode is covered by gauze saturated with a bicarbonate solution.

4. The electrical current is allowed to flow for 5 to 12 minutes.

5. The electrodes are removed, and the arm is washed with distilled water.

6. Paper disks are placed over the test site with the use of clean, dry forceps.

7. These disks are covered with paraffin to obtain an airtight seal, preventing evaporation of sweat.

8. After 1 hour the paraffin is removed. The paper disks are transferred immediately by forceps to a weighing jar and sent for sodium and chloride analysis.

9. A *screening test* may be done to detect sweat chloride levels. For screening, a test paper containing silver nitrate is pressed against the child's hand for several seconds. The test is positive when the excess chloride combines with the silver nitrate to form white-silver chloride on the paper (i.e., the child with cystic fibrosis will leave a "heavy" handprint on the paper).

10. A positive screening test is usually validated by iontophoresis.

• Note that an experienced technologist performs the sweat test in approximately 90 minutes in the laboratory or at the patient's bedside.

PT Inform the patient that the electrical current is small and no discomfort or pain is generally associated with this test.

After

PT Initiate extensive education and counseling for the patient and/or parents if the results indicate cystic fibrosis.

Abnormal findings

Cystic fibrosis

notes

syphilis detection test (Serologic test for syphilis [STS], Venereal Disease Research Laboratory [VDRL], Rapid plasma reagin [RPR], Fluorescent treponemal antibody test [FTA])

Type of test Blood

Normal findings Negative, or nonreactive

Test explanation and related physiology

Serologic tests are used to diagnose and to document successful therapy for syphilis. Syphilis is caused by the spirochete *Treponema pallidum* that cannot be isolated in culture. Two groups of antibodies form the basis for these tests. The first and older of these tests detects a nontreponemal antibody called *reagin*, which reacts to phospholipids similar to lipids in the membrane of *T. pallidum*. The nontreponemal antibody tests are relatively nonspecific and lack sensitivity. These antibodies would be detected by the *Wassermann test, VDRL test,* or *RPR test*. These tests become positive after 2 weeks from the patient's inoculation with *T. pallidum* and return to normal after adequate treatment is administered. The test is positive in nearly all primary and secondary stages of syphilis and in two thirds of patients with tertiary syphilis. Screening for syphilis is usually done during the first prenatal checkup for pregnant women using the VDRL or RPR. VDRL is the only test that can be used on CSF when evaluating neurosyphilis. They are also used to document the success of treatment.

If these nontreponemal serologic tests are positive, the diagnosis must be confirmed by the second type of syphilis test called *Treponema test*, such as the *FTA absorption test (FTA-ABS)* or the *microhemagglutination assay (MHA-TP)*. These tests for a more specific antibody are more accurate than the VDRL and RPR tests. The FTA-ABS and MHA-TP are technically simple to perform, but they are labor intensive and require subjective interpretation by testing personnel. In contrast, the syphilis IgG *enzyme immunoassay (EIA)* is a treponemal test for the detection of IgG class antibodies.

During early primary syphilis, the first antibodies to appear are IgM, with IgG antibodies reaching significant titers later in the primary phase. As the disease progresses into the secondary phase, IgG *T. pallidum* antibodies reach peak titers. *T. pallidum* IgG antibodies persist indefinitely, regardless of the course of the disease. If syphilis IgG and/or IgM is positive, results can be confirmed with FTA or MHA testing. The IgG- and IgM-specific

S

antibodies assist in determining the etiology of neonatal syphilis. IgM does not pass through the placenta and if positive indicates active neonatal infection.

Interfering factors

- Excessive hemolysis and gross lipemia may affect test results.
- Excess chyle in the blood may interfere with the test results.
- Many conditions cause false-positive results when VDRL and RPR tests are used. Some of these conditions include *Mycoplasma* pneumonia, malaria, acute bacterial and viral infections, autoimmune diseases, and pregnancy.
- Recent ingestion of alcohol may alter the test results.

Procedure and patient care

- See inside front cover for Routine Blood Testing.
- Fasting: verify with lab.
- Blood tube commonly used: red.
- Check with the laboratory regarding fasting requirements. Some prefer collecting the specimen before meals. Some laboratories request that the patient refrain from alcohol for 24 hours before the blood test.
- **PT** If the test is positive, instruct the patient to inform recent sexual contacts so that they can be evaluated.
- **PT** If the test is positive, be sure the patient receives the appropriate antibiotic therapy.

Abnormal findings

Syphilis

notes

testosterone (Dihydrotestosterone [DHT])

Type of test Blood

Normal findings

Free testosterone, pg/mL

Male	Female
	Postmenopausal: 0.6-3.8
Tanner Stage I: ≤3.7	Tanner Stage I: <2.2
Tanner Stage II: 0.3-21	Tanner Stage II: 0.4-4.5
Tanner Stage III: 1.0-98	Tanner Stage III: 1.3-7.5
Tanner Stage IV: 35.0-169	Tanner Stage IV: 1.1-15.5
Tanner Stage V: 41.0-239	Tanner Stage V: 0.8-9.2

% Free testosterone:
  Adult male: 1.6%-2.9%
  Adult female: 0.1%-0.3%

Total testosterone, ng/dL

Age	Male	Female
7 months-9 years (Tanner Stage I)	<30	<30
10-13 years (Tanner Stage II)	<300	<40
14-15 years (Tanner Stage III)	170-540	<60
16-19 years (Tanner Stage IV, V)	250-910	<70
20 years and over	280-1080	<70

Dihydrotestosterone:
  Adult male: 240-650 pg/mL
  Adult female: ≤300 pg/mL

Test explanation and related physiology

Testosterone levels are used to evaluate ambiguous sex characteristics, precocious puberty, virilizing syndromes in the female, and infertility in the male. This test can also be used as a tumor marker for rare tumors of the ovary and testicle.

Androgens include dehydroepiandrosterone (DHEA), androstenedione, and testosterone. DHEA is produced in the adrenal glands during cortisol and aldosterone formation, and it is also produced *de novo* by the testes or the ovaries. DHEA is the precursor of androstenedione, which is the precursor of testosterone (and estrogen).

T

Testosterone levels vary by stage of maturity (indicated by Tanner Stage). Serum concentrations of testosterone in both sexes during the first week of life average about 25 ng/dL. In male infants, values increase sharply in the second week to a maximum (the mean is about 175 ng/dL) at about 2 months, which lasts until about 6 months of age. In female infants, values decrease in the first week and remain low throughout early childhood. Levels increase during puberty to adult values.

In the male, most of the testosterone is made by the Leydig cells in the testicle; this accounts for 95% of the circulating testosterone in men. In the female, about half of the testosterone is made by the conversion of DHEA to testosterone in the peripheral fat tissue. Another 30% is made by the same conversion of DHEA in the adrenal gland, and 20% is made directly by the ovaries.

Approximately 60% of circulating testosterone binds strongly to sex hormone–binding globulin (SHBG), which is also called testosterone-binding globulin. Most of the remaining testosterone is bound loosely to albumin, and approximately 2% is free or unbound. The unbound portion is the active component. Most assays for testosterone measure the total testosterone (i.e., bound and unbound portions). The free testosterone can be measured in situations where the testosterone-binding proteins may be altered (e.g., obesity, cirrhosis, thyroid disorders). Free testosterone is estimated in this panel by an indirect method, equilibrium ultrafiltration. It can be reported as a percentage of total testosterone or as an absolute number.

Physiologically, testosterone stimulates spermatogenesis and influences the development of male secondary sex characteristics. Overproduction of this hormone in the young male may cause precocious puberty. This can be caused by testicular, adrenal, or pituitary tumors. Overproduction of this hormone in females causes masculinization, which is manifested as amenorrhea and excessive growth of body hair (hirsutism). Ovarian and adrenal tumors/hyperplasia and medications (e.g., danazol) are all potential causes of masculinization in the female. Reduced levels of testosterone in the male suggest hypogonadism or Klinefelter syndrome.

Dihydrotestosterone (DHT) is the principal androgen made in body tissues, particularly the prostate. Levels of DHT remain normal with aging, despite a decrease in the plasma testosterone, and are not elevated in benign prostatic hyperplasia. Measurement of this hormone is useful in monitoring patients receiving 5 alpha-reductase inhibitor therapy, such as finasteride or chemotherapy, that may affect prostate function. It is also useful in evaluating patients with possible 5 alpha-reductase deficiency.

There are several *testosterone stimulation tests* that can be performed to more accurately evaluate hypogonadism. Human chorionic gonadotropin, clomiphene, and GnRH can be used to stimulate testosterone secretion.

17-ketosteroids (17-KS) are metabolites of the testosterone and nontestosterone androgenic sex hormones that are excreted in the urine.

Interfering factors

✗ Drugs that may cause *increased* testosterone levels include anticonvulsants, barbiturates, estrogens, and oral contraceptives.

✗ Drugs that may cause *decreased* testosterone levels include alcohol, androgens, dexamethasone, diethylstilbestrol, digoxin, ketoconazole, phenothiazine, spironolactone, and steroids.

Procedure and patient care

- See inside front cover for Routine Blood Testing.
- Fasting: no.
- Blood tube commonly used: red.
- Because testosterone levels are the highest in the early morning hours, blood should be drawn in the morning.

T

Abnormal findings

▲ **Increased levels (male)**
Idiopathic sexual precocity
Pinealoma
Encephalitis
Congenital adrenal
hyperplasia
Adrenocortical tumor
Testicular or extragonadal
tumor
Hyperthyroidism
Testosterone resistance
syndromes

▲ **Increased levels (female)**
Ovarian tumor
Adrenal tumor
Congenital adrenocortical hyperplasia
Trophoblastic tumor
Polycystic ovaries
Idiopathic hirsutism

▼ **Decreased levels (male)**
Klinefelter syndrome
Cryptorchidism
Primary and secondary
hypogonadism
Trisomy 21 (Down
syndrome)
Orchidectomy
Hepatic cirrhosis

notes

thoracentesis and pleural fluid analysis (Pleural tap)

Type of test Fluid analysis

Normal findings

Gross appearance: Clear, serous, light yellow, 50 mL
Red blood cells (RBCs): None
White blood cells (WBCs): <300/mL
Protein: <4.1 g/dL
Glucose: 70-100 mg/dL
Amylase: 138-404 units/L
Alkaline phosphatase
    Adult male: 90-240 units/L
    Female: <45 years: 76-196 units/L
    Female: >45 years: 87-250 units/L
Lactic dehydrogenase (LDH): Similar to serum LDH
Cytology: No malignant cells
Bacteria: None
Fungi: None
Carcinoembryonic antigen (CEA): <5 ng/mL

Test explanation and related physiology

Thoracentesis is an invasive procedure that entails insertion of a needle into the pleural space for removal of fluid (Figure 41). Pleural fluid is removed for diagnostic and therapeutic purposes. *Therapeutically*, it is done to relieve pain, dyspnea, and other symptoms of pleural pressure. Removal of this fluid also permits better radiographic visualization of the lung.

Diagnostically, thoracentesis is performed to obtain and analyze fluid to determine the etiology of the pleural effusion. Pleural fluid is classified according to transudate or exudate. This is an important differentiation and is very helpful in determining the etiology of the effusion. *Transudates* are most frequently caused by congestive heart failure, cirrhosis, nephrotic syndrome, and hypoproteinemia. *Exudates* are most often found in inflammatory, infectious, or neoplastic conditions. However, collagen vascular disease, pulmonary infarction, trauma, and drug hypersensitivity also may cause an exudative effusion.

Pleural fluid is usually evaluated for the following features.

Gross appearance

The color, optical density, and viscosity are noted as the pleural fluid appears in the aspirating syringe. Empyema is characterized by the presence of a foul odor and thick, puslike fluid.

T

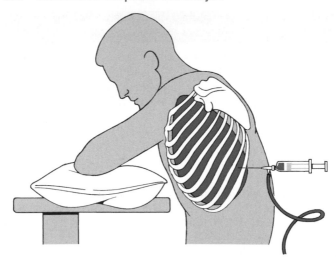

FIGURE 41 Thoracentesis. A needle is placed through the chest wall and into the fluid contained in the pleural cavity. A special one-way valve system is placed between the needle and the syringe to allow aspiration of fluid when the plunger of the syringe is pulled back and diversion of the fluid to a container when the plunger is pushed in.

An opalescent, pearly fluid is characteristic of chylothorax (chyle in the pleural cavity).

Cell counts

The WBC and differential counts are determined. A WBC count exceeding 1000/mL is suggestive of an exudate. The predominance of polymorphonuclear leukocytes usually is an indication of an acute inflammatory condition (e.g., pneumonia, pulmonary infarction, early tuberculosis effusion). When more than 50% of the WBCs are small lymphocytes, the effusion is usually caused by tuberculosis or tumor. Normally, no RBCs should be present. The presence of RBCs may indicate neoplasms, tuberculosis, or intrathoracic bleeding.

Protein content

Total protein levels greater than 3 g/dL are characteristic of exudates, whereas transudates usually have a protein content of less than 3 g/dL. The *albumin gradient* between serum and pleural fluid can differentiate better between the transudate and exudate natures of pleural fluid than can the total protein content. This gradient is obtained by subtracting the pleural albumin value from the serum albumin value. Values of 1.1 g/dL or more suggest a transudate. Values less than 1.1 g/dL suggest an exudate but will not differentiate the potential cause of the exudate (e.g., malignancy from infection or inflammation). The total protein ratio (fluid/serum) has been considered to be another accurate criterion differentiating transudate from exudate. A total protein ratio of fluid to serum of greater than 0.5 is considered to be an exudate.

Lactic dehydrogenase

A pleural fluid/serum LDH ratio greater than 0.6 is typical of an exudate. An exudate is identified with a high degree of accuracy if the pleural fluid/serum protein ratio is greater than 0.5 and the pleural fluid/serum LDH ratio is greater than 0.6.

Glucose

Usually pleural glucose levels approximate serum levels. Low values appear to be a combination of glycolysis by the extra cells and impairment of glucose diffusion because of damage to the pleural membrane. Values less than 60 mg/dL are occasionally seen in tuberculosis or malignancy and typically occur in rheumatoid arthritis and empyema.

Amylase

In a malignant effusion, the amylase concentration is slightly elevated. Amylase levels above the normal range for serum or two times the serum level are seen when the effusion is caused by pancreatitis or rupture of the esophagus associated with leakage of salivary amylase.

Triglyceride

Measurement of triglyceride levels is an important part of identifying chylous effusions. These effusions are usually produced by obstruction or transection of the lymphatic system caused by lymphoma, neoplasm, trauma, or recent surgery. The triglyceride value in a chylous effusion exceeds 110 mg/dL.

Gram stain and bacteriologic culture

These tests are routinely performed when bacterial pneumonia or empyema is a possible cause of the effusion. If possible, these should be done before initiation of antibiotic therapy.

Cultures for *Mycobacterium tuberculosis* and fungus

Tuberculosis is less often a cause for pleural effusion in the United States today than it was. Fungus may be a cause of pulmonary effusion in patients with compromised immunologic defenses.

Cytology

A cytologic study is performed to detect tumor cells in patients with malignant effusions. Breast and lung are the two most common tumors; lymphoma is the third.

Carcinoembryonic antigen

Pleural fluid CEA levels are elevated in various malignant (gastrointestinal, breast) conditions. (See p. 212.)

Special tests

The pH of pleural fluid is usually 7.4 or greater. The pH is typically less than 7.2 when empyema is present. The pH may be 7.2 to 7.4 in tuberculosis or malignancy.

In some instances, the rheumatoid factor (p. 807) and the complement levels (p. 277) are also measured in pleural fluid.

Pleural fluid antinuclear antibody (ANA) levels and pleural fluid/serum ANA ratios are often used to evaluate pleural effusion secondary to systemic lupus erythematosus.

Contraindications

- Patients with significant thrombocytopenia

Potential complications

- Pneumothorax because of puncture of the visceral pleura or entry of air into the pleural space
- Interpleural bleeding because of puncture of tissue or a blood vessel
- Hemoptysis caused by needle puncture of a pulmonary vessel or by inflammation
- Reflex bradycardia and hypotension
- Pulmonary edema
- Seeding of the needle track with tumor when malignant pleural effusion exists

Procedure and patient care

Before

- **PT** Explain the procedure to the patient.
- Obtain informed consent for this procedure.
- **PT** Tell the patient that no fasting or sedation is necessary.
- **PT** Inform the patient that movement or coughing should be minimized to avoid inadvertent needle damage to the lung or pleura during the procedure.

- Administer a cough suppressant before the procedure if the patient has a troublesome cough.

During

- Note the following procedural steps:
  1. The patient is usually placed in an upright position, with the arms and shoulders raised and supported on a padded overhead table. This position spreads the ribs and enlarges the intercostal space for insertion of the needle.
  2. Patients who cannot sit upright are placed in a side-lying position on the unaffected side, with the side to be tapped uppermost.
  3. The thoracentesis is performed under strict sterile technique.
  4. The needle insertion site, which is determined by percussion, auscultation, and examination of a chest x-ray image, ultrasound scan, or fluoroscopy, is aseptically cleansed and anesthetized locally.
  5. The needle is positioned in the pleural space, and the fluid is withdrawn with a syringe and a three-way stopcock.
  6. Various mechanisms to stabilize the pleural needle are available to secure the needle depth during the fluid collection.
  7. A short polyethylene catheter may be inserted into the pleural space for fluid aspiration; this decreases the risk of puncturing the visceral pleura and inducing a pneumothorax.
  8. Also, large volumes of fluid may be collected by connecting the catheter to a gravity-drainage system.
- Monitor the patient's pulse for reflex bradycardia and evaluate the patient for diaphoresis and a feeling of faintness.
- Note that this procedure is performed by a physician at the patient's bedside, in a procedure room, or in the physician's office in less than 30 minutes.
- **PT** Although local anesthetics eliminate pain at the insertion site, tell the patient that he or she may feel a pressure-like pain when the pleura is entered and the fluid is removed.

After

- Place a small bandage over the needle site. Usually turn the patient on the unaffected side for 1 hour to allow the pleural puncture site to heal.
- Label the specimen with the patient's name, date, source of fluid, and diagnosis. Send the specimen promptly to the laboratory.

- Obtain a chest x-ray study as indicated to check for pneumothorax.
- Monitor the patient's vital signs.
- Observe the patient for coughing or expectoration of blood (hemoptysis), which may indicate trauma to the lung.
- Evaluate the patient for signs and symptoms of pneumothorax, tension pneumothorax, subcutaneous emphysema, and pyogenic infection (e.g., tachypnea, dyspnea, diminished breath sounds, anxiety, restlessness, fever).
- Assess the patient's lung sounds for diminished breath sounds, which could be a sign of pneumothorax.
- If the patient has no complaints of dyspnea, normal activity usually can be resumed 1 hour after the procedure.

Abnormal findings

Exudate
Empyema
Pneumonia
Tuberculosis effusion
Pancreatitis
Ruptured esophagus
Tumors
Lymphoma
Pulmonary infarction
Collagen vascular disease
Drug hypersensitivity

Transudate
Cirrhosis
Congestive heart failure
Nephrotic syndrome
Hypoproteinemia
Trauma

notes

thoracoscopy

Type of test Endoscopy

Normal findings Normal pleura and lung

Test explanation and related physiology

This procedure is used to directly visualize the pleura, lung, and mediastinum. Tissue can be obtained for testing. It is also helpful in assisting in the staging and dissection of lung cancers.

With this technique, the parietal pleura, visceral pleura, and mediastinum can be directly visualized. Tumors involving the chest cavity can be staged by direct visualization. Any abnormality can be biopsied. Collections of fluid can be drained and aspirated for testing. Dissection for lung resection can be carried out with the thoracoscope *(video-assisted thoracotomy [VAT])*, thereby minimizing the extent of a thoracotomy incision.

Contraindications

- Patients with previous lung surgery, because it is difficult to obtain access to the free pleural space

Potential complications

- Bleeding
- Infection or empyema
- Prolonged pneumothorax

Procedure and patient care

Before

PT Explain the procedure to the patient.
- Ensure that informed consent for this procedure is obtained.
- Inform the patient that an open thoracotomy may be required because of the possibility of intrathoracic injury.
- Because the procedure is usually performed with the patient under general anesthesia, follow routine general anesthesia precautions.
- Shave and prepare the patient's chest as ordered.
- Keep the patient NPO after midnight on the day of the test. IV fluids may be given.

During
- Note the following procedural steps:
  1. Thoracoscopy is performed in the operating room. The patient is initially placed in the lateral decubitus position.

T

2. After the thorax is cleansed, a blunt-tipped (Verres) needle is inserted through a small incision, and the lung is collapsed.

3. A thoracoscope is inserted through a trocar to examine the chest cavity. Other trocars can be placed as conduits for other instrumentation.

4. After the desired procedure is completed, the scope and trocars are removed.

5. Usually a small chest tube is placed to ensure full reexpansion of the lung.

6. The incision(s) is (are) closed with a few skin stitches and covered with an adhesive bandage.

After

- Assess the patient frequently for signs of bleeding (increased pulse rate, decreased blood pressure). Report any significant findings to the physician.
- Provide analgesics to relieve the minor to moderate pain that may be experienced.
- If a surgical procedure has been performed thoracoscopically, provide appropriate specific postsurgical care.
- A chest x-ray is performed after the procedure to ensure complete reexpansion of the lung.

Abnormal findings

Primary lung cancer
Metastatic cancer to the lung or pleura
Empyema
Pleural tumor
Pleural infection
Pleural inflammation
Pulmonary infection

notes

throat and nose cultures

Type of test Microscopic examination

Normal findings Negative

Test explanation and related physiology

Because the throat and nose are normally colonized by many organisms, cultures of these areas serve only to isolate and identify a few particular pathogens (e.g., streptococci, meningococci, gonococci, *Bordetella pertussis, Corynebacterium diphtheriae*).

Streptococci are most often sought on a throat culture, because beta-hemolytic streptococcal pharyngitis may be followed by rheumatic heart disease or glomerulonephritis. This type of streptococcal infection most frequently affects children between the ages of 3 and 15 years. Throat cultures in adults are indicated only when the patient has a severe or recurrent sore throat often associated with fever and palpable lymphadenopathy.

Rapid immunologic tests *(strep screens)* with antiserum against group A streptococcus antigen are now available and are very accurate. With these kits, the streptococcus organism can be identified directly from the swab specimen without culture. These tests can be performed in about 15 minutes. If the test is negative, no streptococcus infection exists.

Nasal and nasopharyngeal cultures are often done to screen for infections and carrier states caused by various other organisms, such as *Staphylococcus aureus, Haemophilus influenzae, Neisseria meningitidis,* respiratory syncytial virus (RSV), and viruses causing rhinitis. Health care workers in the operating room and newborn nursery may have these cultures to screen potential sources of spread when an outbreak occurs in a hospital setting. These cultures are also used to detect infection in elderly and debilitated patients.

All cultures should be performed before antibiotic therapy is initiated. Otherwise, the antibiotic may interrupt the growth of the organism in the laboratory. Most organisms take approximately 24 hours to grow in the laboratory, and a preliminary report can be given at that time. Occasionally, 48 to 72 hours is required for growth and identification of the organism. Cultures may be repeated on completion of appropriate antibiotic therapy to identify resolution of the infection.

T

Interfering factors

☒ Drugs that may affect test results include antibiotics and antiseptic mouthwashes.

Procedure and patient care

Before

PT Explain the procedure to the patient.

During

- Obtain a *throat culture* by depressing the tongue with a wooden tongue blade and touching the posterior wall of the throat and areas of inflammation, exudation, or ulceration with a sterile cotton swab. Two swabs are preferred. Growth of streptococcus from both swabs is more accurate, and the second swab can also be used in the strep screen. Avoid touching any other part of the mouth. Place the swabs in a sterile container.
- Obtain a *nasal culture* by gently raising the tip of the nose and inserting a flexible swab into the nares. Rotate the swab against the side of the nares. Remove the swab and place it in an appropriate culture tube.
- Obtain a *nasopharyngeal culture* by gently raising the tip of the nose and inserting a flexible swab along the bottom of the nares. Guide this swab until it reaches the posterior pharynx. Rotate the swab to obtain secretions and then remove it. Place the swab in an appropriate culture tube.
- Wear gloves and handle the specimen as if it were capable of transmitting disease.
- Indicate on the laboratory slip any medications that the patient may be taking that could affect test results.

After

- Label all specimens and send them immediately to the microbiology lab.
- Notify the physician of any positive results so that appropriate antibiotic therapy can be initiated.

Abnormal findings

Bacterial pathogens (e.g., streptococci)
Respiratory syncytial virus
H. influenzae bacteria

notes

thromboelastography (Thromboelastometry)

Type of test Blood

Normal findings 5.3-12.4 dynes/cm²

Possible critical value >12.4 dynes/cm²

Test explanation and related physiology

Hemostasis is a balanced process in which the blood forms localized clots when the integrity of the vascular system is breeched. Trauma, infection, and inflammation all activate the blood's clotting system, which depends on the interaction of two separate systems: enzymatic proteins (clotting factors, intrinsic and extrinsic systems; see Figure 42) and platelets. The two systems work in concert to plug defects in the broken vessels. The clots that form in this process need to be of sufficient strength to resist dislodgement. If a particular clotting factor is dysfunctional or absent, as in hemophilia, an insufficient amount of fibrin forms. Similarly, massive consumption of clotting factors in a trauma situation decreases the amount of fibrin formed. Inadequate numbers of platelets resulting from trauma, surgery, or chemotherapy also decrease platelet aggregation, as do genetic disorders, uremia, or medication therapy. Ultimately, reduced fibrin formation or platelet aggregation results in clots of inadequate tensile strength. This *hypo*coagulable state is associated with excessive bleeding. Conversely, endothelial injury, stasis, cancer, genetic diseases, or other *hyper*coagulable states lead to thrombosis formation, causing thromboembolic events.

This test is used to identify patients who are hypercoagulable and may experience a thromboembolic phenomenon when immobile (e.g., after surgery or trauma). It is particularly helpful in cardiac surgery and liver transplantation. It is also used to determine hyperfibrinolysis. This test can evaluate platelet function and determine the percent of platelet inhibition instigated by drugs such as heparin, aspirin, and antiplatelet drugs (Plavix, Ticlid).

Interfering factors

🍷 Drugs that may cause *decreased* thromboelastography include antiplatelet drugs (e.g., ticlodipine), some antibiotics, aspirin, beta-blockers, clofibrate, dextran, ethanol, heparin, nonsteroidal antiinflammatory drugs (NSAIDs), phenothiazines, tricyclics, theophylline, and warfarin sodium (Coumadin).

T

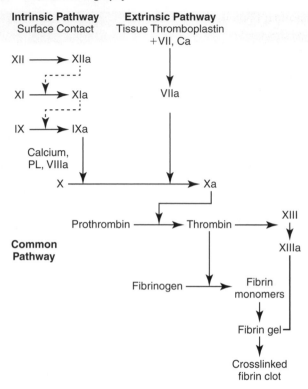

Intrinsic Pathway
Surface Contact

Extrinsic Pathway
Tissue Thromboplastin
+VII, Ca

XII ⟶ XIIa

XI ⟶ XIa

VIIa

IX ⟶ IXa

Calcium,
PL, VIIIa

X ⟶ Xa

**Common
Pathway**

Prothrombin ⟶ Thrombin ⟶ XIII

XIIIa

Fibrinogen ⟶ Fibrin
monomers

Fibrin gel

Crosslinked
fibrin clot

FIGURE 42 Simplified enzymatic cascade of fibrin clot formation.

Procedure and patient care

- See inside front cover for Routine Blood Testing.
- Fasting: no.
- Blood tube commonly used: red.
- If the patient is receiving any drugs that may interfere with normal coagulation or has any diseases such as jaundice, hyperlipidemia, or hemolysis, this should be listed on the laboratory request slip.
- Immediately transfer the specimen to the laboratory.
- Remember that abnormalities in platelet aggregation can prolong bleeding time, and a significant hematoma at the venipuncture site may occur.

Abnormal findings

Hypocoagulability
    Factor deficiency
    Anticoagulation
    Thrombocytopenia
    Platelet function abnormalities
    Increased fibrinolysis
Hypercoagulability
    Factor V-Leiden abnormality
    Protein S/C abnormality
    Genetic hypercoagulability
    Idiopathic hypercoagulability

notes

T

> **thrombosis indicators**
> **fibrin monomers** (Fibrin degradation products [FDPs], Fibrin split products [FSPs])
> **fibrinopeptide A** (FPA)
> **prothrombin fragment** (F1+2)

Type of test Blood

Normal findings

FDP: <10 mcg/mL or <10 mg/L (SI units)
FPA
    Male: 0.4-2.6 mg/mL
    Female: 0.7-3.1 mg/mL
F1+2: 7.4-103 mcg/L or 0.2-2.8 nmol/L

Possible critical values FDP: >40 mcg/mL

Test explanation and related physiology

Identification of FDPs, FPA, and F1+2 is mostly used to document that fibrin clot formation and therefore thrombosis is occurring in patients. These tests support the diagnosis of disseminated intravascular coagulation (DIC). The D-dimer test (p. 335) is more commonly used to identify DIC or other forms of thrombosis. These tests also provide an indication of the effectiveness of anticoagulation therapy. Finally, they are used to support the diagnosis and follow treatment for hypercoagulable states.

F1+2 is liberated when prothrombin is converted to thrombin in reaction 4 of secondary hemostasis (see Figure 10, p. 264). FPA is released into the bloodstream from alpha and beta chains of fibrinogen during its conversion to fibrin.

Measurement of FDPs is an indicator of the activity of the fibrinolytic system. Whenever a fibrin clot or primarily fibrinogen degenerates, fragment monomers called FDPs (X, D, E, and Y) result. These, therefore, are indirect evidence of thrombosis and/or DIC. FDPs also are increased with other secondary fibrinolytic disorders. Thrombolytic therapy used to treat vascular thrombosis is associated with increased FDPs. Streptokinase or urokinase stimulates the conversion of plasminogen to plasmin.

These products of hemostasis and fibrinolysis also may be elevated in patients with extensive malignancy, tissue necrosis, trauma surgery, or gram-negative sepsis. For discussion of D-dimer fibrin degradation products, see p. 335.

Interfering factors

- Traumatic venipunctures may increase FPA levels.
- Surgery or massive trauma is associated with increased levels.
- Menstruation may be associated with increased FDP levels.
- ✗ Drugs that may cause *increased* levels include barbiturates, streptokinase, and urokinase.
- ✗ Drugs that may cause *decreased* levels include warfarin and other oral anticoagulants.

Procedure and patient care

- See inside front cover for Routine Blood Testing.
- Fasting: no.
- Blood tube commonly used: verify with lab.
- Avoid prolonged use of a tourniquet.
- Draw the sample before initiating heparin therapy.
- Avoid excessive agitation of the blood sample.

Abnormal findings

▲ **Increased levels**
DIC
Heart or vascular surgery
Thromboembolism
Thrombosis
Advanced malignancy
Severe inflammation
Postoperative states
Massive trauma
Deficiency in proteins S and C
Antithrombin III deficiency

▼ **Decreased levels**
Anticoagulation therapy

notes

thyroglobulin (Tg, Thyrogen-stimulated thyroglobulin)

Type of test Blood

Normal findings

Age	Male	Female
0-11 months	0.6-5.5 ng/mL	0.5-5.5 ng/mL
1-11 years	0.6-50.1 ng/mL	0.5-52.1 ng/mL
12 years and older	0.5-53.0 ng/mL	0.5-43.0 ng/mL

Test explanation and related physiology

Thyroglobulin is the protein precursor of thyroid hormone and is made by both normal, well-differentiated, benign thyroid cells and thyroid cancer cells. Because thyroglobulin is normally only made by thyroid cells, it serves as a useful readout for the presence or absence of thyroid cells, especially after thyroid cancer surgery. This test is primarily used as a tumor marker for well-differentiated thyroid cancers.

In the treatment of well-differentiated thyroid cancers, it is important to remove as much thyroid tissue as possible so that adjunctive radioactive iodine treatment will not go to residual thyroid gland tissue in the neck but will go instead to any metastatic thyroid cells. If postoperative Tg levels are low, very little thyroid tissue remains.

Tg is also used as a tumor marker in these postoperative patients. Tg is a marker of disease activity and the volume of thyroid tumor. Ideally, the thyroglobulin levels will be low (less than 2 ng/mL) or undetectable after treatment (usually surgery followed by radioactive iodine). Rising levels herald tumor recurrence and progression. Although Tg levels may be elevated in patients with thyroid cancer, a large number of benign thyroid conditions may also be associated with elevated levels of Tg. Therefore, an increased Tg level alone in a patient is not a sensitive or specific test for the diagnosis of thyroid cancer. Simply examining the thyroid or carrying out a thyroid biopsy can produce significant elevations in the circulating blood level of thyroglobulin. Similarly, patients with thyroid inflammation can have very high levels of Tg.

After thyroidectomy, thyroid hormone replacement is required for normal metabolic function. Thyroid-stimulating hormone (TSH) levels are usually very low when thyroid hormone is replaced adequately. Endogenous stimulation of any residual thyroid cells is minimal in these patients. As a result, Tg and endogenous thyroid hormones are low. Until recently, to stimulate Tg production in these patients for cancer surveillance testing, thyroid hormone had to be temporarily discontinued for as long as 6 weeks until the body was depleted of any thyroid hormone. TSH was then maximally stimulated and able to stimulate the production of Tg from thyroid cells. If there were any functioning thyroid cancer cells, Tg would be elevated. During the time of thyroid hormone withdrawal, the patient would be very uncomfortable, lethargic, tired, and slow.

Thyrogen-stimulated testing has eliminated the need for withdrawal of thyroid hormone medications and provides a safe and effective method to elevate TSH levels so that even minimal levels of Tg can be detected. This allows patients to undergo periodic thyroid cancer follow-up evaluations while avoiding the often debilitating side effects of hypothyroidism, which is caused by withdrawal of hormone medication.

Thyrogen is a highly purified recombinant source of human TSH. Thyrogen raises serum TSH levels and thereby stimulates Tg production. Normal thyroid-remnant and well-differentiated thyroid tumors display a greater (>tenfold) serum Tg response to TSH stimulation. If, after thyroid surgery, Thyrogen-stimulated Tg levels are elevated, either a significant amount of normal thyroid gland was left in the neck or metastatic disease exists. If Thyrogen-stimulated Tg levels are elevated after postoperative therapeutic I^{131} (given to destroy any residual thyroid tissue in the neck), metastatic disease certainly exists and will require treatment.

Thyrogen stimulation is also used for patients undergoing I^{131} whole-body scanning for metastatic thyroid cancer. Like Tg testing, in the past these patients had to withdraw from their thyroid hormone–replacement medicine so that their endogenous TSH levels would rise, stimulate any metastatic thyroid cancer cells to pick up I^{131}, and be detected on a nuclear scan of the body. Now, with the use of Thyrogen, the ill effects of hormone withdrawal are not experienced.

T

Interfering factors

- Tg levels are decreased in less well-differentiated thyroid cancers.
- Thyrogen stimulation of Tg levels is less in patients whose tumors do not have TSH receptors or whose tumors cannot make Tg.
- Tg autoantibodies cause either underestimation or overestimation of serum Tg measurements made by immunometric assay (IMA) or radioimmunoassay (RIA) methods, respectively.

Procedure and patient care

- See inside front cover for Routine Blood Testing.
- Fasting: no.
- Blood tube commonly used: serum separator.
- Determine whether the patient is to have a whole-body nuclear scan along with the Tg blood test.
- If *Thyrogen stimulation* is to be used:
  1. Administer Thyrogen intramuscularly to the buttock every 24 hours for two or three doses as ordered.
  2. Collect a venous blood sample in a gold-top (serum separator) tube after 3 days.
- For *radioiodine imaging*:
  1. The nuclear medicine technologist will administer the radioiodine 24 hours following the final Thyrogen injection.
  2. Scanning is usually performed 48 hours after radioiodine administration. Whole-body images are acquired for a minimum of 30 minutes and/or should contain a minimum of 140,000 counts.
  3. Scanning times for single (spot) images of body regions may be obtained.

Abnormal findings

▲ **Increased levels**
Residual thyroid tissue in the neck
Metastatic thyroid cancer

notes

thyroid scanning (Thyroid scintiscan)

Type of test Nuclear scan

Normal findings

Normal size, shape, position, and function of the thyroid gland
No areas of decreased or increased uptake

Test explanation and related physiology

Thyroid scanning allows the size, shape, position, and physiologic function of the thyroid gland to be determined with the use of radionuclear scanning. A radioactive substance, such as technetium-99 m, is given to the patient to visualize the thyroid gland. Planar and pinhole (magnified concentrated) images of the thyroid are obtained.

Thyroid nodules are easily detected by this technique. Nodules are classified as functioning (warm/hot) or nonfunctioning (cold), depending on the amount of radionuclide taken up by the nodule. A functioning nodule could represent a benign adenoma or a localized toxic goiter. A nonfunctioning nodule may represent a cyst, carcinoma, nonfunctioning adenoma or goiter, lymphoma, or localized area of thyroiditis.

Scanning is useful in patients with:
- A neck or substernal mass
- A thyroid nodule. Thyroid cancers are usually nonfunctioning (cold) nodules.
- Hyperthyroidism. Scanning assists in differentiating Graves disease (diffusely enlarged hyperfunctioning thyroid gland) from Plummer disease (nodular hyperfunctioning gland).
- Metastatic tumors without a known primary site. A normal scan excludes the thyroid gland as a possible primary site.
- A well-differentiated form of thyroid cancer. Areas of metastasis may show up on subsequent whole-body nuclear scans.

Thyroid scanning is usually preceded by a thyroid uptake scan. An iodine-123 capsule is given to the patient 6 to 24 hours before measuring iodine uptake. After uptake counts are obtained, Tc 99m^{04} is administered intravenously. Scan images are then obtained as described above.

Another form of thyroid scan is called the *whole-body thyroid scan*. This scan is performed on patients who have previously had a thyroid cancer treated. An iodine-131 capsule/solution, Tc 99m^{04}, or iodine-123 is given orally, and the entire body is scanned to look for metastatic thyroid tissue. A hot spot indicates recurrent tumor. This test is routinely performed (every

T

1 to 2 years) on patients who have had a thyroid cancer larger than 1 cm.

Contraindications

- Patients who are allergic to iodine or shellfish
- Patients who are pregnant, unless the benefits outweigh the risks

Potential complications

- Radiation-induced oncogenesis
  This complication is minimized if technetium or low-radioactive iodine isomers are used instead of iodine-131.

Interfering factors

- Iodine-containing foods
- Recent administration of x-ray contrast agents
- ✗ Drugs that may affect test results include cough medicines, multiple vitamins, oral contraceptives (some), and thyroid drugs.

Procedure and patient care

Before

PT Explain the procedure to the patient.
- Check the patient for allergies to iodine.
PT Instruct the patient about medications that need to be restricted for weeks before the test (e.g., thyroid drugs, medications containing iodine).
- Obtain a history concerning previous contrast x-ray studies, nuclear scanning, or intake of any thyroid-suppressive or antithyroid drugs.
PT Tell the patient that fasting is usually not required. Check with the laboratory.

During

- Note the following procedural steps:
  1. A standard dose of iodine-123 is usually given to the patient by mouth 6 to 24 hours before scanning. The capsule or solution is tasteless.
  2. Iodine uptake is measured. Intravenous technetium is administered, and thyroid imaging is performed 2 hours later.
  3. At the designated time, the patient is placed in a supine position and anterolateral images of the thyroid area are obtained. The whole-body imaging protocol is somewhat different.
  4. The radioactive counts are recorded and displayed.

- Note that this study is performed by a radiologic technologist in less than 30 minutes and is then interpreted by a nuclear medicine physician.
PT Tell the patient that no discomfort is associated with this study.

After

PT Usually the dose of radioactivity used in this test is minimal and considered harmless. No isolation and no special urine precautions are needed. However, if higher doses of radionuclide are used, isolation for 24 hours may be recommended.

Abnormal findings

Adenoma
Toxic and nontoxic goiter
Cyst
Carcinoma
Lymphoma
Thyroiditis
Graves disease
Plummer disease
Metastasis
Hyperthyroidism
Hypothyroidism
Hashimoto thyroiditis

notes

T

thyroid-stimulating hormone (TSH, Thyrotropin, TRH stimulation test)

Type of test Blood

Normal findings

Adult: 2-10 µU/mL or 2-10 mU/L (SI units)
Newborn: 3-18 µU/mL or 3-18 mU/L
Cord: 3-12 µU/mL or 3-12 mU/L
(Values vary among laboratories.)

Test explanation and related physiology

The TSH concentration aids in differentiating primary from secondary hypothyroidism. Pituitary TSH secretion is stimulated by hypothalamic thyroid-releasing hormone (TRH). Low levels of triiodothyronine and thyroxine (T_3, T_4) are the underlying stimuli for TRH and TSH. Therefore, a compensatory elevation of TRH and TSH occurs in patients with primary hypothyroid states such as surgical or radioactive thyroid ablation; patients with burned-out thyroiditis, thyroid agenesis, idiopathic hypothyroidism, or congenital cretinism; or patients taking antithyroid medications.

In secondary hypothyroidism, the function of the hypothalamus or pituitary gland is faulty because of tumor, trauma, or infarction. Thus, TRH and TSH cannot be secreted, and plasma levels of these hormones are near 0 despite low T_3 and T_4 levels.

The *TRH stimulation test* is sometimes used to stimulate low levels of TSH to identify primary from secondary hypothyroidism in cases in which TSH is low. However, this test is not commonly used because extremely low levels of TSH can be identified now with the use of immunoassays.

The TSH test is used as well to monitor exogenous thyroid replacement. The goal of thyroid replacement therapy is to provide an adequate amount of thyroid medication so that TSH secretion is in the low normal range, indicating a euthyroid state. Therefore, doses of medication are given to keep the TSH level less than 2. Even lower TSH levels are preferred if thyroid suppression is the clinical goal. This test is also done to detect primary hypothyroidism in newborns with low screening T_4 levels. TSH and T_4 levels are frequently measured to differentiate pituitary from thyroid dysfunction. A decreased T_4 with a normal or elevated TSH level can indicate a thyroid disorder. A decreased T_4 with a decreased TSH level can indicate a pituitary disorder.

Interfering factors

- Recent radioisotope administration may affect test results.
- Severe illness may cause decreased TSH levels.
- Drugs that may cause *increased* levels include antithyroid medications, lithium, potassium iodide, and TSH injection.
- Drugs that may cause *decreased* levels include aspirin, dopamine, heparin, steroids, and T_3.

Procedure and patient care

- See inside front cover for Routine Blood Testing.
- Fasting: no.
- Blood tube commonly used: red.
- Use a heel stick to obtain blood from newborns.

Abnormal findings

▲ Increased levels

  Primary hypothyroidism
    (thyroid dysfunction)
  Thyroiditis
  Thyroid agenesis
  Congenital cretinism
  Large doses of iodine
  Severe and chronic illnesses
  Pituitary TSH-secreting tumor

▼ Decreased levels

  Secondary
    hypothyroidism
    (pituitary dysfunction)
  Hyperthyroidism
  Pituitary hypofunction

notes

T

thyroid-stimulating hormone stimulation test (TSH stimulation test)

Type of test Blood

Normal findings Increased thyroid function with administration of exogenous TSH

Test explanation and related physiology

The TSH stimulation test is used to differentiate *primary* (or thyroidal) hypothyroidism from *secondary* (or hypothalamic-pituitary) hypothyroidism. Normal people and patients with hypothalamic-pituitary hypothyroidism can increase thyroid function when exogenous TSH is given. However, patients with primary thyroidal hypothyroidism do not; their thyroid gland is inadequate and cannot function no matter how much stimulation it receives. Patients with less than a 10% increase in radioactive iodine uptake (RAIU) or less than a 1.5 mcg/dL rise in thyroxine (T_4) are considered to have a primary cause for their hypothyroid state. If the initially low uptake is caused by inadequate pituitary stimulation of an intrinsically normal thyroid gland, the RAIU should increase at least 10% and the T_4 level should rise 1.5 mcg/dL or more. This is characteristic of secondary hypothyroidism.

Procedure and patient care

- See inside front cover for Routine Blood Testing.
- Fasting: no.
- Blood tube commonly used: verify with lab.
- Obtain baseline levels of RAIU or T_4 (p. 922) as indicated.
- Administer the prescribed dose of TSH intramuscularly for 3 days.
- Repeat the levels of RAIU or T_4 as indicated.

Abnormal findings

Primary (thyroidal) hypothyroidism
Secondary (hypothalamic-pituitary) hypothyroidism

notes

thyroid-stimulating immunoglobulins (TSIs, Long-acting thyroid stimulator [LATS], Thyroid-binding inhibitory immunoglobulin [TBII], Thyrotropin receptor antibody, Thyroid-stimulating hormone receptor [TSHR] antibodies)

Type of test Blood

Normal findings

TSI: <130% of basal activity
TBII: <10% inhibition

Test explanation and related physiology

Thyroid-stimulating immunoglobulins (TSIs) represent a group of immunoglobulin G (IgG) antibodies directed against the thyroid cell receptor for thyroid-stimulating hormone (TSH) and are associated with autoimmune thyroid disease states, such as chronic thyroiditis and Graves disease. These autoantibodies bind and transactivate the TSH receptors (TSHRs). This instigates stimulation of the thyroid gland independent of the normal feedback-regulated TSH stimulation. This, in turn, will stimulate the release of thyroid hormones from the thyroid cells. Some patients with Graves disease also have TSHR-blocking antibodies, which do not transactivate the TSHR. The balance between TSI and TSHR-blocking antibodies, as well as their individual titers, is felt to be a determinant of Graves disease severity.

The use of these antibodies is helpful in the evaluation of patients for whom the diagnosis of Graves disease is confused by conflicting data (e.g., subclinical Graves hyperthyroidism or euthyroid patients with ophthalmopathy). In these cases, the antibodies help determine and support the diagnosis of Graves disease.

The effect of these antibodies on the thyroid may be long-lasting, and titers do not decrease until nearly 1 year after successful treatment of the thyroid disease. However, measurement of these antibodies may be helpful in identifying remission or relapse of Graves disease after treatment. Because TSIs can cross the placenta, they may be found in neonates whose mothers have Graves disease. These infants experience hyperthyroidism (neonatal thyrotoxicosis) for as long as 4 to 8 months. This syndrome must be identified and treated early.

TSI and TSHR antibodies can be measured individually. Other antibodies associated with autoimmune thyroid diseases include thyroglobulin antibodies (p. 101) and antithyroid peroxidase antibodies (p. 102).

T

Interfering factors

- Recent administration of radioactive iodine may affect test results.

Procedure and patient care

- See inside front cover for Routine Blood Testing.
- Fasting: no.
- Blood tube commonly used: red or gold.
- Notify the laboratory if the patient has received radioactive iodine in the preceding 2 days.
- Handle the blood sample gently. Hemolysis may interfere with interpretation of test results.

Abnormal findings

▲ Increased levels

Hyperthyroidism

Malignant exophthalmos

Graves disease

Hashimoto thyroiditis

Neonatal thyrotoxicosis

notes

thyroid ultrasound (Thyroid echogram, Thyroid sonogram)

Type of test Ultrasound

Normal findings Normal size, shape, and position of the thyroid gland

Test explanation and related physiology

Ultrasound examination of the thyroid gland is valuable for distinguishing cystic from solid thyroid nodules. If the nodule is found to be purely cystic (fluid filled), the fluid can simply be aspirated and surgery avoided. If the nodule has a mixed or solid appearance, however, a tumor may be present, and surgery may be required. This study may be repeated at intervals to determine the response of a thyroid mass to medical therapy.

Procedure and patient care

Before

PT Explain the procedure to the patient.

PT Tell the patient that breathing or swallowing will not be affected by the placement of a transducer on the neck.

PT Inform the patient that a lubricant will be applied to the neck to ensure effective transmission of sound waves.

PT Tell the patient that no fasting or sedation is required.

During

- Note the following procedural steps:
  1. The patient is taken to the ultrasonography department and placed in the supine position with the neck hyperextended.
  2. Gel is applied to the patient's neck.
  3. A sound transducer is passed over the nodule.
  4. Photographs are taken of the image displayed.
- Note that an ultrasound technologist usually performs this study in approximately 15 minutes and that a radiologist evaluates the results.

PT Tell the patient that no discomfort is associated with this study.

After

- Assist the patient in removing the lubricant from the neck.

Abnormal findings

Cyst	Thyroid carcinoma
Tumor	Goiter
Thyroid adenoma	

notes

thyrotropin-releasing hormone stimulation test (TRH stimulation test, Thyrotropin-releasing factor stimulation test [TRF stimulation test])

Type of test Blood

Normal findings

Baseline thyroid-stimulating hormone (TSH): <10 µU/mL
Stimulated TSH: more than double the baseline

Test explanation and related physiology

The TRH stimulation test assesses the anterior pituitary gland via its secretion of TSH in response to an IV injection of TRH. After the TRH injection, the normally functioning pituitary gland should secrete TSH. In hyperthyroidism, either a slight or no increase in the TSH level is seen because pituitary TSH production is suppressed by the direct effect of excess circulating thyroxine and triiodothyronine (T_4, T_3) on the pituitary gland. A normal result is considered reliable evidence for excluding the diagnosis of thyrotoxicosis. Since the development of very sensitive radioimmunoassay for TSH, the TRH stimulation test is no longer required to diagnose hyperthyroidism. However, it still has a role in the evaluation of pituitary deficiency.

In addition to assessing the responsiveness of the anterior pituitary gland, this test aids in the detection of primary, secondary, and tertiary hypothyroidism. In primary hypothyroidism (thyroid gland failure), the increase in the TSH level is two or more times the normal result. With secondary hypothyroidism (anterior pituitary failure), no TSH response occurs. Tertiary hypothyroidism (hypothalamic failure) may be diagnosed by a delayed rise in the TSH level. Multiple injections of TRH may be needed to induce the appropriate TSH response in this case.

The TRH test also may be useful in differentiating primary depression from manic-depressive psychiatric illness and from secondary types of depression. In primary depression, the TSH response is blunted in most patients, whereas patients with other types of depression have a normal TRH-induced TSH response.

Interfering factors

- Pregnancy may increase the TSH response to TRH.
- Drugs that may modify the TSH response include antithyroid drugs, aspirin, corticosteroids, estrogens, levodopa, and T_4.

Procedure and patient care

- See inside front cover for Routine Blood Testing.
- Fasting: no.
- Blood tube commonly used: verify with lab.
- **PT** Instruct the patient to discontinue thyroid preparations for 3 to 4 weeks before the TRH test, if indicated.
- Assess the patient for medications currently being taken.
- Administer a prescribed IV bolus of TRH.
- Obtain venous blood samples at intervals, and measure for TSH levels.
- Indicate on the laboratory slip if the patient is pregnant.

Abnormal findings

Hyperthyroidism
Hypothyroidism
Psychiatric primary depression
Acute starvation
Old age (especially in men)
Pregnancy

notes

T

thyroxine, total and free (T₄, Thyroxine screen, FT₄)

Type of test   Blood

Normal findings

Free T₄:

0-4 days: 2-6 ng/dL or 26-68 pmol/L (SI units)
2 weeks-20 years: 0.8-2 ng/dL or 10-26 pmol/L (SI units)
Adult: 0.8-2.8 ng/dL or 10-36 pmol/L (SI units)

Total T₄:

1-3 days: 11-22 mcg/dL or 152-292 nmol/L (SI units)
1-2 weeks: 10-16 mcg/dL or 126-214 nmol/L (SI units)
1-12 months: 8-16 mcg/dL or 101-213 nmol/L (SI units)
1-5 years: 7-15 mcg/dL or 94-194 nmol/L (SI units)
5-10 years: 6-13 mcg/dL or 83-172 nmol/L (SI units)
10-15 years: 5-12 mcg/dL or 72-151 nmol/L (SI units)
Adult male: 4-12 mcg/dL or 59-135 nmol/L (SI units)
Adult female: 5-12 mcg/dL or 71-142 nmol/L (SI units)
Adult >60 years: 5-11 mcg/dL or 64-142 nmol/L (SI units)
Pregnancy: 9-14 mcg/dL or 117-181 nmol/L (SI units)

Test explanation and related physiology

Thyroid hormones regulate a number of developmental, metabolic, and neural activities throughout the body. The two main hormones secreted by the thyroid gland are thyroxine, which contains four atoms of iodine (T_4), and triiodothyronine (T_3, p. 929). More than 90% of thyroid hormone is made up of T_4. Thyroid hormones circulate primarily bound to carrier proteins (e.g., thyroid-binding globulin [TBG], albumin, or transthyretin); a small fraction circulates unbound (free). Only the free forms are metabolically active. Ninety-nine percent of T_4 is bound to proteins (TBG, albumin, or transthyretin). Total T_4 measurements consists of both the bound and unbound fractions. Free T_4 is a measure of unbound metabolically active T_4. Thyroxine tests are used to determine thyroid function. Greater than normal levels indicate hyperthyroid states, and subnormal values are seen in hypothyroid states. T_4 and TSH are used to monitor thyroid replacement and suppressive therapy.

Abnormalities in protein levels can have a significant effect on the results of the total T_4. Pregnancy and hormone replacement therapy increase TBG and may cause total T_4 to be falsely elevated, suggesting that hyperthyroidism exists when in fact the patient is euthyroid. If the free T_4 is measured in these patients, it would be normal, indicating that free T_4 is a more accurate indicator of thyroid function than total T_4. In cases in which TBG is reduced (e.g., hypoproteinemia), the total T_4 is likewise reduced, suggesting hypothyroidism. Measurement of free T_4 would indicate normal levels and thereby discount the abnormal total T_4 as merely a result of the reduced TBG and not as a result of hypothyroidism.

Interfering factors

- Neonates have higher free T_4 levels than older children and adults.
- Prior use of iodinated radioisotopes or iodinated contrast material can alter test results.
- Pregnancy causes increased total T_4 levels.
- ✘ Drugs that *increase* free T_4 levels include aspirin, danazol, heparin, and propranolol.
- ✘ Drugs that *decrease* free T_4 levels include furosemide, methadone, phenytoins, and rifampicin.
- ✘ Exogenously administered thyroxine causes *increased* free T_4.
- ✘ Drugs that may cause *increased* total T_4 levels include clofibrate, estrogens, heroin, methadone, and oral contraceptives.
- ✘ Drugs that may cause *decreased* T_4 levels include anabolic steroids, androgens, antithyroid drugs (e.g., propylthiouracil), lithium, phenytoin, and propranolol.

Procedure and patient care

- See inside front cover for Routine Blood Testing.
- Fasting: no.
- Blood tube commonly used: red.
- Evaluate the patient's medication history.
- **PT** If indicated, instruct the patient to stop exogenous T_4 medication 1 month before testing.
- List on the laboratory slip any drugs that may affect test results.

T

Abnormal findings

▲ **Increased levels**
  Graves disease
  Toxic thyroid adenoma
  Acute thyroiditis
  Familial dysalbuminemic
    hyperthyroxinemia
  Factitious hyperthyroidism
  Struma ovarii
  Pregnancy
  Hepatitis
  Congenital hyperproteinemia
  Thyroid cancer
  Toxic multinodular goiter`

▼ **Decreased levels**
  Cretinism
  Surgical ablation of the
    thyroid
  Myxedema
  Pituitary insufficiency
  Hypothalamic failure
  Iodine insufficiency
  Renal failure
  Cushing syndrome
  Cirrhosis
  Hashimoto thyroiditis
  Thyroid agenesis
  TSH receptor defects

notes

thyroxine-binding globulin (TBG, Thyroid-binding globulin)

Type of test Blood

Normal findings

Age	Male (mg/dL)	Female (mg/dL)
1-5 days	2.2-5.9	2.2-5.9
1-11 months	3.1-5.6	3-5.6
1-9 years	2.5-5	2.5-5
10-19 years	2.1-4.6	2.1-4.6
>20 years	1.2-2.5	1.4-3

Oral contraceptives: 1.5-5.5 mg/dL
Pregnancy (third trimester): 4.7-5.9 mg/dL

Test explanation and related physiology

TBG is the major thyroid hormone protein carrier. When it is elevated, total T_3 and total T_4 are also elevated. This may give the false indication that the patient has hyperthyroidism when in fact the patient just has elevated TBGs. When total T_4 is elevated, one must ascertain whether that elevation is caused by an elevation in TBG or a real elevation in T_4 alone, which is associated with hyperthyroidism.

The most common causes of elevated TBGs are pregnancy, hormone replacement therapy, and the use of oral contraceptives. Elevated TBGs are also present in some cases of porphyria and in infectious hepatitis. Decreased TBGs are commonly associated with other causes of hypoproteinemia (e.g., nephrotic syndrome, gastrointestinal malabsorption, and malnutrition).

Interfering factors

✘ Drugs that *increase* TBG include estrogens, methadone, oral contraceptives, and tamoxifen.
✘ Drugs that *decrease* TBG include androgens, anabolic steroids, danazol, phenytoin, propranolol, and steroids.

Procedure and patient care

- See inside front cover for Routine Blood Testing.
- Fasting: no.
- Blood tube commonly used: red.
- List on the laboratory slip any drugs that may affect test results.

T

Abnormal findings

▲ **Increased levels**

Pregnancy

Estrogen replacement
   therapy

Estrogen-producing tumors

Infectious hepatitis

Genetic increased TBG

Acute intermittent porphyria

▼ **Decreased levels**

Protein-losing enteropathy

Protein-losing nephropathy

Malnutrition

Testosterone-producing
   tumors

Ovarian failure

Major stress

notes

TORCH test

The term *TORCH* (toxoplasmosis, other, rubella, cytomegalovirus, herpes) has been applied to maternal infections with recognized detrimental effects on the fetus. TORCH testing refers to the testing for IgG (indicating past infection) and IgM (indicating recent infection) antibodies to the particular infectious agents described. Included in the category of *other* are such infections as syphilis. All of these tests are discussed separately:

- Toxoplasmosis, p. 920
- Rubella, p. 810
- Cytomegalovirus, p. 333
- Herpesvirus, p. 510

The direct effects of these infections may be immediate or delayed. A majority of infants infected by toxoplasmosis in utero are asymptomatic at birth with neurologic sequelae appearing later in life. Prenatal rubella infections, on the other hand, may severely damage the fetus, causing congenital heart disease and mental retardation. Congenital CMV infections can result in infant death, hearing loss, cerebral palsy, mental retardation, or chorioretinitis. Neonatal herpes infection (can occur in utero or during birth) presents as localized infection to the skin, eye, and mouth (SEM), or as disseminated infection (involving multiple organs, such as the liver, lung, adrenal glands, or brain). The earlier these infections are recognized, the earlier they can be treated or steps can be made to preclude the long-term effects of the disease. Other effects of TORCH infections on the fetus may be indirect and precipitate abortion or premature labor.

The accuracy of prenatal serology testing is variable. TORCH infections can be more accurately diagnosed by direct identification of the organism by PCR testing or culture of amniotic fluid.

notes

T

total blood volume (TBV, Red blood cell [RBC] volume)

Type of test Nuclear scan

Normal findings Approximately 70 mL per kg of body weight

Test explanation and related physiology

Measurement of total blood volume (TBV) has been performed for several years using radionuclides. This measurement is becoming increasingly requested by clinicians as an accurate indicator of true plasma (liquid components of blood) measurement. Based on the patient's height, weight, gender, and body composition, TBV can determine whether the measured volumes are high or low compared to what would be ideal for the particular patient. The report indicates actual volumes for TBV and RBCs that deviate from normal.

Radioiodine-labeled albumin is injected intravenously. Blood is withdrawn every 5 minutes for 5 samples. The radioactivity is counted and compared to what would be considered normal. A lower amount of radioactivity in the sample indicates a higher plasma volume. The hematocrit is then used to derive the RBC volume. The TBV is obtained by adding the plasma volume and the RBC volume.

This information may be useful in the following clinical circumstances:

- *Congestive heart failure.* The actual amount of fluid overload can be calculated, and diuresis can be more appropriately determined.
- *Presurgery.* The patient's fluid status can be accurately determined as can RBC status.
- *Acutely ill patients.* There are often large fluid shifts in these patients, and TBV may help in guiding IV fluid replacement.
- *Azotemia.* Measurement of TBV will indicate if azotemia is pre-renal (hypovolemia) or primary renal.
- *Hypertension.* TBV may indicate plasma volume overload versus vascular constriction.
- *Anemia.* TBV and RBC volumes can indicate accurately the extent of anemia that otherwise could be affected by fluid status, etc.

Before

PT Explain the procedure and tell the patient that no fasting is required.

During
- Obtain venous access.
- Fifteen minutes after radionuclide injection, the first venous blood sample is collected in a red-top tube.
- Similar venous blood samples are obtained every 5 minutes for a total of five samples.

After
- Apply pressure to the intravenous site upon removal after extracting the last sample.

Abnormal findings

▲ **Increased levels**
Hypervolemia
Hypertension
Congestive heart failure
Primary renal disease
Polycythemia vera

▼ **Decreased levels**
Dehydration
Hypovolemia
Acute bleeding
Anemia

notes

toxoplasmosis antibody titer

Type of test   Blood

Normal findings

Ig G titers <1:16 indicate no previous infection

Ig G titers 1:16-1:256 are usually prevalent in the general population

Ig G titers >1:256 suggest recent infection

Ig M titers >1:256 indicate acute infection

Test explanation and related physiology

Toxoplasmosis is a protozoan disease caused by *Toxoplasma gondii*, which is found in poorly cooked or raw meat and in cat feces. Most often, humans are asymptomatic from the infection. When symptoms occur, this disease is characterized by central nervous system lesions, which may lead to blindness, brain damage, and death. The condition may occur congenitally or postnatally. The Centers for Disease Control and Prevention (CDC) recommends that patients who are pregnant be serologically tested for this disease.

The presence of antibodies before pregnancy indicates prior exposure and chronic asymptomatic infection. The presence of these antibodies probably ensures protection against congenital toxoplasmosis in the child. Fetal infection occurs if the mother acquires toxoplasmosis after conception and passes it to the fetus through the placenta. Repeat testing of pregnant patients with low or negative titers may be done before the twentieth week and before delivery to identify antibody converters and determine appropriate therapy (e.g., therapeutic abortion at 20 weeks, treatment during the remainder of the pregnancy, or treatment of the newborn). Hydrocephaly, microcephaly, chronic retinitis, and seizures are complications of congenital toxoplasmosis.

Procedure and patient care

- See inside front cover for Routine Blood Testing.
- Fasting: no.
- Blood tube commonly used: red.

Abnormal findings

Toxoplasmosis infection

notes

transesophageal echocardiography (TEE)

Type of test Endoscopy/ultrasound

Normal findings Normal position, size, and movement of the heart muscle, valves, and heart chambers

Test explanation and related physiology

TEE provides ultrasonic imaging of the heart from a retrocardiac vantage point, avoiding interference with the ultrasound by the interposed subcutaneous tissue, bony thorax, and lungs. In this procedure, a high-frequency ultrasound transducer placed in the esophagus by endoscopy provides better resolution than that of images obtained with routine transthoracic echocardiography (p. 356). For TEE, the distal end of the endoscope is advanced into the esophagus. The transducer is positioned behind the heart (Figure 43). Controls on the handle of the endoscope permit the transducer to be rotated and flexed in both the anteroposterior and right-left lateral planes. TEE images have better resolution than those obtained by routine transthoracic echocardiography because of the higher-frequency sound waves and closer proximity of the transducer to the cardiac structures. (See p. 356 for a discussion of M-mode, two-dimensional, and color Doppler echocardiography.)

TEE is helpful in the evaluation of structures that are inaccessible or poorly visualized by the transthoracic probe approach. It is especially helpful in patients who are obese or have large lung-air spaces.

This test is performed for the following reasons:
- To better visualize the mitral valve
- To differentiate intracardiac from extracardiac masses and tumors
- To better visualize the atrial septum (for atrial septal defects)
- To diagnose thoracic aortic dissection
- To better detect valvular vegetation indicative of endocarditis
- To determine cardiac sources of arterial embolism
- To detect coronary artery disease

Ischemic muscle movement is much different from normal muscle movement; therefore, TEE is a very sensitive indicator of myocardial ischemia. TEE can be used to monitor patients undergoing major abdominal, peripheral vascular, and carotid artery procedures who are at high risk for intraoperative ischemia because of coronary artery disease.

T

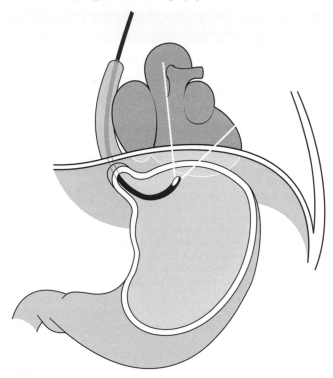

FIGURE 43 Transesophageal echocardiography. Diagram illustrates location of the transesophageal endoscope in the esophagus.

TEE is more sensitive than electrocardiography (ECG) for detecting ischemia. It is also used intraoperatively to evaluate surgical results of valvular or congenital heart disease. Furthermore, TEE is also the most sensitive technique for detecting air emboli, a serious complication of neurosurgery, performed with the patient in the upright position (cervical laminectomy).

Contraindications

- Patients with known upper esophageal pathology
- Patients with known esophageal varices
- Patients with Zenker diverticulum

- Patients with esophageal abnormalities (e.g., stricture diverticula, scleroderma, esophagitis)
- Patients with bleeding disorders
- Patients who have had prior esophageal surgery
- Patients who cannot cooperate with the procedure

Potential complications

- Esophageal perforation or bleeding
- Cardiac arrhythmias

Procedure and patient care

Before

PT Explain the procedure to the patient.

PT Instruct the patient to fast for 4 to 6 hours before the test.

PT Tell the patient to remove all oral prostheses.

- Obtain IV access.

During

- Intravenous sedation is commonly provided.
- Apply ECG leads and continually monitor heart rhythm.
- Apply a blood pressure cuff, and monitor blood pressure periodically.
- Pulse oximetry is monitored to determine oxygen saturation.
- Note the following procedural steps:
  1. The pharynx is anesthetized with a local topical agent to depress the gag reflex.
  2. The patient is placed in the left lateral decubitus position.
  3. Intubation is carried out through the mouth and into the upper esophagus.
  4. The patient is asked to swallow, and the transducer is advanced into position behind the heart.
  5. The room is darkened, and the ultrasound images are displayed on a monitor. Views can be obtained of the ultrasound image after desired images are visualized.
- The procedure is performed by a cardiologist and/or a gastrointestinal endoscopist in approximately 20 minutes in the endoscopy suite. It also can be performed at the bedside.
- Very little discomfort is associated with this test.

After

- Observe the patient closely for approximately 1 hour after the procedure until the effects of sedation have worn off.

T

Abnormal findings

Myocardial ischemia
Myocardial infarction
Valvular heart disease
Intracardiac thrombi
Cardiac valvular vegetation
Ventricular and atrial septal defects
Cardiomyopathy
Marked cardiac chamber dilation
Cardiac tumors
Aortic aneurysm or dissection
Aortic plaque
Pulmonary hypertension
Anomalous pulmonary veins

notes

transferrin receptor (TfR) assay

Type of test Blood

Normal findings

Men: 2-5.0 mg/L
Women: 1.9-4.4 mg/L
(Results vary depending on the testing method.)

Test explanation and related physiology

Both iron metabolism and transport are altered in chronic illness. Differentiation of the anemia of chronic disease (anemia of inflammation or anemia of aging) from iron deficiency anemia may be difficult, and the results of conventional laboratory assessment of iron stores may not be definitive. The most valuable iron-store marker (obtained without direct bone marrow testing) in distinguishing these two entities is the serum transferrin receptor (TfR) concentration.

TfR is a cell surface protein found on most cells and especially those with a high requirement for iron (e.g., immature erythroid and malignant cells). Its function is to internalize absorbed iron into target cells. TfR is increased when erythropoiesis is enhanced (such as often occurs in iron deficiency). The concentration of cell surface TfR is carefully regulated by TfR mRNA, according to the internal iron content of the cell and its individual iron requirements. Iron-deficient cells contain increased numbers of receptors, while receptor numbers are down-regulated in iron-replete cells.

An increased mean TfR concentration is noted in patients with iron deficiency anemia as compared with patients with anemia secondary to chronic disease. Calculation of the ratio of TfR/log ferritin concentration provides an even higher sensitivity and specificity for the detection of Fe deficiency.

TfR is also useful in distinguishing iron deficiency anemia from situations that are commonly encountered in childhood, adolescence, and during pregnancy when iron stores are uniformly low to absent. In these situations, iron-deficient erythropoiesis is not necessarily present, and TfR levels are not elevated. Finally, in situations in which iron deficiency anemia coexists with anemia of chronic disease, TfR concentrations increase secondary to the underlying iron deficiency, thus avoiding the need for a bone marrow examination.

T

Interfering factors

- Individuals who live at high altitudes have a reference range that extends 6% higher than the upper level of this reference interval.
- Results are related to ethnicity. Individuals of African descent can be expected to have higher levels.
- ✘ Drugs that may cause *increased* TfR levels include recombinant human erythropoietins.

Procedure and patient care

- See inside front cover for Routine Blood Testing.
- Fasting: no.
- Blood tube commonly used: red or green.

Abnormal findings

▲ **Increased plasma TfR levels**
Iron deficiency anemia
Reticulocytosis
Erythropoietin therapy

▼ **Decreased plasma TfR levels**
Hemochromatosis

notes

triglycerides (TGs)

Type of test Blood

Normal findings

Adult/elderly
    Male: 40-160 mg/dL or 0.45-1.81 mmol/L (SI units)
    Female: 35-135 mg/dL or 0.40-1.52 mmol/L (SI units)

Child/adolescent

Age	Male	Female
0-5 years	30-86 mg/dL	32-99 mg/dL
6-11 years	31-108 mg/dL	35-114 mg/dL
12-15 years	36-138 mg/dL	41-138 mg/dL
16-19 years	40-163 mg/dL	40-128 mg/dL

Possible critical values >400 mg/dL

Test explanation and related physiology

TGs are a form of fat that exists in the bloodstream. They are transported by very-low-density lipoproteins (VLDLs) and low-density lipoproteins (LDLs). TGs are produced in the liver by using glycerol and other fatty acids as building blocks. TGs act as a storage source for energy. When TG levels in the blood are in excess, TGs are deposited into the fatty tissues. TGs are a part of a lipid profile that also evaluates cholesterol (p. 248) and lipoproteins (p. 587). A lipid profile is performed to assess the risk of coronary and vascular disease.

Interfering factors

- Ingestion of fatty meals may cause increased TG levels.
- Ingestion of alcohol may cause increased levels.
- Pregnancy may cause increased levels.
- ✒ Drugs that may cause *increased* TG levels include cholestyramine, estrogens, and oral contraceptives.
- ✒ Drugs that may cause *decreased* levels include ascorbic acid, asparaginase, clofibrate, colestipol, fibrates, and statins.

Procedure and patient care

- See inside front cover for Routine Blood Testing.
- Fasting: yes (12-14 hours).
- Blood tube commonly used: red.
- **PT** Tell the patient not to drink alcohol for 24 hours before the test.

T

PT Inform the patient that dietary indiscretion for as long as 2 weeks before this test will influence results.

• Mark the patient's age and gender on the laboratory slip.

PT Instruct the patient with increased TG levels regarding diet, exercise, and appropriate weight.

Abnormal findings

▲ **Increased levels**
Glycogen storage disease
Hyperlipidemias
Hypothyroidism
High-carbohydrate diet
Poorly controlled diabetes
Risk of arteriosclerotic occlusive coronary disease and peripheral vascular disease
Nephrotic syndrome
Hypertension
Alcoholic cirrhosis
Pregnancy
Myocardial infarction

▼ **Decreased levels**
Malabsorption syndrome
Malnutrition
Hyperthyroidism

notes

triiodothyronine (T₃ radioimmunoassay)

Type of test Blood

Normal findings

1-3 days: 100-740 ng/dL
1-11 months: 105-245 ng/dL
1-5 years: 105-270 ng/dL
6-10 years: 95-240 ng/dL
11-15 years: 80-215 ng/dL
16-20 years: 80-210 ng/dL
20-50 years: 70-205 ng/dL or 1.2-3.4 nmol/L (SI units)
>50 years: 40-180 ng/dL or 0.6-2.8 nmol/L (SI units)

Test explanation and related physiology

As with the thyroxine (T_4) test, the serum T_3 test is an accurate measure of thyroid function. T_3 is less stable than T_4 and occurs in minute quantities in the active form. Only about 7% to 10% of thyroid hormone is composed of T_3. Seventy percent of that T_3 is bound to proteins (thyroid-binding globulin [TBG] and albumin). Abnormal levels (high or low) of thyroid hormone–binding proteins (primarily albumin and TBG) may cause abnormal T_3 concentrations in euthyroid patients. This test is a measurement of total T_3 (i.e., the free and the bound T_3). Generally, when the T_3 level is below normal, the patient is in a hypothyroid state.

Other severe nonthyroidal diseases can decrease T_3 levels by diminishing the conversion of T_4 to T_3 in the liver. This makes T_3 levels less useful in indicating hypothyroid states. Furthermore, there is considerable overlap between hypothyroid states and normal thyroid function. Because of this, T_3 levels are mostly used just to assist in the diagnosis of hyperthyroid states. T_3 levels are frequently low in sick or hospitalized euthyroid patients. An elevated T_3 level indicates hyperthyroidism, especially when the T_4 is also elevated. There is a rare form of hyperthyroidism called T_3 *toxicosis*, in which the T_4 is normal and the T_3 is elevated.

Interfering factors

- T_3 values are increased in pregnancy.
- ☛ Drugs that may cause *increased* levels include estrogen, methadone, and oral contraceptives.
- ☛ Drugs that may cause *decreased* levels include anabolic steroids, androgens, phenytoin, propranolol, reserpine, and salicylates (high dose).

T

Procedure and patient care

- See inside front cover for Routine Blood Testing.
- Fasting: no.
- Blood tube commonly used: red.
- Determine whether the patient is taking any exogenous T_3 medication, because this will affect test results.
- Withhold drugs that may affect results (with physician's approval).

Abnormal findings

▲ **Increased levels**
Graves disease
Plummer disease
Toxic thyroid adenoma
Acute thyroiditis
Factitious hyperthyroidism
Struma ovarii
Pregnancy
Hepatitis
Congenital
  hyperproteinemia

▼ **Decreased levels**
Hypothyroidism
Cretinism
Thyroid surgical ablation
Myxedema
Pituitary insufficiency
Hypothalamic failure
Protein malnutrition
  and other protein-
  depleted states
  (e.g., nephrotic
  syndrome)
Iodine insufficiency
Renal failure
Cushing syndrome
Cirrhosis
Liver diseases

notes

troponins (Cardiac-specific troponin T [cTnT], Cardiac-specific troponin I [cTnI])

Type of test Blood

Normal findings

Cardiac troponin T: <0.1 ng/mL
Cardiac troponin I: <0.03 ng/mL

Test explanation and related physiology

Cardiac troponins are important biochemical markers for cardiac disease. This test is used to assist in the evaluation of patients with suspected acute coronary ischemic syndromes. In addition to improving the diagnosis of acute ischemic disorders, troponins are also valuable for early risk stratification in patients with unstable angina. They can be used to predict the likelihood of future cardiac events.

Troponins are proteins that exist in skeletal and cardiac muscles and regulate the calcium-dependent interaction of myosin with actin for the muscle contractile apparatus. Cardiac troponins can be separated from skeletal troponins by the use of monoclonal antibodies or enzyme-linked immunosorbent assay. There are two cardiac-specific troponins: cardiac troponin T (cTnT) and cardiac troponin I (cTnI).

Because of their extraordinarily high specificity for myocardial cell injury, cardiac troponins are very helpful in the evaluation of patients with chest pain. Their use is similar to that of creatine kinase-MB (CK-MB). However, cardiac troponins have several advantages over CK-MB. Cardiac troponins are more specific for cardiac muscle injury. CK-MB can be elevated in severe skeletal muscle injury, brain or lung injury, or renal failure. Cardiac troponins will nearly always be normal in noncardiac muscle diseases. Cardiac troponins become elevated sooner and remain elevated longer than CK-MB. This expands the time window of opportunity for diagnosis and thrombolytic treatment of myocardial injury. Finally, cTnT and cTnI are more sensitive to muscle injury than CK-MB. That is most important in evaluating patients with chest pain.

Cardiac troponins become elevated as early as 2 to 3 hours after myocardial injury. Typically, 2 to 3 sets of troponins over the course of a day (every 3 to 6 hours) are required to indicate myocardial infarction. Levels of cTnI may remain elevated for 7 to 10 days after myocardial infarction, and cTnT levels may remain elevated for up to 14 days.

T

Cardiac troponins are used in the following cardiac clinical situations:

- Evaluation of patient with unstable angina. If cardiac troponins are normal, no myocardial injury has occurred, and there will be no lasting cardiac dysfunction. If cardiac troponins are elevated, muscle injury has occurred. Revascularization may be indicated because this latter group is at great risk for a subsequent cardiac event (infarction or sudden death).
- Detection of reperfusion associated with coronary recanalization. A *washout*, or second peak of cardiac troponin levels, accurately indicates reperfusion by way of recanalization or coronary angioplasty.
- Estimation of myocardial infarction size. Late (4 weeks) cardiac troponin levels are inversely related to left ventricular ejection fraction.
- Detection of perioperative myocardial infarction. Cardiac troponins are not affected by skeletal muscle injury.
- Evaluation of the severity of pulmonary emboli. Elevated levels may indicate more severe disease and the need for thrombolytic therapy.
- Congestive heart failure. Persistently elevated troponins indicate continued ventricular strain.

Elevations of troponin T do not necessarily indicate the presence of an ischemic mechanism. Many other disease states are associated with elevations of troponin T via mechanisms different from those that cause injury in patients with acute coronary syndromes. These include cardiac trauma (e.g., contusion, ablation, or pacing), congestive heart failure, hypertension, hypotension (often with arrhythmias), pulmonary embolism, renal failure, and myocarditis.

Interfering factors

- Severe skeletal muscle injury may cause false elevation of cTnT.
- Troponin T levels are falsely elevated in dialysis patients.

Procedure and patient care

- See inside front cover for Routine Blood Testing.
- Fasting: no.
- Blood tube commonly used: yellow.

PT Discuss with the patient the need and reason for frequent venipuncture in diagnosing myocardial infarction.

- After the initial blood sample, blood is collected 12 hours later followed by daily testing for 3 to 5 days and possibly weekly for 5 to 6 weeks.
- Record the exact time and date of venipuncture on each laboratory slip. This aids in the interpretation of the temporal pattern of enzyme elevations.
- If a qualitative immunoassay is to be done at the bedside, whole blood is obtained in a micropipette and placed in the sample well of the testing device. A red or purple color in the read zone indicates that 0.2 ng/mL or more of cardiac troponin is present in the patient's blood.

Abnormal findings

▲ **Increased levels**
Myocardial injury
Myocardial infarction

notes

T

tuberculin skin test (TST, Tuberculin test, Mantoux test, Purified protein derivative [PPD] test)

Type of test Skin

Normal findings

PPD: Negative; reaction <5 mm

Test explanation and related physiology

Tuberculin testing is performed for persons who are:

- Suspected of having active TB
- At increased risk for progression to active TB
- At increased risk for latent TB infection (LTBI) (e.g., health care workers, recent immigrants, or IV drug abusers)
- At low risk for LTBI, but are tested for other reasons (e.g., entrance to college)

For this test, a purified protein derivative (PPD) of the tubercle bacillus is injected intradermally. If the patient is infected with TB (whether active or dormant), lymphocytes will recognize the PPD antigen and cause a local reaction; if the patient is not infected, no reaction will occur. If the test is negative and the physician still strongly suspects TB, a *second-strength PPD* can be used. If this test is negative, the patient does not have TB. (See p. 936 for tuberculosis culture.) A positive reaction usually occurs 6 weeks after infection. If positive, a localized skin reaction will recur with any subsequent testing throughout the person's life. This test is used to detect TB infection but is unable to indicate whether the infection is active or latent.

The PPD test also can be used as part of a series of skin tests to assess the immune system. If the immune system is nonfunctioning because of poor nutrition or chronic illness (e.g., neoplasia, infection), the PPD test will be negative despite the patient having had an active or dormant TB infection. Other skin tests used to test immune function include *Candida*, the mumps virus, and *Trichophyton*. Most people in the United States have been exposed to these organisms.

When a patient known to have active TB receives a PPD test, the local reaction may be so severe that it causes complete skin slough and requires surgical care. When these patients are eliminated from PPD testing, the test has no complications. The PPD test will not cause active TB because no live organisms exist in the test solution.

There is now an alternative to the tuberculin skin test; the QuantiFERON-TB Gold test (p. 938) is a blood test used for diagnosing *Mycobacterium tuberculosis* infection.

Contraindications

- Patients with known active TB
- Patients who have received *bacille Calmette-Guérin (BCG)* immunization against PPD, because these patients will demonstrate a positive reaction to the PPD vaccination even though they have never had TB infection

Procedure and patient care

Before

PT Explain the procedure to the patient.

PT Assure the patient that she or he will not develop TB from this test.

- Assess the patient for a previous history of TB. Report a positive history to the physician.
- Evaluate the patient's history for previous PPD results and BCG immunization.

During

- Prepare the patient's forearm with alcohol and allow it to dry.
- Intradermally inject the PPD. A skin wheal will occur.
- Circle the area with indelible ink.
- Record the time at which the PPD was injected.

After

- Read the results in 48 to 72 hours.
- Examine the test site for induration (hardening). Measure the area of induration (not redness) in millimeters.
- If the test is positive, ensure that the physician is notified and the patient is treated appropriately.
- If the test is positive, check the patient's arm 4 to 5 days after the test to be certain that a severe skin reaction has not occurred.

Abnormal findings

Positive results

Tuberculosis infection
Nontuberculous mycobacteria infections

Negative results

Possible immunoincompetence

notes

T

tuberculosis culture (TB culture, Acid-fast bacillus [AFB] smear)

Type of test Microbiology culture

Normal findings Negative for tuberculosis

Test explanation and related physiology

Diagnosis of TB can be made only by identification and culture of *Mycobacterium tuberculosis* in a specimen. Conventional culture techniques for growth, identification, and susceptibility of acid-fast mycobacteria take 4 to 6 weeks. Because a patient suspected of having TB cannot be isolated for that duration, the disease may spread to many other people while he or she waits for the diagnosis. With the resurgence and increasing incidence of TB in the U.S. population (especially among immunocompromised patients with acquired immunodeficiency syndrome), newer, more rapid culture techniques have been identified and are now being performed.

The *BACTEC* method is a culture technique in which the growth medium for culturing mycobacteria is supplanted with a substrate labeled with radioactive carbon (^{14}C). This substrate is used by mycobacteria; during metabolism, radioactive carbon dioxide ($^{14}CO_2$) is produced from the substrate. The $^{14}CO_2$ is detected and quantitated. This permits quick identification of mycobacterial growth.

Polymerase chain reaction (PCR) culture methods have also been developed. With the addition of a deoxyribonucleic acid (DNA) polymerase, genetic chromosomal parts can be multiplied. This allows amplification of genomes, which then can be detected by genetic DNA probes. With the newer techniques already described, *M. tuberculosis* can be identified in as few as 36 to 48 hours. With this reduction in diagnostic time, treatment can be started earlier.

After identification and growth of mycobacteria, antibiotic susceptibility testing is performed to identify the most effective antimycobacterial drugs. The culture specimen can be performed on sputum, body fluids, cerebrospinal fluid, and even biopsy tissue specimens.

When tuberculosis is suspected, a sputum smear for *acid-fast bacillus (AFB)* can be obtained. After taking up a dye, such as fuchsin, *M. tuberculosis* is not decolorized by acid alcohol (i.e., it is acid-fast). It is seen under the microscope as a red, rod-shaped organism. If this bacillus is seen, the patient may have active TB. Other specimens, such as cerebrospinal fluid, tissue, and synovial fluid, may be used. AFB is also used to monitor treatment for TB. If after adequate therapy (2 months) the sputum still contains AFB (even though the culture may be negative due to anti-TB drugs), treatment failure should be considered.

Interfering factors

☒ Antituberculosis drugs

Procedure and patient care

Before

PT Explain the procedure to the patient.

PT Tell the patient that no fasting is required.

During

- For *sputum* collection, it is best to induce sputum production with an ultrasonic or nebulizing device. Collect three to five early morning sputum specimens. All specimens must contain mycobacteria to make the diagnosis of TB.
- For *urine* collection, obtain three to five single clean-voided specimens early in the morning.
- *Swabs, intestinal washings,* and *biopsy* specimens should be transported to the laboratory immediately for preparation.
- When the specimen is received by the laboratory, a decontamination process is applied to it to kill all nonmycobacteria. The specimen is then cultured in the appropriate medium.
- With the rapid growth techniques, the specimen is evaluated every 24 hours.
- When culture growth is considered adequate, the organisms are stained for AFB and identified.
- With genetic probes, the *Mycobacterium* species is identified.
- At this point, if *M. tuberculosis* is present, the report will read "culture more positive for mycobacteria." If the species has been identified, this also will be reported.
- Drug-susceptibility testing then will be carried out and subsequently reported.

After

PT Instruct the patient as to appropriate isolation of sputum and other body fluids to avoid potential spread of suspected TB.

Abnormal findings

Tuberculosis

Atypical mycobacterial nontuberculosis disease

notes

> **tuberculosis testing** (TB testing, Interferon gamma release assay [IGRA], QuantiFERON-TB Gold [QFT, QFT-G, TB Gold test, TB blood test], Nucleic acid amplification for TB [NAAT], TB antibody)

Type of test Blood, sputum, fluid analysis

Normal findings

IGRA result	Interpretation
Positive	*Mycobacterium tuberculosis* infection likely
Negative	*M. tuberculosis* infection unlikely but cannot be excluded. If TB disease is highly suspected, a negative result does not rule out infection. False-negative results may be seen in immunocompromised patients.
Indeterminate	Test not interpretable. Collection of a new specimen for testing is recommended, if clinically indicated.

Test explanation and related physiology

Interferon gamma release assays (IGRA, e.g., QuantiFERON-TB), nucleic acid amplification test (NAAT), and serologic TB testing are used to diagnose active TB infection. The gold standard for making the diagnosis of active TB is the TB culture (page 936). However, it takes 2 to 6 weeks to obtain results. Identifying acid-fast bacilli in a smear (AFB smear) (page 936) of the body fluid (usually sputum) is a rapid method of identifying TB in 24 hours. Unfortunately, AFB is not very sensitive or specific. It is often positive in nontuberculosis mycobacterial diseases. The IGRA is a whole-blood test used in diagnosing *Mycobacterium tuberculosis* infection. The NAAT is a rapid and accurate test of sputum and is used as corroborative information in the diagnosis of TB. Serology testing on blood is also a rapid test used to identify active TB disease infection.

The value of decreasing the time it takes to make the diagnosis of TB is significant. With an earlier laboratory confirmation of TB disease, treatment can be initiated earlier, patient outcome can be improved, opportunities to interrupt transmission of the disease can be increased, and more effective public health interventions can be instigated. IGRA TB antibody testing and NAAT can provide rapid confirmation of TB infection. These tests, however, cannot indicate anti-TB drug sensitivities.

The diagnosis of active or latent TB still requires additional testing (including chest radiography, sputum smear, and culture). IGRA is a diagnostic aid that measures a component of cell-mediated immune reactivity to *M. tuberculosis* similar to the tuberculin skin testing (TST) (see page 934). IGRA can be performed on patients with prior *bacille Calmette-Guérin (BCG)* vaccination without causing a hypersensitivity response. Similar to TST, false negatives can occur in anergic patients.

IGRA cannot differentiate active from latent TB infection. IGRA results are available in 24 hours. IGRA can be used for serial surveillance testing up to 12 months after a negative purified protein derivative (PPD) result if the initial IGRA is negative. IGRA and NAAT are used in the same patient population as TST. These include contact investigations, evaluation of recent immigrants, and sequential-testing surveillance programs for infection control, such as those for health care workers.

NAAT is designed to identify TB complex DNA in a body fluid (bronchoalveolar lavage, bronchial washing, sputum, stool, pleural or abdominal fluid, tissue, or urine sample). This test provides a rapid result in 24 hours. Similar to the above-described rapid tests, NAAT cannot indicate active infection from a previously treated TB infection. The Centers for Disease Control and Prevention has indicated that NAAT should be performed on at least one respiratory specimen for each patient with signs and symptoms of pulmonary TB for whom a diagnosis of TB is being considered but has not yet been established and for whom the test results would alter case management.

TB antibody serology is designed to identify IgG antibodies to TB mycobacteria in patients with active TB infections. This blood test can be used in previously vaccinated BCG patients. It is particularly useful in evaluating the effectiveness of anti-TB therapy and documenting a response to therapy. Similar to IGRA, serology results may not be positive in immunocompromised patients, making use in HIV-infected patients less helpful.

Interfering factors

- Heterophile (e.g., human antimouse) antibodies in serum or plasma of certain individuals are known to cause interference with immunoassays.
- A false-negative IGRA result can be due to the stage of infection (i.e., specimen obtained before the development of cellular immune response), comorbid conditions that affect immune function, or other individual immunologic factors.

Procedure and patient care

Before
PT Explain the procedure to the patient or the family.

During

- Collect 1 mL of whole blood in each of three lab-specified collection tubes. The accuracy of the IGRA depends on the proper collection and incubation of the blood specimen. Blood should fill the tube as close to the 1-mL mark as possible. Under- or overfilling the tubes outside the 0.8- to 1.2-mL range may lead to erroneous results.
- Immediately after collection, each specimen tube must be shaken vigorously by shaking the tube up and down 10 times to ensure that the entire inner surface of the tube has been coated with blood. This distributes the stimulating antigens, allowing optimal processing and presentation of the antigens to T-cells, which causes release of interferon-γ.
- For NAAT testing, 1 to 3 mL of sputum or body fluid is required. This should be refrigerated in a screw cap sterile container.

After

- Apply pressure or a pressure dressing to the venipuncture site.
- **PT** If the patient's results are positive, educate the patient on the necessary follow-up studies, such as chest radiography and sputum cultures.

Abnormal finding

TB infection

notes

upper gastrointestinal x-ray study (Upper GI series, UGI)

Type of test   X-ray with contrast dye

Normal findings   Normal size, contour, patency, filling, positioning, and transit of barium through the lower esophagus, stomach, and upper duodenum

Test explanation and related physiology

The upper GI study consists of a series of x-ray images of the lower esophagus, stomach, and duodenum, usually with barium sulfate as the contrast medium. When there is concern about leakage of x-ray contrast through a perforation of the GI tract, however, Gastrografin (a water-soluble contrast) is used. This test can be performed in conjunction with a barium swallow or a small bowel series (pp. 136 and 849), which can precede or succeed the upper GI study, respectively.

The purpose of this examination is to detect ulcerations, tumors, inflammations, and anatomic malpositions (e.g., hiatal hernia) in these organs. Obstruction of the upper GI tract is also easily detected.

In this test, the patient is asked to drink barium. As the contrast descends, the lower esophagus is examined for position, patency, and filling defects (e.g., tumors, scarring, varices). As the contrast enters the stomach, the gastric wall is examined for benign or malignant ulcerations, filling defects (most often in cancer), and anatomic abnormalities (e.g., hiatal hernia). The patient is placed in a flat or head-down position, and the gastroesophageal area is examined for evidence of gastroesophageal reflux of barium.

As the contrast leaves the stomach, patency of the pyloric channel and the duodenum is evaluated. Benign peptic ulceration is the most common pathologic condition affecting these areas. Extrinsic compression caused by tumors, cysts, or enlarged pathologic organs (e.g., liver) near the stomach also can be identified by anatomic distortion of the outline of the upper GI tract. The small intestine can then be studied (see discussion of small bowel follow-through, p. 849).

Contraindications

- Patients with complete bowel obstructions
- Patients suspected of upper GI perforation
  Water-soluble Gastrografin should be used instead of barium.

U

- Patients with unstable vital signs
  These patients should be supervised during the time required for this test.
- Patients who are uncooperative because of the necessity of frequent position changes

Potential complications

- Aspiration of barium
- Constipation or partial bowel obstruction caused by inspissated barium in the small bowel or colon

Interfering factors

- Previously administered barium may block visualization.
- Incapacitated patients cannot assume the multiple positions required for the study.
- Food and fluid in the stomach give the false impression of filling defects within the stomach, precluding adequate evaluation of the gastric mucosa.

Procedure and patient care

Before

PT Explain the procedure to the patient. Allow the patient to verbalize concerns.

PT Instruct the patient to abstain from eating for at least 8 hours before the test. Usually keep the patient NPO after midnight on the day of the test.

PT Assure the patient that the test will not cause any discomfort.

During

- Note the following procedural steps:
  1. The patient is asked to drink approximately 16 ounces of barium sulfate. This is a chalky substance usually suspended in milk shake form and drunk through a straw. Usually the drink is flavored to increase palatability.
  2. After drinking the barium, the patient is moved through several position changes (e.g., prone, supine, lateral) to promote filling of the entire upper GI tract.
  3. X-ray images are taken at the discretion of the radiologist observing the flow of barium fluoroscopically.
  4. The flow of barium is followed through the lower esophagus, stomach, and duodenum.
  5. Several x-ray images are taken throughout the course of the test.
  6. In an *air-contrast upper GI study*, the patient is asked to rapidly swallow carbonated powder. This creates carbon

dioxide in the stomach, providing air contrast to the barium in the stomach and increased visualization of the gastric mucosa.

- Note that a radiologist performs this procedure in approximately 30 minutes.

PT Tell the patient that he or she may be uncomfortable lying on the hard x-ray table and may experience the sensation of bloating or nausea during the test.

After

PT Inform the patient that if Gastrografin was used, he or she may have significant diarrhea. Gastrografin is an osmotic cathartic.

PT Instruct the patient to use a cathartic (e.g., milk of magnesia) if barium sulfate was used as the contrast medium. Water absorption may cause the barium to harden and create fecal impaction if catharsis is not carried out.

PT Instruct the patient to watch his or her stools to ensure that all of the barium has been removed. The stools should return to a normal color after completely expelling the barium, which may take as long as a day and a half.

Abnormal findings

Esophageal cancer
Esophageal varices
Hiatal hernia
Esophageal diverticula
Gastric cancer
Gastric inflammatory disease (e.g., Ménétrier disease)
Benign gastric tumor (e.g., leiomyoma)
Extrinsic compression by pancreatic pseudocysts, cysts, pancreatic tumors, or hepatomegaly
Perforation of the esophagus, stomach, or duodenum
Congenital abnormalities (e.g., duodenal web, pancreatic rest, malrotation syndrome)
Gastric ulcer (benign and malignant)
Gastritis
Duodenal ulcer
Duodenal cancer
Duodenal diverticulum

U

notes

urea breath test (UBT, *H. pylori* breath test)

Type of test Other

Normal findings

<50 dpm (if ^{14}C is used)

<3% (if ^{13}C is used)

Test explanation and related physiology

This test is used to detect *Helicobacter pylori (H. pylori)* infections. It is indicated in patients who have recurrent or chronic gastric or duodenal ulceration or inflammation. When the *H. pylori* infection is successfully treated, the ulcer or inflammation will usually heal.

H. pylori is a bacterium that can be found in the mucus overlying the gastric mucosa and in the mucosa (cells that line the stomach). It is a risk factor for gastric and duodenal ulcers, chronic gastritis, or even ulcerative esophagitis. This gram-negative bacillus is also a class I gastric carcinogen. Gastric colonization by this organism has been reported in about 90% to 95% of patients with a duodenal ulcer; in 60% to 70% of patients with a gastric ulcer; and in about 20% to 25% of patients with gastric cancer.

There are several serologic and microscopic methods of detecting *H. pylori* (see *Helicobacter pylori* antibodies test, p. 494). The UBT is the noninvasive test of choice for diagnosis of *H. pylori* infection. It is based on the capability of *H. pylori* to metabolize urea to CO_2 because of the organism's capability to produce a large amount of urease. In the breath test, carbon (^{13}C)-labeled urea is administered orally. The urea is then absorbed through the gastric mucosa. If *H. pylori* is present, the urea will be converted to $^{13}CO_2$. The $^{13}CO_2$ is then taken up by the capillaries in the stomach wall and delivered to the lungs where it is exhaled. The labeled carbon can be measured by gas chromatography or a mass spectrometer.

This test has been simplified to the point that two breath samples collected before and 30 minutes after the ingestion of urea in a liquid form suffice to provide reliable diagnostic information. Labeling urea with ^{13}C is becoming increasingly popular because it is a nonradioactive isotope of ^{14}C and is innocuous. It can be safely used in children and women of childbearing age.

Interfering factors

- Dietary constituents with a natural abundance of ^{13}C, such as maize, cane, and corn flour, can cause increased levels.
- ☙ Bismuth (Pepto-Bismol) or sucralfate (Carafate) will suppress mucosal uptake of the urea and interfere with test results.
- ☙ The concomitant use of a proton pump inhibitor, such as Prilosec, Nexium, Prevacid, or Protonix, will also inhibit urea absorption.

Procedure and patient care

Before

PT Explain the procedure to the patient.

PT Instruct the patient to abstain from oral intake for 6 hours before testing.

- If radioactive carbon (rare) is being used, be sure that female patients are not pregnant.

PT When providing the isotopic urea to the patient, instruct the patient as to proper administration (per local laboratory routine).

During

- Several minutes after the patient has swallowed the carbon dose, provide the patient with 2 oz of water.
- Breath samples are collected in any one of a number of gas collection devices depending on how and when the sample will be analyzed.

After

PT Instruct the patient to resume medications and normal diet.

PT If radioactive carbon was used, instruct the patient to drink plenty of fluids to facilitate excretion of the radioisotope.

Abnormal findings

H. pylori infection

notes

U

urea nitrogen blood test (Blood urea nitrogen [BUN])

Type of test Blood

Normal findings

Adult: 10-20 mg/dL or 3.6-7.1 mmol/L (SI units)
Elderly: may be slightly higher than those of adult
Child: 5-18 mg/dL
Infant: 5-18 mg/dL
Newborn: 3-12 mg/dL
Cord: 21-40 mg/dL

Possible critical values >100 mg/dL (indicates serious impairment of renal function)

Test explanation and related physiology

The BUN measures the amount of urea nitrogen in the blood. Urea is formed in the liver as the end product of protein metabolism. During ingestion, protein is broken down into amino acids. In the liver, these amino acids are catabolized, and free ammonia is formed. The ammonia is combined to form urea, which is then deposited into the blood and transported to the kidneys for excretion. Therefore, BUN is directly related to the metabolic function of the liver and the excretory function of the kidney. It serves as an index of the function of these organs. Patients who have elevated BUN levels are said to have azotemia.

Nearly all renal diseases cause inadequate excretion of urea, which causes the blood concentration to rise above normal. If the disease is unilateral, however, the unaffected kidney can compensate for the diseased kidney, and BUN may not become elevated. BUN also increases in conditions other than primary renal disease. For example, when excess amounts of protein are available for hepatic catabolism (from a high-protein diet or gastrointestinal [GI] bleeding), large quantities of urea are made. BUN levels also may vary according to the state of hydration, with increased levels seen in dehydration and decreased levels seen in overhydration. Finally, one must be aware that the synthesis of urea depends on the liver. Patients with severe primary liver disease will have a decreased BUN. With combined liver and renal disease (as in hepatorenal syndrome), BUN can be normal not because renal excretory function is good but because poor hepatic functioning has resulted in decreased formation of urea.

BUN is interpreted in conjunction with the creatinine test (p. 308). These tests are referred to as *renal function studies*.

The BUN/creatinine ratio is a good measurement of kidney and liver function. The normal adult range is 6 to 25, with 15.5 being the optimal adult value for this ratio.

Interfering factors

- Changes in protein intake may affect BUN levels.
- Advanced pregnancy may cause increased BUN levels.
- Overhydration and underhydration will affect BUN levels.
- GI bleeding can cause increased BUN levels.
- Drugs that may cause *increased* BUN levels include allopurinol, aminoglycosides, cephalosporins, chloral hydrate, cisplatin, furosemide, guanethidine, indomethacin, methotrexate, methyldopa, nephrotoxic drugs (e.g., amphotericin B, aspirin, bacitracin, carbamazepine, colistin, gentamicin, methicillin, neomycin, penicillamine, polymyxin B, probenecid, vancomycin), propranolol, rifampin, spironolactone, tetracyclines, thiazide diuretics, and triamterene.
- Drugs that may cause *decreased* BUN levels include chloramphenicol and streptomycin.

Procedure and patient care

- See inside front cover for Routine Blood Testing.
- Fasting: no.
- Blood tube commonly used: red.

U

Abnormal findings

▲ **Increased levels**

Prerenal causes

Hypovolemia

Shock

Burns

Dehydration

Congestive heart failure

Myocardial infarction

GI bleeding

Excessive protein ingestion

Alimentary tube feeding

Excessive protein catabolism

Starvation

Sepsis

Renal causes

Renal disease
(e.g., glomerulonephritis,
pyelonephritis, acute
tubular necrosis)

Renal failure

Nephrotoxic drugs

Postrenal azotemia

Ureteral obstruction

Bladder outlet obstruction

▼ **Decreased levels**

Liver failure

Overhydration caused
by fluid overload or
syndrome of
inappropriate
antidiuretic hormone
(SIADH)

Negative nitrogen
balance (e.g.,
malnutrition
or malabsorption)

Pregnancy

Nephrotic syndrome

notes

uric acid, blood and urine

Type of test Blood; urine

Normal findings

Blood

Adult
  Male: 4.0-8.5 mg/dL or 0.24-0.51 mmol/L
  Female: 2.7-7.3 mg/dL or 0.16-0.43 mmol/L
Elderly: values may be slightly increased
Child: 2.5-5.5 mg/dL or 0.12-0.32 mmol/L
Newborn: 2.0-6.2 mg/dL

Physiologic saturation threshold: >6 mg/dL or >0.357 mmol/L
Therapeutic target for gout: <6 mg/dL or <0.357 mmol/L

Urine 250-750 mg/24 hr or 1.48-4.43 mmol/day (SI units)

Possible critical values Blood: >12 mg/dL

Test explanation and related physiology

Uric acid is a nitrogenous compound that is a product of purine (a deoxyribonucleic acid [DNA] building block) catabolism. Uric acid is excreted to a large degree by the kidney and to a smaller degree by the intestinal tract. When uric acid levels are elevated (hyperuricemia), the patient may have gout. Gout is a common metabolic disorder characterized by chronic hyperuricemia, defined as serum urate >6.8 mg/dL (>0.360 mmol/L). At this level, uric acid concentrations exceed the physiologic saturation threshold, and monosodium urate crystals may be deposited in the joints and soft tissues. Gout may be managed through urate-lowering therapy with the goal of treatment being uric acid <6 mg/dL or <0.357 mmol/L.

Causes of hyperuricemia can be overproduction or decreased excretion of uric acid (e.g., kidney failure). Overproduction of uric acid may occur in patients with a catabolic enzyme deficiency that stimulates purine metabolism or in patients with cancer in whom purine and DNA turnover is great. Other causes of hyperuricemia may include alcoholism, leukemia, metastatic cancer, multiple myeloma, hyperlipoproteinemia, diabetes mellitus, renal failure, stress, lead poisoning, and dehydration caused by diuretic therapy. Ketoacids (as occur in diabetic or alcoholic ketoacidosis) may compete with uric acid for tubular excretion and may cause decreased uric acid excretion. Many causes of hyperuricemia are undefined and therefore labeled as *idiopathic*.

U

Elevated uric acid in the urine is called uricosuria. Uric acid can become supersaturated in the urine and crystallize to form kidney stones that can block the renal system. Urinary excretion of uric acid depends on uric acid levels in the blood, along with glomerular filtration and tubular secretion of uric acid into the urine. Uric acid is less well saturated in alkaline urine. As the urine pH rises, more uric acid can exist without crystallization and stone formation. Therefore, when a person is known to have high uric acid in the urine, the urine can be alkalinized by ingestion of a strong base to prevent stone formation.

Interfering factors

- Stress may cause increased uric acid levels.
- Recent use of x-ray contrast agents may cause decreased serum levels.
- Recent use of x-ray contrast agents may increase uric acid levels in the urine.
- ✗ Drugs that may cause *increased* serum levels include alcohol, ascorbic acid, aspirin (low dose), caffeine, cisplatin, diazoxide, diuretics, epinephrine, ethambutol, levodopa, methyldopa, nicotinic acid, phenothiazines, and theophylline.
- ✗ Drugs that may cause *decreased* serum levels include allopurinol, aspirin (high dose), azathioprine, clofibrate, corticosteroids, estrogens, glucose infusions, guaifenesin, mannitol, probenecid, and warfarin.
- ✗ Drugs that may cause *increased* urine levels include ascorbic acid, calcitonin, citrate, dicumarol, estrogens, glyceryl, iodinated dyes, phenolsulfonphthalein, probenecid, salicylates, steroids, and outdated tetracycline.

Procedure and patient care

Before

PT Explain the procedure to the patient.

- Follow the institution's requirements regarding fasting.

During

Blood

- Collect a venous blood sample in a red-top tube.

Urine

PT Instruct the patient to begin the 24-hour urine collection after voiding. Discard the initial specimen and start the 24-hour timing at that point. See inside front cover for Routine Urine Testing.

After

Blood
- Apply pressure to the venipuncture site.

Urine
- Transport the urine specimen promptly to the laboratory.

Abnormal findings

▲ **Increased blood levels (hyperuricemia)**
Gout
Increased ingestion of purines
Genetic inborn error in purine metabolism
Metastatic cancer
Multiple myeloma
Leukemia
Cancer chemotherapy
Hemolysis
Rhabdomyolysis (e.g., heavy exercise, burns, crush injury, epileptic seizure, or myocardial infarction)
Chronic renal disease
Acidosis (ketotic or lactic)
Hypothyroidism
Toxemia of pregnancy
Hyperlipoproteinemia
Alcoholism
Shock or chronic blood volume depletion states
Idiopathic

▼ **Decreased blood levels**
Wilson disease
Fanconi syndrome
Lead poisoning
Yellow atrophy of the liver

▲ **Increased urine levels**
Gout
Metastatic cancer
Multiple myeloma
Leukemia
Cancer chemotherapy
High purine diet
Lead toxicity

▼ **Decreased urine levels**
Kidney disease
Eclampsia
Chronic alcohol ingestion
Acidosis (ketotic or lactic)

U

notes

urinalysis (UA)

Type of test Urine

Normal findings

Appearance: clear
Color: amber yellow
Odor: aromatic
pH: 4.6-8.0 (average 6.0)
Protein
    0-8 mg/dL
    50-80 mg/24 hr (at rest)
    <250 mg/24 hr (exercise)
Specific gravity
    Adult: 1.005-1.030 (usually 1.010-1.025)
    Elderly: values decrease with age
    Newborn: 1.001-1.020
Leukocyte esterase: negative
Nitrites: negative
Ketones: negative
Crystals: negative
Casts: none present
Glucose
    Fresh specimen: negative
    24-hour specimen: 50-300 mg/day or 0.3-1.7 mmol/day (SI units)
White blood cells (WBCs): 0-4 per low-power field
WBC casts: negative
Red blood cells (RBCs): ≤2
RBC casts: none

Test explanation and related physiology

A total urinalysis involves multiple routine tests on a urine specimen. This specimen is not necessarily a clean-catch specimen. However, if urinary tract infection is suspected, often a midstream clean-catch specimen is obtained. This urine is then split into two parts. One is sent for urinalysis, and the other is held in the laboratory refrigerator and cultured (p. 968) if the urinalysis indicates infection. Abnormalities detected by urinalysis may reflect either urinary tract diseases (e.g., infection, glomerulonephritis, loss of concentrating capacity) or extrarenal disease processes (e.g., glucosuria in diabetes, proteinuria in monoclonal gammopathies, bilirubinuria in liver disease).

Urinalysis routinely includes remarks about the color, appearance, and odor of the urine. The pH is determined. The urine is tested for the presence of proteins, glucose, ketones, blood, and leukocyte esterase. The urine is examined microscopically for RBCs, WBCs, casts, crystals, and bacteria.

Examination of the urine sediment provides a significant amount of information about the urinary system. Reference ranges have been provided to recognize marked abnormalities.

Appearance and color

Urine appearance and color are noted as part of routine urinalysis. The appearance of a normal urine specimen should be clear. Cloudy urine may be caused by the presence of pus, RBCs, or bacteria; however, normal urine also may be cloudy because of ingestion of certain foods (e.g., large amounts of fat, ureates, or phosphates). The color of urine ranges from pale yellow to amber because of the pigment *urochrome*. The color indicates the concentration of the urine and varies with specific gravity. Dilute urine is straw colored, and concentrated urine is deep amber.

Abnormally colored urine may result from a pathologic condition or the ingestion of certain foods or medicines. For example, bleeding from the kidney produces dark red urine, whereas bleeding from the lower urinary tract produces bright red urine. Dark yellow urine may indicate the presence of urobilinogen or bilirubin. *Pseudomonas* organisms may produce green urine. Beets may cause red urine, and rhubarb can color the urine brown. Many frequently used drugs also may affect urine color (Table 34).

Odor

Determination of urine odor is a part of routine urinalysis. The aromatic odor of fresh, normal urine is caused by the presence of volatile acids. Urine of patients with diabetic ketoacidosis has the strong, sweet smell of acetone. In patients with a urinary tract infection, the urine may have a very foul odor. Patients with a fecal odor to their urine may have an entero bladder fistula.

pH

Urine pH is affected by diet, medications, systemic acid-base disturbances, and renal tubular function. An alkaline pH is obtained in a patient with alkalemia. Also, bacteria, urinary tract infection, or a diet high in citrus fruits or vegetables may cause an increased urine pH. An alkaline urine pH is common after eating. Certain medications (e.g., streptomycin, neomycin, kanamycin) are effective in treating urinary tract infections when

U

TABLE 34 Frequently used drugs that may affect urine color

Generic and brand names	Drug classification	Urine color
Cascara sagrada	Stimulant laxative	Red in alkaline urine; yellow-brown in acid urine
Chloroquine (Aralen)	Antimalarial	Rusty yellow or brown
Chlorzoxazone (Paraflex)	Skeletal muscle relaxant	Orange or purple-red
Docusate calcium (Doxidan, Surfak)	Laxative	Pink to red to red-brown
Doxorubicin (Adriamycin)	Antineoplastic	Red-orange
Iron preparations (Ferotran, Imferon)	Hematinic	Dark brown or black on standing
Levodopa	Antiparkinsonian	Dark brown on standing
Metronidazole (Flagyl)	Antiinfective	Darkening, red-brown
Nitrofurantoin (Macrodantin, Nitrofan)	Antibacterial	Brown-yellow
Phenazopyridine (Pyridium)	Urinary tract analgesic	Orange to red
Phenolphthalein (Ex-Lax)	Contact laxative	Red or purple-pink in alkaline urine
Phenothiazines (e.g., prochlorperazine [Compazine])	Antipsychotic, neuroleptic, antiemetic	Red-brown
Phenytoin (Dilantin)	Anticonvulsant	Pink, red, red-brown
Riboflavin (vitamin B)	Vitamin	Intense yellow
Rifampin	Antibiotic	Red-orange
Sulfasalazine (Azulfidine)	Antibacterial	Orange-yellow in alkaline urine
Triamterene (Dyrenium)	Diuretic	Pale blue fluorescence

the urine is alkaline. Slightly acidic urine is normal. Normal average pH is 7.0, slightly acidic compared to average blood pH of 7.4. However, acidic urine is observed in patients with acidemia, which can result from metabolic or respiratory acidosis, starvation, dehydration, or a diet high in meat products or cranberries. In patients with renal tubular acidosis, however, the blood is acidic, and the urine is alkaline.

The urine pH is useful in identifying crystals in the urine and determining the predisposition to form a given type of stone. Acidic urine is associated with xanthine, cystine, uric acid, and calcium oxalate stones. To treat or prevent these urinary calculi, urine should be kept alkaline. Alkaline urine is associated with calcium carbonate, calcium phosphate, and magnesium phosphate stones; for these stones urine should be kept acidic. See *stone analysis*, p. 966.

Protein

Protein is a sensitive indicator of glomerular and tubular renal function. Normally, less than 30 mg of protein per day is in urine. This is not detectable in the routine protein analysis. Microalbumin can be detected, however (p. 641). If the glomerular filtration membrane is injured, as in glomerulonephritis, the spaces become much larger, and protein seeps out into the filtrate and then into the urine. Renal tubules are a site of protein reabsorption. If tubular disease exists, protein is in the urine. If proteinuria persists at a significant rate, the patient can become hypoproteinemic because of the severe protein loss through the kidneys. This decreases the normal capillary oncotic pressure that holds fluid in the vasculature and causes severe interstitial edema. The combination of proteinuria and edema is known as the nephrotic syndrome.

Proteinuria (usually albumin) is probably the most important indicator of renal disease. The urine of all pregnant women is routinely checked for proteinuria, which can be an indicator of preeclampsia. In addition to screening for nephrotic syndrome, urinary protein also screens for complications of diabetes mellitus, glomerulonephritis, amyloidosis, and multiple myeloma (see test for Bence Jones protein, p. 139).

If significant protein is noted at urinalysis, a 24-hour urine specimen should be collected to measure the quantity of protein. This estimate of 24-hour protein excretion is usually performed with a urine creatinine because hydration status and other factors may influence urine concentration. The normal *protein/creatinine ratio* is less than 0.15.

U

Glucose

This can be an effective screening test for the presence of glucose in the urine that may identify diabetes mellitus or other causes of glucose intolerance (see glucose, p. 479). Although urine glucose tests previously were used to monitor the effectiveness of diabetes therapy, today glucose monitoring is largely done by fingerstick determinations of blood glucose levels.

Glucose is filtered from the blood by the glomeruli of the kidney. Normally, all of the glucose is resorbed in the proximal renal tubules. When the blood glucose level exceeds the capability of the renal threshold to resorb the glucose (normally around 180 mg/dL), it begins to spill over into the urine (glycosuria). As the blood glucose level increases further, greater amounts of glucose are spilled into the urine.

Glucosuria may occur immediately after eating a high-carbohydrate meal in patients with a low tubular maximum for glucose. Similarly, glucosuria can occur with a normal serum glucose level when kidney disease affects the renal tubule. The renal threshold for glucose becomes abnormally low, and glucosuria occurs. Glucosuria is not abnormal, however, in patients receiving dextrose-containing IV fluids. Patients with acute severe physical stress or injury can have a transient glucosuria caused by normal compensatory endocrine-mediated responses.

Osmolality

This is measured during routine urinalysis. See p. 671 for this discussion.

Specific gravity

The specific gravity is a measure of the concentration of particles, including wastes and electrolytes, in the urine. A high specific gravity indicates concentrated urine; a low specific gravity indicates dilute urine. Specific gravity refers to the weight of the urine compared with that of distilled water (which has a specific gravity of 1.000). Particles in the urine give it weight or specific gravity.

The specific gravity is used to evaluate the concentrating and excretory power of the kidney. Renal disease tends to diminish the concentrating capability of the kidney. As a result, chronic renal diseases are associated with a low specific gravity. Nephrogenic *diabetes insipidus* is associated with very little variation in specific gravity of the urine because the kidney cannot respond to such variables as hydration and solute load. The specific gravity is also a measurement of the hydration status of the patient. An overhydrated patient will have a more dilute urine with a lower specific gravity. The specific gravity of the urine in a dehydrated patient can be expected to be abnormally high. The specific gravity correlates roughly with osmolality (p. 671).

Leukocyte (WBC) esterase

Leukocyte (WBC) esterase is a screening test used to detect leukocytes in the urine. When positive, this test indicates a urinary tract infection. This examination uses chemical testing with a leukocyte esterase dipstick; a shade of purple is considered positive. Some laboratories have established screening protocols in which a microscopic examination (p. 968) is performed only if a leukocyte esterase test is positive.

Nitrites

Like the leukocyte esterase test, the nitrite test is a screening test for the identification of urinary tract infections. This test is based on the principle that many, but not all, bacteria produce an enzyme called *reductase*, which can reduce urinary nitrates to nitrites. Chemical testing is done with a dipstick containing a reagent that reacts with nitrites to produce a pink color, thus indirectly suggesting the presence of bacteria. A positive test result would indicate the need for a urine culture. Nitrite screening enhances the sensitivity of the leukocyte esterase test to detect urinary tract infections.

Ketones

Normally no ketones are present in the urine; however, a patient with poorly controlled diabetes who is hyperglycemic may have massive fatty acid catabolism. Ketones (beta-hydroxybutyric acid, acetoacetic acid, and acetone) are the end products of this fatty acid breakdown. As with glucose, ketones (predominantly acetoacetic acid) spill over into the urine when the blood levels of patients with diabetes are elevated. The excess production of ketones in the urine is usually associated with poorly controlled diabetes. This test for ketonuria is also important in evaluating ketoacidosis associated with alcoholism, fasting, starvation, high-protein diets, and isopropanol ingestion. Ketonuria may occur with acute febrile illnesses, especially in infants and children.

Bilirubin and urobilinogen

Bilirubin is a major constituent of bile. If bilirubin excretion is inhibited, conjugated (direct) hyperbilirubinemia will result (p. 142). Unlike the unconjugated form, conjugated bilirubin is water soluble and can be excreted into the urine. Therefore, bilirubin in urine suggests disease affecting bilirubin metabolism after conjugation or with defects in excretion (e.g., gallstones). Unconjugated bilirubin caused by prehepatic jaundice will not be excreted in the urine because it is not water soluble.

U

Bilirubin is excreted by way of the bile ducts into the bowel. There, some of the bilirubin is transformed into *urobilinogen* by the action of bacteria in the bowel. Most of the urobilinogen is excreted from the liver back into the bowel, but some is excreted by the kidneys.

Crystals

Crystals found in urinary sediment on microscopic examination indicate that renal stone formulation is imminent, if not already present. Urea crystals occur in patients with high serum uric acid levels (gout). Phosphate and calcium oxalate crystals occur in the urine of patients with parathyroid abnormalities or malabsorption states. The type of crystal found varies with the disease and the pH of the urine (see prior discussion on urinary pH).

Casts

Casts are rectangular clumps of materials or cells that are formed in the renal distal and collecting tubules, where the material is maximally concentrated. These clumps of material and cells take on the shape of the tubule, thus the term *cast*. Casts are usually associated with some degree of proteinuria and stasis in the renal tubules. There are two kinds of casts: hyaline and cellular.

Hyaline casts are conglomerations of protein and indicate proteinuria. A few hyaline casts are normally found, especially after strenuous exercise or dehydration.

Cellular casts, which are conglomerations of degenerated cells, are described in the following paragraphs.

Granular casts result from the disintegration of cellular material into granular particles within a WBC or epithelial cell cast. Granular casts are found after exercise and in patients with various renal diseases.

In some diseases, the epithelial cells desquamate into the renal tubule. As the cells degenerate, fatty deposits in the cells coalesce and become incorporated with protein into *fatty casts*. These casts are all associated with glomerular disease or the nephrotic syndrome/nephrosis. Free oval fat bodies may also be associated with fatty emboli that occur in patients with bone fractures.

Waxy casts may be cell casts, hyaline casts, or renal failure casts. Waxy casts probably represent further degeneration of granular casts. They occur when urine flow through the renal tubule is diminished, giving time for granular casts to degenerate. Waxy casts are found especially in patients with chronic renal diseases and are associated with chronic renal failure. They also occur in patients with diabetic nephropathy, malignant hypertension, and glomerulonephritis.

Epithelial cells can enter the urine anywhere along the process of urinary excretion. The presence of occasional epithelial cells is not remarkable. Large numbers, however, are abnormal and can conglomerate into *tubular (epithelial) casts*. These are most suggestive of renal tubular disease or toxicity.

Normally, few WBCs are found in urine sediment on microscopic examination. The presence of five or more WBCs in the urine indicates a urinary tract infection involving the bladder, kidney, or both. A clean-catch urine culture should be done for further evaluation. *WBC casts* are most commonly found in infections of the kidney, such as acute pyelonephritis or interstitial nephritis.

Any disruption in the blood-urine barrier, whether at the glomerular, tubular, or bladder level, will cause RBCs to enter the urine. The bleeding can be microscopic or gross hematuria. Patients with more than three RBCs per high-power field in 2 out of 3 properly collected urine specimens should be considered to have microhematuria, and hence be evaluated for possible pathologic causes. *RBC casts* suggest glomerulonephritis. RBC casts are also seen in patients with acute tubular necrosis, pyelonephritis, renal trauma, or renal tumor.

Interfering factors

Appearance and color

- Sperm in the urethra can cause the urine to appear cloudy.
- Urine that has been refrigerated for longer than 1 hour can become cloudy.
- Certain foods affect urine color: carrots may cause dark yellow urine; beets may cause red urine; rhubarb may cause reddish or brownish urine.
- Urine darkens with prolonged standing because of oxidation of bilirubin metabolites.
- Many drugs, given the right environment, can alter the color of urine. See Table 34, p. 954.

Odor

- Some foods (e.g., asparagus) produce a characteristic odor.
- When urine stands for a long time and begins to decompose, it has an ammonia-like smell.

pH

- Urine pH becomes alkaline on standing, because of the action of urea-splitting bacteria, which produce ammonia.
- The urine pH of an uncovered specimen will become alkaline because carbon dioxide vaporizes from the urine.
- Dietary factors affect urine pH. Ingestion of large quantities of citrus fruits, dairy products, and vegetables produces

alkaline urine, whereas a diet high in meat and certain foods (e.g., cranberries) produces acidic urine.

- Drugs that *increase* urine pH include acetazolamide, bicarbonate antacids, and carbonic anhydrase inhibitors.
- Drugs that *decrease* urine pH include ammonium chloride, chlorothiazide, and mandelic acid.

Protein

- Transient proteinuria may be associated with severe emotional stress, excessive exercise, and cold baths.
- Radiopaque contrast media administered within 3 days may cause false-positive results for proteinuria.
- Urine contaminated with prostate or vaginal secretions commonly causes proteinuria.
- Diets high in protein can cause proteinuria.
- Highly concentrated urine may have a higher concentration of protein than more dilute urine.
- Hemoglobin may cause a positive result with the dipstick method.
- Bence Jones protein may not appear with the dipstick method.
- Drugs that may cause *increased* protein levels include acetazolamide, aminoglycosides, amphotericin B, cephalosporins, colistin, griseofulvin, lithium, methicillin, nafcillin, nephrotoxic drugs, oxacillin, penicillamine, penicillin G, phenazopyridine, polymyxin B, salicylates, sulfonamides, tolbutamide, and vancomycin.

Specific gravity

- Recent use of radiographic dyes increases specific gravity.
- Cold temperatures cause falsely high specific gravity.
- Drugs that may cause *increased* specific gravity include dextran, mannitol, and sucrose.

Leukocyte esterase

- False-positive results may occur in specimens contaminated by vaginal secretions (e.g., heavy menstrual discharge, *Trichomonas* infection, parasites) that contain WBCs.
- False-negative results may occur in specimens containing high levels of protein or ascorbic acid.

Ketones

- Special diets (carbohydrate-free, high-protein, high-fat) may cause ketonuria.
- Drugs that may cause false-positive results include bromosulfophthalein, isoniazid, isopropanol, levodopa, paraldehyde, phenazopyridine, and phenolsulfonphthalein.

Bilirubin and urobilinogen

- Bilirubin is not stable in urine, especially when exposed to light.
- pH can affect urobilinogen levels. Alkaline urine indicates higher levels; acidic urine may show lower levels.

- ✘ Phenazopyridine colors the urine orange. This may give the false impression that the patient has jaundice.
- ✘ Cholestatic drugs may *decrease* urobilinogen levels.
- ✘ Antibiotics reduce intestinal flora, which in turn *decreases* urobilinogen levels.

Crystals
- Radiographic contrast media may cause precipitation of urinary crystals.

WBCs
- Vaginal discharge may contaminate the urine specimen and factitiously cause WBCs in the urine.

RBCs
- Strenuous physical exercise may cause RBC casts.
- Traumatic urethral catheterization may cause RBCs.
- Overaggressive anticoagulant therapy or bleeding disorders tend to cause RBCs in the urine without concomitant disease.

Procedure and patient care

Before

PT Explain the procedure to the patient.

During
- Collect a fresh urine specimen in a urine container.
- If the urine specimen contains vaginal discharge or bleeding, a clean-catch or midstream specimen will be needed. This requires meticulous cleaning of the urinary meatus with an antiseptic preparation to reduce contamination of the specimen by external organisms. The cleansing agent then must be completely removed or it will contaminate the specimen. For the *midstream collection*, use the following procedural steps:
  1. Have the patient begin urinating in a bedpan, urinal, or toilet and then stop urinating (this washes the urine out of the distal urethra).
  2. Correctly position a sterile urine container into which the patient voids 3 to 4 ounces of urine.
  3. Cap the container.
  4. Allow the patient to finish voiding.
- For ketones, this test can be performed immediately after collection with a dipstick.
- With a Ketostix, dip the reagent into the urine specimen and remove it. Read the strip in 15 seconds by comparing it with the color chart.
- For urine specific gravity, a first-voided specimen is the best.
- For protein, the first-voided specimen is the best; however, occasionally a 24-hour urine collection (See inside front cover for Routine Urine Testing) is preferred.

U

After

- Transport the urine specimen to the laboratory promptly.
- If the specimen cannot be processed immediately, refrigerate it. If the urine cannot be tested within 2 hours of collection, a preservative should be used.
- If a 24-hour urine collection is requested, the specimen should be refrigerated or a preservative should be used during the collection time.
- Casts will break up as urine is allowed to sit. Urine examinations for casts should be performed on fresh specimens.

Abnormal findings

Appearance and color

Bacteria
Pus
Red blood cells
Certain foods (e.g., beets, carrots)
Drug therapy (see Table 34, p. 954)
Pathologic conditions (e.g., bleeding from the kidney)

Dehydration
Overhydration
Diabetes insipidus
Fever
Excessive sweating
Jaundice

Odor

Infection
Ketonuria
Urinary tract infection
Rectal fistula

Maple syrup urine disease
Phenylketonuria
Hepatic failure

pH

▲ **Increased levels**
  Respiratory alkalosis
  Metabolic alkalosis
  Urea-splitting bacteria
  Vegetarian diet
  Renal failure with inability to form ammonia
  Gastric suction
  Vomiting
  Diuretic therapy
  Renal tubular acidosis
  Urinary tract infection

▼ **Decreased levels**
  Metabolic acidosis
  Diabetes mellitus
  Diarrhea
  Starvation
  Respiratory acidosis
  Sleep
  Pyrexia

Protein

▲ **Increased levels**

Nephrotic syndrome
Diabetes mellitus
Multiple myeloma
Preeclampsia
Glomerulonephritis
Congestive heart failure
Malignant hypertension
Polycystic kidney disease
Diabetic glomerulosclerosis
Amyloidosis
Systemic lupus
  erythematosus
Goodpasture syndrome
Renal vein thrombosis
Heavy-metal poisoning
Galactosemia
Bacterial pyelonephritis
Nephrotoxic drug therapy
Bladder tumor

Glucose

▲ **Increased levels**

Diabetes mellitus
Pregnancy
Renal glycosuria
Hereditary defects in metabolism of other reducing substances
  (e.g., galactose, fructose, pentose)
Nephrotoxic chemicals (e.g., carbon monoxide, mercury, lead)

Specific gravity

▲ **Increased levels**

Dehydration
Pituitary tumor or trauma
  that causes syndrome of
  inappropriate antidiuretic
  hormone (SIADH)
Decrease in renal blood flow (as in
  heart failure, renal artery stenosis,
  or hypotension)
Glycosuria and proteinuria
Water restriction
Fever
Excessive sweating
Vomiting
Diarrhea
X-ray contrast dye

▼ **Decreased levels**

Overhydration
Diabetes insipidus
Renal failure
Diuresis
Hypothermia
Glomerulonephritis
Pyelonephritis

U

Leukocyte esterase

Possible urinary tract infection

Nitrites

Possible urinary tract infection

Ketones

Uncontrolled diabetes mellitus
Starvation
Excessive aspirin ingestion
Ketoacidosis of alcoholism
Febrile illnesses in infants and
  children
Weight reduction diets

Following anesthesia
Prolonged vomiting
Anorexia nervosa
Fasting
High-protein diets
Isopropanol ingestion
Dehydration

Crystals

Renal stone formation
Drug therapy
Urinary tract infection

Granular casts

Acute tubular necrosis
Urinary tract infection
Glomerulonephritis
Pyelonephritis
Nephrosclerosis

Chronic lead poisoning
Reaction after exercise
Stress
Renal transplant rejection

Fatty casts

Nephrotic syndrome
Diabetic nephropathy

Glomerulonephritis
Chronic renal disease

Epithelial casts

Glomerulonephritis
Eclampsia
Heavy-metal poisoning

Ethylene glycol intoxication
Acute renal allograft
  rejection

Waxy casts

Chronic renal disease
Chronic renal failure
Diabetic nephropathy
Malignant hypertension

Glomerulonephritis
Renal transplant rejection
Nephrotic syndrome

Hyaline casts

Proteinuria
Fever
Strenuous exercise
Stress

Glomerulonephritis
Pyelonephritis
Congestive heart failure
Chronic renal failure

Red blood cells and casts

▲ **Increased RBC levels**
  Glomerulonephritis
  Interstitial nephritis
  Acute tubular necrosis
  Pyelonephritis
  Renal trauma
  Renal tumor
  Renal stones
  Cystitis
  Prostatitis
  Traumatic bladder catheterization

▲ **Increased RBC cast levels**
  Glomerulonephritis
  Subacute bacterial endocarditis
  Renal infarct
  Goodpasture syndrome
  Vasculitis
  Sickle cell anemia
  Malignant hypertension
  Systemic lupus erythematosus

White blood cells and casts

▲ **Increased WBC levels**
  Bacterial infection in the urinary tract

▲ **Increased WBC cast levels**
  Acute pyelonephritis
  Glomerulonephritis
  Lupus nephritis

notes

U

urinary stone analysis (Renal calculus analysis)

Type of test Urine

Normal findings All urinary stones are pathologic.

Test explanation and related physiology

Urinary stone analysis is performed to identify the chemicals that make up a kidney stone and to treat any underlying disease that may have caused the stone formation. This information is also used to determine the most effective methods to diminish the chance of another stone.

About 5% of American women and 12% of American men will develop a kidney stone at some time in their lives. Approximately 80% of stones are composed of calcium oxalate (CaOx) and calcium phosphate (CaP); 10% of struvite (magnesium ammonium phosphate produced during infection with bacteria that possess the enzyme urease); 9% of uric acid (UA); and the remaining 1% are composed of cystine or ammonium acid urate or are diagnosed as drug-related stones. Stones ultimately occur because of a supersaturated phase of these substances from liquid to solid state.

A kidney stone can be as small as a grain of sand or as big as 1 inch (2.5 cm) or larger in diameter. Sometimes a stone can leave the kidney and move down a ureter into the bladder. From the bladder, the stone passes through the urethra and out of the body in urine. Stone passage produces renal colic that usually begins as a mild discomfort and progresses to a plateau of extreme severity over 30 to 60 minutes. If the stone obstructs the ureteropelvic junction, pain localizes to the flank; as the stone moves down the ureter, pain moves downward and anterior. Colic is independent of body position or motion and is described as a boring or burning sensation.

Stones less than 5 mm in diameter have a high chance of passage; those of 5 mm to 7 mm have a modest chance (50%) of passage; and those greater than 7 mm almost always require urologic intervention. Analysis is done on a kidney stone that has been passed in the urine or removed from the urinary tract during surgery to determine its chemical makeup. People who have had a kidney stone have a risk for having another one. Therefore, prevention measures are important. Analysis includes an evaluation of the size, shape, color, and weight of the stone.

Urinary stones can be partially prevented by altering the composition of the urine. In a simplified format, the following types of stones are often treated as follows:

- Hyperuricuria and predominately uric acid stones: alkalinize urine to increase uric acid solubility with potassium alkali 2 or 3 times daily.
- Hypercalciuria and predominately hydroxyapatite stones: acidify urine to increase calcium solubility. However, treatment also depends on urine pH and urine phosphate, sulfate, oxalate, and citrate concentrations. Thiazide diuretics reduce urinary calcium and increase urinary volume.
- Hyperoxaluria and calcium oxalate stones: increase daily fluid intake and consider reduction of daily calcium.
- Magnesium ammonium phosphate stones (struvite): investigate and treat urinary tract infection.

Interfering factors

- Tape used to attach a stone to paper may affect the ability to accurately identify the composition of the stone.

Procedure and patient care

Before

PT Explain the procedure to the patient.
- Ensure pain relief if the patient is having ureteral colic.
- Obtain a history of any previous urinary stones.
PT Explain that there are no dietary restrictions for this test.
PT Provide and explain the use of a strainer into which the patient is to urinate.

During

PT Instruct the patient to urinate into the strainer provided.
PT Tell the patient to transfer any particulate matter to a container for laboratory analysis.

After

- Transport the specimen to the laboratory promptly.

Abnormal findings

Urinary stones

notes

U

urine culture and sensitivity (C&S)

Type of test Urine; microscopic

Normal findings

Negative: <10,000 bacteria per milliliter of urine
Positive: >100,000 bacteria per milliliter of urine

Test explanation and related physiology

Urine cultures and sensitivities are obtained to determine the presence of pathogenic bacteria in patients with suspected urinary tract infections. Most often, urinary tract infections are limited to the bladder. However, the kidneys, ureters, bladder, or urethra can be the source of infection. All cultures should be performed before antibiotic therapy is initiated; otherwise the antibiotic may interrupt the growth of the organism in the laboratory. Most organisms require approximately 24 hours to grow in the laboratory, and a preliminary report can be given at that time. Usually 48 to 72 hours is required for growth and identification of the organism. Cultures may be repeated after appropriate antibiotic therapy to assess for complete resolution of the infection.

To save money, urine cultures are usually done only if the urinalysis suggests a possible infection (e.g., increased number of white blood cells [WBCs], bacteria, high pH, positive leukocyte esterase). The urine is collected and divided. One half is sent for urinalysis; the other is held in the laboratory refrigerator and evaluated only if the urinalysis indicates a possible infection.

An important part of any routine culture is to assess the sensitivity of any bacteria that are growing in the urine to various antibiotics. The physician can then more appropriately recommend the correct antibiotic therapy.

Interfering factors

- Contamination of the urine with stool, vaginal secretions, hands, or clothing will cause false-positive results.
- ☤ Drugs that may affect test results include antibiotics.

Procedure and patient care

Before

- ᴾᵀ Explain to the patient the procedure for obtaining a clean-catch (midstream) urine collection.
- Hold antibiotics until after specimen collection.
- Provide the patient with the necessary supplies.

During

- Note that a *clean-catch* or *midstream urine* collection is required for C&S testing. This requires meticulous cleansing of the urinary meatus with an antiseptic preparation to reduce contamination of the specimen by external organisms. Then the cleansing agent must be completely removed or it will contaminate the urine specimen. The midstream collection is obtained by:
  1. Having the patient begin to urinate in a bedpan, urinal, or toilet and then stop urinating (this washes the urine out of the distal urethra)
  2. Correctly positioning a sterile urine container, into which the patient voids 3 to 4 ounces of urine
  3. Capping the container
  4. Allowing the patient to finish voiding
- Note that *urinary catheterization* may be needed for patients unable to void.
- For patients with an *indwelling urinary catheter*, obtain a specimen by aseptically inserting a syringe into the sampling port on the catheter. (Usually the catheter tubing distal to the puncture site needs to be clamped for 15 to 30 minutes before the aspiration of urine to allow urine to fill the tubing. After the specimen is withdrawn, the clamp is removed.)
- Note that *suprapubic aspiration* of urine is a safe method of obtaining urine in neonates and infants. The abdomen is prepared with an antiseptic, and a 25-gauge needle is inserted into the suprapubic area 1 inch above the symphysis pubis. Urine is aspirated into the syringe and then transferred to a sterile urine container.
- Collect specimens from infants and young children in a disposable pouch called a *U bag*. This bag has an adhesive backing around the opening to attach to the child.
- Note that for patients with a *urinary diversion* (e.g., an ileal conduit), catheterization should be done through the stoma.
- Urine should *not* be collected from an ostomy pouch.

After

- Transport the specimen to the laboratory immediately (at least within 30 minutes).
- Notify the physician of any positive results so that appropriate antibiotic therapy can be initiated.

Abnormal findings

Urinary tract infection

notes

urine flow studies (Uroflowmetry, Urodynamic studies)

Type of test Urodynamic

Normal findings Depend on the patient's age, gender, and volume voided

Test explanation and related physiology

Uroflowmetry is the simplest of the urodynamic techniques, being noninvasive and requiring uncomplicated and relatively inexpensive equipment. This study measures the volume of urine expelled from the bladder per second. This test is indicated to investigate dysfunctional voiding or suspicious outflow tract obstruction. It is also done before and after any procedure designed to modify the function of the urologic outflow tract.

The urine flow depends greatly on the volume of urine voided. The flow rates are the highest and most predictable in the urine volume range of 200 mL to 400 mL. When the bladder contains more than 400 mL of urine, the efficiency of the bladder muscle is greatly decreased. Nomograms of maximal flow versus voided volume may be used for accurate test result interpretation, taking into account the patient's gender and age. If the flow rates are abnormally low, the test should be repeated to check for accuracy.

Modern urine flowmeters provide a permanent graphic recording. If flowmeters are not available, the patient can time the urinary stream with a stopwatch and record the voided volume; from this, the average flow is calculated.

In some cases it is more valuable to analyze several voided volumes and flow rates rather than a single flow rate. If this is to be done, the patient is taught to use a flowmeter. A graph of flow versus volume can be plotted. Together with clinical observation, this provides very valuable information on the severity of outflow obstruction, the likelihood of urinary retention, and the state of compensation or decompensation of the detrusor muscle.

Procedure and patient care

Before

PT Explain the procedure to the patient.

PT Instruct the patient on how to void into the urine flowmeter.

• Determine the number of flow rates that will be needed.

During

- Note that this test should be performed when the patient has a normal desire to void and in conditions suitable for privacy. The bladder should be adequately full. Essentially, all the patient must do is urinate into the flowmeter.
- **PT** Tell the patient that no discomfort is associated with this test.
- Note that the duration of this test is several seconds.

After

- Record the position of the patient, the method of filling the bladder (it should be natural), and whether this study was part of another evaluation.

Abnormal findings

Dysfunctional voiding
Urethral stricture
Prostate cancer
Prostatic hypertrophy

notes

uroporphyrinogen-1-synthase

Type of test   Blood

Normal findings   1.27-2 mU/g of hemoglobin or 81.9-129.6 units/mol Hgb (SI units)

Test explanation and related physiology

Porphyria is a group of genetic disorders characterized by an accumulation of porphyrin products, usually in the liver. This group of disorders results from enzymatic deficiencies in synthesis of heme (a part of hemoglobin). Acute intermittent porphyria (AIP) is the most common form of the liver porphyrias; it is caused by a deficiency in uroporphyrinogen-1-synthase (also called porphobilinogen deaminase). This enzyme is necessary for erythroid cells to make heme.

Most patients with AIP have no symptoms (latent phase) until the acute phase is precipitated by medication or some other factor. The acute phase is highlighted by symptoms of abdominal and muscular pain, nausea, vomiting, hypertension, mental confusion, sensory loss, and hemolysis.

This enzyme is significantly reduced during the acute and latent phases of this disorder. It is important to identify this deficiency to prevent acute bouts of porphyria.

Procedure and patient care

- See inside front cover for Routine Blood Testing.
- Fasting: no.
- Blood tube commonly used: purple.
- Because this test is based on the hemoglobin measurement, concurrently obtain a hemoglobin level on the patient.
- Indicate on the laboratory slip if the patient is having symptoms of acute porphyria.

Abnormal findings

▼ **Decreased levels**

Acute intermittent porphyria

notes

vanillylmandelic acid (VMA), homovanillic acid (HVA), and catecholamines (Epinephrine, Norepinephrine, Metanephrine, Normetanephrine, Dopamine)

Type of test Urine (24-hour)

Normal findings

VMA

Adult/elderly: <6.8 mg/24 hr or <35 µmol/24 hr (SI units)
Adolescent: 1-5 mg/24 hr
Child: 1-3 mg/24 hr
Infant: <2 mg/24 hr
Newborn: <1 mg/24 hr

HVA

≥15 years (adults): not applicable
10-14 years: <12 mg/g creatinine
5-9 years: <9 mg/g creatinine
2-4 years: <13.5 mg/g creatinine
1 year: <23 mg/g creatinine
<1 year: 35 mg/g creatinine

Catecholamines

Free catecholamines
<100 mcg/24 hr or <590 nmol/day (SI units)
Epinephrine
Adult/elderly: <20 mcg/24 hr or <109 nmol/day (SI units)
Child
    0-1 year: 0-2.5 mcg/24 hr
    1-2 years: 0-3.5 mcg/24 hr
    2-4 years: 0-6 mcg/24 hr
    4-7 years: 0.2-10 mcg/24 hr
    7-10 years: 0.5-14 mcg/24 hr
Norepinephrine
Adult/elderly: <100 mcg/24 hr or <590 nmol/day (SI units)
Child
    0-1 year: 0-10 mcg/24 hr
    1-2 years: 0-17 mcg/24 hr
    2-4 years: 4-29 mcg/24 hr
    4-7 years: 8-45 mcg/24 hr
    7-10 years: 13-65 mcg/24 hr

V

Dopamine
Adult/elderly: 65-400 mcg/24 hr
Child
    0-1 year: 0-85 mcg/24 hr
    1-2 years: 10-140 mcg/24 hr
    2-4 years: 40-260 mcg/24 hr
    >4 years: 65-400 mcg/24 hr
Metanephrine
<1.3 mg/24 hr or <7 μmol/day (SI units)
Normetanephrine
15-80 mcg/24 hr or 89-473 nmol/day (SI units)

Test explanation and related physiology

This 24-hour urine test is a screening test for the diagnosis of catecholamine-producing tumors, such as neuroblastoma, pheochromocytoma, and other rare adrenal and neural crest tumors. A *pheochromocytoma* is a tumor of the chromaffin cells within the adrenal medulla that frequently secretes abnormally high levels of epinephrine and norepinephrine. Likewise, neural crest tumors such as neuroblastoma can also hypersecrete catecholamines. These hormones cause episodic or persistent severe hypertension by producing peripheral arterial vasoconstriction. Dopamine is the precursor of epinephrine and norepinephrine. HVA is a metabolite of dopamine. Metanephrine and normetanephrine are catabolic products of epinephrine and norepinephrine, respectively. VMA (3-methoxy-4-hydroxymandelic acid) is the product of catabolism of both metanephrine and normetanephrine. In pheochromocytoma, one or all of these substances will be present in excessive quantities in a 24-hour urine collection. These hormones may be measured singularly in the urine, but the collective metabolic end products, HVA and VMA, are more easily detected because their concentrations are much higher than any one catecholamine component.

VMA and HVA are primarily used as a screening test for neural crest tumors. These urinary tests can also be used to monitor tumor activity. HVA levels may also be altered in disorders of catecholamine metabolism. For example, monoamine oxidase-A deficiency can cause decreased urinary HVA values, and a deficiency of dopamine beta-hydrolase (the enzyme that converts dopamine to norepinephrine) can cause elevated urinary HVA values.

A 24-hour urine test is preferable to a blood test because catecholamine secretion from the tumor may be episodic and potentially could be missed at a random time during the day. A

24-hour urine reflects catecholamine production over an entire day. Nevertheless, urine testing is cumbersome and time consuming. With high pressure liquid chromatography (HPLC), measurement of plasma free metanephrines (see page 636) has nearly replaced urine testing for pheochromocytoma. It is best to perform testing when symptoms (hypertension) of the potential adrenal tumor are significant. At that time, catecholamine production is greatest and can be more assuredly identified.

Interfering factors

- Increased levels of VMA may be caused by certain foods (e.g., tea, coffee, cocoa, vanilla, chocolate).
- Vigorous exercise, stress, and starvation may cause increased VMA levels.
- Falsely decreased levels of VMA may be caused by uremia, alkaline urine, and radiographic iodine contrast agents.
- ✗ Drugs that may cause *increased* VMA levels include caffeine, epinephrine, levodopa, lithium, and nitroglycerin.
- ✗ Drugs that may cause *decreased* VMA levels include clonidine, disulfiram, guanethidine, imipramine, monoamine oxidase inhibitors, phenothiazines, and reserpine.
- ✗ Drugs that may cause *increased* catecholamine levels include alcohol (ethyl), aminophylline, caffeine, chloral hydrate, clonidine (chronic therapy), contrast media (iodine containing), disulfiram, epinephrine, erythromycin, insulin, methenamine, methyldopa, nicotinic acid (large doses), nitroglycerin, quinidine, riboflavin, and tetracyclines.
- ✗ Drugs that may cause *decreased* catecholamine levels include guanethidine, reserpine, and salicylates.

Procedure and patient care

Before

- **PT** Explain the procedure to the patient.
- **PT** Explain the dietary restrictions and the 24-hour urine collection procedure to the patient.
- **PT** For 2 or 3 days before the 24-hour collection for VMA and throughout the collection, place the patient on a VMA-restricted diet. Generally, instruct the patient to avoid coffee, tea, bananas, chocolate, cocoa, licorice, citrus fruit, all foods and fluids containing vanilla, and aspirin. Obtain specific restrictions from the laboratory.
- **PT** Inform the patient of the need to avoid taking antihypertensive medications, and sometimes all medications, during this period and possibly even longer.

V

During

- Collect the 24-hour urine specimen using a preservative.
- **PT** Instruct the patient to begin the 24-hour urine collection after voiding. See inside front cover for Routine Urine Testing.
- Identify and minimize factors contributing to patient stress and anxiety. Excessive physical exercise and emotion may alter catecholamine test results by causing an increased secretion of epinephrine and norepinephrine.

After

- Send the specimen to the laboratory as soon as the test is completed.
- Allow the patient to have foods and drugs that were restricted in preparation for the test.

Abnormal findings

▲ **Increased levels**
   Pheochromocytomas
   Neuroblastomas
   Ganglioneuromas
   Ganglioblastomas
   Severe stress
   Strenuous exercise
   Acute anxiety

notes

vascular ultrasound studies (Venous Doppler ultrasound, Venous duplex scan)

Type of test Ultrasound

Normal findings

Venous

A normal Doppler venous signal with spontaneous respiration

Normal venous system without evidence of occlusion

Arterial

Normal arterial Doppler signal with systolic and diastolic components

No reduction in blood pressure in excess of 20 mm Hg compared with the normal extremity

A normal ankle-to-brachial arterial blood pressure index of 0.85 or greater

No evidence of arterial occlusion

Test explanation and related physiology

Vascular ultrasound studies are used to identify occlusion or thrombosis of the veins or arteries of an extremity. Patency is demonstrated with Doppler ultrasound by detecting moving red blood cells (RBCs) in the vein. The patency of the venous system can also be identified by evaluating the degree of venous reflux (backward blood flow in the veins of the lower extremities in patients with venous valvular insufficiency).

Vascular duplex scanning is called duplex because it combines the benefits of Doppler with B-mode scanning. With the use of the transducer, a B-mode ultrasound gray-scale image of the vessel is obtained. A pulsed Doppler probe within the transducer is used to evaluate blood flow velocity and direction in the artery and to measure the amplitude and waveform of the carotid arterial pulse. A computer combines that information and provides a two-dimensional image of the vessel along with an image of blood flow. With this technique, one is able to directly visualize areas of vascular narrowing or occlusion. The degree of occlusion is measured as percentage of the entire lumen that is occluded. Venous thrombosis is suspected when the vein is not easily compressible by the ultrasound probe.

Color Doppler ultrasound (CDU) can be added to arterial duplex scanning. CDU assigns color for direction of blood flow within the vessel, and the intensity of that color is dependent on the mean computed velocity of blood traveling in the vessel. This allows visualization of stenotic areas based on velocity or direction of blood flow in a particular area of the artery.

Duplex scanning is routinely used to identify venous thrombosis in patients suspected of having deep vein thrombosis (DVT) in an extremity. It is more rapidly performed and interpreted than venography (p. 980). In general, venous duplex scanning is less accurate than venography in identifying DVT in the calf or in the iliac veins.

With a single-mode transducer, venous blood flow can be heard audibly and is augmented by an audio speaker as a swishing noise. If the vein is occluded, no swishing sounds are detected. With single-mode arterial Doppler studies, peripheral arteriosclerotic occlusive disease of the extremities can be easily located. By slowly deflating blood pressure cuffs placed on the calf and ankle, systolic pressure in the arteries of the extremities can be accurately measured by detecting the first evidence of blood flow with the Doppler transducer. The extremely sensitive Doppler ultrasound detector can recognize the swishing sound of even the most minimal blood flow. Normally systolic blood pressure is slightly higher in the arteries of the arms than in the legs. If the difference in blood pressure exceeds 20 mm Hg, occlusive disease is believed to exist immediately proximal to the area tested. Lower extremity arterial bypass graft patency can also be assessed with Doppler ultrasound.

Interfering factors

- Venous or arterial occlusive disease proximal to the site of testing
- Cigarette smoking, because nicotine can cause constriction of the peripheral arteries and alter the results

Procedure and patient care

Before

PT Explain the procedure to the patient.

PT Inform the patient that this is a painless procedure.

- Remove all clothing from the extremity to be examined.

PT Instruct the patient to abstain from cigarette smoking for at least 30 minutes before the test.

During

- Note the following procedural steps:

Venous studies

1. A conductive gel is applied to the skin overlying the venous system of the extremity in multiple areas.
2. Usually, for the lower extremity the deep venous system is identified in the ankle, calf, thigh, and groin.

3. The characteristic "swishing" sound of the blood flow indicates a patent venous system.
4. Usually both the superficial and deep venous systems are evaluated.

Arterial studies
1. These are performed with the use of blood pressure cuffs, which are placed around the thigh, calf, and ankle.
2. A conductive paste is applied to the skin overlying the artery distal to the cuffs.
3. The proximal cuff is inflated to a level above systolic blood pressure in the normal extremity.
4. The Doppler ultrasound transducer is placed immediately distal to the inflated cuff.
5. The pressure in the cuff is slowly released.
6. The highest pressure at which blood flow is detected by the characteristic "swishing" Doppler signal is recorded as the blood pressure of that artery.
7. The test is repeated at each successive level.
8. When the ankle pressure is divided by the arm (brachial artery) pressure, this is known as the *AB index*. If the AB index is less than 0.85, significant arterial occlusive disease exists within the extremity.

- Note that these studies are usually performed in the vascular laboratory or radiology department and take approximately 30 minutes.

After
- Encourage the patient to verbalize his or her fears.
- Remove the transducer gel from the extremity.
- **PT** Inform the patient that the physician must interpret the studies and that results will be available in a few hours.

Abnormal findings

Venous occlusion secondary to thrombosis or thrombophlebitis
Venous varicosities
Small or large vessel arterial occlusive disease
Spastic arterial disease (e.g., Raynaud phenomenon)
Small vessel arterial occlusive disease (as in diabetes)
Embolic arterial occlusion
Arterial aneurysm

V

notes

venography of lower extremities (Phlebography, Venogram)

Type of test X-ray with contrast dye

Normal findings No evidence of venous thrombosis or obstruction

Test explanation and related physiology

Venography is an x-ray study designed to identify and locate thrombi within the venous system (most commonly in the extremities). During this study, dye is injected into the venous system of the affected extremity. X-ray images are then taken at timed intervals to visualize the venous system. Obstruction to the flow of dye or a filling defect within the dye-filled vein indicates that thrombosis exists. A positive study accurately confirms the diagnosis of venous thrombosis; however, a normal study, though not as accurate, does make the diagnosis of venous thrombosis very unlikely. Venography is also used to identify venous stenosis caused by external obstruction or indwelling catheter-induced thrombosis.

Often both extremities are studied, even though only one leg is suspected of containing deep vein thrombosis. The normal extremity is used for comparison with the involved extremity. Venography is more accurate than venous Doppler (p. 977) for thrombosis below the knee or in the femoral veins.

Contraindications

- Patients with severe edema of the legs
- Patients who are uncooperative
- Patients who are allergic to iodinated dye or shellfish
- Patients with renal failure, because the iodinated dye is nephrotoxic

Potential complications

- Allergic reaction to iodinated dyes
- Renal failure, especially in elderly people who are chronically dehydrated or may have a mild degree of renal failure
- Subcutaneous infiltration of the dye, causing cellulitis and pain
- Venous thrombophlebitis caused by the dye
- Bacteremia caused by a break in a sterile technique
- Venous embolism caused by dislodgment of a deep vein clot induced by the dye injection

- Lactic acidosis may occur in patients who are taking metformin and receiving iodine contrast. The metformin should be held the day of the test to prevent this complication.

Procedure and patient care

Before

PT Explain the procedure to the patient.

PT Obtain informed consent for this procedure.

- Assess the patient for allergies to iodinated dyes and shellfish.
- If needed, provide appropriate pain medication.

PT Ensure that the patient is appropriately hydrated before testing. Injection of the iodinated contrast may cause renal failure, especially in the elderly.

During

- Note the following procedural steps:
    1. The patient is taken to the radiology department and placed in a supine position on the x-ray table.
    2. Catheterization of a superficial vein on the foot is performed. This may require a surgical cutdown.
    3. An iodinated, radiopaque dye is injected into the vein.
    4. X-ray images are taken to follow the course of the dye up the leg.
    5. A tourniquet is frequently placed on the leg to prevent filling of the superficial saphenous vein. As a result, all of the dye goes toward filling the deep venous system, which contains the most clinically significant thrombosis that can embolize.
- Note that a radiologist performs this study in approximately 30 to 90 minutes.

PT Tell the patient that the venous catheterization is only as uncomfortable as a cutaneous heel stick.

PT The dye may cause the patient to feel a warm flush. Occasionally, mild degrees of nausea, vomiting, or skin itching also may occur.

After

- Continue appropriate hydration of the patient.
- Observe the puncture site for infection, cellulitis, or bleeding.
- Assess the patient's vital signs for signs of bacteremia.

Abnormal findings

Obstructed venous systems
Acute deep vein thrombosis

notes

viral cultures

Type of test Blood; urine; stool; throat; skin lesions

Normal findings No virus isolated

Test explanation and related physiology

Viral infections are the most common infections affecting children and adults. Viruses are subdivided by the nucleic acid material they contain (RNA or DNA). Infections from viruses are often indistinguishable from bacterial infections. Definitive diagnosis of viral disease is made by culture of the virus (discussed here). Other methods used to identify viral disease include:

- Serologic methods of identifying antibodies to a specific virus
- Serologic methods of identifying antigen parts of a virus
- Direct detection by electron microscopy
- Detection by nucleic acid probes/viral load

The ability to isolate a virus in culture depends on many aspects of the culture process. The first is determining the correct specimen for culture. That depends on the organ involved and the type of virus suspected (Table 35). Timing is important. Viral load is always the greatest in the early stages of the disease. This can now be measured by direct quantification of viral DNA/RNA. Cultures obtained in the first few days after symptoms appear offer the best chance of identifying the infective culture. Viruses are grown in tissue/cell cultures. Different viruses vary greatly in their ability to grow in specific cell cultures. Viral cultures take 1 to 2 days to be reported.

Interfering factors

- An inadequate specimen, the timing, or the choice of culture medium will cause false-negative tests.
- The use of a cotton swab or wooden applicator for specimen collection may destroy the virus.

Procedure and patient care

Before

PT Explain the method of collection of the specimen to the patient.

- Obtain a history regarding the timing of symptoms.
- Accurately record the source of the specimen.

During

- Use a closed specimen system to obtain and transport the specimen to the laboratory.

TABLE 35 Specimen culture for common viruses and diseases

Common viruses	Specimens	Diseases
Adenovirus, influenza, respiratory syncytial, rhinovirus	Throat culture, bronchoscopic aspiration, nasopharyngeal swab	Influenza, pneumonia, pharyngitis
Rubella, rubeola, coxsackie, varicella	Throat culture, skin vesicle	Skin rash, zoster
Arbovirus, enterovirus, herpes simplex, cytomegalovirus	Throat culture, cerebrospinal fluid, blood	Meningitis, encephalitis
Influenza A	Throat culture	Flu syndrome

- Transport the specimen immediately to the laboratory. Viruses in specimens quickly lose their vitality.
- Place samples on ice if delivery to the laboratory is not immediate.
- Small-volume specimens, such as tissue aspirates, are often best transported in viral transport medium. If bacterial cultures are to be performed, collect as a separate specimen.
- If blood is the specimen, obtain 5 mL to 7 mL of blood in a lavender- or blue-top tube.

After

PT Explain that the patient may still be infectious and should minimize exposure to others.

Abnormal findings

Viral infectious disease (see Table 35).

notes

V

virus testing

Type of test Blood; miscellaneous

Normal findings Negative for viral antibody

Test explanation and related physiology

Testing for a virus is indicated when a person with viral symptoms lives in or has traveled to an area harboring the virus. Testing is done in the clinical setting when a patient has severe symptoms contributing to significant morbidity. Testing is also performed for epidemiologic reasons to identify a viral outbreak and its extent. Finally testing can indicate immunity after exposure to the virus or a vaccination.

Viral testing is performed by identifying antibodies to viral particles in the blood or in other body fluids. Virus can be cultured in special media and subsequently identified. Finally viral RNA or DNA can be identified in body fluids (e.g., nasopharyngeal mucus) heavily contaminated by the live virus. Epstein-Barr (p. 388), hepatitis (p. 505), respiratory syncytial, herpes, parainfluenza, HIV (p. 521), Dengue fever, coxsackie, choriomeningitis, mumps, West Nile, arbovirus, equine, cytomegalovirus, rubella, and influenza A and B (including H_1N_1) can all be detected by identifying antibodies to some part of the viral particle.

Most viral infections have common symptoms that are flu-like and include fever, lethargy, headache, and neck/body aches. In some cases, the disease can progress to cause considerable morbidity. Furthermore, when the diagnosis is confirmed, where possible, aggressive antiviral treatment can be instigated and isolation can be carried out.

Front-line testing measures IgM or IgG antibodies to the virus that may or may not be specific to that particular virus. If the front-line testing is positive, confirmatory tests may be carried out. This testing may be particularly important for public health officials and researchers. Some viruses (e.g., West Nile virus [WNV]) can be transmitted through donated blood or blood components. For that reason, WNV testing kits for WNV antibodies are routinely performed on all donated blood.

Interfering factors

• Other viral infections will cause elevations of serologic testing, especially when combined total immunoglobulin IgM and IgG are tested.

Procedure and patient care

- See inside front cover for Routine Blood Testing.
- Fasting: no.
- Blood tube commonly used: red.
- Obtain other samples for testing as directed. These may include nasopharyngeal swabs, sputum, or other body fluids.

PT Explain to the patient and family that, in most circumstances, testing is carried out at a referral laboratory.

PT Inform patients that they should observe isolation precautions until results are negative. Explain that results may not be available for 2 weeks.

Abnormal findings

Viral infections (acute and chronic)

notes

V

vitamin B$_{12}$ (Cyanocobalamin) and methylmalonic acid (MMA)

Type of test Blood; urine

Normal findings

Vitamin B$_{12}$: 160-950 pg/mL or 118-701 pmol/L (SI units)
MMA: <3.6 μmol/mmol creatinine

Test explanation and related physiology

Vitamin B$_{12}$ is necessary for conversion of the inactive form of folate to the active form. This function is most notable in the formation and function of red blood cells (RBCs). Vitamin B$_{12}$ deficiency, like folic acid deficiency, causes anemia. The RBCs formed in light of these deficiencies consist of large megaloblastic RBCs. These RBCs cannot conform to the size of small capillaries. Instead they fracture and hemolyze. The shortened life span ultimately leads to anemia.

In the stomach, gastric acid detaches vitamin B$_{12}$ from its binding proteins. Intrinsic factor (IF), which is necessary for vitamin B$_{12}$ absorption in the terminal ileum, is made in the stomach mucosa. Without IF, vitamin B$_{12}$ cannot be absorbed. Deficiency of IF is the most common cause of vitamin B$_{12}$ deficiency (pernicious anemia [PA]). The next most common cause of vitamin B$_{12}$ deficiency is lack of gastric acid to separate the ingested vitamin B$_{12}$ from its binding proteins. This is common in patients who have had gastric surgery. A third cause of vitamin B$_{12}$ deficiency is malabsorption caused by diseases of the small terminal ileum. Vitamin B$_{12}$ deficiency is common in the poorly nourished elderly and in vegetarians. The clinical picture of advanced B$_{12}$ deficiency is mental confusion, neurologic defects, or even mental illness.

Serum B$_{12}$ is a measurement of recent B$_{12}$ ingestion. More prolonged B$_{12}$ deficiency is better and more easily measured by *urinary methylmalonic acid (MMA)* measurement. Elevated serum MMA levels and urinary excretion of MMA are direct measures of tissue vitamin B$_{12}$ activity. The active form of B$_{12}$ is essential in the intracellular conversion of L-methylmalonyl coenzyme A (MMA CoA) to succinyl CoA. Without B$_{12}$, MMA CoA metabolism is diverted to make large quantities of MMA. MMA is then excreted by the kidneys. MMA testing is the most sensitive test for B$_{12}$ deficiency.

Procedure and patient care

- See inside front cover for Routine Blood Testing.
- Fasting: verify with lab.
- Blood tube commonly used: red.
- **PT** Instruct the patient not to consume alcoholic beverages before the test. Check the time period with the physician or laboratory.
- Draw the specimen before starting vitamin B$_{12}$ therapy.

Abnormal findings

▲ **Increased levels**
Leukemia
Polycythemia vera
Severe liver dysfunction
Myeloproliferative disease

▼ **Decreased levels**
Pernicious anemia
Malabsorption syndromes
Inflammatory bowel disease
Intestinal worm infestation
Atrophic gastritis
Zollinger-Ellison syndrome
Large proximal gastrectomy
Resection of terminal ileum
Achlorhydria
Pregnancy
Vitamin C deficiency
Folic acid deficiency

notes

V

vitamin D (25-hydroxy vitamin D$_2$ and D$_3$; 1,25-dihydroxyvitamin D [1,25(OH)$_2$D])

Type of test Blood

Normal findings

Total 25-hydroxy D (D$_2$+D$_3$): 25-80 ng/mL
1,25(OH)$_2$D
    Males: 18-64 pg/mL
    Females: 18-78 pg/mL

Test explanation and related physiology

Vitamin D levels are calculated to ensure that postmenopausal women have adequate vitamin D levels to absorb dietary calcium. Because of the increased number of research studies investigating the role of vitamin D in osteoporosis and cancer prevention, more and more patients are having this blood test.

Vitamin D is a fat-soluble vitamin. The two major forms of vitamin D are vitamin D$_2$ (or ergocalciferol) and vitamin D$_3$ (or cholecalciferol). Vitamin D$_2$ is provided by dietary sources. Because only fish is naturally rich in vitamin D, most of the vitamin D$_2$ intake in the industrialized world is from fortified products, including milk, soy milk, and breakfast cereals or supplements.

Vitamin D$_3$ is produced in skin exposed to sunlight, specifically ultraviolet B (UVB) radiation. In this scenario, 7-dehydrocholesterol reacts with UVB light at wavelengths between 270 nm and 300 nm to produce vitamin D$_3$. These wavelengths are present in sunlight at sea level when the UV index is greater than 3. These wavelengths occur on a daily basis in the tropics, daily during the spring and summer seasons in temperate regions, and almost never in the arctic circles. Adequate amounts of vitamin D$_3$ can be made in the skin after only 10 to 15 minutes of sun exposure at least 2 times per week to the face, arms, hands, or back without sunscreen.

After vitamin D is produced in the skin or consumed in food, it is converted in the liver and kidney to form 1,25-dihydroxyvitamin D (1,25[OH]$_2$D), the physiologically active form of vitamin D. Following this conversion, the hormonally active form of vitamin D is released into the circulation. Vitamin D regulates the calcium and phosphorus levels in the blood by promoting their absorption from food in the intestines, and by promoting reabsorption of calcium in the kidneys. This enables normal mineralization of bone needed for bone growth and bone remodeling. Vitamin D inhibits parathyroid hormone secretion from the parathyroid gland. Vitamin D promotes the immune system by increasing phagocytosis, antitumor activity, and other immunomodulatory functions.

Vitamin D deficiency can result from inadequate dietary intake, inadequate sunlight exposure, malabsorption syndromes, liver or kidney disorders, or by a number of metabolic hereditary disorders. Deficiency results in impaired bone mineralization and leads to bone softening diseases (rickets in children and osteomalacia in adults). Vitamin D deficiency may also contribute to the development of osteoporosis. Recently, it has been observed that vitamin D deficiencies are associated with cancers in the colon, breast, and pancreas. Several recent reports indicate a beneficial correlation between vitamin D intake and prevention of cancer. Vitamin D deficiency is associated with an increase in high blood pressure and cardiovascular risk.

Vitamin D levels can be measured in the blood. Usually 25-hydroxy vitamin D_2 and D_3 are measured and added to obtain the total 25-hydroxy vitamin D level. They are usually reported individually and as a total. Therapy is based on the measurement of total 25-hydroxy vitamin D levels. 1,25-dihydroxyvitamin D (the active metabolite of vitamin D) can be measured and is helpful in patients who have signs of vitamin D deficiency yet have normal levels of total vitamin D.

Dietary guidelines for Americans recommend that older adults, people with dark skin, and those exposed to insufficient ultraviolet radiation (i.e., sunlight) consume extra vitamin D from vitamin D–fortified foods (e.g., milk) and/or supplements. Vitamin D requirements increase with age; however, the ability of skin to convert 7-dehydrocholesterol to vitamin D_3 decreases. At the same time, the ability of the kidneys to convert D_2 to its active form also decreases with age, prompting the need for increased vitamin D supplementation in elderly individuals. Others particularly at risk for vitamin D deficiency include:

- Breastfed infants, because human milk alone does not have adequate vitamin D levels
- People with limited sun exposure
- Women who wear long robes and head coverings
- People with occupations that prevent sun exposure
- Individuals with a body mass index (BMI) ≥30 because vitamin D_2 is trapped in the subcutaneous fat
- Individuals who have a reduced ability to absorb dietary fat because, as a fat-soluble vitamin, vitamin D requires some dietary fat in the gut for absorption

V

- Patients with liver or renal disease because they cannot convert vitamin D to its active metabolic forms

Interfering factors

☒ Corticosteroid drugs can *decrease* vitamin D levels by reducing calcium absorption.

☒ The weight-loss drug orlistat and the cholesterol-lowering drug cholestyramine can *decrease* vitamin D levels by reducing the absorption of vitamin D and other fat-soluble vitamins.

☒ Barbiturates and phenytoin *decrease* vitamin D levels by increasing hepatic metabolism of vitamin D to inactive compounds.

Procedure and patient care

- See inside front cover for Routine Blood Testing.
- Fasting: no.
- Blood tube commonly used: red or green.
- **PT** If the patient has a vitamin D deficiency, educate him or her about dietary food sources and about the importance of sunlight.

Abnormal findings

▼ **Increased levels**
William syndrome
Excess dietary supplements

▼ **Decreased levels**
Rickets
Osteomalacia
Osteoporosis
Gastrointestinal
  malabsorption syndromes
Renal failure
Liver disease
Familial hypophosphatemic
  rickets (X-linked
  hypophosphatemic
  rickets)
Acute inflammatory disease
Inadequate dietary intake
Inadequate exposure to
  sunlight

notes

white blood cell count and differential count
(WBC and differential, Leukocyte count)

Type of test Blood

Normal findings

Total WBCs

Adult/child >2 years: 5000-10,000/mm³ or 5-10×10⁹/L (SI units)
Child ≤2 years: 6200-17,000/mm³
Newborn: 9000-30,000/mm³

Differential count

	(%)	Absolute (per mm³)
Neutrophils	55-70	2500-8000
Lymphocytes	20-40	1000-4000
Monocytes	2-8	100-700
Eosinophils	1-4	50-500
Basophils	0.5-1	25-100

Possible critical values WBCs <2500 or >30,000/mm³

Test explanation and related physiology

The WBC count has two components. The first is a count of the total number of WBCs (leukocytes) in 1 mm³ of peripheral venous blood. The other component, the differential count, measures the percentage of each type of leukocyte present in the same specimen. An increase in the percentage of one type of leukocyte means a decrease in the percentage of another. Neutrophils and lymphocytes make up 75% to 90% of the total leukocytes. These leukocyte types may be identified easily by their morphology on a venous blood smear. The total leukocyte count has a wide range of normal values, but many diseases may induce abnormal values.

An increased total WBC count (leukocytosis: WBC >10,000) usually indicates infection, inflammation, tissue necrosis, or leukemic neoplasia. Trauma or stress, either emotional or physical, may increase the WBC count. A decreased total WBC count (leukopenia: WBC <4000) occurs in many forms of bone marrow failure (e.g., after antineoplastic chemotherapy or radiation therapy, marrow infiltrative diseases, overwhelming infections, dietary deficiencies, and autoimmune diseases).

W

The major function of the WBCs is to fight infection and react against foreign bodies or tissues. Five types of WBCs may easily be identified on a routine blood smear. These cells, in order of frequency, include neutrophils, lymphocytes, monocytes, eosinophils, and basophils. All of these WBCs arise from the same pluripotent stem cell in the bone marrow, as do red blood cells (RBCs). Beyond this origin, however, each cell line differentiates separately. Most mature WBCs are deposited into the circulating blood.

WBCs are divided into granulocytes and nongranulocytes. Granulocytes include neutrophils, basophils, and eosinophils. Neutrophils have multilobed nuclei and are sometimes referred to as polymorphonuclear leukocytes (PMNs or *polys*). The normal ranges for absolute counts depend on age, sex, and ethnicity. For example, normal range for absolute neutrophils for adult African American males is 1400 to 7000 cells/microliter.

Neutrophils, the most common granulocyte, are produced in 7 to 14 days, and exist in the circulation for only 6 hours. The primary function of the neutrophil is phagocytosis (killing and digestion of bacterial microorganisms). Acute bacterial infections and trauma stimulate neutrophil production, resulting in an increased WBC count. Often when neutrophil production is significantly stimulated, early immature forms of neutrophils enter the circulation. These immature forms are called *band* or *stab* cells. This occurrence, referred to as a *shift to the left* in WBC production, is indicative of an ongoing acute bacterial infection.

Basophils (also called mast cells), especially *eosinophils*, are involved in the allergic reaction. Parasitic infestations also are capable of stimulating the production of these cells. These cells are capable of phagocytosis of antigen-antibody complexes. As the allergic response diminishes, the eosinophil count decreases. Eosinophils and basophils do not respond to bacterial or viral infections.

Nongranulocytes (mononuclear cells) include lymphocytes, monocytes, and histiocytes. *Lymphocytes* are divided into two types: T-cells and B-cells. T-cells are primarily involved with cellular-type immune reactions, whereas B-cells participate in humoral immunity (antibody production). The primary function of the lymphocytes is fighting chronic bacterial and acute viral infections. The differential count does not separate the T- and B-cells but rather counts the combination of the two.

Monocytes are phagocytic cells capable of fighting bacteria in a way very similar to that of neutrophils. However, monocytes can be produced more rapidly and can spend a longer time in the circulation than neutrophils.

The WBC and differential counts are routinely measured as part of the complete blood count (p. 280). Serial WBC counts and differential counts have both diagnostic and prognostic value. For example, a persistent increase in the WBC count (particularly the neutrophils) may indicate a worsening of an infectious process (e.g., appendicitis). A dramatic decrease in the WBC count below the normal range may indicate marrow failure. In patients receiving chemotherapy, a reduced WBC count may delay further chemotherapy.

The absolute count is calculated by multiplying the differential count (%) by the total WBC count. For example, the *absolute neutrophil count (ANC)* is helpful in determining the patient's real risk for infection. It is calculated by multiplying the WBC count by the percent of neutrophils and percent of bands; that is,

$$\text{ANC} = \text{WBC} \times (\% \text{ neutrophils} + \% \text{ bands})$$

If the ANC is less than 1000, the patient may need to be placed in protective isolation because he or she could be severely immunocompromised and at great risk for infection.

Interfering factors

- Physical activity and stress may cause an increase in WBC and differential values.
- Pregnancy (final month) and labor may cause increased WBC levels.
- Patients who have had a splenectomy have a persistent, mild elevation of WBC counts.
- ✍ Drugs that may cause *increased* WBC levels include adrenaline, allopurinol, aspirin, chloroform, epinephrine, heparin, quinine, steroids, and triamterene.
- ✍ Drugs that may cause *decreased* WBC levels include antibiotics, anticonvulsants, antihistamines, antimetabolites, antithyroid drugs, arsenicals, barbiturates, chemotherapeutic agents, diuretics, and sulfonamides.

Procedure and patient care

- See inside front cover for Routine Blood Testing.
- Fasting: no.
- Blood tube commonly used: lavender.

W

Abnormal findings

▲ **Increased WBC count (leukocytosis)**
Infection
Leukemic neoplasia
Trauma
Stress
Tissue necrosis
Inflammation

▼ **Decreased WBC count (leukopenia)**
Drug toxicity
Bone marrow failure
Overwhelming infections
Dietary deficiency
Autoimmune disease
Bone marrow infiltration (e.g., myelofibrosis)
Congenital marrow aplasia

▲▼ **Increased/decreased differential count**
See Table 36.

TABLE 36   Causes of abnormalities in WBC and differential counts

Type of WBC	Increased	Decreased
Neutrophils	*Neutrophilia* Physical or emotional stress Acute suppurative infection Myelocytic leukemia Trauma Cushing syndrome Inflammatory disorders (e.g., rheumatic fever, thyroiditis, rheumatoid arthritis) Metabolic disorders (e.g., ketoacidosis, gout, eclampsia)	*Neutropenia* Aplastic anemia Dietary deficiency Overwhelming bacterial infection (especially in the elderly) Viral infections (e.g., hepatitis, influenza, measles) Radiation therapy Addison disease Drug therapy: myelotoxic drugs (i.e., chemotherapy)
Lymphocytes	*Lymphocytosis* Chronic bacterial infection Viral infection (e.g., mumps, rubella) Lymphocytic leukemia Multiple myeloma	*Lymphocytopenia* Leukemia Sepsis Immunodeficiency diseases Systemic lupus erythematosus

TABLE 36 Causes of abnormalities in WBC and differential counts—cont'd

Type of WBC	Increased	Decreased
	Infectious mononucleosis Radiation Infectious hepatitis	Later stages of human immunodeficiency virus infection Drug therapy: adreno-corticosteroids, antineoplastics Radiation therapy
Monocytes	*Monocytosis* Chronic inflammatory disorders Viral infections (e.g., infectious mononucleosis) Tuberculosis Chronic ulcerative colitis Parasites (e.g., malaria)	*Monocytopenia* Aplastic anemia Hairy-cell leukemia Drug therapy: prednisone
Eosinophils	*Eosinophilia* Parasitic infections Allergic reactions Eczema Leukemia Autoimmune diseases	*Eosinopenia* Increased adrenosteroid production
Basophils	*Basophilia* Myeloproliferative disease (e.g., myelofibrosis, polycythemia rubra vera) Leukemia Uremia	*Basopenia* Acute allergic reactions Hyperthyroidism Stress reaction

notes

W

white blood cell scan (WBC scan, Inflammatory scan)

Type of test Nuclear scan

Normal findings No signs of WBC localization outside the liver or spleen

Test explanation and related physiology

This test is based on the fact that WBCs are attracted to an area of infection or inflammation. When a patient is suspected of having had infection or inflammation yet the site cannot be localized, the injection of radiolabeled WBCs may identify and localize the area of inflammation or infection. This is especially helpful in patients who have a fever of unknown origin, suspected occult intraabdominal infection, or suspected (yet radiographically inapparent) osteomyelitis. The scan can differentiate infectious from noninfectious processes. For example, it is used to indicate whether an abnormal mass (e.g., a pancreatic pseudocyst) is infected. Areas of noninfectious inflammation (e.g., inflammatory bowel disease) also take up radiolabeled WBCs.

This scan requires drawing blood from the patient, separating out the WBCs, labeling the WBCs with technetium or indium, and reinjecting them back into the patient. Imaging of the whole body 4 to 24 hours later may show an area of increased radioactivity suggestive of accumulation of the radiolabeled WBCs in an area of infection or inflammation.

The liver, spleen, and bone marrow normally tend to accumulate radiolabeled WBCs, thereby obscuring vision behind these organs.

Procedure and patient care

Before

PT Explain the procedure to the patient.

PT Assure the patient that he or she will not be exposed to large amounts of radioactivity, because only tracer doses of the isotope are used.

PT Tell the patient that no preparation or sedation is required.

During
- Note the following procedural steps:
  1. Approximately 40 to 50 mL of blood is withdrawn from the patient, and the WBCs are extracted from the rest of the blood cells. This is usually done by centrifugation. With leukopenia, the WBC count is so low that separating WBCs out from the other blood cellular components would be very difficult. In these instances, donor WBCs are used instead of autologous WBCs. Donor WBCs are also used for human immunodeficiency virus–positive patients to minimize the risk to laboratory workers.
  2. The WBCs are suspended in saline and tagged with ^{99m}technetium (^{99m}Tc) or ^{111}indium (^{111}In) lipid-soluble product. ^{99m}Tc is preferable to ^{111}In because its half-life is longer. Therefore it is cheaper and more readily available for the infrequent times this scan is requested.
  3. The tagged WBCs are reinjected into the patient.
  4. At 4, 24, and 48 hours after injection, a gamma ray detector/camera is placed over the body.
  5. The patient is placed in supine, lateral, and prone positions so that all surfaces of the body can be visualized.
  6. The radionuclide image is recorded on film.

After

PT Inform the patient that because only tracer doses of radioisotopes are used, no precautions need to be taken against radioactive exposure.

Abnormal findings

Infection (e.g., abscess or osteomyelitis)
Inflammation (e.g., inflammatory bowel disease, arthritis)

notes

W

wound culture and sensitivity (C&S)

Type of test   Microscopic examination

Normal findings   Negative

Test explanation and related physiology

Wound cultures are obtained to determine the presence of pathogens in patients with suspected wound infections. Wound infections are most often caused by pus-forming organisms.

All cultures should be performed before antibiotic therapy is initiated. Otherwise, the antibiotic may interrupt the growth of the organism in the laboratory. More often than not, however, the physician will want to institute antibiotic therapy before the culture results are reported. In these instances a *Gram stain* of the specimen smeared on a slide is most helpful and can be reported in less than 10 minutes. All forms of bacteria are grossly classified as gram-positive (blue staining) or gram-negative (red staining). Knowledge of the shape of the organism (e.g., spheric, rod-shaped) also may be very helpful in the tentative identification of the infecting organism. With knowledge of the Gram stain results, the physician can institute a reasonable antibiotic regimen based on experience of the organism's possible identity.

Most organisms require approximately 24 hours to grow in the laboratory, and a preliminary report can be given at that time. Usually 48 to 72 hours is required for growth and identification of the organism. Cultures may be repeated after appropriate antibiotic therapy to assess for complete resolution of the infection.

Interfering factors

☒ Drugs that may alter test results include antibiotics.

Procedure and patient care

Before

PT Explain the procedure to the patient.

During

- Aseptically place a sterile cotton swab into the pus of the patient's wound, and then place the swab into a sterile, covered test tube. (Culturing specimens from the skin edge is much less accurate than culturing the suppurative material.)
- If an anaerobic organism is suspected, obtain an anaerobic culture tube from the microbiology laboratory.

- If wound cultures are to be obtained on a patient requiring wound irrigation, obtain the culture before the wound is irrigated.
- If any antibiotic ointment or solution has been previously applied, remove it with sterile water or saline before obtaining the culture.
- Handle all specimens as though they were capable of transmitting disease.
- Indicate on the laboratory slip any medications the patient may be taking that could affect test results.

After

- Transport the specimen to the laboratory immediately after testing (at least within 30 minutes).
- Notify the physician of any positive results so that appropriate antibiotic therapy can be initiated.

Abnormal findings

Wound infection

notes

W

D-**xylose absorption test** (Xylose tolerance test)

Type of test Blood; urine

Normal findings

Age	60-min plasma (mg/dL)	120-min plasma (mg/dL)	Urine (g/5 hr) [%]
Child	>15-20	>20	>4 [16-32]
Adult	20-57	30-58	>3.5-4 [>14]

Test explanation and related physiology

D-Xylose is a monosaccharide that is easily absorbed by the normal intestine. In patients with malabsorption, intestinal D-xylose absorption is diminished; as a result, blood levels and urine excretion are reduced. D-Xylose is the monosaccharide chosen for the test because it is not metabolized by the body. Its serum levels directly reflect intestinal absorption.

This particular monosaccharide is used because absorption does not require pancreatic or biliary exocrine function. Its absorption is directly determined by the small intestine. This test is used to separate patients with diarrhea caused by maldigestion (pancreatic/biliary dysfunction) from those with diarrhea caused by malabsorption (sprue, Whipple disease, Crohn disease).

In this test, the patient is asked to drink a fluid containing a prescribed amount of D-xylose. Blood and urine levels are subsequently evaluated. Excellent gastrointestinal absorption is documented by high blood levels and good urine secretion of D-xylose. Poor intestinal absorption is marked by decreased blood levels and urine excretion.

Contraindications

- Patients with abnormal kidney function
- Patients who are dehydrated

Interfering factors

☒ Drugs that may affect test results include aspirin, atropine, and indomethacin.

Procedure and patient care

Before

PT Explain the procedure to the patient.

PT Instruct the adult patient to fast for 8 hours before testing.

PT Tell the pediatric patient or the parents that the patient should fast for at least 4 hours before testing.

During

- Collect a venous blood sample in a red-top tube before the patient ingests the D-xylose.
- Collect a first-voided morning urine specimen and send it to the laboratory.
- Ask the patient to drink the prescribed dose of D-xylose dissolved in 8 ounces of water. Record the time of ingestion.
- Calibrate pediatric doses according to body weight.
- Repeat venipunctures to obtain blood in exactly 2 hours for an adult and 1 hour for a child.
- Collect urine for a designated time, usually 5 hours. Refrigerate the urine during the collection period.
- Observe the patient for nausea, vomiting, and diarrhea, which may occur as side effects of D-xylose.

PT Instruct the patient to remain in a restful position. Intense physical activity may alter digestion and affect results.

After

- Apply pressure to the venipuncture site.

PT Inform the patient that normal activity may be resumed after completion of the study.

Abnormal findings

▼ **Decreased levels**

Sprue

Lymphatic obstruction

Enteropathy (e.g., radiation)

Crohn disease

Whipple disease

Small intestine bacterial overgrowth

Hookworm

Viral gastroenteritis

Giardia lamblia infestation

Short-bowel syndrome

notes

X

zinc protoporphyrin (ZPP)

Type of test   Blood

Normal findings   0-69 μmol ZPP/mol heme

Test explanation and related physiology

ZPP is used in screening for iron deficiency anemia or lead poisoning. It is also used in monitoring treatment of chronic lead poisoning. ZPP is found in red blood cells when heme production is inhibited by lead toxicity. Lead prevents iron, but not zinc, from attaching to the protoporphyrin. If there is iron deficiency, instead of incorporating a ferrous ion to form heme, protoporphyrin (the immediate precursor of heme) incorporates a zinc ion, forming ZPP. In addition to lead poisoning and iron deficiency, zinc protoporphyrin levels can be elevated as the result of a number of other conditions (e.g., sickle cell anemia).

Procedure and patient care

- See inside front cover for Routine Blood Testing.
- Fasting: yes (12 hour).
- Blood tube commonly used: verify with lab.

Abnormal findings

▲ **Increased levels**
   Lead poisoning
   Iron deficiency
   Anemia of chronic illness
   Sickle cell anemia
   Sideroblastic anemia
   Vanadium exposure

notes

appendix A: list of tests by body system

Tests in this list are grouped by the following: cancer studies; cardiovascular, endocrine, gastrointestinal, hematologic, hepatobiliary, and immunologic systems; miscellaneous studies; and nervous, pulmonary, renal/urologic, reproductive, and skeletal systems.

CANCER STUDIES

Acid phosphatase, 7
Antibody tumor imaging, 752
Bence Jones protein, 139
Beta$_2$-microglobulin, 643
Bladder cancer markers, 152
Bone scan, 171
Breast cancer genetic testing, 463
Breast cancer genomics, 182
Breast cancer tumor analysis, 184
Breast ductal lavage, 187
CA 15-3 and CA 27.29 tumor markers, 196
CA 19-9 tumor marker, 197
CA-125 tumor marker, 199
Carcinoembryonic antigen, 212
Cathepsin D, 184
Cell culture drug resistance testing, 231
Cervical biopsy, 237
Colon cancer genetic testing, 464
Colon cancer tumor analysis, 269
DNA ploidy status, 184
Ductoscopy, 353
Early prostate cancer antigen, 757

Estrogen receptor assay, 408
Gallium scan, 450
HER 2 protein, 184
Ki67 protein, 184
Mammography, 624
Melanoma genetic testing, 466
Microglobulin, 643
Neuron specific enolase, 653
Octreotide scan, 667
Ovarian cancer genetic testing, 463
p53 protein, 184
Papanicolaou smear, 680
Progesterone receptor assay, 748
ProstaScint scan, 752
Prostate-specific antigen, 756
Salivary gland nuclear imaging, 812
Sentinel lymph node biopsy, 821
Serotonin, 827
S-phase fraction, 184
Sputum cytology, 860
Squamous cell carcinoma antigen, 861
Thyroid cancer genetic testing, 467

CARDIOVASCULAR SYSTEM

ENDOCRINE SYSTEM

GASTROINTESTINAL SYSTEM

HEMATOLOGIC SYSTEM

HEPATOBILIARY SYSTEM

IMMUNOLOGIC SYSTEM

MISCELLANEOUS STUDIES

NERVOUS SYSTEM

PULMONARY SYSTEM

RENAL/UROLOGIC SYSTEM

REPRODUCTIVE SYSTEM

SKELETAL SYSTEM

appendix B: list of tests by type

Tests in this list are grouped by the following types: blood, electrodiagnostic, endoscopy, fluid analysis, manometric, microscopic examinations, nuclear scans, other studies, sputum, stool, ultrasound, urine, and x-ray.

BLOOD TESTS

ELECTRODIAGNOSTIC TESTS

ENDOSCOPY

FLUID ANALYSIS

MANOMETRIC TESTS

MICROSCOPIC EXAMINATIONS

NUCLEAR SCANS

OTHER STUDIES

SPUTUM TESTS

STOOL TESTS

Apt test, 108
Bioterrorism infectious
  agents, 146
Clostridial toxin assay, 259
Culture, 862
Fecal fat, 419

Helicobacter pylori
  antibody, 494
Lactoferrin, 573
Occult blood, 864
Ova and parasites, 862
Viral cultures, 982

ULTRASOUND TESTS

Abdominal ultrasound, 1
Amniotic fluid index, 424
Breast sonogram, 189
Carotid artery duplex
  scanning, 229
Echocardiography, 356
Endourethral urologic
  ultrasound, 1
Fetal, 423
  Biophysical profile, 423
  Nuchal translucency, 697
Intravascular
  ultrasound, 558
IUD localization, 698
Kidney sonogram, 1

Liver and pancreaticobiliary
  system ultrasonography, 2
Obstetric ultrasonography, 697
Pelvic ultrasonography, 697
Prostate/rectal sonogram, 754
Scrotal ultrasound, 816
Testicular ultrasound, 816
Thyroid ultrasound, 909
Transesophageal
  echocardiography, 921
Transrectal ultrasonography, 754
Transthoracic
  echocardiography, 356
Vascular ultrasound
  studies, 977

URINE TESTS

Adrenocorticotropic hormone
  stimulation test with
  metyrapone, 16
Aldosterone, 25
Amino acid profiles, 44
Amylase, 56
Appearance and color, 953
Bence Jones protein, 139
Beta$_2$-microglobulin, 643
11 Beta-prostaglandin
  F(2), 141
Bioterrorism infectious
  agents, 146
Bladder cancer markers, 152
Bone turnover markers, 174
Calcium, 203

Cortisol, 301
Creatinine clearance, 315
Crystals, 958
Culture and sensitivity, 968
Delta-aminolevulinic
  acid, 337
Dexamethasone suppression
  test, 339
Epithelial casts, 959
Estimated glomerular filtration
  rate, 315
Estriol excretion, 405
Estrogen fractions, 405
Ethanol, 410
Fatty casts, 958
Flow studies, 970

X-RAY EXAMINATIONS

appendix C: disease and organ panels

This appendix includes groupings of tests commonly used either for screening or to evaluate disease situations. These panels may be modified or expanded in different clinical settings.

Anemia

Complete blood count (CBC), 280
Macrocytic anemia
    Folate, 443
    TSH, 907
    Vitamin B$_{12}$, 986
Microcytic anemia
    Reticulocyte index, 805
    Iron panel, 561
Normocytic anemia
    Reticulocyte index, 805
    Hemolysis profile, 491
Red blood cell (RBC) indices, 788
Reticulocyte count, 805

Arthritis

Antinuclear antibody (ANA), 86
C-reactive protein, 306
ESR (sedimentation rate), 393
Rheumatoid factor, 807
Uric acid, 949

Basic metabolic panel

Blood urea nitrogen (BUN), 946
Calcium, 203
Carbon dioxide, 208
Chloride, 246
Creatinine, 312
Glucose, 474
Potassium, 736
Sodium, 852

Bone/joint

Albumin, 760
Alkaline phosphatase, 29
Calcium, 203
Osteocalcin, 174
Phosphorus, 706
Protein, total, 760
Uric acid, 949

Cardiac injury

Creatine kinase (CK), 308
CK-MB, 308
Myoglobin, 650
Troponin I, 931

Coagulation screening

Partial thromboplastin time (PTT), 693
Platelet count, 718
Prothrombin time (PT), 767

Coma

Alcohol, 410
Ammonia, 47
Anion gap, 62
Arterial blood gases, 109
Basic metabolic panel, 1026
Calcium (total and ionized), 203
Ethyl alcohol, 410
Lactic acid, 569
Osmolality (serum), 669
Salicylate, 348
Toxicology screen, 869

disease and organ panels

Hepatitis, acute

Hepatitis A antibody IgM, 505
Hepatitis B, 506
  Core antibody IgM, 506
  Surface antigen, 506
Hepatitis C antibody, 508

HIV

CD4 and CD8, 234
Complete blood count
  (CBC), 280
HIV antibody with Western
  blot confirmation, 521

Hypertension

Basic metabolic panel, 1026
Cortisol, urinary free, 301
Metanephrines, urinary, 636
Renin, 800
Thyroid screening panel, 1029
Urinalysis, 952

Lipid panel

HDL cholesterol, 248
Total cholesterol, 248
Triglycerides, 927

Obstetric

Blood
  Screen, 159
  Type, 159
Complete blood count
  (CBC), 280
Hepatitis B surface antigen, 506
Rubella antibody, 810
Syphilis test (RPR, VDRL), 877

Pancreatic

Amylase, 56
Calcium (total and ionized),
  203
Glucose, 474
Lipase, 584
Triglycerides, 927

Parathyroid

Albumin, 760
Alkaline phosphatase, 29
Calcium (total and
  ionized), 203
Calcium, urinary, 203
Creatinine, 312
Magnesium, 625
Parathyroid hormone
  (PTH), 689
Phosphorus, 706
Protein, total, 760
PTH, 689

Prenatal

ABO and Rh
  typing, 159
Antibody screen, 299
Blood urea nitrogen
  (BUN), 946
Cervical cultures for
  sexually transmitted
  diseases, 828
Complete blood count
  (CBC), 280
Creatinine, 312
Cytomegalovirus
  (CMV), 333
Glucose, 474
Hepatitis B surface
  antigen, 506
Herpes simplex I and
  II, 510
Pap smear, 680
Rubella titer, 810
Thyroxine, free T_4, 912
Toxoplasmosis
  antibody, 920
Uric acid, 949
Urinalysis, 952
Urine culture, 968
VDRL, 877

Renal panel

Albumin, 760
Blood urea nitrogen
 (BUN), 946
Calcium, 203
Carbon dioxide, 208
Chloride, 246
Complete blood count
 (CBC), 280
Creatinine
 Blood, 312
 24-hour urine, 315
Glucose, 474
Magnesium, 625
Phosphorus, 706
Potassium, 736
Sodium, 852

Thyroid screening panel

Thyroid-stimulating hormone
 (TSH), 904
Thyroxine (free T_4), 912

TORCH antibody panel

Cytomegalovirus
 antibody, 333
Herpes simplex
 antibody, 510
Rubella antibody, 810
Toxoplasmosis
 antibody, 920

Toxicology screening (urine)

Amphetamines, 870
Barbiturates, 870
Benzodiazepines, 870
Cocaine metabolites, 870
Marijuana metabolites,
 870
Methadone, 870
Methaqualone, 870
Opiate metabolites,
 870
Phencyclidine, 870
Propoxyphene, 870

appendix D: symbols and units of measurement

<	less than
≤	less than or equal to
>	greater than
≥	greater than or equal to
c (prefix)	centi (10^{-2})
C	celsius
Cc	cubic centimeter
cg	centigram
cm	centimeter
cm H_2O	centimeter of water
cu	cubic
d (prefix)	deci (10^{-1})
dL	deciliter (100 ml)
fL	femtoliter
fmol	femtomole
g	gram
hr	hour
IU	international unit
ImU	international milliunit
IμU	international microunit
k (prefix)	kilo (10^3)
kat	katal
kg	kilogram (1000 grams)
L	liter
m (prefix)	milli (10^{-3})
m	meter
m^2	square meter
m^3	cubic meter
mcg	microgram
mEq	milliequivalent
mEq/L	milliequivalent per liter
mg	milligram (1/1000 gram)
min	minute
mL	milliliter
mm	millimeter (1/10 centimeter)
mm^3	cubic millimeter
mM	millimole
mm Hg	millimeter of mercury
mm H_2O	millimeter of water
mmol	millimole

mol	mole
mOsm	milliosmole
mμ	millimicron
mU	milliunit
mV	millivolt
μ (prefix)	micro (10^{-6})
μ^3	cubic micron
μkat	microkatal
μL	microliter
μm	micrometer
μm^3	cubic micrometer
μmol	micromole
μU	microunit
n (prefix)	nano (10^{-9})
ng	nanogram
nkat	nanokatal
nm	nanometer
nmol	nanomole
p (prefix)	pico (10^{-12})
Pa	pascal
pg	picogram
pL	picoliter
pm	picometer
pmol	picomole
sec	second
SI units	International System of Units
U	unit
yr	year

bibliography

Ashoor G, Syngelaki A, Nicolaides KH, et al: Trisomy 13 detection in the first trimester of pregnancy using a chromosome-selective cell-free DNA analysis method, Ultrasound Obstet Gynecol 41(1):21–25, 2013.

Bain LJ, Barker W, Loewenstein CA, Duara R: Towards an earlier diagnosis of Alzheimer disease (Proceedings of the 5th MCI Symposium, 2007), Alzheimer Dis Assoc Disord 22:99–110, 2008.

Barr Fritcher EG, et al: A multivariable model using advanced cytologic methods for the evaluation of indeterminate pancreatobiliary strictures, Gastroenterology 136:2180–2186, 2009.

Beta J, Bredaki FE, Calvo JR, Akolekar R, Nicolaides KH: Maternal serum α-fetoprotein at 11-13 weeks' gestation in spontaneous early preterm delivery, Fetal Diagn Ther 30:88–93, 2011.

Bettstetter M, et al: Distinction of hereditary nonpolyposis colorectal cancer and sporadic microsatellite-unstable colorectal cancer through quantification of MLH1 methylation by real-time PCR, Clin Cancer Res 13:3221–3228, 2007.

Braun L: How inflammatory markers refine CV risk status, Am Nurse Today 5(5):30–31, 2010.

Bredaki FE, Wright D, Matos P, et al: First-trimester screening for trisomy 21 using alpha-fetoprotein, Fetal Diagn Ther 30:215–218, 2011.

Brenner DJ, Hall EJ: Computed tomography—An increasing source of radiation exposure, N Engl J Med 357(22):2277–2284, 2007.

Brenner H, et al: Protection from colorectal cancer after colonoscopy, Ann Intern Med 154:22–30, 2011.

Castle PE, et al: Five year experience of human papilloma virus DNA and Papanicolaou test co-testing, Obstet Gynecol 113:595–600, 2009.

Cavert W, Balfour HH: Detection of antiretroviral resistance in HIV-1, Clin Lab Med 23:915–928, 2003.

Centers for Disease Control and Prevention: *Seasonal influenza.* http://www.cdc.gov/flu.

Christenson RH, Duh SH, Wu AH, et al: Multi-center determination of galectin-3 assay performance characteristics: Anatomy of a novel assay for use in heart failure, Clin Biochem 43:683–690, 2010.

Cooper D, Heera J, Goodrich J, et al: Maraviroc versus efavirenz, both in combination with zidovudine-lamivudine, for the treatment of antiretroviral-naive subjects with CCR5-tropic HIV-1 infection, J Infect Dis 201:803–813, 2010.

Danesh J, et al: C-reactive protein and other circulation markers of inflammation in the prediction of coronary heart disease, N Engl J Med 350(14):1387–1397, 2004.

de Boer RA, Lok DJ, Jaarsma T, et al: Predictive value of plasma galectin-3 levels in heart failure with reduced and preserved ejection fraction, Ann Med 43:60–68, 2011.

deVos T, et al: Circulating methylated SEPT9 DNA in plasma is a biomarker for colorectal cancer, Clin Chem 55(7):1337–1346, 2009.

DiNisio M, et al: Diagnostic accuracy of D-dimer test for exclusion of venous thromboembolism: a systematic review, J Thromb Haemost 5:296–304, 2007.

Dirkmann D, Hanke AA, Görlinger K, Peters J: Hypothermia and acidosis synergistically impair coagulation in human whole blood, Anesth Analg 106:1627–1632, 2008.

Felker GM, Fiuzat M, Shaw LK, et al: Galectin-3 in Ambulatory patients with heart failure: results from the HF-ACTION study, Circulation 5(1):72–78, 2012.

Ferlay J, et al: Is a worldwide burden of cancer in 2008, Int J Cancer 127:2893–2917, 2010.

Finn JP, et al: Cardiac MR imaging: state of the technology, Radiology 241(2):338–354, 2006.

Foster G, Stocks C, Borofsky S: *Emergency department visits and hospital admissions for kidney stone disease*, 2009. Healthcare Cost and Utilization Project Statistical. Agency for Healthcare Research and Quality 139:July 2012.

Halsey D, et al: Implications for educating the next generation of nurses on genetics and genomics in the 21st century, J Nurs Schol 43(1):3–12, 2011.

Hecht HS, et al: Coronary artery calcium scanning: clinical paradigms for cardiac risk assessment and treatment, Am Heart J 151:1139–1146, 2006.

Hirsch MS, Gunthard HF, Schapiro JM, et al: Antiretroviral drug resistance testing in adult HIV-1 infection: 2008 Recommendations of an International AIDS Society-USA Panel, Clin Infect Dis 47:266–285, 2008.

Hirsch R, et al: NGAL is an early predictive biomarker of contrast-induced nephropathy in children, Pediatr Nephrol 22(12):2089–2095, 2007.

Hoffmann U, Ferencik M, Cury R, Pena A: Coronary CT angiography, J Nucl Med 47:797–806, 2006.

Kamstrup PR, et al: Genetically elevated lipoprotein a and increased risk of myocardial infarction, JAMA 301:2331–2339, 2009.

Kägi G, Bhatia KP, Tolosa E: The role of DAT-SPECT in movement disorders, J Neurol Neurosurg Psychiatry 81(1):5–12, 2010.

Kim DH, et al: CT colonography versus colonoscopy for the detection of advanced neoplasia, N Engl J Med 357(14):1403–1412, 2007.

Kitchener HC, et al: Comparison of HPV DNA testing and liquid base cytology, European Journal cancer 47:864 to 871, 2011.

Kragelund C, et al: N-terminal pro-B-type natriuretic peptide and long-term mortality in stable coronary heart disease, N Engl J Med 352(7):666–674, 2005.

Levin B, et al: Screening and surveillance for the early detection of colorectal cancer and adenomatous polyps, CA Cancer J Clin 58(3):130–160, 2008.

Li N, et al: HPV distribution in 30,848 invasive cervical cancers worldwide, Int J Cancer 128:927–935, 2011.

Lok DJ, Van Der Meer P, de la Porte PW, et al: Prognostic value of galectin-3, a novel marker of fibrosis, in patients with chronic heart failure: data from the DEAL-HF study, Clin Res Cardiol 99:323–328, 2010.

Lorenz MW, et al: Prediction of clinical cardiovascular events with carotid intima-media thickness: a systematic review and meta-analysis, Circulation 115(4):459–467, 2007.

Maiz N, Nicolaides KH: Ductus venosus in the first trimester: Contribution to screening of chromosomal, cardiac defects and monochorionic twin complications, Fetal Diagn Ther 28:65–71, 2010.

Maiz N, Wright D, Ferreira AF, et al: A mixture model of ductus venosus pulsatility index in screening for aneuploidies at 11-13 weeks' gestation, Fetal Diagn Ther 31:221–229, 2012.

Manson JE, et al: Estrogen therapy and coronary artery calcification, N Engl J Med 356(25):2591–2602, 2007.

Maryand M, et al: Human papillomavirus DNA versus Papanicolaou screening tests for cervical cancer, N Engl J Med 357(16):1579–1588, 2007.

Montalto N, et al: Validation of self-reported smoking status using saliva cotinine: a rapid semiquantitative dipstick method, Cancer Epidemiol Biomarkers Prev 16(9):1858–1862, 2007.

Nicolaides KH, Syngelaki A, Ashoor G, et al: Noninvasive prenatal testing for fetal trisomies in a routinely screened first-trimester population, Am J Obstet Gynecol 207:374–376, 2012.

Nicolaides KH, Wright Poon DLC, Syngelaki A, Gil MM: First-trimester contingent screening for trisomy 21 by biomarkers and maternal blood cell-free DNA testing, Ultrasound Obstet Gynecol 42:41–50, 2013.

Nordberg A: Amyloid plaque imaging in vivo: current achievement and future prospects, Eur J Nucl Med Mol Imaging 35(suppl 1):S46–S50, 2008.

Norton M, Brar H, Weiss J, et al: Non-Invasive Chromosomal Evaluation (NICE) Study: results of a multicenter, prospective, cohort study for detection of fetal trisomy 21 and trisomy 18, Am J Obstet Gynecol 7(2):137–138, 2012.

Novel H1N1 Flu (Swine Flu). http://www.cdc.gov.

O'Brien JT: Role of imaging techniques in the diagnosis of dementia, Br J Radiol 80(spec no, 2):S71–S77, 2007.

Pagana KD: BNP: rapid detector of heart failure, Am Nurse Today 2(5):17–18, 2007.

Pagana KD: Laboratory and diagnostic testing: a perioperative update, AORN J 85(4):754–762, 2007.

Pagana KD: Microalbumin: little test, big payoff, Am Nurse Today 1(1):57–58, 2006.

Pagana KD: Sleeping in the danger zone, Am Nurse Today 2(9):14–15, 2007.

Pagana KD: Virtual colonoscopy: a noninvasive look at the colon, Am Nurse Today 1(3):20–21, 2006.

Pagana KD: What's the latest on lipoproteins? Am Nurse Today 2(11):41–42, 2007.

Pagana KD, Pagana TJ: Mosby's manual of diagnostic and laboratory tests, ed 5, St Louis, 2014, Mosby.

Pandya P, Wright D, Syngelaki A, Akolekar R, Nicolaides KH: Maternal serum placental growth factor in prospective screening for aneuploidies at 8-13 weeks' gestation, Fetal Diagn Ther 31:87–93, 2012.

Parente DB, et al: Potential role of diffusion tensor MRI in the differential diagnosis of mild cognitive impairment and Alzheimer's disease, Am J Roentgenol 190:1369–1374, 2008.

Pickhardt PJ, et al: Computed tomographic virtual colonoscopy to screen for colorectal neoplasia in asymptomatic adults, N Engl J Med 349(23):2191–2200, 2005.

Preisman S, Kogan A, Itzkovsky K, et al: Modified TEG evaluation of platelet dysfunction patients undergoing coronary artery surgery, Eur J Cardiothorac Surgery 37:1367–1374, 2010.

Quintero E, et al: Colonoscopy versus fecal immunochemical testing in colorectal cancer screening, J Med 336:697–706, 2012.

Richards SJ, et al: The role of flow cytometry in the diagnosis of paroxysmal nocturnal hemoglobinuria in the clinical laboratory, Clin Lab Med 27(3):577–590, 2007.

Rosenthat DL, et al: The PapSpin: a reasonable alternative to other, more expensive liquid-based Papanicolaou tests, Cancer 108: 137–143, 2006.

Saraiya M, et al: Cervical cancer screening, Int Med 170:977–985, 2010.

Smith RA, Cokkinides V, Brawley OW: Cancer screening in the United States, 2008: a review of current American Cancer Society guidelines and cancer screening issues, CA Cancer J Clin 58(3):161–179, 2008.

Stevens LA, et al: Estimating GFR using serum cystatin C alone and in combination with serum creatinine: a pooled analysis of 3418 individuals with CKD, Am J Kidney Dis 51(3):395–406, 2008.

Strander B, et al: Liquid-based cytology versus conventional Papanicolaou smear in an organized screening program: a prospective randomized study, Cancer 111:285–291, 2007.

Swenson L, Mo T, Dong W, et al: Deep sequencing to infer HIV-1 co-receptor usage: application to three clinical trials of maraviroc in treatment-experienced patients, J Infect Dis 203:237–245, 2011.

Swenson L, Mo T, Dong W, et al: Deep V3 sequencing for HIV type 1 tropism in treatment-naive patients: a reanalysis of the MERIT trial of maraviroc, Clin Infect Dis 53:732–742, 2011.

Thompson MA, Aberg JA, Cahn P, et al: Antiretroviral treatment of adult HIV infection: 2010 Recommendations of the International AIDS Society-USA Panel, JAMA 304:321–333, 2010.

VanMeurs JB, et al: Homocysteine levels and the risk of osteoporotic fracture, N Engl J Med 350(20):2033–2041, 2004.

Wagner J, et al: Noninvasive prenatal paternity testing from maternal blood, Int J Legal Med 123:75–79, 2009.

Weintraub NL, Collins SP, Pang PS, et al: Acute heart failure syndromes: emergency department presentation, treatment, and disposition: current approaches and future aims: a scientific statement from the American Heart Association, Circulation 122:1975–1996, 2010.

Yeh E, et al: Evaluation of urinary cotinine immunoassay test strips used to assess smoking status, Nicotine Tob Res 13(11):1045–1051, 2011.

index

Note: Page numbers followed by *b* indicate boxes, *f* indicate figures, and *t* indicate tables.

abbreviations for diagnostic and laboratory tests

A	AAT	Alpha$_1$-antitrypsin
	ABGs	Arterial blood gases
	ACE	Angiotensin-converting enzyme
	ACT	Activated clotting time
	ACTH	Adrenocorticotropic hormone
	ADH	Antidiuretic hormone
	AFB	Acid-fast bacilli
	AFP	Alpha-fetoprotein
	A/G ratio	Albumin/globulin ratio
	AIT	Agglutination inhibition test
	ALA	Aminolevulinic acid
	ALP	Alkaline phosphatase
	ALT	Alanine aminotransferase
	AMA	Antimitochondrial antibody
	ANA	Antinuclear antibody
	ANCA	Antineutrophil cytoplasmic antibody
	ANP	Atrial natriuretic peptide
	APCA	Antiparietal cell antibody
	APTT	Activated partial thromboplastin time
	ASMA	Anti–smooth muscle antibody
	ASO	Antistreptolysin O titer
	AST	Aspartate aminotransferase
B	BE	Barium enema
	BMC	Bone mineral content
	BMD	Bone marrow density
	BNP	Brain natriuretic peptide
	BRCA	Breast cancer (gene)
	BSAP	Bone-specific alkaline phosphatase
	BTA	Bladder tumor antigen
	BUN	Blood urea nitrogen
C	C&S	Culture and sensitivity
	CBC	Complete blood count
	CC	Creatinine clearance
	CEA	Carcinoembryonic antigen
	CK	Creatine kinase
	CMV	Cytomegalovirus
	CO	Carbon monoxide
	CO$_2$	Carbon dioxide
	COHb	Carboxyhemoglobin test
	CPK, CP	Creatine phosphokinase
	CRP	C-reactive protein
	CSF	Cerebrospinal fluid
	CST	Contraction stress test
	CT	Computed tomography
	cTnI	Cardiac troponin I
	cTnT	Cardiac troponin T
	CVB	Chorionic villus biopsy
	CVS	Chorionic villus sampling
	CXR	Chest x-ray

D	D&C	Dilation and curettage
	DEXA	Dual-energy x-ray absorptiometry
	DSA	Digital subtraction angiography
	DSMA	Disodium monomethane arsonate
	DST	Dexamethasone suppression test
E	ECG, EKG	Electrocardiography
	EEG	Electroencephalogram
	EGD	Esophagogastroduodenoscopy
	EIA	Enzyme immunoassay
	ELISA	Enzyme-linked immunosorbent assay
	EMG	Electromyography
	ENG	Electroneurography
	EP	Evoked potential
	EPCA	Early prostate cancer antigen
	EPO	Erythropoietin
	EPS	Electrophysiologic study
	ER	Estrogen receptor
	ERCP	Endoscopic retrograde cholangiopancreatography
	ESR	Erythrocyte sedimentation rate
	EUG	Excretory urography
F	FBS	Fasting blood sugar
	FDPs	Fibrin degradation products
	%FPSA	Percent free PSA
	FSH	Follicle-stimulating hormone
	FSPs	Fibrin split products
	FT_4	Thyroxin, free
	FTA-ABS	Fluorescent treponemal antibody absorption test
	FVL	Factor V Leiden
G	GE reflux	Gastroesophageal reflux scan
	GGT	Gamma-glutamyl transferase
	GGTP	Gamma-glutamyl transpeptidase
	GH	Growth hormone
	GHb, GHB	Glycosylated hemoglobin
	GI series	Gastrointestinal series
	GTT	Glucose tolerance test
H	HAA	Hepatitis-associated antigen
	HAI	Hemagglutination inhibition
	Hb, Hgb	Hemoglobin
	HCG	Human chorionic gonadotropin
	HCO_3	Bicarbonate
	Hct	Hematocrit
	Hcy	Homocysteine
	HDL	High-density lipoprotein
	5-HIAA	Hydroxyindoleacetic acid
	HIDA	Hepatic iminodiacetic acid
	HIV	Human immunodeficiency virus
	HLA-B27	Human lymphocyte antigen B27
	HTLV	Human T-cell lymphotrophic virus
I	IAA	Insulin autoantibody
	ICA	Islet cell antibody
	Ig	Immunoglobulin
	INR	International normalized ratio
	IV-GTT	Intravenous glucose tolerance test
	IVP	Intravenous pyelography
	IVU, IUG	Intravenous urography

K	KS	Ketosteroid
	KUB	Kidney, ureter, and bladder
L	LAP	Leucine aminopeptidase
	LATS	Long-acting thyroid stimulator
	LDH	Lactic dehydrogenase
	LDL	Low-density lipoprotein
	LFTs	Liver function tests
	LH	Luteinizing hormone
	LP	Lumbar puncture
	L/S ratio	Lecithin/sphingomyelin ratio
	LS spine	Lumbosacral spine
M	MA	Microalbumin
	MCH	Mean corpuscular hemoglobin
	MCHC	Mean corpuscular hemoglobin concentration
	MCV	Mean corpuscular volume
	MEG	Magnetic encephalography
	M/E ratio	Myeloid/erythroid ratio
	MMA	Methylmalonic acid
	MPG	Mean plasma glucose
	MPV	Mean platelet volume
	MRI	Magnetic resonance imaging
	MUGA	Multigated acquisition cardiac scan
N	NMP 22	Nuclear matrix protein 22
	NST	Nonstress test
	NT_x	N-telopeptide
O	O&P	Ova and parasites
	OB	Occult blood
	OCT	Oxytocin challenge test
	OGTT	Oral glucose tolerance test
	17-OHCS	17-Hydroxycorticosteroids
P	PAB	Prealbumin
	PAI-1	Plasminogen activator inhibitor-1
	PAP	Prostatic acid phosphatase
	pCO_2	Partial pressure of carbon dioxide
	PCR	Polymerase chain reaction
	PET	Positron emission tomography
	PFTs	Pulmonary function tests
	pH	Hydrogen ion concentration
	PKU	Phenylketonuria
	PMN	Polymorphonuclear
	PNH	Paroxysmal nocturnal hemoglobinuria
	pO_2	Partial pressure of oxygen
	PO_4	Phosphate
	PPBS	Postprandial blood sugar
	PPD	Purified protein derivative
	PPG	Postprandial glucose
	PR	Progesterone receptor
	PRA	Plasma renin assay
	PSA	Prostate-specific antigen
	PT	Prothrombin time
	PTH	Parathormone, parathyroid hormone
	PTHC, PTC	Percutaneous transhepatic cholangiography
	PTT	Partial thromboplastin time
	PYD	Pyridinium crosslink